Memoirs of a
Cancer Researcher

Other Related Titles from World Scientific

The Training of Cancer Researchers
by Jose Russo
ISBN: 978-981-3203-14-3
https://www.worldscientific.com/worldscibooks/10.1142/10343

The Tools of Science: The Handbook for the Apprentice of Biomedical Research
by Jose Russo
ISBN: 978-981-4293-16-7
https://www.worldscientific.com/worldscibooks/10.1142/7583

Memoirs of a Cancer Researcher

Jose Russo
*The Fox Chase Cancer
Center-Temple Health,
Philadelphia, USA*

W‍‌ World Scientific

NEW JERSEY · LONDON · SINGAPORE · BEIJING · SHANGHAI · HONG KONG · TAIPEI · CHENNAI · TOKYO

Published by

World Scientific Publishing Co. Pte. Ltd.

5 Toh Tuck Link, Singapore 596224

USA office: 27 Warren Street, Suite 401-402, Hackensack, NJ 07601

UK office: 57 Shelton Street, Covent Garden, London WC2H 9HE

Library of Congress Cataloging-in-Publication Data
Names: Russo, Jose, 1942–   author.
Title: Memoirs of a cancer researcher / by Jose Russo.
Description: New Jersey : World Scientific, 2019. | Includes bibliographical references.
Identifiers: LCCN 2018040047 | ISBN 9789813271197 (hardcover : alk. paper)
Subjects: | MESH: Oncologists | Breast Neoplasms | Research Personnel |
    Biomedical Research | Argentina | United States | Autobiography
Classification: LCC RC267 | NLM WZ 100 | DDC 362.19699/40072--dc23
LC record available at https://lccn.loc.gov/2018040047

British Library Cataloguing-in-Publication Data
A catalogue record for this book is available from the British Library.

Cover photo by Ronald W. Waite

For any available supplementary material, please visit
https://www.worldscientific.com/worldscibooks/10.1142/11012#t=suppl

Typeset by Stallion Press
Email: enquiries@stallionpress.com

To Patricia

Preface

These are my memoirs of a long career as a physician-scientist doing cancer research. I wrote them because I do not want to be forgotten by my daughter and descendants or by the next generation of cancer researchers. I want to leave a testimony that I have existed and used my life to contribute to a better understanding of what cancer is. I want my memoirs to tell my story, a story that could have many points in common with the stories of thousands of other cancer researchers. We have a communality despite the variations in our nationalities, our genders, our languages, and the color of our skin, but I believe that the story described in this book — of my childhood, my development in college, my medical studies, my training as a researcher, my small successes, and my frustrations — could be mirrored in the lives of other cancer researchers. I share with all of them the truthful realization that although our names will be forgotten, our accomplishments have added to the ever-growing pyramid of cancer knowledge. These memoirs are not a reproach that I was not recognized with a great scientific prize, or that my name is not on the front of large medical buildings or research facilities, rather my memoirs are intended to remind all the cancer researchers that at the end of the race there is not a visible prize but only a story to tell. This story tells those who will come after me that the most important reward has been the work well done and the knowledge that the fruit of my research endeavor has contributed to our understanding of what cancer is and that the secret for overcoming the human need for recognition is to work for the intrinsic value of the action of creation and not because we are expecting a reward.

Prof. Jose Russo, MD, FACP
March 13, 2018
Philadelphia, PA, USA

Contents

Chapter 1
My Childhood (1942–1954)

1.1. My parents

On March 24, 1942, the midwife who took care of my delivery from my mother, Teresa Pagano, announced to my father, Felipe Russo, that he had a son. The place that I was born was Rivadavia, a small town to the east of the city of Mendoza, which in those days had less than ten thousand inhabitants. I was baptized in the local church, and my godfather was Natalio, the younger brother of my mother. The name Jose was given to me at my mother's request in honor of my grandfather, who was loved and admired by her for his rectitude and gentleness. Unfortunately, my grandfather Jose Russo passed away when I was two years old, and although he knew me and held me in his arms, I do not remember his face.

My place of birth was a small town, yet it was not lacking in historical importance and character. Before the Spaniards arrived in the sixteenth century, the place was already a thriving farming community due to the ingenuity of the Huarpe Indians, who dug canals across the lands of Mendoza and neighboring states, providing water to the small farms. The original inhabitants had very well-established farming practices and grew potatoes and corn that, with the addition of the horses and cows the Spaniards brought, allowed them to develop a strong agricultural society. In 1853, the first public school opened, and local parents were required to send their children to receive an education; those who did not comply were fined by the government. In 1900, the immigration influx that populated Argentina

1

reached Rivadavia and spurred the development of the local economy, further enhanced by the connection of the town to the main railroad, allowing the products generated there to be transported to the port of Buenos Aires and then on to the rest of the world.

My father was the eleventh of the thirteen children that my grandmother Maria Belfiore brought into this world in Laboulaye, a small town in the province of Cordoba. She was a pious woman involved in the local church, and all her children were basically good Christians but to her dismay, the practicing of Catholicism was not a priority in their lives.

The inhabitants of Laboulaye speak differently than the rest of the province of Cordoba because they do not have the gliding vowels that cause a word to be pronounced with a sluggish intonation similar to that of the American South. Their Castellan, or Spanish, more closely resembles the dialect spoken in Buenos Aires and Santa Fe than the rest of the province of Cordoba. However, they have a particular way of speaking their Castellan that is more clear and musical and without the high pitch that is often noticed in those coming from Buenos Aires. The name Laboulaye came in honor of Edouard Rene de Laboulaye, a French jurist, poet, author, and anti-slavery activist. He was the one who initiated the idea of a gift from the French people to the United States, eventually resulting in presentation of the Statue of Liberty. Laboulaye was a zealous advocate for the abolition of slavery. This remarkable man inspired the founders to give his name to that small town in Argentina.

The Russos, together with other Italian families, arrived at this particular place in Argentina under the auspicious action of the Argentinean government that at the end of the nineteenth and beginning of the twentieth centuries facilitated immigration to those areas with low population density. I never could find out exactly what kind of incentives my ancestors received from the Argentinean government, but probably the lure was a piece of land at a very low price. Whatever the conditions, my grandfather got fifteen acres of land, and this was the way in which bakeries, butcher shops, tailors, and general stores were built all across Argentina at that time. The "1880s generation," as they are called, designed the ports, the railroads, and the roads that were opening and connecting the east with the west and the north with the south for the first time. My grandparents' family grew not only in wealth but in business and in number (provided by my lovely aunts who attracted good suitors). This was also a way of introducing a new influx of blood and tastes, most notably an interest in politics, which was added to their special inclination to music. Most of my uncles and my father played musical instruments, and they had a band that was the center of any gathering in Laboulaye, as well as in the surrounding small towns.

My mother, Teresa, the fourth of five children born to my grandmother Dominga Pelleriti and my grandfather Sebastian Pagano, was raised in the town of San Martin, a short distance from Rivadavia. Both were located east of the city of Mendoza. My grandparents were in the exportation business, and my grandfather Sebastian was very successful. My grandmother Dominga was fourteen when she first met Sebastian. The encounter was a very special one because Dominga and her parents had been visiting from Messina, Italy, and they were staying with some members of the Pelleriti family who were already in San Martin and ran a general store. It was in that store that Sebastian met Dominga, and she eventually decided not to return to Italy with her parents but instead stayed in San Martin and married Sebastian. In fact, she never went back to Italy or saw her parents again. My grandmother Dominga was very close to us until she died at 94. She was a person with an extraordinary valor and willpower. I loved her, and she was an integral part of our childhood, participating in very important moments of our lives.

My grandfathers, Jose Russo and Sebastian Pagano, had been friends in Italy as both were from Catania. Sebastian was an opera lover and traveled to Buenos Aires often to enjoy good opera at the Colon Theatre. Because Laboulaye had become a main stop on the railroad from Mendoza to Buenos Aires, it was also a common stop for Sebastian to visit his friend Jose. This friendship meant that both families were known to each other, and it was common custom for the Russos to visit the Paganos family and vice versa.

However, my father, Felipe, was unknown to the Paganos because in a certain way he was an irritation to his family. He was the only one of the Russos who did not embrace the liberal political ideas held by most of the town. To easily understand this difference, extrapolate that Argentina's Democratic Party is akin to the United States' Republican Party, and the Radical Party is similar to the Democratic Party. Political ideas ran very strong in the Argentina of those days.

The Democratic Party, or in Spanish "Partido Democrata," started as early as 1852 but became known as PD in 1931. The party supported the idea of preserving and promoting traditional values and social institutions in the context of culture and civilization and mainly social hierarchy by emphasizing stability and continuity. The PD governed Argentina for almost four decades, and with the help of Great Britain, Argentina maintained neutrality in both world wars. This allowed Argentina to provide grains and beef to the rest of the world that was struggling with wars. In the early 1940s, the PD started to lose energy and was overtaken by Radicalism and Peronism. However, it maintained hegemony in a few places like Mendoza, which was a stronghold for their conservative ideas. The province eventually became a showcase for a nation in crisis by showing that conservative ideals, and not the populism of the Radicals, were the right path.

The Republican Party, or Union Civica Radical (UCR), was founded by Leandro N. Alem in 1891, and although it had gone through different periods, it was fundamentally based in "laicism," a political system characterized by the exclusion of ecclesiastical control and influence, an egalitarian society believing in the principle that all people are equal and deserve equal rights and opportunities. The UCR helped to establish the obligatory vote and a liberal populist position. The spark of the UCR was to oppose the predominance of the Democratic Party and the conservative vision for the development of Argentina as a nation.

In 1940, in the middle of the Second World War, there was a confrontation between both Conservatism and Radicalism, and the newly emerging ideas of Peronism, which used the populist basis of Radicalism to create a new party and put forward Domingo Peron as a predominant player in Argentinean politics. The nationalist and populist vision of Peron convinced many Radicals to leave their party and embrace Peronism.

The important point is that in 1941 my father had a political dispute not only with his family but with the whole town, which was Radical. The main issue was that my father accused them of being "pancistas," meaning opportunistic and parasites, because they changed their ideologies and principles to get a political position created by the collusion between Radicals and Peronists. The Russos now had two sons-in-law who were Radical politicians, each running for a different position. My father was a thorn for the family. He could not accept Radicalism easily, and in the new collusion between Radicals and Peronists, he saw a lack of principles evidenced by how they changed their views in order to get a place in the government. He never accepted this lack of principles, which went even deeper and in fact, had been the root of Argentina's political corruption, getting a favor to be paid by another favor to reach their aims. In this environment of favoritism, *the merit of a person was lost along the way* and *favor was the passport for obtaining things*. This process became so deeply rooted that even small things were obtained using this exchange of favors. My father was against all of that, and it was natural that he turned to be an irritation to more than one person. It was in this situation that my grandfather Jose decided that his son needed some breathing space to ventilate his brain, and for that reason, Felipe was sent to the Paganos in San Martin. The Paganos did not care too much about politics as they were more interested in business; they were basically merchants. My mother and godfather, Natalio, the youngest of the family, were the only ones that received formal training in the craft of tailoring women's and men's clothes. My father's visit to the Paganos was unexpected but accepted because he was from a family known to them, but they had never heard about him. This is an indication of how rebellious my father must have been considered by the rest of the family and was probably the reason why my grandfather Russo never talked about his son Felipe. But the history of my life starts with these small, unrelated but interwoven stories because my father met my mother, Teresa, on that visit, and both of them felt an immediate attraction. My mother used to tell us that the first thing that caught her notice was his voice. She said it didn't hurt that Felipe was slim and good-looking, but it was the way he spoke Castellan that attracted her the most. They had a short engagement and married in May of 1941. My mother was only 18 and my father 28 years old. My father established himself as a cabinetmaker in Rivadavia, and I was born there. Although the family that he and my mother established was never wealthy, and we belonged to the middle class in Argentina, he never lost his belief in the conservative ideals and turned a vociferous anti-Peronist.

My father was a carpenter and a cabinetmaker, and in his own right a special man who knew how to dress and carry himself as a gentleman while never afraid to express his opinions. The older I became the more I understood his conduct, and I inherited from him a distaste and profound aversion to asking favors of my friends, especially for nominations for prizes or positions of honor. My distaste for lobbying has resulted in many cases where I have been passed by others with less merit and credentials. The root of my position became clearer to me later in my life, and it will be discussed in Chapter 2. The most painful thing for me is to ask somebody to write a recommendation letter, which is a common practice even in the research environment these days. Personally, I never pay any attention to the recommendation letters that I receive in grant or employment applications. Only my personal evaluation in the interviews gives me the moral compass of a candidate. Coming back to my father, I want to clarify that his aversion to favoritism did not mean that he didn't help people — on the contrary, he never left a friend in need but he did so without expecting anything in return. He had a sense of moral obligation toward his entire family, although I was not sure that it was reciprocated, but for him it was important to keep the bonds with his family until he died at 92. He maintained a continuous communication with his family, and he used to travel to Laboulaye twice a year to see his mother and then after she passed to stay in contact with his brothers and sisters that still lived there. He declined his share of their inheritance because he felt one of his younger brothers was more in need than him, and that our family did not need the extra money, even though I know now that we did not have much in those days. In certain ways, he was a real conservative man who was confident in his own hard work and great ability to craft things. Those were his assets.

The best demonstration of my father's character was how he sustained the family when my mother became very sick with tuberculosis (TBC) after my sister was born. In that period of our family, we were in need of money, and my father worked 12–14 hours a day to keep the money flowing for my mother's treatment. He even sold some of his tools while still maintaining his shop, and he started over and over again without despairing or giving up. In those days, very few people in Argentina had health insurance, and there was no social welfare system to provide a safety net for those who were in need. The treatment of TBC today is basically two months of taking isoniazid, rifampin, and pyrazinamide, followed by four months of isoniazid and streptomycin, but this treatment was unknown by practicing physicians in 1944 — even penicillin was an experimental drug at that time. Although streptomycin was first isolated on October 19, 1943, by Albert Schatz, a PhD student in the Waksman laboratory at Rutgers University [1,2], it was not marketed until many years later. In 1952, Waksman was the recipient of the Nobel Prize in Physiology or Medicine in recognition for his discovery of streptomycin, the first antibiotic active against TBC.

But back in 1944 when my mother contracted TBC, one of the most promising treatments was a salt of gold that was marketed by a firm in Copenhagen. It was called "Sanacrysin," and was extremely expensive due to the nature of the compound and the cost of importing it. This salt was first tested on thirty patients who showed a significant improvement, spurring demand for it. Gold compounds were initially introduced based on the reputation of Robert Koch, who had found gold cyanide effective against *M. tuberculosis* in cultures, but not in experimentally infected animals. Yet, treatment of pulmonary tuberculosis with these compounds was popular, particularly with Danish physicians, in the mid-1920s, despite consistently negative experimental results [3,4]. So that was the treatment that my mother received, and she recovered but maintained a frail appearance all her life, although she saw us grow and accomplish our dreams and was 77 years old when she passed away. Probably because of her illnesses, she was more contemplative than my father; she had a compassionate soul and was a good listener and companion to those who were in need. *She was the balm that made our lives sweeter and was my confidante for life.*

1.2. Memories of my early childhood

I have few memories of my early childhood before I was 7 years old, but they are vivid ones — not the collection of facts told by my parents.

When I was a small child, I remember sleeping in my father's arms, and that I placed my hands on his neck or held his hand as I fell asleep. My father was an anchor of safety and protection against the many ghosts that permeated my mind as a child.

The other memory that comes to me often is when I was walking in the house of my grandmother Dominga in San Martin. The house had an indoor patio surrounded by the living quarters, and at the end of the patio was a garden, and in the garden, hanging from a wire, was the dried skin of a goat that had been slaughtered, probably for a special occasion. I must have been very small because I remember that my mother was walking behind me to be sure that I did not wander off or fall. But what's interesting is that I was fascinated by the way the goat skin looked suspended in the air, clearly delineated against the sky and illuminated by the strong sun of the summer and me extending my hands to reach and touch it. The meaning is still unknown to me, but it has been fixed in my memory.

Another vivid memory is when I was probably 5 years old. We were in the house of my grandmother Maria in Laboulaye, and I was fascinated by the large central garden, which contained fruit trees, among them pomegranates — the "apple of Grenada" — and several paths ending in a rain well, known in Spanish as "aljibe," an Arabic name. In Laboulaye, most of the houses collected the rainwater in those wells, which were also used for bathing and washing clothes due to the low salt concentration. The garden was surrounded by a gallery containing several rooms; most were used as bedrooms although the largest one was the dining room and the adjacent was a large kitchen that was the meeting place for the family. The dining room contained oak furniture, and on the wall hung several photo portraits of members of the family.

In one of the corners of the garden was a swing that my sister and I mastered early. The whole place emanated serenity and comfort, and in that space of the earth, all the members of the Russo family had been born and raised. In a certain way, every room was telling a story, and even though I was too small to see all of these things, probably the perception that I was a part of something bigger than me, that the voices, the laughter, and the cries of my aunts and uncles were a part of my physical surroundings, created in me a special feeling that was engraved in my memory.

Another patent image in my memory, from when I was probably still 5 years of age, is my fascination with glass bottles of different sizes and shapes. I had amassed quite a varied collection. It was so pleasurable to see all of them in lines on the shelves and in my mind; these were the makings of a laboratory, each one holding a different imaginary chemical or solution. It is difficult to explain the why of my affection for those collectible items, because neither my father nor my mother was fond of collecting things. I am sure that I did not inherit this affection from any of my ancestors, this much I know.

I need to introduce at this point my sister. She is 2 years younger than me, and she was called Maria del Carmen but my father gave her the nickname of Pitty. We never found out from where the name came from, but that is the name that everybody still calls her. Pitty was the treasure of my father, and she received most of the attention because she was younger, very social and outgoing, and also a cute girl (Figure 1.1). My mother made all her dresses, and when she reached school age, she was sent to the private school of the Dominican nuns, and I was her chaperone until she could manage by herself. My mother's sickness kept us very close, and we used to help each other with the household chores when my mother could not do them. We

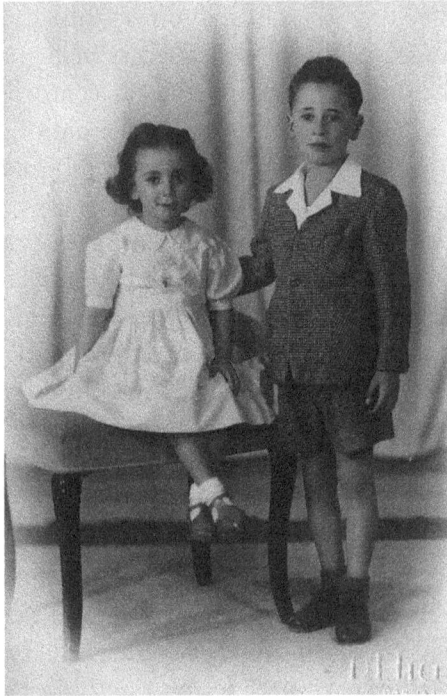

Figure 1.1:   My sister Maria del Carmen and I in Mendoza. She was 5 and I was 7 years old.

played, laughed, and cried together and have maintained a very tight closeness until the present day.

1.3. My school years

1.3.1. *The place of my home*

Before my 7th birthday my parents moved from Rivadavia to Mendoza, to a place called the San Jose Parish. We moved into the house where I lived until I left to marry Irma. The San Jose Parish was the head of a municipal region called Guaymallen. That was separated physically from the city of Mendoza by the Guaymallen Canal, an artificial waterway constructed by the Huarpe Indians to convey water for irrigation. The water comes from the Mendoza River, which has its origin in the Andes Mountains, and the amount of water is directly related to how much snow accumulates in the winter. Therefore, when the melting takes place in early spring, the canals are the only way to control the volume, otherwise overflow occurs, causing human and property damage. The Huarpes constructed the canal to redirect the water using "acequias," small waterways that border all the streets of Mendoza and provide a watering system for the trees planted by the colonizers of the region. The Spaniards and Italians that arrived in this region planted the *Platanus occidentalis,* also known as American sycamore. These trees have dense, green foliage and are perfect for adding shade or leafy lushness to a place like Mendoza, which is hot and dry in midday summer. The dense foliage is also a great nesting place for the sparrows; their chirping is a wake-up call in the Mendoza morning.

The acequias are built in such a way that the amount of water can be controlled using sluice gates, which are basically floodgates that redirect the water to different purposes. The municipal government regulates fair distribution of how much water every neighborhood or farm receives in their parcels according to how much land they have.

When I arrived at my new home, the broad sidewalks that separated the houses from the street caught my attention, and the separation was even more marked by the acequias and the perfect line of sycamore trees. The sidewalks were covered by tiles that each household was responsible for keeping clean and sparkling using "lampazos," or floor mops, that were impregnated with kerosene, left to dry, and then used. This treatment facilitated absorption of the small particles of dust that were produced by the dry nature of the place, and although the water of the acequias and shade of the trees created some moisture, it was not enough to conquer the dust. Of course for children, the sidewalks, or "veredas," were for playing with other kids or riding bikes or roller-skating, meaning that in front of every house was a playground for the neighborhood kids, and that had been my main concern when I arrived in Mendoza — who would be my playmates, besides my sister.

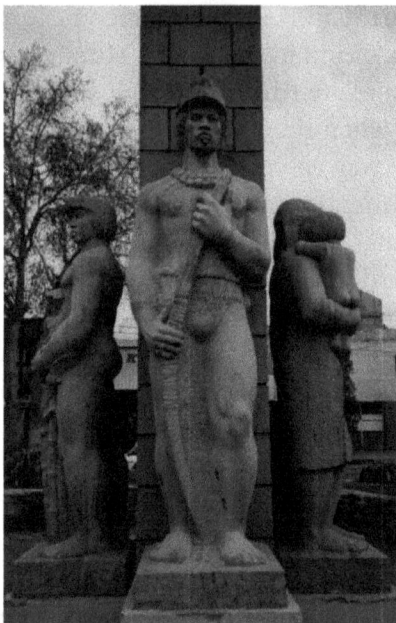

Figure 1.2: Statues in the Guaymallen Square representing the Indian Chief Guaymallen. These statues were designed and carved by T. Pages, a local artist who lived in the neighborhood.

Our house was located in the middle of the block, and on the western corner of the block was the Guaymallen Square, with monuments of the Indian chief called Guaymallen (Figure 1.2), and in the eastern corner was the main square called Plaza San Jose, or San Jose Square. The San Jose Church was at its southern border, and the chapel of the Dominican nuns was at the north side. Six blocks to the east was the elementary school Leandro N. Alem. Those were the borders of my world during my elementary school years, and the place in which I grew up.

Part of this new world was the "tramvia," or streetcar. The name tramvia was probably taken from the English word "tram" and Argentines added "via" to make it more Spanish. Whatever the reason, the tramvia was the friendly way to go places in the Mendoza of my childhood.

1.3.2. *My elementary school*

We arrived to this new place in early February 1949 with plenty time to get acquainted with the area before I began attending school in March — which would coincide with my 7th birthday. I was registered by my mother at the local elementary public school, Leandro N. Alem. It was the only one in the neighborhood and just a few blocks from my home. Thus, when classes started a couple of weeks later, I was able to walk to school by myself in a safe neighborhood. The school was located in an old building that 156 years after its inauguration had been remodeled and rebuilt again. For me, the yellow stone bust of Leandro N. Alem that was placed at the entrance of the gated school was only that, a bust of a bearded man wearing a top hat, as was fashionable among men from the latter part of the eighteenth to the middle of the twentieth centuries (Figure 1.3).

Later on, I learned more about this distinguished person. He had been born in 1842, almost 100 years before me, and he was a political revolutionary and distinguished member of the Masonic Order of Argentina. He was a political revolutionary in all senses of the word, and a manifestation of his rebellious nature was that he changed his original name from Alen to Alem, and while not completely

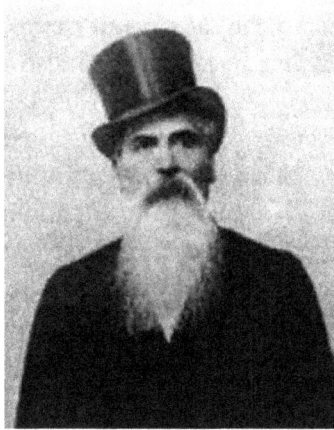

Figure 1.3: Photograph of Leandro N. Alem from which the bust at the school was sculptured.

confirmed, it's rumored he kept the *N* as a middle name, although other historians believe that his middle name was Nicephorus. He committed suicide when he was 54 years old after a terrible defeat in the 1893 insurrection organized by him against the conservative government. He left a letter to be published after his death that confessed that "*he had finished the race and his mission was not anymore and he prefers to die than to bend to his enemy*" [5]. That period of Argentina was a turbulent one, and my father narrated to us many times the insurgency and the role of Hipolito Yrigoyen, another Radical leader in those days. Yrigoyen was the only one of the Radicals that my father had some small respect for. It is not doubted that Leandro N. Alem was a man truthful with himself who lived and fought for his ideals.

Knowing all of this, I realized later on that it had been natural for my father, with his concerns, to send me to that school. Leandro N. Alem was the founder of the Union Civica Radical (UCR), an organization in complete ideological opposition to his ideas. Basically, he did not want me to be influenced by those ideologies, which the teachers may have held as they were a part of that school, and he wanted me to be a part of another school that was more conservative. However, the good sense and logic of my mother prevailed. She made her point by bringing very strong arguments like the Alem school's nearness to our home and the safeness of the place, and that I could be independent by walking by myself and also that it would be less costly than if I needed to take public transportation to go to another school that was farther away. My father accepted the situation, and I started and finished my elementary education in the Alem school. In retrospect, I admit that my father was right about the influence of the teachers due to their political orientation but what was unexpected to him was that they were as furiously anti-Peronist as he was. Facts that I discovered many years later when I realized that they had not used Eva Peron's *La Razon de mi Vida* (Figure 1.4) as a textbook.

During Peronism, this book, by executive order, replaced the other textbooks in the country. This was the only book that we were supposed to read in the lecture classes. In my recollection, we read only one page of it, and the teachers never again brought the book to our

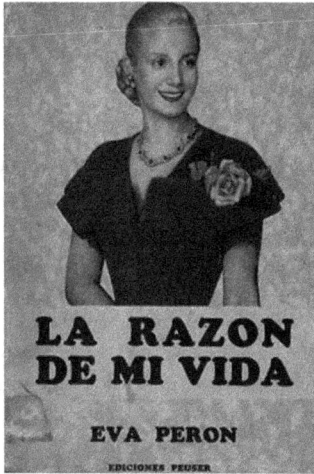

Figure 1.4:   Cover of the book *La razon de mi vida* or *The reason of my life.*

attention. That was an extremely courageous position for them to take because Peronism was a very repressive regime. Besides this, I do not recall any incident that indicated the political ideas of my elementary school teachers had permeated my education or influenced me.

1.3.3. *Small little things*

There are small little things that make my schooling years memorable. In the second grade, we were introduced to writing with ink, and that was a gigantic step in our learning process. The teacher only allowed us to use either a pen with a bottle of ink that was held in a special hole to the right side of each school desk or, for those that could afford it, a fountain pen. My father gave me his old Parker fountain pen, which I treasured for many years until the ink container could no longer be replaced and the tip was not available anymore for that model. My father had a nice cursive calligraphy that I admired when he wrote to his family or friends, and I really liked that fountain pen.

It was also in that period that my father built for me a viewer that was a wooden box with an electric bulb and on the top a frosted glass that allowed transparency but made the light subdued yet still strong enough to make common paper transparent. That was the way that I copied my maps and how I used the China ink that was also a new tool in my scholarly repertoire.

When my aunt Carmen, one of my father's sisters, came to visit us, she brought me as a gift a beautiful metal box containing German-made Faber-Castell color pencils. Those pencils were precious and so well-crafted that they lasted many years before they were exhausted and too difficult to keep hold of. I used them for constructing a Compendium of Zoology later on in college. The value of this gift was that it was not the utilitarian type that I usually received from my aunts, in general socks or underwear. This was like she had thought about it.

Another memorable thing from those days was the *Billiken*. This was a magazine for school-age children created by Constancio C. Vigil in 1919 and still available. It was called to my attention that *Billiken* was part of the pop art of Argentina, and it was displayed in an exhibit at the Philadelphia Museum of Art in 2016. The *Billiken* was the source of information for the kids of those days.

In the fourth grade, we had a book called *Horizontes Abiertos*, or *Open Horizons*, and in particular, there was a reading called "Never Postpone Till Tomorrow What You Can Do Today." It was the story of a gaucho who was working in the field and had to repair a fence to stop the cattle from escaping the hacienda. A *gaucho* was a migratory horseman, very experienced in traditional livestock farming, but this particular gaucho postponed day after day the repair of the barbed wire fence until one day the cattle ran away using the opening in the fence. The lesson was very graphic and produced a significant impression in me. Even now when I am tired and not ready to face a problem, I laugh to myself and the story comes to me — *never postpone till tomorrow what you can do today*. At the end of fourth grade, my teacher, Ms. Simon, gave me the special assignment of finding out if the name Luis Russo was cited in the list of people that have done something significant. She knew that the only way that I could find out about this was to go to the San Martin Public Library. The library was located in an old building on Gutierrez Street in downtown Mendoza. The building belonged to the National Schools and had been constructed in 1822 as part of the legacy of General Jose de San Martin under the auspices of Bernardino Rivadavia. These Argentinians saw the future before anybody else and understood that the best legacy was to provide a cultural environment for their citizens. As a matter of fact, the San Martin library is the only public library in Mendoza. The request of Ms. Simon was really a challenge for me because it was something unusual that she had not asked to the other kids, and it was something that I had not done before. I went to the library and found that the name Luis Russo was the only one listed in the *Enciclopedia Espasa-Calpe,* which the clerk, an old man, helped me to locate. For a child, a person in his fifties was old, but the point is that I discovered that the encyclopedia had 72 volumes and it was considered one of the greatest encyclopedias in the world, together with the Italian and Britannica.

This Mr. Luis Russo turned out to be a writer who was born in 1890, and among his writings was an essay about the principles of Machiavelli and the art of government. His biography was small. I took all the notes and handed the report to Ms. Simon the following day. She only asked me if I had enjoyed the experience. I told her that it had been fabulous and I would probably go back again. She never made any comments to me about whether or not my report on Luis Russo was acceptable. I never found out what she'd wanted to know or if she'd used that information, but in my analysis of the assignment I realized that the goal was not to find out about Luis Russo, it was an excuse to push me to a different world. She succeeded because when I saw the library, with the walls covered from top to bottom by shelves with books of different sizes and colors, it was a dream coming to fruition. There was also a central table with lamps and leather chairs worn by the daily use of hundreds of people through the years (Figure 1.5). The magical environment and the feeling of discovering a new world still persist in me. That day was the beginning of more frequent visits that helped me to unveil what I was looking for. That was the library that I had been dreaming to have around me. The building was an old one, and the number of books made the place overcrowded. As a matter of fact, a few years later, the library was moved to a new building in *Remedios Escalada de San Martin,* in the

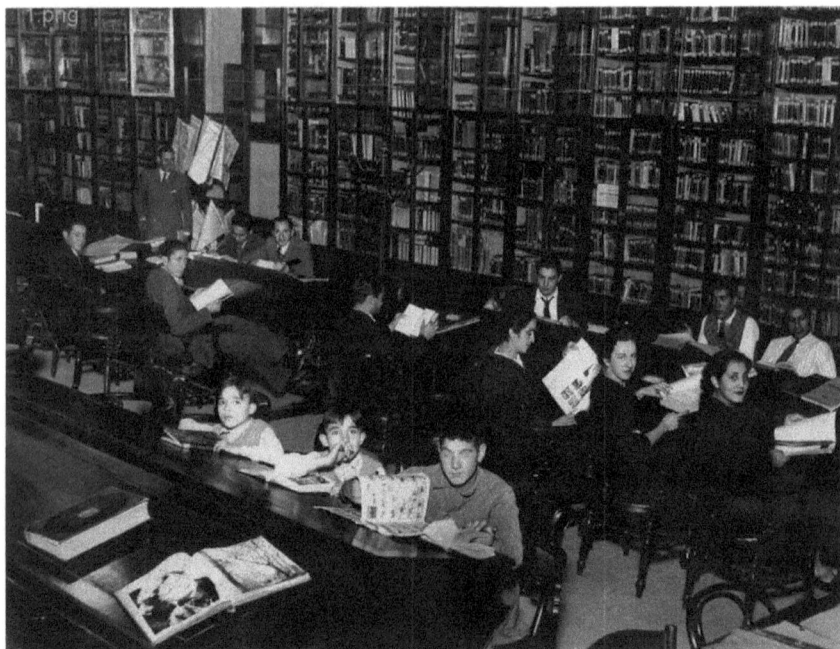

Figure 1.5: View of the San Martin library in 1952. This photograph was provided by Ms. Cristina from the San Marin Public Library in February 2017 from the archives of the library.

southern portion of the city. The reading rooms were less crowded and more illuminated with new modern leather chairs, but the display bookcases were not there any longer.

Why Ms. Simon assigned this task to me I only can guess. Probably she knew more about me from talking with my father, who'd done a carpentry job for her, and I am sure that my father talked more about me than he ever told me. I am also sure that he told her about my chemistry cabinet, and my desire to be surrounded by books and to be a scientist and my plays with my friend Angel, who was also her pupil. Whatever the reason, that first visit to the library was a small thing that opened my mind to a new world. *It was in that library that I learned about the existence of the word "cancer" and the beginning of my quest.*

1.4. The character of my father and mother

Our home was not luxurious but we had everything that we needed, and we never had an empty table and our family was never deprived of going together to the movies in the open movie theater during the summer nights, which was something unique in our neighborhood. The weekly family visits to my aunts and uncles and cousins were a rigorous ritual during the weekends and special holidays that was never interrupted. My father also used to take my sister and me to the San Martin Park (Figure 1.6) followed by the special treat of ice cream at *The Confiteria Colon* on San Martin Avenue. He was really proud to show us off and to be with us.

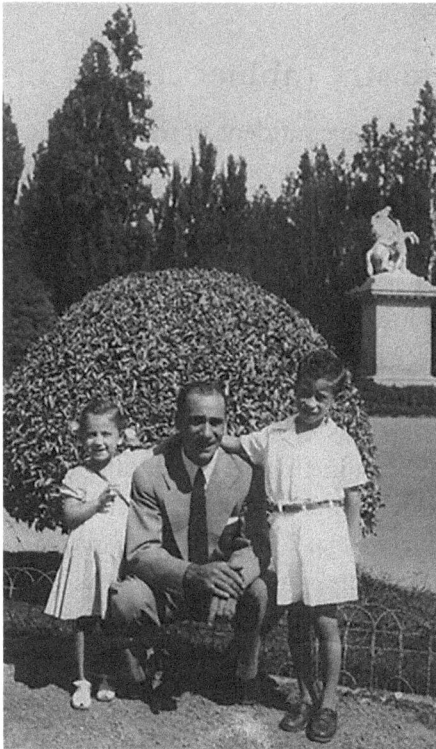

Figure 1.6: My father, my sister Maria del Carmen (Pitty) and I in the San Martin Park. Behind us are the Marly Horses.

My childhood was full of paternal and maternal care and doing what children do, learning and playing. My playing was related to being a scientist or a doctor, using the dolls of my sister and making imaginary incisions and surgical procedures, and applying all sort of unguents that were not longer used but still kept in the bottom shelf of my mother's night table.

The only thing that disturbed my childhood was the sickness of my mother. She carried the TBC contracted after my sister's birth, and although cured, it gave her a permanent weakness that even her strong will could not overcome. I was afraid that she would die and we would be orphans. For me, coming home from school and finding her alive was the most miraculous act. The feeling that I could lose her made me feel weak.

1.5. The chemistry cabinet and my first friend

I started to become more confident of myself in the second grade and that was the year that I met my best childhood friend, Angel Francisco Fisichella. Our friendship surged spontaneously because he also had the dream to be a scientist, and together we built our first laboratory in an empty dove henhouse that his father and aunt did not use any longer. Angel had lost his mother at birth, and he was raised by his aunt, who had never married, and his father, a highly spirited Italian man who loved his son and blessed our friendship. Our families met and a long friendship was established between them. Angel's father and aunt had been born in Palermo, Italy, and they were so proud to show me photos of the cathedral and the statue of Verdi in front of the opera house, places that I later visited, bringing my memories to life. They had a special celebration of Saint Joseph's Day on March 19, also called the "day of the poor." On that day, they prepared a lot of varied food and distributed it among the poor people of the neighborhood. A few years ago, I found a Sicilian community in Philadelphia that also celebrates the day of the poor on March 19 each year. In my childhood, on that day the Fisichella's would open their house for all those most in need or the ones that they could gather, and I was the guest of honor because of my name.

Angel eventually replaced my sister as a playmate and companion during my elementary school years. His interest in science was rooted in his desire to invent things to improve our chances of survival in case of an atomic disaster. The atomic bombs had been dropped when we were 3 years old. The war never touched our existence, nor that of most Argentineans, directly but we started learning about what was happening in Europe, the persecution of the Jewish people, the concentration camps, the Nazis, the American role in the conflict, and the ending with Hiroshima and Nagasaki. I remember that Angel found a way to create a plastic sealed container for water that could be stored in safe place and used when needed. This was a way that we could survive in case of another atomic conflict. He perfected the technique of sealing, but the plastic materials that we have now were unknown to us then and the only available material was rubber-like sheets that were used in repairing old car tires. The rubbery sheets smelled bad, and also the water tasted awful after a few weeks. However, he made a point. Other pursuits that we had were more biologically oriented and spurred us to venture to the San Martin Park, thanks to the safety of the tramvia, which could be taken in front of my house and after 45 minutes of riding through all the neighborhoods, we would finally arrive at the gates of the park. In the park, we started to collect frogs — more difficult than we'd expected the first time but it got easier later on. The problem that we faced was a simple one: what to do with the frogs and how to kill them so we could study their insides. Finally, we decided that we did not know how to do it, and we released them near the acequias of our homes. Because we were so secretive that we did not allow anybody to know what we were doing, we decided to stop the frog hunting and started to collect insects instead. I made a box with a glass cover and a bottom that was not cork but plywood that I got from my father's shop. We learned that the vapor of alcohol killed them and also facilitated their preservation. My incipient laboratory gained more stature when, at the age of 8, my parents gave me a chemistry set that came from the USA. With the chemistry set, I discovered the amazing power of phenolphthalein, a chemical compound used as an indicator in acid-based titrations. The marvelous thing was that you could change the color of a colorless solution to red or blue, depending on whether they were acid or alkaline. I learned how to create black powder with sodium hydroxide and potassium permanganate, and extracted chlorophyll from plants using an alcohol solution. We followed all the experiments in the instruction books — which apparently were translated in Mexico because we did not understand many words — but that was not important. The tragedy for us was when we were short of drugs or we wanted additional elements; the address and phone number to reorder were in the USA. That was a great limitation until later on I found that most of these materials could be purchased in any of the many laboratories of enology in Mendoza, abundant due to the local wine industry. But it took several years and other friends in college to help us venture in those lines. The chemistry set was the beginning of what we considered a serious enterprise. We designed a special card stating that we were the only members of the lab; it was signed by both of us and divided in two parts. On one half I would have Angel's name and signature, and the other would have my name and signature. The idea was that this would be our countersign. We were scarcely 9 years old and that was our world. When we could no longer keep the henhouse for our enterprise, my parents gave me permission to use a portion of a long gallery to build a small laboratory that I called my "chemistry cabinet," imagining a setup like the one assembled by Grand Duke Peter Leopold in the late eighteenth century so he could pursue his scientific passions.

A major addition to my chemistry cabinet was the acquisition of a monocular microscope with 10× magnification that I purchased at Lutz Ferrando, an optical store in Mendoza, with money that I saved from helping my father with his carpentry work (Figure 1.7). The chemistry cabinet was large enough to allow two people to work in it and had all the elements of a laboratory; it also had a door so we could keep our work private.

On December 28, 1957, Angel and I signed an agreement that this day we would start a new phase of our research (Figure 1.8). The words now sound so grandiloquent and pretentious, but that was our way to express our commitments in those days.

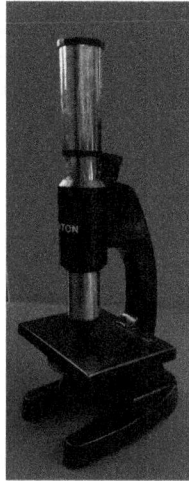

Figure 1.7: The monocular microscope that was the main acquisition with the money that I saved working in the shop of my father.

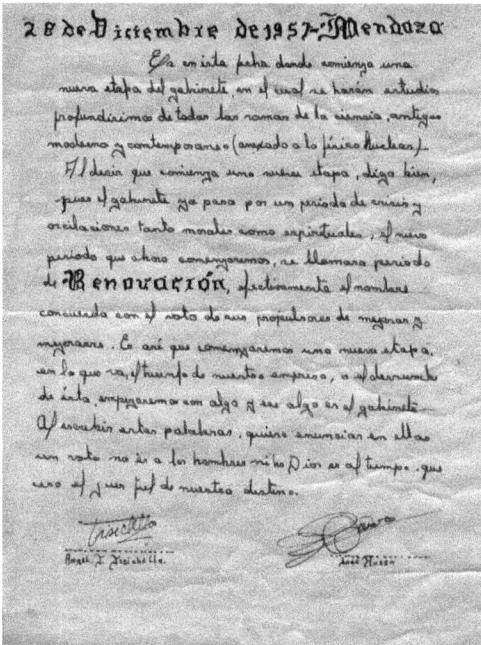

Figure 1.8: Statement that my friend Angel and I wrote indicating the new phase of our research enterprise.

1.6. An average student with secret ambitions

Going back to my elementary school years, I admit that I was not the best student of the class; I was an average kid at that school. There were others who surpassed me in grammar and mathematics. I was all the time very conscious of my deficiencies and shortcomings. But at that age, I did not know how to overcome my deficiencies and improve my level of knowledge. This only took place when I started college. In Argentina of those days, the elementary school lasted 6 years, starting at age 7 and ending at 12. At 13, it was assumed that you would go to college and receive a bachelor's degree, or become licensed to practice some level of accounting or an account controller, or become a technical person in an enology laboratory or a teacher in an elementary school. Generally, college finished at 17 years of age, and the next step was the university or professional level. Less than 10% of my schoolmates went to college and less than 25% of those who finished college with me went on to the university for professional education.

I was the only kid in my elementary school who became a medical doctor and the only one in my college class to enter the medical school at the University of Cuyo in Mendoza, and the only one of my classmates from my elementary school, college, and medical school to become a medical researcher or a physician scientist.

I remember very vividly my first day of first grade. I cried in panic when I saw a lot of writing on the blackboard — I did not know how to read or to write. The teacher, Miss DeMarco, was a seasoned woman who understood my anxiety, and she told the class that we were in school to learn how to read and write. She started from the beginning, how to read the first letters of the alphabet and the numbers, and day after day I was conquering my ignorance. There were other kids that already knew how to write or read, but not me. In elementary school, I never received high praise from the teachers or made the honor roll, but I knew there was something powerful in me, there was faith in myself and a great willpower. My teachers probably saw this because on my last day of elementary school I received a book dedicated to me that said *To José for his perseverance.* The book was *Yanquis in Marte* by Hipolito Jerez. The translation is

Yankees on Mars. It is the story of American scientists traveling to the planet Mars. The most important thing is that this was a prize for my constancy and perseverance, that probably was the best characterization of my persona, because I had the secret fantasy that I would make it, and I knew that I needed to persevere.

I discovered some traits in my personality that made me different from the other kids. For example, I needed to be surrounded by an intellectual environment when I was doing homework, and I craved having books and a real library that I could consult for my work. My father built for me a three-shelve bookcase in cedar, but most of the shelves were empty because my family, like most of the family in our neighborhood, did not have books, and the books that I needed in elementary school were few. When I was in third grade, my father gave me as a birthday gift a three-volume encyclopedia bound in leather. It was called *Enciclpedia Ilustrada de la Lengua Castellana*, published by Editorial Sopena Argentina. This was a treasure that I still keep which has a special place in my library in Rydal. In those days, I needed to be surrounded by something that looked like books so I took from my father's shop pieces of wood the size of an average book and covered them with paper of different textures and colors so they looked like books. Of course they were useless for reading, but fulfilled my fantasy to create an intellectual environment where I could pursue a world that I did not have. Later on, I learned to make book-like boxes when I started to collect pieces of journals or newspaper notes that I further used for my work. It was an interior need to organize the world and the knowledge around me. *This fantasy and my chemistry cabinet set me apart.*

I was hungry to be surrounded by an environment that I did not have — books, oil paintings, photographs, beautiful furniture in hard and expensive wood — like those things that my father built but we did not have at home. The portrait of great scientists that reached my attention in the San Martin Public Library gave me the framework of the intellectual life and how the great intellectual environment was. Although, the scarcity of those things did not affect my happiness, but on the contrary, gave me the determination of being the founder of my own enterprise. For me, the present was a path to a future that I was constructing in my mind. Although I was almost 9 years old,

I visualized what I wanted and what was the surrounding media that a creative mind needed for pursuing its work. I do not think that I developed a master plan, but I realize that what I have achieved to the present day was not more than an extension of what I wanted to be when I was a child. My dearest possession in my childhood was not what I had or achieved at that moment but the *secret in me of what I wanted to be*. The only one that I dared to share this secret ambition with was my mother when I was 10 years old. She turned out to be my confidante and remained so until her death.

I never felt envy or great admiration for what others possessed. In those days, I was constructing the person that I wanted to be, although my real awakening and the centering of my life came later on. But probably this was possible because the germ started in my early schooling years.

How all these were germinating in me can only be explained because of my parents who, although economically poor, were rich in love and confidence in us. They gave us freedom and with that the wisdom of knowing how to use it. It was a freedom that made me extremely responsible for my own work and destiny. My sister, Maria del Carmen, suffered her inequality with other friends that had more material things around them. She felt the social impact of inequality more closely to her. She suffered most of her life for that, but now she has found harmony and peace in her readings and writings. I took from my mother to be more silent and observe the world that need to be conquered.

Our schooling hours were from eight to noon, which gave us a full afternoon and part of the evening to pursue the goals of our childhood — doing homework, socializing with our friends, playing, and in my case, either observing what my father was working on in his shop or doing errands for both my father and mother.

1.7. The apprentice of carpentry and cabinetmaking

I passed a great deal of my childhood watching my father make furniture or doors or windows or anything that a carpenter and a cabinetmaker might do. Observing him working made me learn enough to start helping him. The duties of a carpenter's apprentice begin with holding things and sanding. Sanding was boring and laborious, but in the end I learned how to measure and use the different saws and cut straight, how to use the different planes, and even how to sharpen the knives of the plane and align it with the main surface of the plane. The angle needed to be right to produce an even and smooth surface. I learned how to make different cuts and glue them together, how to make them dovetail for building drawers, and how to adjust them for perfect sliding. Preparing the carpenter's glue was also a job done by the apprentice. First, I learned how to buy from a special store in the city; that was the best excuse to use the tramvia. The hardware store was a dream for those workers in the carpentry and cabinetmaking business due to the variety of hardware and tools on display. The glue was sold in small bars that contained basically animal proteins like gelatin obtained from the cartilage and connective tissues of the feet of slaughtered cows or horses. The bars were mixed with an equal part of water and then heated until they melted and maintained in a receptacle with hot water to keep the glue fluid. My father used a secret ingredient that gave strength to the gluing properties — garlic. The glue smelled awful but I admit that none of the furniture glued with it ever separated. Learning the size of the nails and screws also introduced me to the English measuring system in which inches and feet were mixed with the metric system. This was a practical application of the mathematical knowledge that I received in school.

I also learned how to do the wood veneer; that is, to glue thin slices of wood, thinner than 3 mm (1/8 inch) onto core panels to produce flat surfaces that have a different appearance. It was really a lot of heavy work because everything needed to be done fast and by applying an even pressure to the thin wood while the glue was still fresh, so it would spread evenly underneath. If a bubble of air was trapped, a special cut must be done in the thin wood to release the trapped air or the job must be done again. The end results were beautiful. The thin wood came in large rolls of up to 3 m in length and up to 75 cm in width. The rolls came in oak, cedar, walnut, or mahogany. The latter was most often used. The price of the furniture was determined by the type of wood. Mahogany and guantambu, or ivory maple, were the most expensive and the hardest to work with. I made a desk in guantambu when I was in my final grade elementary school, and I used it until I graduated from medical school. I know that it is still around and used by one of the sons of my closest cousin.

The evaluation of which type of wood to use for each job was also essential. We used poplar for common stuff like windows and doors as it was well suited for the Mendoza weather, but cedar wood was preferred for the front doors of the houses. To learn to select them from the yard and to know how to buy and calculate the amount that was needed for each specific piece of furniture was also an art in itself. For the hardest woods, the best finishing was obtained when a shellac was applied. Learning how to prepare the shellac was also a special experience. The name in Spanish is *goma laca*. The shellac came in red scales that were obtained by purification of the resinous secretion produced by a small insect called *Laccifer lacca* that in those days came from Sri Lanka. My father never wanted to use the varnish that he considered cheap and unpleasant to the eye. To prepare shellac was also a special procedure because it needs to be dissolved at a concentration of 200 grams per liter of 96% alcohol, and it took 24 hours for the shellac to dissolve and form a homogenous solution. The shellac was applied with a piece of cloth, in general, pieces of old cotton shirts; it needed to be rubbed in a circle on the finished wood. The art was in letting it dry before the next layer was applied. After several passes, a beautiful patina of smoothness and brilliance is created. A well applied shellac lasts a lifetime. My father had big biceps that helped him to apply the shellac with mastery.

From my father, I also learned how to create doors and window panels and how to install them with their vises and locks. By the time I was 12, I had learned and mastered the process of carpentry and cabinetmaking. Knowledge that I still use when I need to construct something around the house.

Many of my neighbors and those near to our family circle were expecting that I would follow my father's footsteps, but also they suspected that I might be a priest. The importance of that apprenticeship was that it gave me a real appreciation of hand labor and blue-collar work in general. As a matter of fact, I never discuss the price when I need their work, and also I must confess that my heart warms up with emotions and those memories when I see a carpenter working or when I see carpenters in a yard or hardware store selecting wood or hardware for the doors or furniture.

Helping my father in the shop and doing small jobs for the neighbors, like repairing doors, furniture, or making small toys, helped me earn some money that I used to buy laboratory supplies and the microscope of my chemistry cabinet.

1.8. Knowing my neighborhood; doing errands for my parents

To be a boy also means to do errands for your parents. Doing the errands put me in touch with merchants and my neighborhood. The interesting part was that in the process I learned the value of money and how to make better use of it and also got to know the people of my neighborhood. For example, the butcher was a social person, but he tried as much as he could to trick his customers by stealing few grams of meat. If you asked him for 500 grams of rib eye, for example, he cut a piece that was almost 500 grams, but he used to throw the piece of meat with a very deliberate speed and strength in such a way that the impact made the meat initially weigh 500 grams, but when the needle of the balance stabilized was only 450 grams. Knowing his trick, you needed to give a gentle reminder to Mr. Rupi that was his name, "I wanted 500 grams not 450 grams." He would then fairly give you the right amount or in some occasions, due to remorse, a little extra for the money.

The owners of the grocery store were three Spanish brothers, but only one of them used to take care of the public and his name was Ramon. He was very friendly with everybody, and he liked to joke with young girls. On one occasion a girl called Angelica, who lived near my home and was extremely shy, went to buy vinegar. Don Ramon said to her that the vinegar he had was sour, and the girl said that if that was the case she did not want it, and she headed toward the door. The joke was that vinegar is acidic or sour, but Angelica understood that it was spoiled. He laughed and called her back and told that he was joking. Then poor Angelica was red all over as she took the vinegar and left. Another interesting character was the saddle maker; he was Lebanese, a tall and thin man. He made beautiful saddles that he kept on display; they were really lovely to the touch and to the eyes. However, he made his money by doing smaller things like repairing belts or suitcases made of heavy and thick leather that the cobbler could not repair. He was basically a complainer, although in reality he was not complaining about anything in particular but gave the impression that everything he was doing for you would be extremely difficult and beyond your means. At the end, the price was more than reasonable, but it was the way that he conducted his trade that made him memorable. For every place like the pharmacy, the noodle factory, the bakery, the shoe store, the haberdasher's shop, where articles for sewing were sold, the bookstore, the photography studio, and all the other neighbors living among them, the proprietors were basically recognized by their nationality, the Polish, the German, the Jewish, the Galician, the Italian, the French, the Turkish or by their surname, the Cortez, the Greco, the Guardia, the Carmona, and the Pages. The Pageses were interesting people because there were three brothers and all were artists. One of them was a sculptor, another a movie star, and the third one a photographer. My father used to do work for them, and my mother was friends with the wife of the sculptor. They were friendly and accomplished in their respective crafts. The sculptor, T. Pages, was the one that designed and carved the statues of the Guaymallen chief shown in Figure 1.2. A remarkable coincidence was that later on in my work I received a medal from the Argentinean Society of Gynecology and Obstetrics in appreciation of my work and the medal says "Al Maestro" or to "The teacher" and the artist that carved that medal was T. Pages.

With the photographer, I learned to do photography, which was very important for my research work. For all of those who were my neighbors and a part of my surroundings during the 18 years that I lived in that neighborhood, I had the experience of seeing their evolution as merchants as well as their losses, triumphs, and moments of happiness, and they saw me growing from a little boy to a college student, medical school attendee, and then a medical doctor who left the place to immigrate to the United States. And when I returned, I was always the son of Don Felipe, the carpenter.

1.9. My first encounter with religion

I was 9 years old when my parents sent my sister and I to catechism at the parish of San José, which was scarcely a block from our home. That was my first encounter with the Catholic Church. The pastor was Father Moreira, a very unorthodox priest who was not afraid to fight against the Peronists or the leftists that were emerging in the parish in those days. I did not interact with him too much, but I remember his impressively large figure which was magnified by his black cassock and the biretta, a stiff square-shaped hat with silk trim and tuft. The biretta is a sign of authority, and he wore it all the time. Anyway, he was an impressively big man with a very loud voice that reverberated from one corner to another in the Church. He was the one that finished the construction of the Church, and I met one of the neighbors, a mason who had been working with him in the final construction of the building. He told me that "without Moreira, the church would never be finished." Father Moreira was a fighter who probably would have been a crusader in the sixteenth century. The catechist teachers were two ladies, one a motherly type of around 35 years of age, and the other could not have been more than 24. Although I do not remember their names, the important point is that they taught us the principles of the Catholic faith, and I must confess that took a while to understand, until I realized that the basic catechism of the Catholic faith is in the Gospels. Later on, I realized that many people get away from the Church because of the dissociation of the Gospel from the Church, as if they were two separate things, and they are not. At the end of our catechism, my sister and I took our First Communion.

In common terms, I was hooked by the curiosity to know more about what was in the Church, and it was coincidental that a new pastor came and replaced Father Moreira. The name of the new pastor was Father Donati; he was born in Italy but spoke perfect Spanish and was a person who changed the spirituality of the parish and made a significant impression in my life. He used to say in mass, "If I am not living a life of sanctity I cannot expect that my parishioner be saints." That concept was really brave to say and to teach.

I was accepted to be an altar boy, and that helped me to learn every single part of the mass and its meaning. We used to wear a red or black cassock depending on whether it was a festive liturgical day or an ordinary time. Part of the learning was also how to keep the cassock clean and erase the paraffin of the candles — that was some kind of universal law, as we used to say, that the candles always dripped on the cassock. In the process of becoming an altar boy, I learned the meaning of the different parts of the vestments that the priest wears during the Mass. Although the vestments were originally ordinary garments in the ancient Church, they have been, with small changes, continuously used to the present day. It constitutes a witness to the historical continuity of the Catholic Church, which was started by St Peter. The most important part of this period of my life was that it allowed me to be close to the life of many priests and helped me to erase from my mind the false conceptions that most of the people have, including myself, about the Church and its ministers.

I spent many hours as an altar boy in the Church, and many of my relatives believed that I would be a priest. Curiously, people have their own ideas of what others should be, like those who speculated that I would follow the footsteps of my father and be a carpenter and a cabinetmaker. The reality was that neither ever crossed my mind — to be a carpenter or a priest. My parents always knew what I wanted to be.

1.10. The attraction for fencing and the movies

My friend Angel and I had, in addition to the common interest of pretending to be scientists, a fascination with fencing, and we rarely missed the serial of *El Zorro* in the Sunday matinee at our neighborhood movie theater. A week without the Sunday dose of fencing was incomplete. We practiced fencing with wooden swords so that we improved with time, until I found that the hardest wood we could get was one that my father used in making furniture, called guantambu. That made the most durable swords, but it was difficult to shape because of the hardness of the wood. Angel started making small knives, but we could not make swords with metal. However, Angel achieved the mastery to make beautiful knife handles with leather and wood. Fencing made our childhood more normal to the eyes of our parents, and after all, we were normal kids. However, fencing was something that interested me, and in college I took fencing classes and there I learned how to use the floret and real swords.

1.11. Facing mortality

I had already celebrated my 7th birthday when, walking home from one of my errands, I saw on the ground a dead bird. Its intestines were exposed, open probably because some predators wanted to eat it. This was my first realization of death; I remember that all my being was moved with pity for the animal and also a tremendous sadness for the loss of life. It was my first awakening that life was limited, and that it was so unique that when it is gone only the decay of the flesh is visible to our eyes. This awakening had a more profound effect when my grandfather Sebastian came to visit us one year later, and he developed cardiac insufficiency and died. He was the first person that I saw dying, and he was a part of us. This highly spirited man suddenly was silent and unresponsive, and when the funeral was over, he was no longer among us, the living. I remember new faces like his brother Ignacio and his sister-in-law Josephine, that was the first time that I met them, and also the other sons and daughter of Sebastian together with my grandmother Dominga. All the Paganos were for the first time in my life together in one room. They were so different to each other but all of them had the warm appeal of human beings who had been suffering and who knew their place in this earth. They stayed for a couple of days and left. However, the emptiness that I felt was not because all the family had returned to their normal activities, but the vacuum that my grandfather left in which there were no more stories about Italy or the sound of his singing arias of the operas he loved. Mortality became real to me.

1.12. My cousin

I have dozens of cousins coming from both sides of the family, but the one that was closest to me during my childhood remained like that until his recent death. He was the son of my aunt Antonia, the sister of my mother. Jorge Sebastian Castillo was 4 years older than me, and we were completely opposed in personality and intellectual interests, but we were very congenial and enjoyed the other's company. He was generous and well intentioned with a jovial character and the propensity to make jokes and laugh. He had a great affection for my father. We used to see each other almost every weekend by our family going to San Martin or them coming to our home. Because he was older than me, he knew things that I did not know, and he was ready to teach me. One of them was how to work with the raw iron. He grew up watching his blacksmith father make shoeing forges, and in those days, his father was still shoeing horses, and that was a show in itself, to see my uncle managing the horse and molding the horseshoe to the right size, and then nailing it to the hoof in the right position; it was a great thing to watch. But when the number of horses decreased as they were replaced by cars, my uncle started using his skills from the shoeing forge to create more artistic work like garden chairs, tables, and other iron garden decorations. Therefore, my cousin Jorge Sebastian also learned the proficiency of this new craft, and he helped me or did for me all the ring stands that I used to suspend beakers, flasks, and other glassware that I gathered in my chemistry cabinet.

When he entered puberty, he was obsessed with seeing girls, and I often accompanied him to San Martin Avenue, Saturday afternoons and Sunday mornings, where there was a good display of girls. Although later on I understood his interest, when I was 10, I preferred to do other things; but for a 14-year-old boy that was a good exercise for the eyes.

1.13. The selection of college

Just a few months after my 10th birthday, I learned the meaning of the word "cancer," which in my rudimentary understanding, meant an abnormal growth of cells that could kill a person. In those days, the Internet did not exist, so the public library was the only source of knowledge. It was in searching those great, dusty science books — which apparently did not appeal to the general public since I was often the only one using them — that my intellectual horizons started to broaden and the desire to be a physician-scientist crystallized in my mind. At that point, it became clear to me that studying medicine was my only option. This was an important realization because then I had to choose the right college when I finished elementary school. When I was in sixth grade, or my last year of elementary school, one of the main tasks was deciding what to do next. I had already chosen the Colegio Nacional Agustin Alvarez, which I will refer to as Agustin Alvarez National College. However, the friends of my family as well as many close relatives felt this was not a good decision for me because that college was selected by those who were planning to go on to the university, pursuing a higher education, and if I did not do that my chances of finding useful employment with a bachelor of science degree would be very limited. Instead, if I selected another college, such as the Commerce College, I would be qualified to work in an accountant's office or perhaps be a clerk in a bank or an insurance company. On the other hand, if I went to the Normal School, I could become certified to be a teacher and teach in an elementary school. The province and the nation in general were short of teachers in those days, and a male teacher would also be highly appreciated in a discipline disproportionately populated by women. Others even suggested that I could also teach individually for those that need additional schooling and work from my home or even work in private academies. Other family friends suggested that my best option would be to go to agronomy and get the title of "certified enology technician." This was considered by some of them the best option because there was so much need for skilled workers in a growing economy like Mendoza's, in which wine was the main export. Still other relatives suggested seriously that due to my proclivity to be so near to the Catholic Church, entering the Lulunta Seminary in Mendoza was a good option. Cynically, they indicated that priests would never be poorer than us.

The sad part of all these good, well-meant, and seriously intentioned opinions was that they saw two main aspects of me, the economic part and my personal capabilities. The reality was that our family friends and many relatives considered that as the son of a carpenter, I would need to start working soon to earn more money that could either help my parents or help myself. The other way to see those opinions was that, to their eyes, probably I did not seem impressive enough to become a medical doctor or a lawyer or an engineer. Even for me, it was difficult to explain that I wanted to be a physician-scientist with the intention of becoming a cancer researcher. At that age, it was too complex for me to explain all my internal evolution and living experiences; it would sound like a foreign language to them. For all these reasons, their opinions and suggestions did not matter to me. My parents, who knew my aspirations, answered those many suggestions by saying that at 12 years I was big enough to start making my own decisions. Many of them volunteered to get the application for those different suggestions, and when I told them that I would go to the Agustin Alvarez National College, they rolled their eyes and changed the subject.

I had made my decision that the only way to become a cancer researcher was to go to the medical school. Thus, in that pursuit, I should be very focused because I had learned that entering the medical school in Mendoza was not easy; there was an exhaustive selection process in which only 80 students were accepted per year, and the examination included a written and an oral test of mathematics, physics, chemistry, biology, and medical English. Therefore, it was clear that the best post-elementary school option for me was the Agustin Alvarez National College, which would provide the solid basis of science that I needed to enter the medical school — and so that is what I did.

References

[1] Comroe, J. H. Jr. Pay dirt: the story of streptomycin. Part I: from Waksman to Waksman. *Am. Rev. Respir. Dis.* 117: 773–781, 1978.

[2] Kingston, W. Streptomycin, Schatz v. Waksman, and the balance of credit for discovery. *J. Hist. Med. Allied Sci.* 59: 441–462, 2004.

[3] Benedek, T. G. The history of gold therapy for tuberculosis. *J. Hist. Med. Allied Sci.* 59: 50–89, 2004.

[4] The gold treatment of Tuberculosis. *Am. J. Public Health* (*NY*) 15: 631, 1925.

[5] Yunque, A. *Alem, el hombre de la multitud*, Ediciones Biebel, Buenos Aires. 1945.

Chapter 2

Agustin Alvarez National College (1955–1959)

2.1. The Agustin Alvarez National College

This chapter covers the years from 1955 to 1959 and narrates the changes that I experienced in my life during that time, as well as my vision of the college education that I received. I will also compare my views with how others perceived the college education and elaborate on the political turmoil that took place in those days. I will emphasize how this education impacted me and remains an integral part of the man that I am today. My experiences could be unique, and I do not know if they can be extrapolated to those students before or after me. Even more, I do not know if my classmates have had the same vital experiences and saw what I saw. *These are my memories.*

2.1.1. Defining the college

The college was an icon in Mendoza holding the name of Agustin Alvarez, a man born in Mendoza in 1857 who belonged to the group of Argentineans called the "generation of the '80s" [1]. The college (Figure 2.1) is still there today, a massive structure with a typical French architecture, occupying 1.7 acres, facing east toward Independence Square.

The college was an expression of Mendoza's conservative society. Agustin Alvarez was a military-educated man, a sociologist and

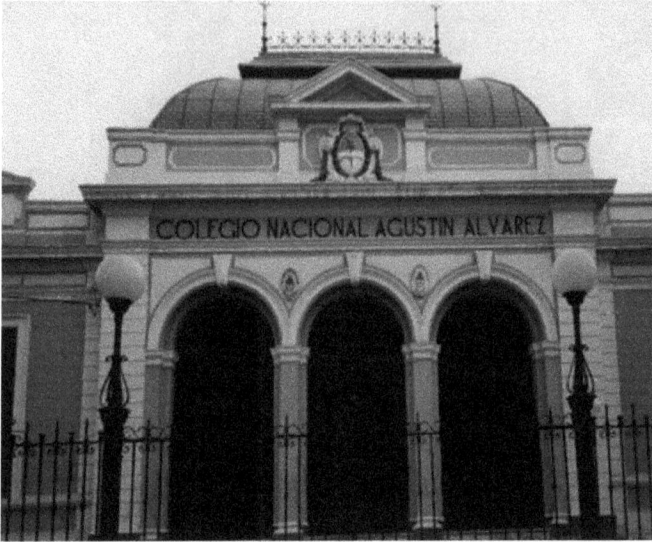

Figure 2.1:   Agustin Alvarez National College in the city of Mendoza. Photo taken in 2006.

educator; although his parents and immediate relatives died in the earthquake of 1861, in 1870, he was able to attend the college that would later hold his name. After enrolling in the Military School of the Nation, Alvarez studied law and dedicated most of his time to teaching in the National College, producing a significant amount of literary and journalistic work. His writing and teaching left a mark in Argentina, making him one of the so-called generation of the '80s. The generation of the '80s [1] has been criticized and is considered to represent the oligarchy, mainly in the provinces of Mendoza and Buenos Aires. Their ideology was basically to keep the country in peace and make it attractive to foreign investment by concentrating on economic growth through their agricultural products, which would help to maintain the importation of manufactured goods. Radicalism and later on Peronism [2] criticized this generation because the positive international balance of trade of Argentina that they achieved was not reinvested in the modernization and industrialization of the country's basic production. However, in their defense, they expended the trade surplus and developed the infrastructure of the country, building roads, ports, bridges, the railroad system, universities, and colleges. They also favored immigration, mainly from Europe, and the idea of free education. The ones who benefited from this free elementary, college, and university education were those who could understand the long-term benefits of it. The generation of the '80s imitated the migratory policies of the USA and advocated developing the country by improving the infrastructure, hoping that the people would be resourceful enough to use those tools to create more wealth. Unfortunately, that did not happen. That generation maintained political power for almost 40 years, but they could not quench the socialist movement and the political forces of a populism brought by radicalism [3] and later, by Peronism [2]. Another thing that they did not correctly calculate was that the wave of European immigration brought, in addition to hard-working immigrants like my grandparents, intellectuals full of anarchistic and socialist ideas that helped generate the populism that surged in Argentina after the Second World War. These positions were completely opposed to each other because in one vision the wealth of a nation must be invested in creating an adequate environment that in turn will help the creation of more wealth by its citizens; instead, the other vision on how to build a nation believed that the government must be the custodian and provider of wealth to its citizens.

Whatever the forces that contributed to the political evolution of Argentina as a nation, the Agustin Alvarez National College was the result of the '80s generation. The college was the embodiment of their vision of how college-age boys and girls should have a humanistic education. This humanistic education required that the students have an understanding of two languages besides Castellan, either English and French, or English and Italian. The college must provide a solid basis of the Castellan language. After all, the way in which you speak is the one that determines your level of education. Not only for the right articulation of the words, but also for avoiding dialectic expressions. Mathematics, trigonometry, geometry, and all the branches of biology, like botany, zoology, anatomy, and hygiene, were emphasized and taught. Part of this humanistic education was also the learning of history, comprised of antiquity, medieval, modern, and contemporary, and ending with Argentinean history; and the same applied to geography and its social and economic implications. Understanding of European, Spanish, and Argentinean literature was emphasized by requiring students to read and comment on the most important original literary works, such as Miguel de Cervantes, Francisco de Quevedo, Baltasar Gracian, and Fernando de Rojas, to name just a few [4–7]. The concept was that this knowledge made a person an educated one. Psychology, logic, accounting, drawing, music, and physical education were also part of the curriculum. This humanistic education was considered by many as elitist, out of fashion or out of touch with the needs of the nation, because it was not a practical background to find and hold a job, but whatever had been the intention of the '80s generation in creating that humanistic education, it was exactly what I was looking for.

2.1.2. *My discovery of the college*

In March 1955, when I was 13 years old, I had my first day of college. The concept of college in the Argentina of those days was different from the American concept of college. It was more comparable to a European high school, which prepares students for the university. In those days, there were four different curriculums functioning in the same building. The Normal School operated from 8 a.m. to noon, and it was the only coed school in the province, otherwise all the schools, with the exception of the university, were separated by gender. The Normal School was oriented toward certification as schoolteachers. They were using the edifice on a temporary basis until the permanent one was built on a nearby street. The second was the girls of the National College, also called lyceum that basically had the same curriculum as the Agustin Alvarez National College. They occupied the same building from noon to 4 p.m. The third turn was the Agustin Alvarez National College for boys that I attended, and we had classes until 8 p.m. followed by a technical school for adult men that lasted until midnight.

The college, in addition to the classrooms and administrative offices, had an "aula magna," or auditorium, that easily held five hundred students, with well-kept leather chairs lining a center aisle that accentuated the polished wooden floor of the room. The ceiling had several lamps with the already generous light enhanced in the early afternoon by the sunlight coming from the sets of French doors at both sides of the auditorium. Those doors were also used by the students entering and exiting the classroom. The auditorium was the main setting for academic gatherings as well as for conferences, musical recitals, and movies. In addition, the "aula magna" had a place for a choir and a concert piano that was used also for our music lessons.

The college had a beautiful library almost 80 × 40 feet in size with wall-to-wall glass doors, covered bookcases, and many desks for reading. The collection of books was significant. The ones that called to me the most were related to chemistry, and I found volumes in Spanish, French, English, and Russian. The majority were in French. My first reading was about inorganic chemistry, and I became fascinated by the discovery of phosphorus and its properties. The library was well kept and had a beautiful oak floor.

A massive mahogany case held a grandfather clock which stood near the entrance as an impartial witness, counting the minutes in the lives of the hundreds of students that passed in front of it. In a society with tardiness as a rule, the clock was a stoic reminder that punctuality was still important. It marked the time and made sure that each class was not one minute too long or too short.

The other main discovery of my first year was that the college had three laboratories, one for physics, another for chemistry, and the third one that contained a large collection of birds, rodents, and other embalmed animals, from felines to small primates. Each of them had a small brass plaque engraved with the Latin names and the common name in French. There were also insectariums, glass jars containing some marine species, and other ones with anatomical organs. All these collections were preserved on wooden oak shelves, and some were covered by doors made of glass framed in oak wood. In a compendium (Figure 2.2) that I prepared for the zoology class in my second year,

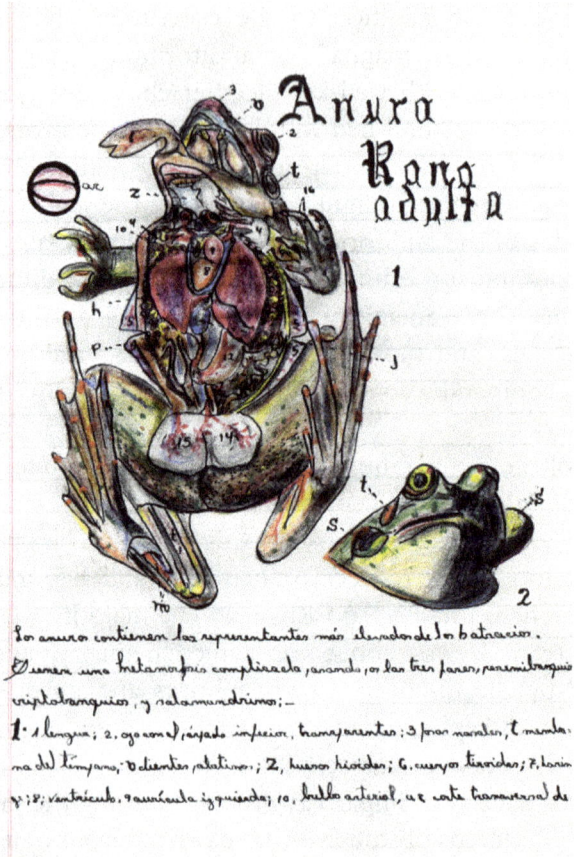

Figure 2.2: Drawing of an adult frog (Bufo arenarum) as part of the Compendium of Zoology that I wrote in my second year of college in 1956. The drawing was in ink and colored with Faber-Castell color pencils.

I used details of some of these specimens to make my drawings, in which I also put to work my mastery of China ink and coloring.

The physics laboratory held an assortment of many devices, like cathetometers, which are telescopes on a graduate scale for accurate measurement of small vertical distances; balances of different vintages and precisions, pulleys of different sizes to study the use of forces and surfaces for studying action and reaction forces. There were also densitometers, vacuum pumps, centrifuges, hydraulic presses, communicating tubes, barometers of different sizes and shapes, pneumatic pumps, and the most beautiful of all were the optical instruments, like microscopes. It would be a long list if I enumerated all the equipment that was used and explained the basics of magnetism and electricity, but they were also part of the physics laboratory. I used some of these instruments in a compendium that I wrote for my physics classes in my first years of college (Figure 2.3).

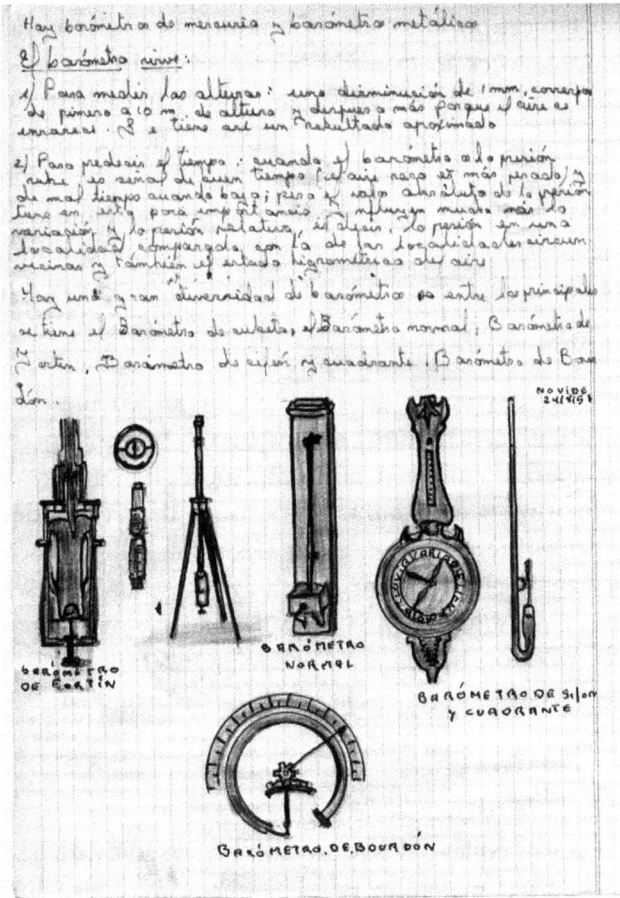

Figure 2.3: Drawing of different types of barometers, as part of the Compendium of Physics, that I wrote in my first year of college, 1955.

The chemistry laboratory was made of different cabinets containing glassware of many varied sizes and shapes, beakers, Erlenmeyer flasks, graduated cylinders, distillation serpentines, and glass balloons. There was an entire wall containing shelves displaying different drugs, most of them powders showing the original German brands. My chemistry cabinet looked so insignificant when compared to this one. The three laboratories were joined by an amphitheater that held sixty students and where the chemistry or physics classes were held at least once a month.

Physical education class, or gymnastics, was given early in the morning once a week in different places around the city, mainly in sports clubs. The most attractive part was that each student could choose a sport to study, and I chose fencing. Those were great classes given to us by Captain Arias, which was the way he wanted to be addressed. We were only eight students in my class, and one of them was Manuel Carmona who, although not in my division, was an alumnus of the college. He was also a neighbor but we had never met before; fencing made us friends and we expended many hours practicing the use of the foil. In Spanish, the foil is called "floret," and is one of the three weapons used in the sport of fencing. The foil was not heavy, less than a pound, and it had a capped tip that, when properly connected, allowed a fencer to score, giving an electric sound or lighting a red light every time that you touched the opponent. I liked fencing because it is a sport full of grace and art. Fencing was the melting of our childhood into our adolescence, and by practicing fencing we learned to apply the rules of the sport instead of the skirmish of the Three Musketeers or El Zorro [8,9]. From my perspective, college had more than I had ever imagined.

2.1.3. *The college environment*

On my first day of college, I wore a dark brown suit with a white shirt and a well-knotted matching tie. The shoes were also brown. The jacket and tie were the dress code for students of the National College. That was our uniform. For the boys of those days, we learned very fast what the uniform was and was not. First you could not wear sneakers because they were only for the gymnastic, or physical education, class. The shoes needed to be the right color to match the rest of the attire. If you wore another not matching color it would be considered in bad taste. For example, you could not wear brown shoes with gray or blue pants. The same applied to the socks, which needed to match the color of the shoes. To wear white socks with the uniform signified that you were a "nerd" or a careless person. A white shirt went well with every ensemble. But the collar was what truly determined your taste and refinement. It should be starched and ironed. The right collared shirt allowed wearing the right tie, which must never be of flashy color or with silly motifs. A common dress code of gray pants with a blue blazer was the most frequent attire of college students, and also Argentinean men's wear in general. This kind of dress code was not difficult for me to implement because my mother and father knew how to dress, and they had a good knowledge of fabrics and styles. My mother tailored women's dresses, and she had a very good sense also of men's fashion. Even though I did not have a great assortment of clothes, she was proud that my shirts were perfectly starched and ironed, and the crease of my pants was always right. I never felt uneasy with my dress code and followed it to my present days. At the National College, the tie was a central piece of our uniform; as a matter of fact, in the last day of our promotion, we cut our ties and shared small pieces of them with the rest of our classmates. We were supposed to keep the scraps forever as a sign of the permanent link between all of us.

The 150 students of my first year were divided into five divisions with around 30 students each. The number of divisions decreased at the end of the 5 years, meaning that from the approximately 150 who started, around 60 of them either dropped out of college or moved to other ones, which is what happened to my best friend, Angel. After the first year, he moved to a private school in the city. My class started with 34 students and only 23 were my classmates at the end of college (Figure 2.4).

Every day we had five different "signatures"; in that first year, they ranged from Castellan, mathematics, chemistry, physics, botany, history, geography, social studies, music, English, and drawing. Each

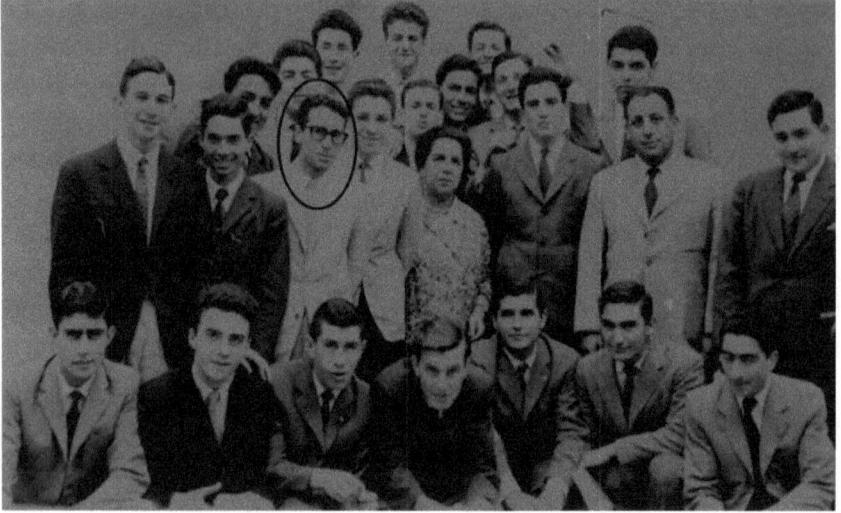

Figure 2.4:   Promotion of 1959. Circled is the author.

signature had a professor specialized in those subjects, and their personalities and ways of teaching were as different as the subjects that they taught. For example, the drawing class was under Professor Jose Estrella, who had a master's degree in fine arts. He was a short but energetic and highly spirited man that also gave special classes to the students who were willing on the third Sunday morning of each month. In those classes, we practiced free drawing in the fresh air of San Martin Park. I remember that I used to take the tramvia number 5/3 that had a special Start = Estrella (in honor of the drawing professor) in the top. This tramvia had the longest route and covered almost all the neighborhoods around the city where the students of the National College lived. All my first concepts of perspective, composition, and the use of light and shadows came from those days.

I continued developing my drawing abilities through college, and I applied that knowledge in the compendiums that I prepared for zoology class (Figures 2.5–2.10).

The first year of college was difficult for me, because I needed to adapt from one teacher to 11 different ones and also to be disciplined enough to prepare for the classes that were evaluated every single day.

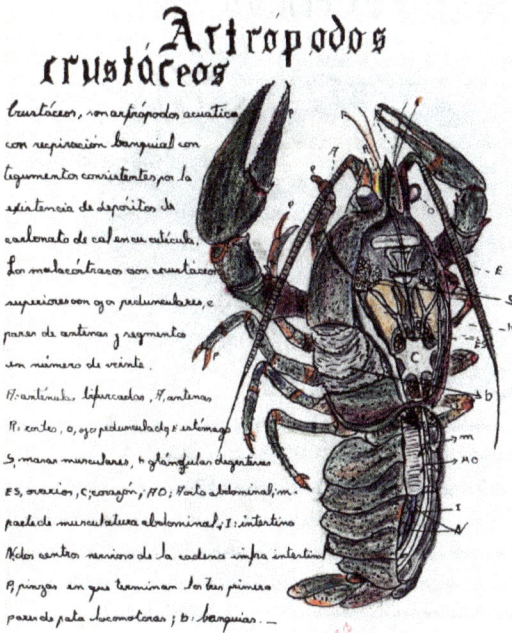

Figure 2.5: Drawing of a lobster (crustaceous), as part of the Compendium of Zoology that I wrote in my second year of college, 1956. The drawing was in ink and colored with Faber-Castell color pencils.

In general, the classes were 45 minutes in length, and in the first 25 minutes, the professor called the students to the front of the class to be interrogated. This process was at random and as a consequence it was very difficult to predict who would be called, because some of the professors called the same student two or three times in a row or started at the beginning or the end of the list. Whatever the method they used, it was difficult for us to predict, and before each class speculations arose as to who was the most probable candidate to be in the front. Therefore, theoretically, you must be prepared all the

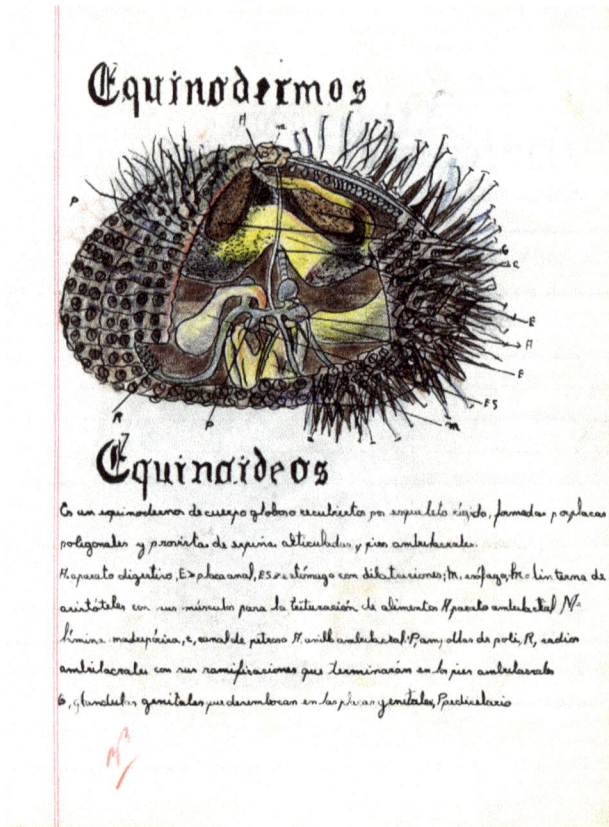

Figure 2.6:   Drawing of a sea urchin, as part of the Compendium of Zoology that I wrote in my second year of college, 1956. The drawing was in ink and colored with Faber-Castell color pencils.

time and in all the subjects. In these oral presentations, also called "being in the front," you must answer specific questions about the topic of the day, meaning that you could not recite by memory the topic, but you needed to know the subject in order to answer specific questions that again were at random. For example, in the geography class, you needed to show on the map — which the monitor of each division brought to the class before the professor arrived — and to be very precise as you indicated the path of a river or the location of a city. In mathematics class, usually one student was called to the front and assigned a problem to solve. The student was expected to explain how he was solving the equation, not only the correct answer. Those calls to the front are unforgettable, and we used to say that the professor made us sweat ink or "*sudar tinta.*" In any of the biology classes, "to be in the front" was to explain using a model or a drawing or the part of a plant or a bird in the case of zoology. After these 25 dramatic minutes, the professor explained a new concept that would be discussed or presented by the students in the next class. It was understood that in 20 minutes the professor could hardly cover the whole topic, and so they only emphasized those concepts that were not well described in the textbook. Therefore, you were expected to take notes from what they said and then to study in the book or books for that signature. If you did not follow this sequence, you paid the consequences when you were chosen. From these experiences, "in the front" originated the most extraordinary stories that we as a group remembered through the years. There were two standout ones. The first took place during our first year of botany class; one of the students was told to come to the front and the professor asked him to describe the *Solanum tuberosum*. The student did not have even a remote idea of what the word *Solanum tuberosum* meant, but instead of saying, "Sorry, Professor, I have not studied the lesson," he just started inventing based on what he believed was *Solanum tuberosum*. He said that it was a plant that grew in tropical areas and that required a lot of light, and from there derived the *Solanum* name, because in Spanish "sol" is the sun, which produces a lot of light. The professor was a massive six and a half feet tall, weighed at least 240 pounds with a red, round face and red hair in a crew cut. He was so furious that we were expecting him to die of an apoplexy. He commanded the student to sit and gave him a fail, or a zero. The reason that he was so upset was because *Solanum tuberosum* refers to the "potato," which is not only native to the Andes but the most abundant and frequent food, something we ate every day, and also the fourth largest food crop in the world, meaning that the question of the professor was pertinent and not skewed; it was something that all of us were supposed to know. The other story took place in anatomy class when we were in our third year. The professor asked the student called to the front a simple question: what was the size of the human testicle? The student intuitively put his hand in the pocket of his trouser, and the professor quickly saw what was coming and sent him back to his seat because he was cheating. The more I recall those days, the more memories come to me, but describing all the demonstrations of our ignorance is not the objective of this chapter. At the same time, all the foolishness, or really bullshitting, was created as part of the drama; "to be in the front" was an important part of college education.

At least once every two weeks, we had a surprise test. The professor would arrive and after greeting the students, used to say, "Please, gentlemen, get a piece of paper and write" the assignment for the day or a portion of the assignment, for example, "write on the consequences of the Second Punic War and the role of Hannibal." Every time that the professor came and called us "gentlemen" or "caballeros," we knew that the test was coming. The point was that if you were not prepared there was a 100% chance of failing, or getting a zero on the test. That fail would be averaged with all the other grades that you had and if your score was less than 5, or "good," then you did not pass or need to take the examination for that signature at the end of the semester. If you failed that examination, you were not allowed to pass to the following year. That was the main reason why, of the 150 students that started in the National College, only around 90 reached the end.

During my first year of college, an additional pressure was the political environment provided by the Union of Students, also called *UES*, which in Spanish means *Union de Estudiantes Secundarios*, which was managed by the Peronist party. The Peronists were deeply interested in hooking new party members and enticing them with attractions like dancing, social meetings with girls, and of course, if needed, some financial aid. For a boy in college, girls were a magnetic attraction. The moral reputation of this group was extremely bad for both boys and girls; however, many were attracted to them. For the UES college was the place to have fun and to do everything that you could not do before. For them college was a liberation and a time to be young before you faced the serious place that was the university, assuming you were able to do it, or got a job and started an independent life.

Another disturbing signal that I received from many of my classmates was that they were not expecting to learn too much in college, because according to them, the professors did not teach anything. Rationally, it was impossible to expect that they covered the entire textbook. The objective was that they provided the salient issues and described those areas that were not well covered in the textbooks, and then you completed the picture with their notes and by studying in the books. In those days, computers did not exist in the classroom and the Internet was unknown, meaning that the notes taken in class and the textbooks were the main sources for acquiring knowledge. Therefore, the philosophy was not to learn but to pass like a laxative from one year to another. In this new environment, first, I was not interested in any political ideology and less in Peronism; second, I wanted to learn; third, the subjects were extraordinarily interesting, and finally the professors really knew their subjects and were not the morons that many of my classmates thought them to be.

In order to be truthful, a few professors were very sketchy and additional explanations would have been of great help. However, in subjects like mathematics, Castellan, chemistry, and physics, they practically explained everything step by step, and in my perspective, that was invaluable. In other areas like history, geography, and literature, for example, the latitudes were broader and it was natural that they only covered the most salient points. One example was the professor of Argentinean history who was also teaching at the University National of Cuyo and was a historian revisionist who had authored several papers on the subject; this was an asset in my view. He explained to us points that were not clearly treated in the book. One of them was the biography of Juan Manuel de Rosas. The version in the textbook as well as in many publications was that he was a brutal tyrant [10,11], and although he is still a controversial figure in Argentinean history, he brought to us another perspective. He showed us that he was the one who developed the concept of federal government and contributed to developing the autonomies of the provinces in Argentina. These were positive points of his government that were lost to the conventional historian. He was criticized for his nationalistic position, being the first one to try to stop foreign influences and develop an Argentinean sense of nation that brought as a consequence two blockades during his government, one by the French and the other from the British [11]. Independently, that Argentinean historian revisionist had been criticized [10,11]; this professor introduced, at least in me, the ability to challenge what is written because what reaches us is not always the correct version, and so we must start seeing things in a broader context and evaluate the different opinions. He used to tell us that the reason why we should see historical events critically is because "history cannot be written in the present, and journalists are the ones that are narrating the present because their function is to show what happens, and the historian instead will use those documents and other acts or events to write history." Therefore, I felt there was an inconsistency in what I was seeing, what the UES tried to depict that college was, a place and time for having fun, and that for many of my classmates, college was a waste of time. They cannot say waste of money because it was free and 99% of them did not work at all and were family sustained. Without sounding dogmatic, I knew that college was not a waste of time; on the contrary, it was a specific time in our lives meant to help us organize and learn what and who we are. Therefore, I believed that I was right, and the other positions were completely wrong.

2.1.4. *The political event*

The most important political event that took place in the first year of college was the military coup that ended in the removal of Domingo Peron from the government, but was not the end of Peronism [12]. On September 16, 1955, I knew the real political colors of the rector, the professors, and the administrators. It was almost 6 p.m. when the alarm sounded in the middle of one of our classes, and we were not expecting that the class would end so soon. We saw the rector and many of the Professors that were not in class at that moment running through the patios of the college holding the Argentinean flag and shouting, "We are free." The next step was soldiers, with their Mausers that had attached bayonets as a remnant of the German army and were still in use by the militaries in Argentina in those days, asking the students to leave in a single file and guarding us in case something might happen outside the building. I remember that I ran to my home with another kid, Manuel Carmona; he was my classmate in fencing and his house was four houses apart from mine. The streets were deserted and when I arrived home, I saw the desperation painted in the faces of my parents. They were worried about what could happen to me because they could not leave the house due to the curfew dictated by the new military government. Although in Mendoza, the military coup or, Freedom Revolution as it was called, was without major incident; in other parts of the country and in Buenos Aires, the military coup was not without violence and shedding of blood. A week after this turmoil, we came back to class and from my perspective nothing changed in my student life. I do not recall any change in the behavior of my professors, but the big change was that the UES disappeared and those who had been promoting it were either silent enough to be inconspicuous or had changed college.

2.1.5. *Looking at myself in the mirror*

My first year of classes ended in November of 1955, and the many events that had taken place at the political level were now in the news, which was full of stories and graphic pictures of terrors and destruction, describing the abuses and corruption of the Peronists during the last 10 years of their rule. In brief, the country was in a mix of happiness, mourning, and shock. There are significant amounts of excellent work detailing the pros and cons of these events [2,12,13], and it is not the place of these memoirs to describe them.

The big change in my family was that my father no longer had the Peronists to attack, and he had a renewed hope for the revival of his Democratic Party. This also was a source of relief for my mother, who had been afraid all the time that something could happen to my father due to his vociferous criticisms of the Peronist government. Besides that, our family life remained like before.

For me, the first year of college was a painful realization of what I was. I finished with an average score, and I saw myself as a mediocre student. My gap of knowledge and education was even higher that I'd believed it was when I'd started. I didn't compare with other students who surpassed me in every single aspect. They spoke better than me, they had better knowledge of a second language, they knew more history and literature, they had read books that I had never heard of before, and they had better social skills than I did. It is true that there were many schoolmates equal to and others worse than me. But this time, I compared myself with those who were significantly brighter or more educated than me. This time all the secret ambitions of my elementary school and my chemistry cabinet were not enough for me to quench the sadness and mortification that I felt at being average.

The only person who knew what was going inside me was my mother, who had been my confidant for the previous 2 years and would continue to be. She did not have an answer for me, and I did not expect that she would have one either, but talking with her, palpating her love, was soothing for me.

The situation that I saw in those days was not of any interest on my part to compete with anybody to be better than them, but the Gordian knot of the conflict was how to be the best not by comparison but because I was "good," the most knowledgeable and educated, able to manage any conversation, debate and produce logical conclusions. I wasn't interested in being the best competitor but instead that my entire person should emanate qualities of knowledge and goodness. Why those feelings? I did not know, but I felt that was a transforming force, emerging like a giant inside of me, although I did not know what to do. It was like my experiences in the elementary school were emerging again but this time magnified.

In trying to be rational, I approached the problem like an equation. In the left side of the equation were all the elements needed to equalize with the right side, which was the final product. The final product was to be a better man or a man that lived in greatness. Therefore, the first step was to define the components needed in the left side of the equation. It was clear to me that I must eliminate any feeling that could skew the result. For example, those students who were the most educated also came from wealthy families that had provided them with the advantage of knowing more, either because they were raised in a more intellectual environment, coming from parents who were professionals, like lawyers, accountants, engineers, or physicians; or they had had the opportunity of traveling or attending language schools; and also an environment that allowed them to have better social skills and manners. They already were used to going to the opera or assisting in music concerts, whereas I was not. I realized that I could not reproduce those things in my life, therefore, I could not turn these disadvantages in my favor, and they must be eliminated from my equation. If I considered those factors, it could be an indication that I was trying to skew the results by considering that those small disadvantages or lack of experiences would give me an excuse to self-justify the factors that must be listed in the left side of the equation. Therefore, the only factors that should be considered for making me the best student and the best man must be outside of that economic and social advantage. I should not use those as an excuse for my ignorance because I did not want to have the sentiments that many of my communist or socialist classmates had.

2.2. The awakening

The reality was that I had sparked a flame for my own awakening. For starters, I decided that I would not change colleges, because that could modify my curriculum and affect my admission to medical school. The option to go to a private school that had similar curriculum was also out of the question because my parents could not afford it, and the other, most important reason was that I was not interested in being part of that pond.

I physically concentrated all my study material in one corner of my room, adding a larger bookcase to the desk that I'd built one year earlier, and I kept my room out of the noise and activities of the house. That turned out to be my room and my study corner until I left my home. I also established a plan for my daily activities starting at 5 a.m. and ending around 11 p.m. I pushed myself to endure 14–16 hours of study a day to prepare for medical school.

In that summer, my method was systematically to use the morning and part of the late afternoon and evening for studying, and then I left the early afternoon for other activities, like helping my father in the carpentry shop or reading. Applying this strict schedule that I imposed on myself, I reviewed all the signatures that I'd had in my first year and located were my deficiencies were most obvious, like my Castellan and my knowledge of history and literature. I also started to study by reading out loud authors like Demosthenes [14] and listening myself so I could improve the speed, intonation, and accent of each word. I went twice a week to the library to borrow books that could supplement my textbooks and started reading voraciously every single minute that I had free so I could catch up where I was deficient. I will say that I had covered a significant amount of literary work [15–30], and one book that flamed my heart was *Cuerpos y Almas,* or *Bodies and Souls,* by Maxence van der Meersch [31].

By the end of the summer of 1956, I started feeling better about myself and realized that my brain network had been improving significantly, and I was able to recall and associate dates and facts faster and more accurately, meaning that I learned at the end how to study consciously and not waste my time.

In addition to this, I must record in these memories the influence of Father Donati, the spiritual leader of the Catholic movement in the San Jose Parish. I'd been admitted to this group one year earlier. The group had acquired a new vigor with Father Donati, and although I did not participate in the multiple activities of the group, I was specially attracted by Donati. He had impressed me by his faith, his commitment to priesthood, and his charity toward others. Another interesting aspect about his person was his impeccable presence and his vast knowledge.

I was not and am not a person who easily finds other human beings to admire, but Father Donati, at that moment of my life, touched the fibers that had started vibrating in me. Much later, when I was already in medical school, he died in a tragic car accident coming from Buenos Aires after having an audience with the Pope in Rome; I felt devastated and it took me a while to accept his passing.

Father Donati understood my thirst for knowledge, and he went to the root of my faith and introduced me to the Gospels. I discovered that the only model of my life was there. He allowed me to understand that in order to be a real man, my life must be centered in Christ. A big relief was to know that this did not mean that I had to embrace priesthood. Basically, the message of the Gospel and the Church is that to be a Christian is to accept and be a *co-creator with God of this world*, and if I wanted to be a researcher, it was a part of the role of a Christian to create knowledge and open a new understanding of what surrounds us. The concept of co-creators put Christians in another dimension that separated us from other philosophical ideas or religions that I will not touch in these memoirs. Among the things that I was able to understand at that moment was the creative activity of the Renaissance [32], in which the artistic and scientific creation of that period was a profound manifestation of the belief that they were creating beauty and knowledge as co-creators of the universe and also made me understand the Counter Reformation [33] that triggered so much intellectual rebirth in the Church.

We have been created in God's spiritual image, and every human being counts and therefore the concept of charity, love, and even self-respect makes sense. The important part of this is that if we are truly centered in this, unchasteness, greed, malice, deceit, envy, blasphemy, arrogance, folly, and even unpunctuality or lying to others or to ourselves do not have a place in our lives. Every time that we fail to do this, we become selfish and that is the real sin for God. If we center our lives in selfishness, we will not face life in a constructive manner. The selfishness or self-gratification of intellectual pursuits could make us obnoxious, arrogant, and cynical, whereas instead the conquering of knowledge must make us humble at heart.

Father Donati was also instrumental in my joining a new group approved by the bishop. This group was directed by Father Arroyo, one of the professors of theology at the seminary, and together with Father Lloret from the Jesuit Order started this new group for boys my age called "Guide Movement." This group had three basic objectives that we focused on: to be a man, to be a saint, and to be a leader. I remained a part of this group until my last day in college.

This was the best thing that could have happened to me because it put me in the right intellectual framework. I understood what was behind St. Thomas [34], St. Augustine [35], St. Francis [36], and also the inner vision of the Jesuits in St. Ignacio's spiritual exercises [37]. I must say that these teachings were the glue that put all my life together, and after I tasted those teachings, my life evolved into what I am today. All of these things that I learned contributed to a very powerful understanding not only of my religious life, but also that if *I wanted to be a medical researcher, it must be in this Christian framework.* Lastly I understood that I do not need to preach or proclaim what I am and what I have done. If I was centered in these concepts of *being a man, being a saint, and being a leader,* meaning greatness, I do not need to proclaim it, *I only need to be and it will show up. That was my quest in those days.*

From the first day of my second year in college in March 1956, I passed from being a low-average student to being one of the best students of the class of 1959 and became one of the two flag-bearers — the most distinguished honor that a student could receive in the Agustin Alvarez National College of those days.

2.3. My walk to be the best student

How did I achieve this transition from being an average student to being the best in my class? Using the principles of the equation, in my second year, I started to apply what I'd been practicing in the summer of 1956, applying all the guidance of my new learning. I studied each signature with attention and care, and I never went to class without studying each of the signatures for that day. That produced a tremendous confidence in me, which was easily observed by my professors and my classmates who saw my answers were all the time sharp and appropriate.

One of the professors that I need to mention in my memoirs is Professor Nallin, because he also impacted me that year. Professor Nallin was a graduate of the University National of Cuyo, and he taught us Castellan II. Castellan was considered different from Spanish. Spanish was the language that other South American countries spoke, or the accent and intonation that the Spaniards had outside of Castilla. Therefore, Castellan was the language spoken in Castilla. There is evidence that the Castellan language, or the Castellan way of speaking Spanish, started in a place called Santo Domingo de Silos Abbey [38], a Benedictine monastery in the village of Santo Domingo de Silos in the southern part of Burgos Province in northern Spain. The monastery dates back to the seventh century, and its library contains the Missal of Silos, the oldest Western manuscript on paper — where the first indication of the language has been recorded. In summary, the Castellan language was the way that the educated Argentinean was supposed to talk. Professor Nallin had recently finished his doctoral thesis on Pío Baroja y Nessi [39], a Spanish writer distinguished by many literary works such as *The Struggle for Life*, the *Memories of a Man of Action*, and *The Tree of Knowledge*. Although he discussed his work briefly with us, he dedicated his classes to teaching us the best Castellan that we could learn. He had a diction that was so beautiful to listen to that he inspired me even more to better master my mother tongue. One of the most important things for me from his teaching was to eliminate the slang that was the sign of the unlearned person. For example, in Argentina, it is very common to address the other person using the word "che" instead of "usted," or "you." The nickname "Che" Guevara came from this slang; because he was from Argentina, his comrades call him "Che." Another kind of slang is the improper use of articles in front of names; for example, the use of the article "la" in front of a name, calling someone "La Maria" instead of "Maria," the first version is incorrect while the latter one is correct. These, like many other vagaries of the language, were stimulating to learn and correct. It took me 2 years to master a great proficiency of my native Castellan but by the end of my third year I felt very confident that I was correctly using words. I also found it extremely easy to formulate complex ideas and I found pleasure in knowing how to express them.

One of the things that Father Donati persistently told me in those days was to be careful of something that he called *Intellectual Snobbery*, the equilibrium between the pleasure of knowing and at the same time being humble and conscious that I had only mastered a minuscule part of the knowledge. All of these made me keep that Christian value all the time in front of me.

I put the same dedication into other disciplines like chemistry, mathematics, history, literature, and even in languages, like Italian. This language of my ancestors introduced me to the original work of Dante Alighieri [40], Boccaccio [41], and other more modern writers like Romano Guardini [42]. I took special pleasure in reading passages of those works out loud in the corner of my room. At the end of college, I spoke conversational Italian and I was able to understand native Italians speaking their mother tongue. In time, this proficiency in Italian was displaced by my need to master English, and now when I speak Italian, the English words jump up when my brain does not quickly retrieve the right Italian word. Other disciplines that I was especially dedicated to were zoology and anatomy. I mention them because I created a Compendium of Zoology and another for anatomy. For me, those compendiums were a preparatory exercise for writing a book or a scientific article, and that was the way that I thought I would do it when I became a Research Scientist and wrote books containing the knowledge that I would generate. In my intellectual awakening, I wanted to make books that people would read. In other words, I wanted to create and be the source of new knowledge. I must emphasize that the Internet did not exist and computers were not available to any of us in those days.

Therefore, the only way to put a compendium together was using a typewriter or writing it out by hand. I did not have a typewriter until 1958, when my parents bought me a secondhand portable Olivetti typewriter from one of the neighbors who was a sales representative for those machines.

The Compendium of Zoology illustrated the main genera of the animal kingdom, and I drew them in China ink and then matched the natural colors as much as possible (Figures 2.3 and 2.5–2.9).

The reason why these drawings are cherished by me is because I used models from different sources, like library books, the college's laboratory, samples from the Cornelio Moyano Museum, and some of them from the dissection that we had started to do in my chemistry cabinet.

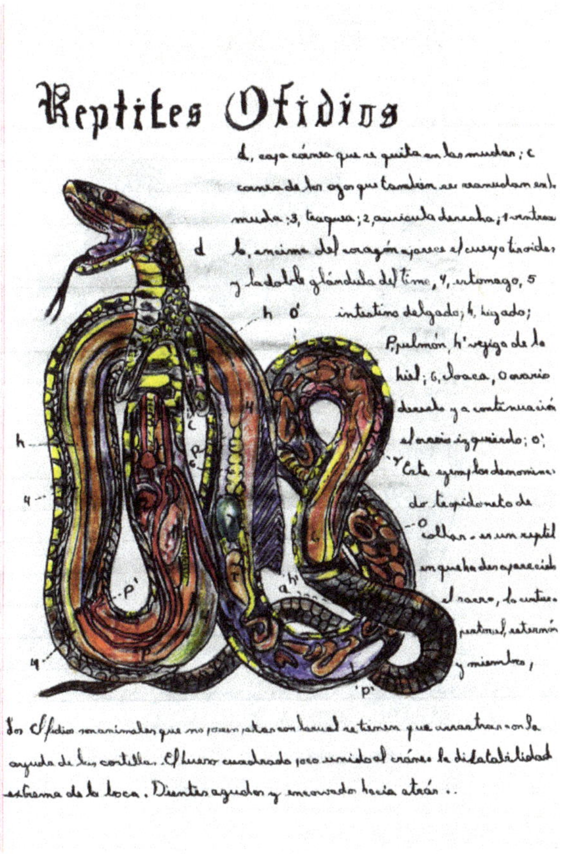

Figure 2.7: Drawing of a snake. These species are a part of the Ophidia family (also known as Pan-Serpentes). This was one of the drawings in my Compendium of Zoology, which I wrote in my second year of college in 1956. The drawing was in ink and colored with Faber-Castell color pencils.

The central market of Mendoza was also a good source of marine specimens like the sea urchin and lobsters depicted in Figures 2.5 and 2.6. The sea urchin was not always available at the market and most of them came from Chile. According to the owner of the fish store, it was considered a delicacy — mainly their eggs to which some attributed aphrodisiac properties. I procured them not for the latter but to learn how they looked inside.

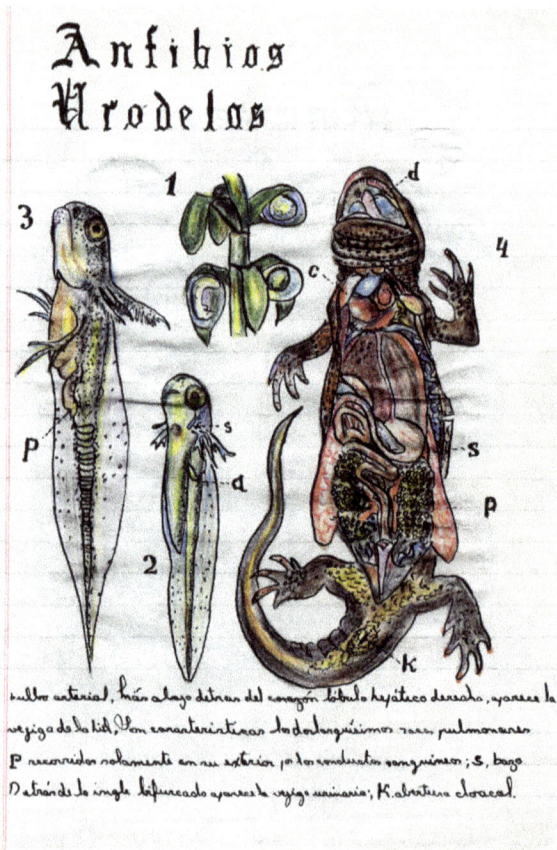

Figure 2.8:   Drawing of a salamander from the Urodela family. Reprinted from my Compendium of Zoology that I wrote in my second year of college in 1956.

Among the reptiles that I drew, there is a group of amphibians typically characterized by a lizard-like appearance, such as the salamander. All present-day salamander families are grouped together under the scientific name of Urodela (Figure 2.8). In Mendoza, it was called Andean lizard, or lagartija andina or *Liolaemus andinus*, these specimens were found easily in the San Martin Park.

Another type of reptile included in the compendium belongs to the Saurios, of which the species most frequently found in Mendoza is the *Iguana iguana,* depicted in Figure 2.9. The figure was constructed

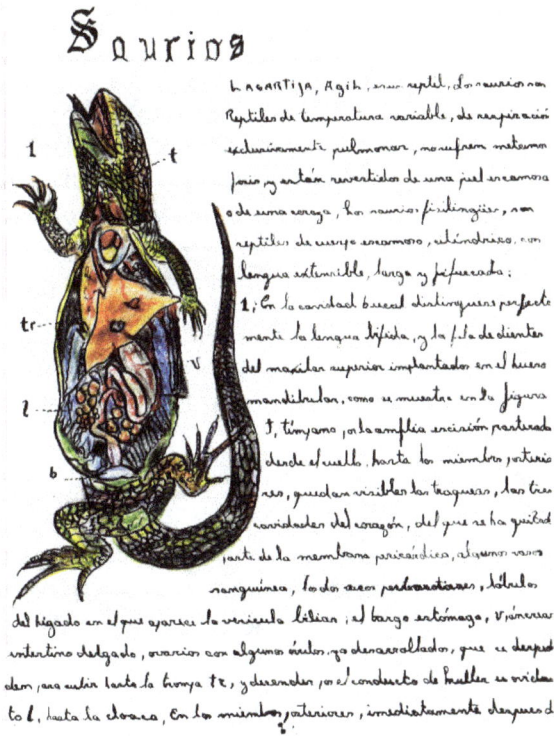

Figure 2.9: Drawing of *Iguana iguana*. Reprinted from my Compendium of Zoology, 1956.

from a sample exposed in Mendoza's unique natural history museum, the Cornelio Moyano. This museum was founded in 1858 and contained more than 150,000 exhibits. The Cornelio Moyano Museum was located in different locations in the city, so not all their material was exposed all the time; their exhibited material was constricted or expanded, depending upon the space available. During my college years, the museum was in the building centrally located in Independence Square at the east side of the Agustin National College. I spent many hours in that museum, and its anthropological section was admirable to me.

Fortunately, from that restricted space the museum now seems to have found its permanent place in the south portion of the San Martin Park and is part of the regional center of the Argentina CONICET.

Another compendium that I created was for my anatomy classes in the third year of college. I drew the diagrams from the books that I borrowed from the San Martin Library, which is now located in a new building in the southern portion of downtown Mendoza.

The coziness of the old library of my childhood was not there anymore, but the books were efficiently found and the librarians were as helpful as before. In Figures 2.10 and 2.11, I depict some of the anatomical figures that I drew for my compendium and that I used to understand the human body. The study of anatomy made me feel closer to medical school.

Although my dedication and the way that I was studying were important factors in my learning process, it was the reinforcement of my learning by teaching others that gave me the plasticity to use that knowledge. My classmates came spontaneously to me for help in the beginning asking me to explain the topics of the day, and eventually even those who had been at the top before started to approach me, at first testing if I was fake or not and later on with legitimate questions. The fact that I was teaching what I was learning reinforced my knowledge and my reasoning; it was like I was logarithmically increasing my brain by associating facts that I retrieved ever faster and more easily. I was challenged every single day in almost every subject, and I understood that was a natural reaction for those who had been at the top of the class, probing me not only in the daily subjects that we discussed in class but also in general history or literature and most of all in sciences like chemistry and physics. Of interest was also that I was known to be Catholic, and that was a magnetic attraction for those who called themselves socialists, communists, liberals, or atheists because challenging me was an intellectual exercise. I am so grateful to them because that increased my principles, and I became extremely skilled in those discussions. They challenged me about everything related to Catholicism — that was the main target, because the problem at the end was their

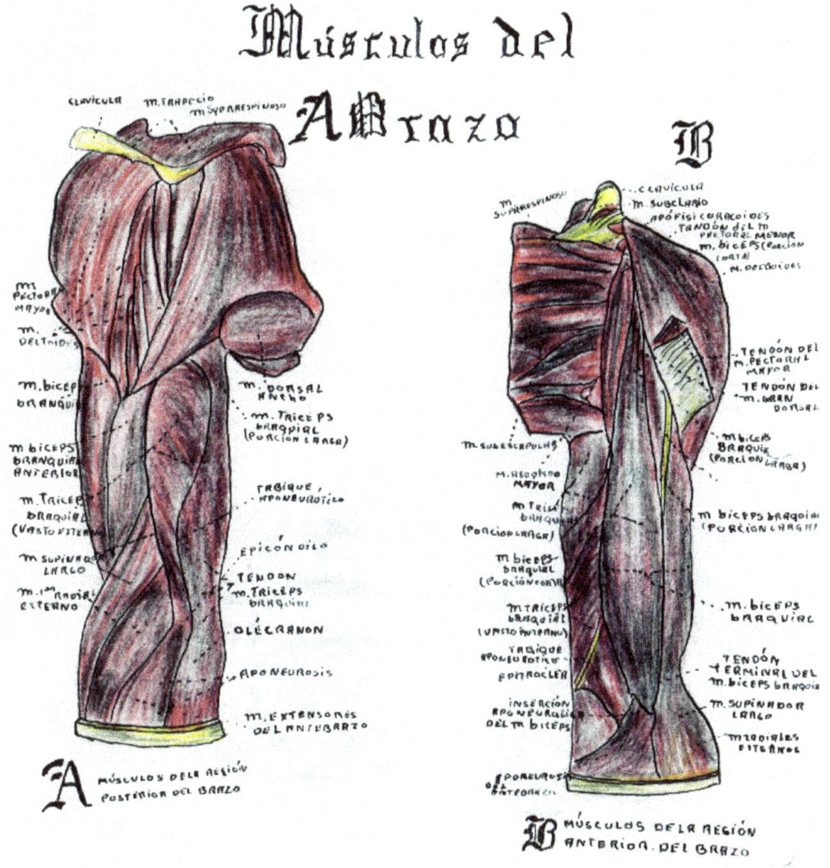

Figure 2.10: Drawings of the upper arm. Reprinted from the Compendium of Anatomy that I wrote in my third year of college in 1957. The drawing was in ink and colored with Faber-Castell color pencils.

resentment of the Church and its human frailty through history. Instead, I was bringing the Gospel to our discussion of their arguments and backing it up by the rational arguments of Thomas Aquinas, which I was starting to understand, or Saint Augustine or

válvulas sigmoideas y situado en la base del ventrículo derecho, nace la arteria pulmonar, que a pesar de ser una arteria lleva sangre venosa. En la aurícula izquierda existen cuatro orificios avalvulares, por donde desembocan las venas pulmonares; y en la aurícula derecha dos orificios; uno para la embocadura de la vena cava superior y otro para la embocadura de la vena cava inferior. El corazón se halla modelado de un saco fibroso, que lo protege, llamado pericardio e interiormente está tapizado por una serosa llamada endocardio, denominándose miocardio al músculo cardii es propiamente dicho.

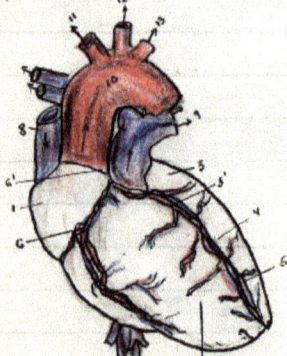

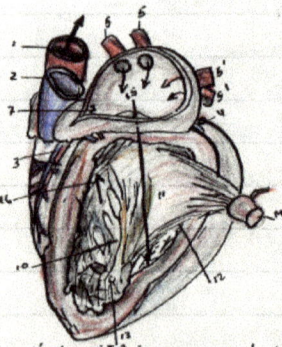

EL CORAZÓN CARA ANTERIOR 2
1 AURÍCULA DERECHA - 2 VENTRÍCULO
DERECHO - 3 AURÍCULA IZQUIERDA
4 VENTRÍCULO IZQUIERDO 5, 6 VASOS
CORONARIOS - 7 VENA CAVA INFERIOR
8 VENA CAVA SUPERIOR 9 ARTERIA
PULMONAR 10 CAYADO AÓRTICO - 11 TRONCO
BRAQUIOCEFÁLICO DERECHO 12 ARTERIA
CARÓTIDA PRIMITIVA IZQUIERDA 13 ARTERIA
SUBCLAVIA IZQUIERDA

SECCIÓN LONGITUDINAL DEL CORAZÓN IZQUIERDO
1 ARTERIA AORTA - 2 ARTERIA PULMONAR - 3 y 4 VASOS
CORONARIOS. 5 VENAS PULMONARES. S. d
IZQUIERDO. 6 CAVIDAD DE LA AURÍCULA IZQUIERDA
CON 7 ID ORÉJUELA CORRESPONDIENTE 10
CAVIDAD DEL VENTRÍCULO 11 VÁLVULA INTERNA DE LA
MITRAL 12 ID INTERNA DE LA MITRAL 13 PILAR
POSTERIOR 14 PILAR ANTERIOR 15 FLECHA QUE
RECORRE EL ORIFICIO AURÍCULO VENTRICULAR 16
FLECHA QUE SE DIRIGE AL ORIFICIO AÓRTICO

Figure 2.11: Drawings of the heart. Reprinted from my Compendium of Anatomy.

Saint Francis, or the writings of Romano Guardini, among others. There were also many philosophical and theological pieces that passed through my hands in those days [43–48], which gave me a strong position from which to deal with the challenges, and I felt

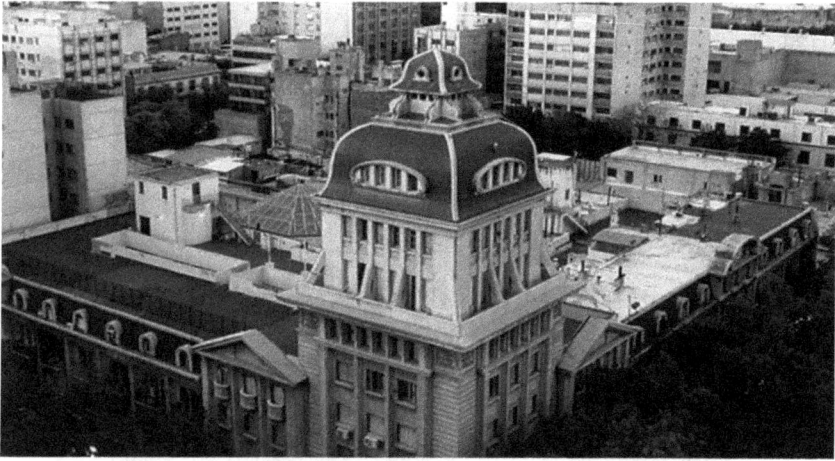

Figure 2.12: Passage San Martin in Mendoza, photo taken in 2006.

very secure knowing that these intellectual giants were behind me. Interestingly enough, those who argued the most were the students with whom I developed a singular link.

As I mentioned before, one of them was Hochman and the other closest challenger was Isgut, who lived in the center of downtown in one of the oldest buildings in Mendoza, called "Pasaje San Martin" (Figure 2.12). I enjoyed visiting it because of the beautiful Vitraux, or stained glass, in the ceiling of the main halls (Figure 2.13).

Isgut came from Buenos Aires and was living with his mother and, according to him, his father was not with them. Even though he only stayed at our college for 2 years, he was attached to me, and I did not see him talking with other students at the college. He came to my home, and I also visited him several times at his place. His mother was a very nice, warm lady who prepared tea and biscuits for both of us. Both Hochman and Isgut challenged many intellectual issues but the basic ones were around my Christian view of science, the creation of the world, the existence of God, and the icing on the cake was Darwin's theories of evolution. I brought to the light of our discussion the works of the recent publications that were available to me from Teilhard de Chardin [49–51]. It would be out of context to describe the details of those discussions here, so I will only say that those were honest questions and answers from both parts, and I do not know if

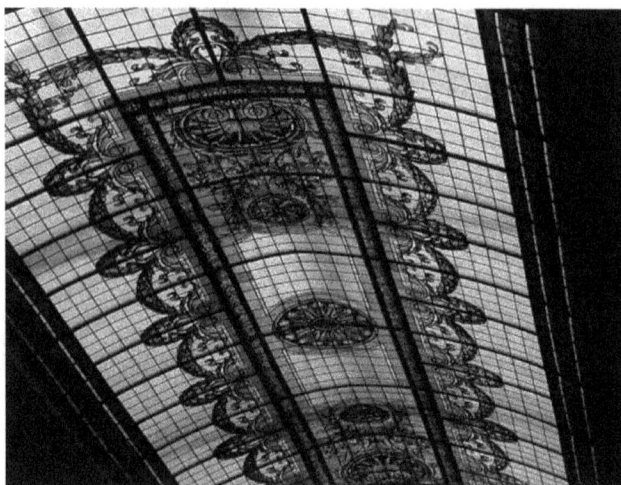

Figure 2.13:   Stained glass in the ceiling of the main halls of Pasaje San Martin in Mendoza. Photo taken in 2006.

I have changed their positions but at least I demonstrated that their arguments were not as solid as they pretended they were. Isgut left the National College in the fourth year and I lost track of him but I still remember his dark framed glasses and his intellectual posture. He was so opposite to Bernardo, who was more highly spirited and, because he was taller than both of us, reminded me of Innocent Smith, one of the characters of the *Manalive* written by Chesterton [52]. With Bernardo we kept having our lively discussions until 1965.

The important part of all these experiences was that I did not need to show up; I was there and they came to me. It was a realization that the way that I was solving the equation was the right one. My classmates came to my home in order to have special explanations of mathematics or trigonometry or other subjects, and that added an extra pressure for me to keep my hours of study. I have kept a journal since 1958 and each day I registered my experiences and the content of each visit that I received and the topics of our conversations. It would be exhausting for the reader to know all about those days of my college life. One thing that I want to mention is that sometimes I even needed to start my day at 4.30 a.m. to compensate for the time that my friends and classmates took from me in their morning visits. I emanated the attraction that I was the person who knew and could be asked. I felt that I had put all the right variables in the left side of the equation, and so in the right side of the original equation, I started to turn myself into the student that I wanted to be. I maintained my first-place position as the best student not only during college but also during my medical studies. Although when I arrived in the USA in 1971, all the rules changed and I needed to start all over again.

2.4. My friends

From my classmates in college, I developed more affinity for those who also had the goal of medical school; among them were Morales, Hochman, Fisichella, Abatte, Lopez, Barone, and Fara. Although I do not recall their first names, I follow the Argentinean custom of referring to your classmates by their surnames and only when you are very close friends do you use first names or even sometimes call a person for the main physical appearance. For example, if a person was overweight they were called Gordo, or if too thin, Flaco. I made friends with other classmates like Miguel Angel Guisasola who, although not interested in pursuing medical school, wanted to be an architect. He was close to me mainly in the second year of college. With Guisasola, we shared our interest in making models of airplanes. He was very knowledgeable in the history of aviation and the making of planes. It was nice to listen to him give passionate descriptions of the types of jets that were used in the Korean War or recently developed in the U.S. Air Force. Using my father's shop, I became proficient in reproducing models of the Argentinean air force, like the *Pulqui I* and *Pulqui II*, which were the first fighter planes developed in South America, and I was proud to know that Argentina was the sixth in the world in developing jet fighters. Also I crafted the latest models from the U.S. Air Force in those days, like the Sabre F86 and the F100. We shared models and compared notes. He had a great ability in making replicas in a very small scale, and he was definitely a very good crafter, which was an early indication of his architectural skills. I left some of the aircraft models that I made in my second year of college in the hands of Paulo and Gustavo, the sons of my cousin Sebastian Jorge, when I immigrated to the USA.

Another close person was Santilli with whom I discussed optical equipment, and I recall that he gave me beautiful glossy print photos of micro-photographies of cells in mitoses taken from the anion roots; one day I visited his home and he gave me as a gift a small magnifier that he had. Alighieri was another classmate. We used to walk together most of the time from the National College to his home, which was halfway to mine, and we shared books and journals, and once I received from him a beautiful gift of several issues of the first 10 years of the *Reader's Digest,* which in Argentina was branded as *Seleciones* and started its circulation in 1939. It was a great collection that depicted the USA before and during the Second War World. From those series, I learned how the world was when I was born in 1942. I treasured that collection but unfortunately it was lost when I moved to the USA.

Fara was another classmate who became a close friend because he was also part of the Catholic Movement [53]. He was the son of a Syro-Lebanese family, and I ate the raw meat called Kibbeh for the first time in their home, but more importantly we discussed the economic situation that we needed to face when studying medicine. Mainly how we would be able to afford it if we were not admitted to the Medical School of the University National of Cuyo in Mendoza, and if we needed to relocate to Cordoba, the nearest city 500 km to the east, or Buenos Aires, 1100 km from Mendoza.

From the group that was aiming to go to medical school, Bernardo Hochman and Jose Roberto Morales (Gordo Morales) were the only friends that shared my interest in scientific research, and it was with them that I spent great moments either in my chemistry cabinet or in their homes. The plan was that they would also construct their own laboratories and the three of us could create a consortium of research laboratories. Although this did not work as we had planned, we made great work together. It was with Gordo Morales that I dissected our first snake, similar to the one depicted in Figure 3.4 in Chapter 3, and from there I got some of the colors and shadows that are depicted in that figure. With Gordo and Bernardo, we dissected lizards and frogs that were part our weekly enterprise. We collected frog eggs and observed how they developed to small tadpoles. It was with both of them that I wandered among the enologist laboratories in Mendoza, searching for bargains in glassware, like test tubes, distillation serpentines and glass balloons, latex tubes, and rubber stoppers for our laboratories. Bernardo had a special eye for detecting those laboratories that were closing because the owner had died and the widow was trying to sell everything that was left. From those places, we got a great variety of drugs and reagents at very low prices. Some of them were still unopened with their original labels, most of those from Germany, and some as old as 1914. It was a unique experience, and I still have vivid memories of those ventures. Bernardo knew who every wealthy or poor Jew in the city was, and he was aware of what was going on in the Jewish community. The only thing that separated us was our religion, but we were growing together and we were neighbors. He was more aware than I was of how wealth was managed, and he had the idea that we should get some seed money from wealthy people in Mendoza. We tried but we never even got an interview, however that was not important. The experience that we had and the time we spent together making plans did not have a price. Bernardo and Gordo Morales were my only two friends in college that really were infected by the curiosity of scientific research; I really missed both of them.

Although the entire college group of aspirants to medical school took the test to be admitted to the Medical School of the University National of Cuyo (UNC), I was the only one who passed it. In the case of Bernardo, he chose agronomy but later went to Israel, and I lost track of him. I deeply wish that he is still alive in some part of this world. Gordo Morales also entered in agronomy but after one year he was admitted into the medical school. He succeeded, and he was the attendant physician who was with me when my mother died in 1991. He was already a professor of infectious diseases in the medical school. He accomplished what he wanted. All my other classmates from the National College ended up in the University of Cordoba or Buenos Aires, and I never saw them again.

I lost contact with my childhood friend Angel after the first years of college when he changed to a private school, and it took almost 60 years for us to meet again. Our friendship was as fresh as it had been when we were 14 years old.

2.5. My research endeavors during my college years

My chemistry cabinet still was my special world that, although I shared it with Bernardo and Gordo Morales, was in a certain way my small enterprise. Even though Angel and I had pledged to make our research endeavor a unique one in our 1957 co-signed document (Figure 1.9 in Chapter 1), it never germinated, and the main reason was that his change of college pushed us farther apart.

He was also attracted by the existentialism of Paul Sartre, and when I opened my eyes, the friend of my childhood was no longer there. When I encountered him 60 years later, our friendship was still there and the unanswered questions that I had about him were explained. The most important thing is that he also accomplished his dreams and became a real healer, not of cancer but of mental diseases. In 1958, I was in my fourth year of college, and my chemistry cabinet, laid out in Figure 2.14, was my small universe. In my records, I described my experiments. One of them was trying to keep my lip's epithelial cells alive *in vitro* (Figure 2.15), and I checked every day to see how they grew or swelled until they got spoiled. Of course I had no way to keep them in sterile conditions, and many other things grew in my elementary culture medium; it contained albumin that was obtained from a chicken egg, and sodium chloride and glucose from a syrup solution that I bought from those enology laboratories that were my suppliers.

In those days, I was reading Alexis Carrel [54,55] and was fascinated by his work and obsessed with the growing of cells and anything that could grow. Paul de Kruif's book *Microbe Hunters* [56] was exhilarating and then Fleming's discovery of penicillin and all the surrounding stories about him entered my mind like flashes of

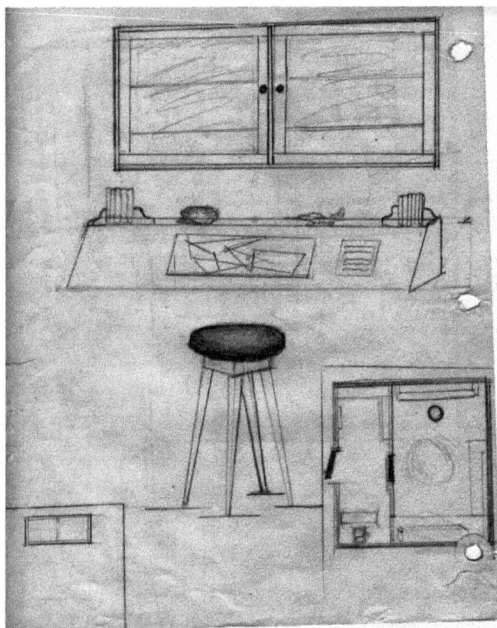

Figure 2.14: Blueprint of the chemistry cabinet in 1958. In the lower corner is a layout of the space, and the desk drawing depicts the one that I built and used for writing my notes.

inspiration. I wanted to reproduce all these discoveries in my small laboratory. The *ascomycetous* fungi *Penicillium notatum* were easy to replicate in my primitive culture media, and I started like Fleming did, using a rotten orange.

The embryologic process was even more fascinating because I intuitively thought that this could be more related to cancer than the microbiology experiments. Going back to the San Martin library, I discovered a fascinating book about *The Frog: Its Reproduction and Development,* by Robert Rugh published in 1951 [57]. Although there were concepts that escaped me, and I could not have in my laboratory, by imitating what I saw, I started studying the larval development of the *Periplaneta americana,* also called the American cockroach. They lay a large egg that contains up to twenty embryos which can become small roaches (Figure 2.16), although observing

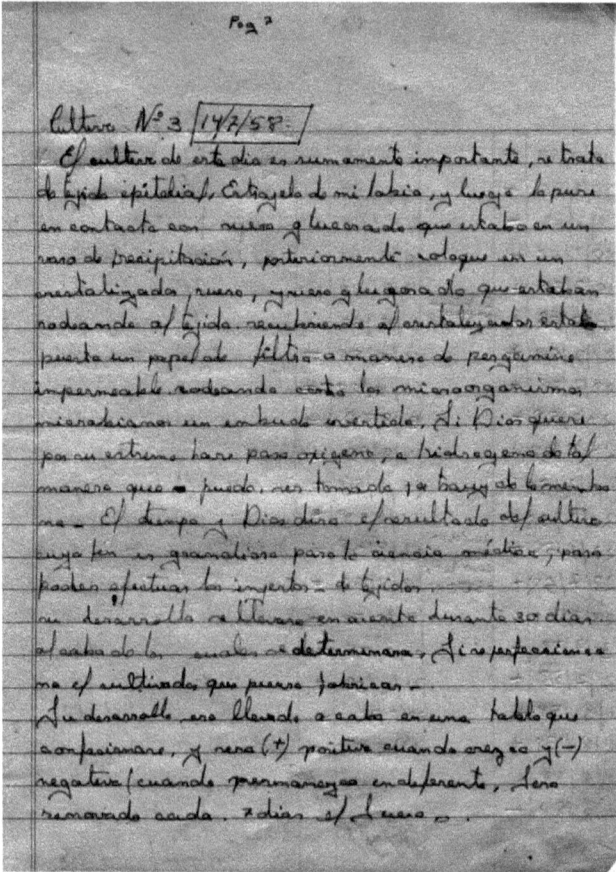

Figure 2.15: Page of my logbook describing my culture number 3 (Cultivo Nro3) to grow epithelial cells from my lips.

carefully I realized that I missed the most important phase of embryogenesis, which started between the gelatinous mass until the small formed insects appeared. It was a fascinating process that took place but I could not see more with my tools at hand.

Another beautiful experiment was the development of the silk cocoons of the larvae of the moth caterpillars. I saw the full metamorphosis ending in the final formation of the butterfly coming out of the cocoon. I kept the yellow silk cocoons for many years. The moth caterpillars were given to me by another classmate from college interested in biology, but he never pursued medicine.

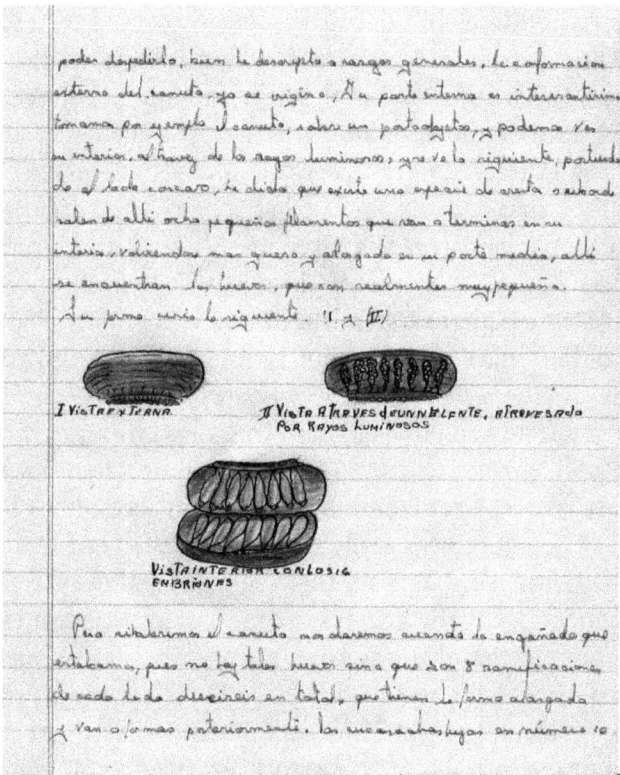

Figure 2.16: Drawing of my observations of the egg of the *Periplaneta americana*. November 27, 1958.

The experiment that I repeated several times was the use of the common frog. I knew more about what could be done with frogs from the work of Robert Rugh [57]. None of the frogs mentioned by Rugh were found in our place, and the most abundant was the autochthonous variety called *Bufo arenarum*. I used the frog eggs that were collected near the lake in San Martin Park. Those eggs were attached to small rocks around the border of the lake, and using the same water, I saw how they went through the larval state to a tadpole and then the formation of limbs and bronchi. The eggs from the female frog were obtained from the massive ovary that filled the abdomen of this amphibian. They were released by the embrace of the male frog that stimulated the brain of these animals and allowed the release of hundreds of oocytes in a chain covered by a gelatinous material. Those fertilized eggs were attached or floating near the rock of the ponds. I wanted to use urethane in this aquatic model. The idea came from reading the translation that was available in 1959 of a book by Jesse P. Greenstein titled *Biochemistry of Cancer*. This was a treasured book that later on, in 1962, I acquired and still have in my library today. Anyway, I read in Greenstein's book that urethane was water soluble and induced tumors in mice. Therefore, my reasoning for using it in the aquatic system that I had was simple. The problem was that I did not have urethane but I thought if I used my chemistry knowledge, urethane, or ethyl carbonate, could be produced by heating urea nitrate and ethyl alcohol. In short, I thought that I could synthesize it. I already had urea in powder but when I started the process of synthesis, I realized that I would not be able to figure out if what I was obtaining was really urethane. Whatever I had obtained made all the larvae die. I am sure that the doses and the way I handled that experiment were the main reasons. To my consolation, many years later I found that this was not a bad idea, and a similar approach is used as a system for testing environmental carcinogens. Because frogs as amphibians live outdoors on land and water, and their skin, larvae, and unshelled eggs are constantly exposed and in contact with the substances in their surroundings, they are good indicators of stressors on the environment. Their extinction and declining population has been considered confirmation that they are indicators of environmental changes [58]. It was coincidental that when I started working in the Experimental Pathology Department under Professor Julian Echave Llanos in 1963, one of the first experiments that he assigned to me was to determine if urethane was a carcinogenic agent in the lung of C3H mice (a special strain of mice that he was maintaining in his animal colony) (see Chapter 3). Today, cancer biologists are using the zebra fish as a model for testing what I wanted to do in my frog system. Evidence that my use of this aquatic model was not farfetched, but in those days it was difficult for me to envision the use of an aquatic system like the zebra fish to make several transgenic models of cancer [59]. This was also another lesson: that ideas, brilliant or not, may occur to more than one person, and in fact, many co-discoveries occurred in this way. Only those who are alert and succeed in publishing first get the main recognition, and that is what happened between Darwin and Wallace with the theory of evolution [60].

Another species that also called my attention was the leech. Leeches are basically worms that belong to the Annelida phylum. They fascinated me because they were easily obtained in the margins of the "acequias" in front of my home, and most intriguing was that they had been used in medicine since the earliest times. This was mainly because it was widely thought that most diseases were caused by an excess of blood, the process of bloodletting from a patient was believed to cure or prevent an illness and disease. Therefore, I thought that maybe leeches could be used for the treatment of blood cancer, and although I spent hours observing the behavior of these creatures, I never did any experiments to demonstrate or deny my assumptions.

I also caught mice, and their litters were subject to my anatomical interest. Studying the mouse, I was interested in the whiskers, or vibrissae, hair located near the nostril of these rodents which is not developed in humans. What called my attention was that a careful dissection of the whiskers led to a large follicle, or oval body, almost 0.5 mm in length and 0.25 mm in diameter. When I dissected it, it was apparently formed by several layers of tissue. What was a curiosity for me in those days turned out to be a specialized anatomical organ with an extremely complex somatosensory structure and a special connection to the brain. Basically, a whisker is a special hair follicle incorporating a capsule of blood called a blood sinus which is heavily innervated by sensory nerves. The total number of sensory nerve cells present in some of these structures could be up to 25,000 [61–63]. This delicate structure was unimaginable to me when I saw them in 1958. However, it has an important significance in my memoirs, because I shared that observation with Ramon Piezzi, who was already a medical student interested in medical research and working in the medical school's Department of Pathology. I knew him through the Catholic Movement, and that was how our long-term friendship began. Ramon was impressed by my description of these structures as well as all that I shared with him of the work that I was doing and had done in my chemistry cabinet. As a matter of fact, he was the only outsider with whom I shared the particulars of my work in the cabinet. As I will describe in the next chapter, he was instrumental in my interview with Professor Julian Echave Llanos, who became my first mentor in my scientific career.

Collection of bones and assembling of skeletons were also part of the work that I was doing in the chemistry cabinet. I used lime or calcium carbonate that in aqueous solution produces calcium hydroxide which is caustic and destroys any organic residual material. Using this solution, I cleaned up the bones of cats and dogs that I found in my Pre-Andean mountain excursions, and using the same technique, I was able to clean up and assemble several skeletons. There are some that I recall vividly, one a Chilean bass corvine fish that I bought in the central market. The other two were the silvery pigeons (*Columba argentina*), also known as silvery wood-pigeons or grey wood-pigeons, and the one that I considered in those days my masterpiece was the skeleton of a *Cavia porcelis* or a guinea pig. In all the cases, the skeletons were supported by a wooden base which I painted red. I left these skeletons in the hands of my cousin's sons when I came to the United States, and I do not know what their final destination was.

These biological pursuits were also interspersed with other chemistry experiments like deposition of silver in glass to create mirrors or the electrolysis experiment. The difference with the biological experiments was that I could be more original, or at least that was what I thought; with chemistry, my work was repetitions of classic experiments. The electrolysis experiment was a great one to get the separation of water in oxygen and hydrogen (Figure 2.17).

With Angel, I also performed other experiments using lenses and natural and artificial light. We used the Morse apparatus for communicating with each other, and created a wooden robot with a human likeness, but even with our arsenal of small engines and electric batteries, we were unable to make it move. When I contemplate how many of the robots this new generation of apprentices of science has with their reach, I see with nostalgia my days of robot-making, and I see in them the future of what science can achieve. The important thing is

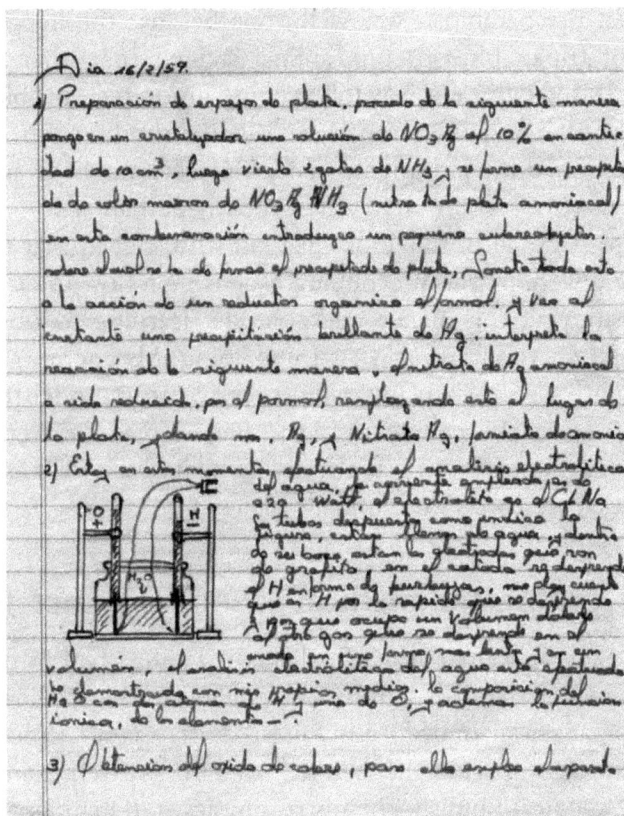

Figure 2.17: Electrolysis experiment performed in February of 1959.

not what I see in them, though, but what they see in their inner selves of what they want to achieve.

Most of these experiments were done with an open question, mainly curiosity awakened from the learning of organic chemistry and anatomy as well as the unknown that could result from the experiment and lead to something novel. What I did not know in those days was that the research process needs more than simple curiosity. However, this was my initial kick for being a researcher.

My last recorded experiment in the chemistry cabinet was a parabiosis with two Sprague Dawley rats. The experiment was a success, and I was able to do it and the animals survived the surgery.

I knew that the parabiosis was well done because the injection of a solution of tripan blue to one animal stained the other. But the success of this experiment was followed by unforeseen problems that I had in maintaining the animals, and it was the first time that my family questioned my judgment. I ended up returning the animals to the medical school where they were properly euthanized.

In retrospect, all of this looks like kid stuff, but in that period of my life these were important training exercises on how to do research and also enjoying the silence and solitude, learning to observe, to describe and try to interpret what I was doing. My chemistry cabinet was kept until 1963 when my parents started to remodel the house and taking apart the cabinet was the first step in the remodeling phase. But in that period, I was already in medical school, and the real laboratories of research were under my eyes.

2.6. Preparing for medical school entrance tests

At the end of my fourth year of college in 1958, I had in my hands the program and the instructions for applying to the medical school. The examinations had been administered. It was an almost three-week examination period that started with five written examinations in biology, medical English, chemistry, physics, and mathematics. The last two were basically for eliminating half of the applicants. After a few days of rest, the oral examinations started with biology, chemistry, physics, and mathematics. I needed to pass those tests if I wanted to accomplish my goal, and if I couldn't enter medical school, all my dreams of being a Research Scientist would vanish.

I had been visiting the medical school in Cordoba with Fara, a friend from the Catholic Movement who was also a classmate from college, and when I saw the rooms that I would need to share as well as the living conditions of the students with similar economic resources to mine, I easily realized that I would not survive that environment and most importantly even in those living conditions it would be a tremendous burden for my family. Working outside of the medical environment during the medical school curriculum was also out of question. The study of medicine was a full-time job, and those that I met, who needed to work to pay for even elementary things or those who already had a family, did not make it through the program. However, it was a group of students that were working in the medical school as instructors who were remarkable achievers.

Realizing that I had to be accepted at the medical school in Mendoza, I started to study as hard as I could. During the summer, I spent every afternoon in the San Martin library reading the book of De Robertis, Nowinski, and Saez [64]. This book was a treasury of new knowledge opening my eyes to what was known in cell biology as the emergence of molecular biology. I started to see every organelle of the cell as a new universe, besides the structure was the emerging knowledge of its function. Chromatin was not only a spot in the cell but a complex composition of DNA that made sense with the newly discovered double strand helix of Watson and Crick. After all, this had been discovered few years before and was already blowing the minds of cell biologists. New organelles were discovered using the electron microscope and were starting to be purified using ultracentrifugation, and the free cells system of their biochemical functions started to emerge. The functions of the endoplasmic reticulum, the mitochondria, the centrioles, the lysosomes, and all the microfilaments in cells and their roles in mitosis, meiosis, and locomotion were like an orchestra performing the complex composition of life. That summer was a great one, and I was digesting knowledge that was part of the curriculum of the second year of medical school. This understanding of cell biology facilitated my study of the general biology that was required for admission to the medical school. That explained my high scores on the admission tests and why the professors on the examining table, Dr. Mario H. Burgos and Dr. Julian Echave Llanos, were so impressed by my performance in the written and oral tests. They even remembered my examination when I started to work with one of them, and this will be part of another chapter. I am not bragging about it, but all this was also a part of another incident that took place many years later when I was already an established cancer researcher in the United States and Dr. Eduardo de Robertis was another speaker at the same meeting as I was. At the end of my talk, which was about the endocrine control of breast cancer, he approached and asked me about the role of tamoxifen, and I explained its function at a molecular level and the secondary effects in patients, like osteoporosis. He asked me about a particular case. But the encounter reminded me of the summer of 1959 that I spent learning cell biology from his book. At the end of our talk, I thanked him for all the work that he had been doing in teaching and writing about the biology of the cell. We finished by talking about the latest book of Umberto Eco, *The Name of the Rose* [65], and the realization that in the book was a monk called George who characterized the Argentinean poet Jorge Luis Borges [66]. Cytology was part of the curriculum of the second year of medical school. Therefore, learning this new frontier for the study of general biology, required for the admissions test, was easy stuff.

When I started my final year of college, in addition to the classes, I dedicated all the spare time that I had to prepare myself for the test. Some other students also hoped to enter the medical school, and these schoolmates took special classes with me in chemistry, physics, and mathematics from 8.30–11 p.m. every night and Saturday mornings. The classes were taught by a retired navy engineer and targeted students who wanted to take the admission tests for medical school. The *tour de force* was to leave the National College at 8 p.m. and in half an hour get some dinner and arrive at the place where the classes started at 8.30 p.m. This was made possible by my friendship with another classmate called Barone who had a bike called "Puma," and he gave me a ride so we could complete all the tasks on time. The group was formed by 20 students, and many of them were later on my classmates in the medical school, but unfortunately my friend Barone did not make it. We made hundreds of equations and problems of physics and mathematics, including complex polynomial equations. We made as many exercises in inorganic and organic chemistry, preparing solutions and solving the entire list of old questions and problems compiled from previous tests. Suffice to say that I kept this rhythm of study until I took my last test on March 9, 1960. This last examination was in mathematics, and with the successful passing of that test, I was admitted to the medical school. I had the highest score of all the applicants, and even in mathematics,

I was the only one that had the highest score of 9, 10 being the maximum.

The last test was in the old amphitheater, where the biochemistry classes would be given in the first year. It was located in the west wing of the Central Hospital, where the medical school functioned in those days. I remember the exhilarating feeling of walking to my home afterward to share this great news with my family.

Later on, I realized that none of my classmates from the National College had been admitted, and I was the only one in that class of 1959 who had been accepted to the medical school. My college period of life had finished, and I had won the race. I was going to the medical school.

References[a]

[1] Levene, R., Rodriguez, A. G., Palcon, A., Heras, A., Braun Menendez, A., Caillet-Bois, R. R., Ruiz-Guinazu, E., Allende, A. R. and Levillier, R. Historia Argentina Contemporanea. *Librería "El Ateneo" Editorial*, Vol. 1, Buenos Aires, 1965, 1862–1930.

[2] Karush, M. B. and Chamosa, O., (eds). *The New Cultural History of Peronism: Power and Identity in Mid-Twentieth-Century Argentina*, Duke University Press. 2010.

[3] Anderson, L. E. *Social Capital in Developing Democracies: Nicaragua and Argentina Compared*, Cambridge University Press. 2010.

[4] Cervantes Saavedra, M. *El Ingenioso Hidalgo Don Quijote de la Mancha*. Editorial Alfredo Ortells, Madrid. 2006.

[5] Walter, P. and Bleznick, D. *Representative Spanish Authors: Volume I*, Oxford University Press Inc. 1971.

[6] Bleznick, D. *Representative Spanish Authors*, Vol. II, 3rd edn., Oxford University Press Inc. 1971.

[7] Gies, D. T., (ed). *The Cambridge History of Spanish Literature*, Cambridge University Press. 2008.

---

[a]The references listed are suggested readings to provide additional documentation of the information provided by the author. The references are not the original material, editorial or publications that the author had access to during the period of 1955–1959.

[8]   Dumas, A. *The Three Musketeers*, The Easton Press, Norwalk. 1978. Penguin Classics Deluxe Editions, New York. 2006.

[9]   *The Mark of Zorro* (1940), American Film, with Tyrone Power based on the original novel of Johnston McCulley's original magazine serial, *The Curse of Capistrano* from *All-Story Weekly*, was published in 1924 as a novel by Grosset & Dunlap under the title *The Mark of Zorro*. It was reprinted by MacDonald & Co. in 1959.

[10] Bethell, L. *Argentina Since Independence*, Cambridge University Press, Cambridge. 1993.

[11] Lynch, J. *Argentine Dictator: Juan Manuel De Rosas, 1829–1852*, Oxford University Press, Oxford. 1981.

[12] Potash, R. A. *The Army and Politics in Argentina, 1945–1962: Peron to Frondizi*, Stanford University Press, Stanford, California. 1980.

[13] Spinelli, M. E. *Los vencedores vencidos: el antiperonismo y la "Revolucion Libertadora"*, Biblos, Buenos Aires. 2005.

[14] Durant, W. *The life of Grece in The Story of Civilization*, Vol. II, The Easton Press, Norwalk. 1992.

[15] Hemingway, E. *Fiesta*. Plaza G Janes S.A., Barcelona. 1966.

[16] Hesse, H. *Viaje A Oriente*. Plaza G Janes S.A., Barcelona. 1966.

[17] Darwin, C. *On the Origin of Species*, Gryphon Editions Inc., Birmingham, Alabama. 1987.

[18] Hamsum, K., *El Juego de la Vida*. Plaza G Janes S.A., Barcelona. 1966.

[19] Mann, T. *Tristan*. Plaza G Janes S.A., Barcelona. 1966.

[20] Melville, H. *Moby-Dick or, The Whale*, The Easton Press, Norwalk. 1977.

[21] Dostoevsky, F. *Crime and Punishment*, The Easton Press, Norwalk. 1980.

[22] Buck, P. S. *Cerca y Lejos*. Plaza G Janes S.A., Barcelona. 1966.

[23] Defoe, D. *A Journal of the Plague Year*, The Easton Press, Norwalk. 1978.

[24] Kipling, R. *Stalky i Cia*. Plaza G Janes S.A., Barcelona. 1966.

[25] Milton, J. *Paradise Lost*, The Franklin Library, Franklin Center, Pennsylvania. 1979.

[26] Mauriac, F. *Nudo de Viboras*. Plaza G Janes S.A., Barcelona. 1966.

[27] Mann, T., *Vision*. Plaza G Janes S.A., Barcelona. 1966.

[28] Tolstoy, L. *War and Peace*, The Easton Press, Norwalk. 1981.

[29] Faulkner, W. *En la Ciudad*. Plaza G Janes S.A., Barcelona. 1966.

[30] Steinbeck, J. *El Linchamiento*. Plaza G Janes S.A., Barcelona. 1966.

[31] van der Meersch, M. *Bodies and Souls*, William Kimber, London. 1857.

[32] Durant, W. A history of Civilization in Italy. In: *The Story of Civilization*, Vol. V, The Easton Press, Norwalk. 1992.

[33] Durant, W. and Durant, A. A history of European Civilization. In: *The Story of Civilization*, Vol. VII, The Easton Press, Norwalk. 1992.

[34] Aquina, St Thomas. Summa Theologica. In: *Christian Classics*, Notre Dame, Indiana. 1948.

[35] St Augustine. *The Confessions*, The Easton Press, Norwalk. 1979.

[36] Spoto, D. *Francisco de Asis*, Bergara, Barcelona. 2004.

[37] Loyola, I. St. The Spiritual Exercises of St Ignatius or Manresa. In: *Tan Classics*. 1999.

[38] Foley O.F.M., Leonard. *Saint of the Day, Lives, Lessons, and Feast* (revised by Pat McCloskey O.F.M.) Franciscan Media.

[39] Azurmendi, J. Pio Baroja: esencia española, cultura vasc. In: *Espainiaren arimaz*, Elkar, Donostia. 2006.

[40] Alighieri, D. *La Divina Comedia*, Middletown, Delaware. 2017.

[41] Boccaccio, G. *The Decameron*, The Easton Press, Norwalk. 1980.

[42] Anthony Krieg, R. A. *Romano Guardini: A Precursor of Vatican II*, University of Notre Dame Press. 1997.

[43] Rahner, K. *Espiritu en el Mundo*, Editorial Herder, Barcelona. 1963.

[44] Pieper, J. *El Ocio y la vida Intelectual*, Ediciones Ralph, S.A., Madrid. 1962.

[45] Maritain, J. *The Peasant of the Garonne*, Holt, Rinehart and Winston, New York. 1966.

[46] van der Meer de Walcheren, P. *Nostalgia de Dios*, Ediciones Carlos Lohle, Buenos Aires. 1955.

[47] Sheen, F. J. *Eleva tu Corazon*, Editorial Difusion, Buenos Aires. 1956.

[48] Maritain, J. *Filosofia de la Historia*, Ediciones Troquel, Buenos Aires. 1960.

[49] Teilhard de Chardin, P. *El Medio Divino*, Taurus, Madrid. 1965.

[50] Teilhard de Chardin, P. *El Grupo Zoologico Humano*, Taurus, Madrid. 1965.

[51] Teilhard de Chardin, P. *La vision del Pasado*, Taurus Ediciones, S.A., Madrid. 1967.

[52] Cherterton, G. K., *Manalive*, Thomas Nelson and Sons, London. 1912.

[53] Truman, T. *Catholic Action and Politics*, The Merlin Press, London. 1960.

[54] Carrel, A. On the Permanent Life of Tissues Outside of the Organism. *J. Exp. Med.* 15: 516–528, 1912.

[55] Hayflick, L. Mortality and Immortality at the Cellular Level: A Review. *Biochemistry* 62: 1180–1190, 1997.

[56] de Kruif, P. *Microbe Hunters*, Q Harvest Book, Harcourt Publishing Company, New York. 1996.

[57] Rugh, R. *The Frog: Its Reproduction and Development*, Blakiston, Philadelphia. 1951.

[58] Stuart, S. N., Chanson, J. S., Cox, N. A., Young, B. E., Rodrigues, A. S. L., Fischman, D. L. and Waller, R. W. Status and trends of amphibian declines and extinctions worldwide. *Science* 306: 1783–1786, 2004.

[59] Liu, S. and Leach, S. D. Zebrafish models for cancer. *Annu. Rev. Pathol.* 6: 71–93, 2011.

[60] Russo, J. *The Apprentice of Science: A Handbook for the Budding Biomedical Researchers*, World Scientific, Singapore. 2010.

[61] Brecht, M., Preilowski, B. and Merzenich, M. M. Functional architecture of the mystacial vibrissae. *Behav. Brain Res.* 84: 81–97, 1997.

[62] Rice, F. L., Mance, A. and Munger, B. L. A comparative light microscopic analysis of the sensory innervation of the mystacial pad. I. Innervation of vibrissal follicle-sinus complexes. *J. Comp. Neurol.* 252: 154–174, 1986.

[63] Ebara, S., Kumamoto, K., Matsuura, T., Mazurkiewicz, J. E. and Rice, F. L. Similarities and differences in the innervation of mystacial vibrissal follicle–sinus complexes in the rat and cat: A confocal microscopic study. *J. Comp. Neurol.* 449: 103–119, 2002.

[64] De Robertis, E. D. P., Nowinski, W. W. and Saez, F. A. *Citologia General*, Libreria El Ateneo Editorial, Buenos Aires. Tercera edición. 1957.

[65] Eco, U. *The Name of the Rose*, The Folio Society, London. 2001.

[66] Borges, J. L. *Labyrinths: Selected stories & other writings*, The Folio Society, London. 2007.

Chapter 3
The Medical School and My Research in Experimental Pathology (1960–1966)

3.1. The medical school

On March 16, 1960, I started the 10th promotion of the medical school and my first class of human anatomy given by Dr. Gumersindo Sánchez Guisande. The medical school was created on December 26, 1950, and began functioning in the Central Hospital of the city of Mendoza. The basic portion of the medical curriculum that comprised the first 3 years was housed in the Central Hospital, and later on in two additional hospitals: the Emilio Civit, for the pediatric and the obstetric portions, and the hospital Lagomaggiore, where infectious diseases were taught.

The history of the medical school in Mendoza was written by all the people that had the vision to create a center of knowledge where the students were rigorously selected and where they would receive a research-oriented education. Some of them, like Drs. G. Sánchez Guisande, J. Garate, F. Bagda, J. M. Cei, and J. Ferreira Márques, were born in Europe. The other founders were J. Echave Llanos, R. Morel, M. H. Burgos, J. C. Fasciolo, J. Suárez, E. Viacava, and R. Suarez; all were born in Argentina and came to Mendoza from the University of Buenos Aires. All of them were basic or clinical researchers, and they created departments that not only taught their specialties but also had research laboratories that created new knowledge and made the school grow in prestige. Those were my teachers and that was the environment that they had created and in which I started my medical studies. They were *physician scientists*, and I wanted to be one of them.

The founders of the medical school realized that the Central Hospital could not be the final location of the medical school, and that for research to grow the school must have more space for laboratories and for the construction of new buildings to facilitate the research enterprise. The opportunity was seized in 1955 when the President of Argentina transferred the still-in-construction Children's Hospital to the Health Department of Mendoza, and through the dedication and effort of Professor Roger Zaldivar, an ophthalmologist and later on by the Dean of the medical school when I took my Hippocratic oath (Figure 4.4 in Chapter 4), the building was transferred to the Department of Education, and as a consequence to the University National of Cuyo in Mendoza. Finishing the construction of the building was made possible by a donation of 300,000 USD by the Rockefeller Foundation. In 1965, the building started to admit administrative and a few departments of the basic sciences. When I left Mendoza in 1971, most of the basic sciences were already functioning in the actual building of the medical school that is part of the University City located on the northwest side of San Martin Park. There are many other people who contributed to the formation of the medical school at the time when I started my studies, and it would be out of place to narrate their stories here, but it is important to recognize that the medical school where I was accepted had an environment that nurtured and fostered my ambitions and dreams to be a physician scientist.

3.2. The medical curriculum

The medical studies took 6 years plus one additional year of internship divided equally in internal medicine, surgery, obstetrics, and pediatrics. Successful completion of all 7 years earned the graduate the titles of physician and surgeon, and allowed him to practice medicine. The medical doctor degree is only possible after a presentation of a thesis consisting of original pieces of research followed by a dissertation, and only after the approval of these two conditions was the title of medical doctor, or MD, given. This title had been conferred to only nine before my doctoral thesis degree in 1968.

The first 3 years of medical studies were considered basic sciences, and only in the third year did the white coat "ceremony" take place; for the first 2 years, the medical students wore khaki coats. The basic disciplines were anatomy, biophysics, biochemistry, physiology, physio-pathology, pathology, microbiology, parasitology, pharmacology, psychology, and English. Internal medicine and surgery started in fourth year and lasted 3 years; in those last 3 years, specialties like gynecology, infectious diseases, neurology, obstetrics, pediatrics, psychiatry, and forensic medicine were taught. My research endeavor was meshed with the learning of all these disciplines, helping me to develop my basis as a physician which added to my final goal of being a researcher.

3.3. My transition from the chemistry cabinet to a research laboratory

Anatomy was the center of the first year of medical school and comprised 32 weeks, four-hour sessions three times a week, totaling 384 hours of practice and theoretical classes that allowed students to digest the four volumes of the textbook written by Testut and Latarjet, translated to Spanish and published by Salvat [1], that presented a detailed description of each organ, its embryology and histology, plus other information narrated by the authors, for example, anomalies and the functional aspects of each organ. I read the four volumes cover to cover three times. I still keep these four volumes as testimony to the many hours that I was behind those books. Around this gigantic task were other classes like topographical anatomy, taught by a surgeon in order to give a practical vision of the anatomy in the way that surgeons see it, like the inguinal region, for example, and for that were two additional volumes of Henri Rouvière that also we needed to know. Radiologic anatomy was taught to us by a radiologist, and we saw in black and white the images of the bones and the contrasting images of the different organs that the practitioner sees in an X-ray film. In the middle of the anatomy classes were the 32 laboratory practices in biochemistry and biophysics.

My most remarkable memory of the anatomy classes was when during one of the tests Dr. Sanchez Guisande flicked a bone of the hand in front of me and I needed to identify it before it landed back in his hand. It was the scaphoid bone. Anatomy was the baptism into medical school, and in all the subjects, I got high scores and praise. In our final test in anatomy, Professor Sanchez Guisande, with his Aragon accent, congratulated three students, and I was one of them, for our dedication and performance in the first year.

The quest for my research enterprise was ongoing in my mind, and besides the chemistry cabinet I was desperate to find a path to begin doing research in cancer. The door started to open to me when talking with Ramon Piezzi, who knew my interest in cancer research and with whom I had shared what I was doing in my chemistry cabinet (see Chapter 2). He invited me to visit the Institute for General and Experimental Pathology where he was an instructor and doing research on the circadian rhythm of the mammary gland. He was in his last year of the medical courses. It was May 8, 1960, when I visited the institute for the first time, and I was impressed by the animal colony that had several strains of mice, like C3H and Balb/c, and many hybrids that the director was crossing, plus the histology and microscopy laboratory that they had. The director was Professor Julian Echave Llanos, and he was also the chairman of the department of pathology, comprising the Institute for General and Experimental Pathology and the two Laboratories of Anatomic Pathology in the Central and Emilio Civit hospitals, directed by Dr. J. Oliva Otero and M. Moll, respectively. The Institute for General and Experimental Pathology was located on the sixth floor of the Central Hospital and was impeccably run by Echave Llanos. The teaching and research was around three mayor pathological processes, namely degenerative, inflammatory, and neoplastic diseases, that were also taught to third year medical students. The students participated in an experimental protocol where they could visualize, for example, how the hydro-nephrosis of the kidney was produced by a ligature in the ureter, mimicking a stone obstruction, or how gastric cancer was produced if a strain of C57L mice was injected in the gastric submucosa with an oil suspension of 20-methylcholanthrene, or how the fat necrosis of the liver was induced by administration of carbon tetrachloride or tetrachloromethane. Other experimental procedures were also performed to show kidney infarction, inflammation, and tumors xenograft.

What I understood from that first visit was that experimental pathology was the discipline that studied the etiology and the pathogenesis of diseases. Using experimental methodologies, the discipline aimed to demonstrate the etiology and pathogenesis of an illness by mimicking human diseases, meaning that if I wanted to understand how cancer was produced, that was the discipline that I needed to master. I concluded that I could not treat or prevent cancer without at least understanding how the disease is produced.

The Institute of General and Experimental Pathology was founded on September 5, 1958, and the philosophy was based on one of the writings of Francis Bacon from his book *Philosophy of Science*:

Observations and experience to assemble materials, induction and deduction to elaborate them, these are the only good intellectual machines.

Echave Llanos was the first to establish an institute of this type in Argentina, and as a medical discipline it would be part of the curriculum of anatomic pathology. This put him apart, not only intellectually but professionally, from the other practicing anatomic pathologists, who were doing autopsies and surgical pathology. Those laboratories were in charge of teaching systemic and descriptive anatomic pathology to the students of the third year medical curriculum.

The main objective of the Institute for General and Experimental Pathology was to understand the etiology and pathogenesis of the disease processes using experimental models that require special methodologies and a unique training for those that are culturing this science. The institute was founded from a small experimental section that had been organized one year earlier in the medical school's Institute for Cancer Research. The model of the institute was taken from the laboratories that Echave Llanos visited in the best Institutes of General and Experimental Pathology in Germany, France, and England. Using the main European schools as models, the animal facility was created maintaining five strains of mice — the C3H Mza, C3H/He, C3He/De, Balb/c De, and C57L/Mza — and two strains of rats — Wistar and AxC. Because a great part of the research was on circadian rhythm, a special section of the animal facility was organized for those specific studies. In addition to the animal facility, the institute had a section for histology and another for experimental surgery in small animals. There was also a section of microscopy and photography and a section for biochemical studies. The institute also had six laboratories that were used by the instructors and researchers. One of them was the laboratory that I used.

In the Institute of General and Experimental Pathology, besides Ramon Piezzi, there were four other researchers, E. Bade, A. Badran, C. Vilchez, and I. Saffe. All of them worked in different but related areas of liver regeneration. C. Vilchez was the only one working on the pathogenesis of gastric cancer. They were older than me and they were either ending their medical courses or starting their internships. In the case of E. Bade, he had received the Humboldt fellowship to go to Dusseldorf Patologischen Institute der Medizinischen Akademie, with Prof. Dr. Meessen. After me, two other research assistants joined the institute, I. L. Sadnik and C. Bordin.

I had a better chance to see the members of the institute in action on October 7 of that year when Ramon Piezzi invited me to assist my first meeting of the Biology Society of Cuyo, where the son of Dr. Bernard Houssay was the plenary speaker and discussing the role of the pituitary gland in adrenal tumors. In the other presentations of that day, I learned in more detail what Carlos Vilchez, Ernesto Bade, and Ramon Piezzi were doing. I met or rather I saw and started to recognize all the other physician scientists, like Cei, Fasciolo, Suarez, and other young investigators working with them. This was my first scientific meeting where real results were presented and discussed. I saw all of them in action, and I liked it and wanted to be part of this group. More importantly, I had understood that to be an experimental pathologist was a pivotal step in my quest to be a cancer researcher.

After all these experiences and my success with my examination in anatomy, I felt empowered to think in a bigger context, and so on November 15 of that year I wrote in my journal that *I should consider the possibility of speeding up my process by taking anatomic pathology as a free student.* In the meantime, I took the examination for biophysics and biochemistry, and in the latter I had 10/10 and praise for my performance. On December 22, 1960, I completed my first year of medical studies.

During that summer, I periodically visited Ramon at the institute, and on January 25, 1961, he told me that he had been talking with Professor Echave Llanos about my interest in research and the possibility of admitting me to the institute. On Wednesday, March 1, 1961, I had my interview with Professor Echave Llanos. I met him in his office, which had a large desk surrounded by a massive bookcase and a photomicroscope and a drawing table. I sat down in front of him, and he listened to me very attentively as I told him that I wanted to be a cancer researcher and that I wanted to be part of his group and if needed I would take anatomic pathology as a free student to speed up the process. He was very forceful but at the same time there was a warmth in his eyes and in his words as he indicated that I needed to have a strong background in histology and also in normal and pathological physiology in order to understand anatomic pathology. He also told me that I would need to have a very good management of the histo-techniques, photography, animal handling, and surgery of small animals. He wanted me to learn all the processes that take place in a research laboratory, because knowing how to do even the most elemental things like handling the mice in the animal facilities would allow me to have the authority later on to teach others and know how the work must be done. He indicated that he would mentor me for everything from the small tasks to the experimental design, data collection, and analysis, and how to interpret them and write a paper. Finally, he told me that I could start on March 3 in the morning, and I followed him as he introduced M. G. Torres and Mrs. E. V de Coria, who were in charge of the laboratories; and Mr. J. Coria and Mr. L. Castro, who were the technical personnel working in the animal facilities. He also introduced me to Mrs. R. Cavoura, his special assistant in animal surgery. That was the way that I started my apprenticeship in experimental pathology.

Echave Llanos was my only real mentor, and he did what he promised that day. I am in debt for all the things he taught me in my formative years; Julian Echave Llanos was my real mentor, and I was told many years later by Carlos Vilchez that I was the only one that he really mentored.

3.4. My quest

My quest was to pass the examination of anatomic pathology that would give me the credentials to be admitted as a full Research Assistant and Instructor of pathology. This also could provide me a paid position, which would help me pay for my studies and also alleviate the stringent economic situation that my family was going through. The little income that I generated using my carpentry knowledge was too meager to make a difference in the tight situation that my parents had at that moment of our life.

The situation was complex because anatomic pathology was taught in the third year of medical school and the course lasted a whole year, meaning if I was successful in passing all the examinations I would be in a position to have the credential in November of 1962. This process would take almost 19 months plus the time that I would need to wait for the position to be opened for competition, but even if I wanted to take the examination of anatomic pathology as a free student, I must first pass the subjects of the second year curriculum, meaning that my earliest target to take the examination would be December of 1961. But more importantly I did not have the basic knowledge of normal histology and physiology needed to understand the even more complex process of human diseases. Therefore, I decided to continue working *ad honorem* in the Institute of General and Experimental Pathology under the guidance of Echave llanos and be trained as a Research Assistant while at the same time conquering my ignorance in the basic discipline of cell morphology and physiology.

In my second year of medical school, which started in March of 1961, I had in front of me three giants that needed to be conquered: histology, embryology, and normal human physiology. I submerged myself in understanding these disciplines with passion, and I enjoyed every minute of each. The Institute of Histology and Embryology was near the San Martin Park and had, under the direction of Professor Dr. Mario H. Burgos, an excellent group of young researchers. The technology that they were handling was very sophisticated, like electron microscopy, and the modern techniques of cell biology, such as ultracentrifugation, tissue culture, and the beginning of molecular biology, were budding in their laboratories. They were interested in solving basic biological problems more than the understanding of diseases. They even laughed at the primitive techniques that pathologists were using, like the simple techniques of hematoxylin and eosin, whereas they were using more sophisticated histo-techniques and cyto-chemistry in frozen and paraffin embedded tissues. The laboratories of histology and embryology were using the same technology that was state-of-the-art at Harvard at that time. Definitely it was another research setting than the one available in the Institute for General and Experimental Pathology. However, statistical significance and statistical power were not required because experimentation was not the main tool for research, as it was in the experimental pathology laboratory. The philosophy of the Institute of Histology and Embryology was to have a thorough understanding of the normal process before asking how the disease emerges.

On July 20, 1961, I passed with flying colors in histology and embryology, and the examiners, Dr. Oliva-Oteros and Dr. Mario H. Burgos, gave me a 10 with congratulations. Dr. Burgos said that there was not any need to ask me questions, and that he would like to tell me the importance of basic research. It was an exhilarating experience to have acquired a grasp of everything that was new up to that day concerning the nature of our histological fabric, like Vesalius [2] *would say if he were living in our time.*

The understanding of the normal morphological process as well as the functionality of each organ was a real treat considering the individualized teaching that we received in all three disciplines. In physiology, we were using frogs, rats, and dogs to measure cardiac activity, the kidney regulation of blood pressure, or the role of psycho estimations in gastric secretion, to mention a few of the many functions in how the human body works. Our professors and instructors were physician scientists doing research in the many areas that we were taught. All of them had already completed their research training in the United States or were ready to go abroad. There was an optimistic environment full of intellectual energy emanating from young and promising scientists, as many of them demonstrated they were.

In October of that year, I passed all the courses with the highest score among the second year students and finally started to study anatomic pathology. I decided to take anatomic pathology in March of 1962 instead of December of 1961 and spent the whole summer in the museum of the Anatomic Pathology Laboratory. Professor Oliva-Oteros was the director of those laboratories, and he gave me his support to do this. Practically, the whole museum, which contained hundreds of well-preserved lesions, was at my disposal. In that summer, I attended and helped Dr. J. Motta with autopsies done in the morgue of the Central Hospital. Dr. Motta was a quiet man devoted to his work and in charge of forensic pathology. He taught me the basics of autopsy procedures, which was the part of the specialty that I never enjoyed. However, I felt like Michel Doutreval in Van der Meersch's novel *Bodies and Souls* when I was assisting Motta in his autopsies. The microscopic anatomy was available to me in the Institute of General and Experimental Pathology, and I still preserve those 120 slides containing the most characteristic lesions in pathology. Carlos Vilchez and Ramon Piezzi helped me by answering questions when I was having trouble understanding the lesions. It was a real *tour de force* but worth doing. It was amazing how little by little every day, I was assembling in my mind the pathological processes. In one of those summer Saturdays when I was in the institute studying my histopathology, I had for the first time the chance to talk with Ernesto Bade on personal matters, and he spontaneously mentioned that he also had been Catholic like me when he was younger but later on he lost faith and moved away from the Church. I also knew from him that he had arrived in Mendoza very young after his parents died in Germany during WWII, and had been raised by his aunt. Ernesto was a smart person and very focused on his future. But because we were at different generational ages, I was not able to befriend him like I had done with Carlos Vilchez, Ramon Piezzi, and Irma Saffe; those older than me were more social and able to share their time with me. Ernesto Bade later left Mendoza and took a research position in Germany where he continues to flourish in his research.

On Friday, March 16, 1962, I took the examination for anatomic pathology and passed with a 10 and congratulations from Dr. Moll and Dr. Oliva-Otero. Dr. Echave Llanos also congratulated me, and then I asked him if the 10 and the congratulations were deserved, and he told me that the 10 and congratulations were from the other professors but that I fully deserved them. I was then duly qualified to apply for the position of Instructor in pathology. On September 19 of that year, I won the competitive position and began as an Instructor in pathology. *That position entitled me to a salary, and from there on all the income that I have generated in my life came by doing research work.* The other more important aspect was that this would help me pay for my studies, and in addition allowed me to give a part of my salary to my parents, who were in great need of economic help. From that day until they passed away in 2005, I was able to help them every single month with a percentage of my earnings. The only thing that I regret was not being able to help them more.

3.5. The election

Another opportunity came to me in the middle of 1961. Dr. Mario H. Burgos, Director of the Institute of Histology and Embryology that now holds his name at the University National of Cuyo in

Mendoza, Argentina, was my professor of histology and embryology. He had been working with Bernard Houssay and came to the medical school after a traineeship in electron microscopy with Dawn Fawcett at Harvard University. This special training and his publications allowed him to have support from the Rockefeller Foundation and obtain the first electron microscope for the medical school. It is not doubted that I was fascinated by the structure of the cell and the modern concepts of cell biology that were available in those days. The double helix was still the big discovery of the century, so were the new findings of cell organelles and their functions, such as the role of the rough endoplasmic reticulum in the synthesis of protein, the world of the mitochondria and the lysosomes. These discoveries were to provide the basis for the functions and the localization of molecules in every part of the cell. I already knew *The Book of Cell Biology* by Eduardo De Robertis [3] by heart; I had been reading it with fascination since my fourth year in the National College when I was taking my preparatory examinations to enter medical school. Burgos was an excellent teacher and had an extraordinary talent for drawing and painting that he transmitted in his classes. I think I must have somewhat impressed him too with my enthusiasm — I was the one ready to ask the questions that were posed by my previous readings in *Cell Biology*. I still remember those days with great fondness. The wonderful world of science was opening itself to me completely, and showed a beauty far more brilliant than I could have ever expected. Professor Burgos asked me to join his group that year. The institute, short for Institute for Histology and Embryology, was a nest of young scientists, working in various areas of cell and structural biology, and each one enthusiastically tackled their project with the fervent energy transmitted by Burgos.

It was a great honor that Burgos wanted me to be part of his research group, but I was already accepted at the Experimental Pathology Institute and Echave Llanos had confided to me that he had accepted me to his team because my person oozed dedication and an obsessive passion for research. This plus the fact that he was already mentoring me and shaping my mind in the use of experimentation as a way to answer questions made my situation even more conflicted.

I laid awake many nights pondering who to choose as a mentor. The trouble was, while I respected and admired Burgos, the Institute for General and Experimental Pathology was where the process of "normal and neoplastic growth" was studied, and this, more than anything else was what fascinated me. Despite the beauty of histology and embryology, I eventually said no to Burgos's invitation, although I kept a good connection with him and the researchers in his group. In retrospect, it was a good decision to become an experimental pathologist first.

3.6. Becoming an experimental pathologist

I started as a Research Assistant in experimental pathology on March 3, 1961, and as I have been told by Echave Llanos, I learned even the simplest tasks from him like sharpening the knives for doing perfect microtome sections to the final task of publishing a paper. For me, learning the basic steps in experimental pathology came in the middle of learning histology, cell biology and human physiology of my second year of medical school.

One important area of research that Echave Llanos had, and that everybody there was working in, related subjects that were the mechanisms of liver regeneration and the role of the circadian rhythm in the process. From my contributions in this area, four publications originated [4–7].

3.6.1. *Studies in liver regeneration*

The topic of cell regeneration was a way to understand the normal and neoplastic growth at that specific time of my life, and at that stage of my learning process, it was a good start in understanding the growth of cells and tissue that is basically the main driving characteristic of cancer cells. The book that I used for understanding this process was written by A. E. Needham and titled *Regeneration and Wound Healing* [8]. The process of regeneration is an important biological event in nature, allowing renewal, restoration, and growth. Although every species is capable of regeneration, the main difference is that either it is complete, where the new tissue is the same as the lost tissue, or incomplete, where the necrotic tissue is afterward replaced by fibrosis, for example. Among the coelenterates, the hydra is a good model of regeneration and also among the urodeles, the salamander is the best example of regeneration in the vertebrate, given their capability to regenerate limbs, tails, jaws, eyes, and a variety of internal structures [9–12].

Coming back to 1961, it was known that the process of regeneration in humans was limited, and one of the most studied regenerative responses in humans was the hypertrophy of the liver following liver injury [8]. For example, the original mass of the liver is re-established in direct proportion to the amount of liver removed following partial hepatectomy [8,13,14], which indicates that signals from the body regulate liver mass precisely, both positively and negatively, until the desired mass is reached. This response is considered cellular regeneration or a form of compensatory hypertrophy, where the function and mass of the liver is regenerated through the proliferation of existing mature hepatic cells, mainly hepatocytes, but the exact morphology of the liver is not regained. Therefore, understanding the mechanism of liver regeneration was a good theme of research, and it was the main subject of study in the Institute for General and Experimental Pathology.

My first scientific presentation was in the II Scientific Session of Biology, organized by the Biology Society of Cordoba in 1962. In that meeting, I presented the work on the variations in dry matter and water in regeneration in the liver. Those were the preliminary data that I had from the paper that I published later on in 1964.

My first paper was published in 1963, and I was one of the coauthors, sharing authorship with Ernesto Bade and Irma Saffe. For these studies, we used a strain of mice called C3H/Mza, a line derived in 1957 of C3H/HeJ from the Roscoe Jackson Memorial Laboratory. The animals were hepatectomized using a technique described by Brues *et al.* in 1936 [15]. Most of the experiments were large, with 205 mice divided in different groups for controlling sex and weight, and our first experiment was to determine if the humoral factors released during hepatectomy might have an effect on other organs.

Partial hepatectomy induced hypertrophy of the kidney as shown by the histological pattern and increase in the dry weight of the organ. The interesting part was that the hypertrophy was observed after 72 hours post-hepatectomy, and it was maintained up to the eight-month follow-up. The hepatic mass was restored to almost 70% of its original value after 72 hours. This was the same time in which the effect was observed in the kidney. The explanation of this effect was not clear, and we postulated several growth factors released during hepatectomy could be responsible for this systemic factor. Among the postulated mechanisms that we wrote about in the discussion of the manuscript was that the hypertrophy of the kidney was producing an inhibitory growth factor to compensate for the rapid growth of the liver. The factors released by the liver during the compensatory hypertrophy was due to the increase in production of secretion of growth hormone by the pituitary gland [16–18], and we cited Houssay, who in 1947 [19] demonstrated that hypophisectomized mice decrease the kidney weight and it is restored by the injection of pituitary extract, meaning that our data were supporting that line of thinking. That first paper was followed by two additional ones that I published with Professor Echave Llanos in 1964 and in 1965. These two successive publications were short, but they were interesting because they indicated that there was a relationship between the pituitary gland and the regeneration process in the liver. In between these two publications, I made my first international presentation at the VI Congress of the Latin American Society of Physiological Sciences, which took place in Vinia del Mar, Chile, in September of 1964. The presentation was on the effect of the pituitary gland in the hepatectomized liver. This presentation was followed by a publication in the same year in *Die Naturwissenschaten*. In these experiments, we used the pituitary glands of AxC rats that were obtained from Dr. Lipschutz from Santiago de Chile. The glands were homogenized in aseptic conditions and diluted with a saline solution. The recipient targets were C3H mice/Mza that had been hepatectomized 32 hours earlier. The mice were killed 16 hours later, and the liver was extracted and the dry weight and mitotic activity were determined. We found that the pituitary extract raised the dry weight of the liver and reduced the mitotic activity. This dual effect was interpreted in part by the data published by N. N. Swann, showing that there was a competitive relation between protoplasmic reproduction and cell division [20], but we speculated that the circadian rhythm of the pituitary hormones was also responsible for this effect. This line of thinking originated in the paper published in 1965. We used the data of Ungar and Halberg [21] on the study of the circadian rhythm of the adrenocorticotrophic activity of the pituitary gland to choose the time of killing the donors and that of injecting the receivers. In this experiment, we again used AxC rats that were hepatectomized and killed 72 hours after the surgery when the ACTH was at its peak, and therefore the right time to remove their pituitary gland. We again took the pituitary glands and homogenized them in a sterile saline solution and injected eight groups of Balb/cDc mice that had been hepatectomized 28 hours before. In this experiment, we demonstrated that the hepatectomy modified the pituitary gland and inhibited the increase in the dry weight of the liver when compared with the effect of the pituitary gland of non-hepatectomized rats. This effect intrigued me, and I wanted to pursue another venue of research. In my laboratory notes (Figure 3.1), I considered that a parabiosis experiment would help to better understand the correlation between the pituitary gland and liver regeneration.

However, parabiosis surgery was not in the general protocol of the laboratory, so I tried to demonstrate that the idea could work. That was the motivation that I'd had to do the parabiosis experiment in my chemistry cabinet that I described in Chapter 2. The idea was not appealing to Dr. Echave llanos but I want to document it anyway because it was based on the experiment reported by W. U. Gardner in *Advances in Cancer Research* in 1953 [22]. In that experiment, he had shown that pituitary gonadotropin was increased by ovariectomy in an animal that was not castrated. The parabiotic experiments could show the effect on the pituitary induced by the liver in regeneration. I took two AxC rats from the laboratory, with the help of Mr. Luis Castro, the person in charge of the animal facility, and in my chemistry cabinet I joined them (see Chapter 2). The parabiosis worked because an injection of tripan blue solution at 1% in one of the pair colored

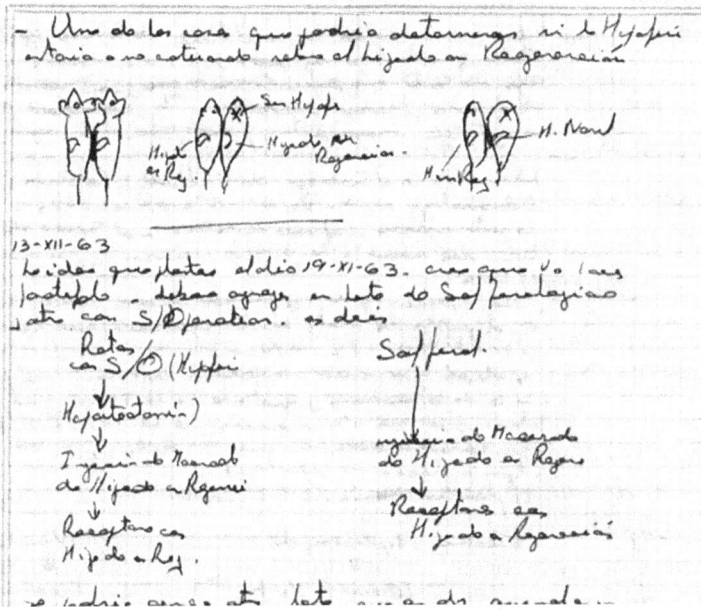

Figure 3.1: Notes in my 1963 laboratory book on the idea of pursuing experiments using a parabiotic system.

the other one, meaning that the system worked. However, that experiment brought significant problems into my home, and finally I returned the animals to the laboratory and they were properly euthanized. In retrospect, the idea was an excellent one, but it would have disrupted the line of research experiments that Echave Llanos had established, and although I did not understand in those days, today I am sympathetic with his reaction but also with my idea.

The mechanisms of cell and tissue regeneration were not known in those days, and presently we have a better idea that the process of regeneration is regulated by genetic induction factors that put cells to work after damage has occurred [14,23–29]. In nerve regeneration growth-associated proteins, such as GAP-43, tubulin, actin, and an array of novel neuropeptides, cytokines induce a cellular physiological response to regenerate from the damage [30]. Many of the genes that are involved in the original development of tissues are reinitialized during the regenerative process. Cells in the primordia of zebra fish fins, for example, express four genes from the homeobox *msx* family during development and regeneration [31–33]. If I started that line of research now, the approach would definitely be more molecular oriented than those primitive experiments in 1962.

3.6.2. *Studies on the role of circadian rhythm in liver regeneration*

An area of research that was of great interest in those days at the institute was the role of circadian rhythm and its implications in biological processes; in this case, in liver regeneration. This area of research was completely unheard of by me, and I learned fast that a *circadian rhythm* is a biological process that displays an endogenous oscillation of about 24 hours. The circadian rhythm has been shown to be present in practically all life forms [34]. The word *circadian* has a Latin origin, meaning "around the day," and although they are endogenously controlled, they are adjusted (entrained) to the local environment by external cues called *zeitgebers* (from German, "time giver"), which include light and temperature, for example [35]. The first observations of a circadian rhythm were described in the diurnal leaf movement of the tamarind tree by Androsthenes in the fourth century BC. Jean-Jacques d'Ortous de Mairan in 1729 observed a 24 hour pattern in the movement of the leaves of the plant *Mimosa pudica* that continued even when the plants were kept in constant darkness. The term *circadian* was coined by Franz Halberg in the 1950s [36]. In order to determine that an organ or a function has a circadian rhythm, it must persist in constant conditions, for example, constant darkness, as was observed in *Mimosa pudica*. Another criterion is that the rhythm be entrainable, meaning that it can be reset by exposure to external stimuli such as light, for example, and finally the rhythm must exhibit temperature compensation and maintain circadian periodicity over a range of physiological temperatures [37]. These 24 hour rhythms are now known to be driven by clock genes [38–42].

In September of 1961, I was assigned my own research project, Experiment 83, to study the circadian rhythm in liver regeneration. The importance of that experiment was that I was involved from its inception and planning until it was finished and resulted in my first publication as a senior author (Figure 3.2). The fact that many organs have rhythmic variations was already known [36,43–45] and the liver was one of those organs [46,47]. The rhythm of the mitotic activity was not observed in the epidermal cells lying within a millimeter of the edge of the wound [48], but it was detected in many tissues [48–52] and also in the liver [52]. *Therefore, the question was whether the mitotic activity during liver regeneration was maintained like in the normal liver or if it was lost as shown in the wound healing of the skin* [48,49]. For this purpose, we used 73 male mice of a line obtained by inbreeding black

()

Zeitschrift für Zellforschung 61, 824—828 (1964)

Instituto de Patología General y Experimental, Facultad de Ciencias Médicas,
Universidad Nacional de Cuyo, Mendoza, Argentina

TWENTY-FOUR-HOUR RHYTHM IN THE MITOTIC ACTIVITY
AND IN THE WATER AND DRY MATTER CONTENT
OF REGENERATING LIVER*

By

JOSE RUSSO and JULIAN M. ECHAVE LLANOS

With 1 Figure in the Text

(Received July 7, 1963)

Figure 3.2:   Paper published in the journal *Zeitschrift fur Zellfoschung* in 1964.

dominants in F1 of a cross between a female C3H/Mza and a male C57L/Mza when they were 90 days old. They had a rhythm of artificial illumination from 5 to 7 a.m. and 5 to 7 p.m. The mice were maintained from weaning up to 90 days in groups of eight animals per cage. When they were 90 days old, they were hepatectomized [15] at noon, and 24 hours later I started the collection of the liver every 24 hours for 48 hours, meaning that I collected 13 groups of mice and I was there for almost two days working continuously. Among the parameters that I studied were the dried matter, water content, and mitotic activity by counting 3,000 nuclei per animal and expressing the number of mitosis per 1,000 nuclei. We found that the three parameters studied followed a perfect circadian rhythm (Figure 3.3). The data were published in the journal *Zeitschrift fur Zellfoschung* in 1964 [5] (Figure 3.2).

The relevance of this work was that the dry matter, water, and mitotic activity in the regenerating liver is not continuous, and that

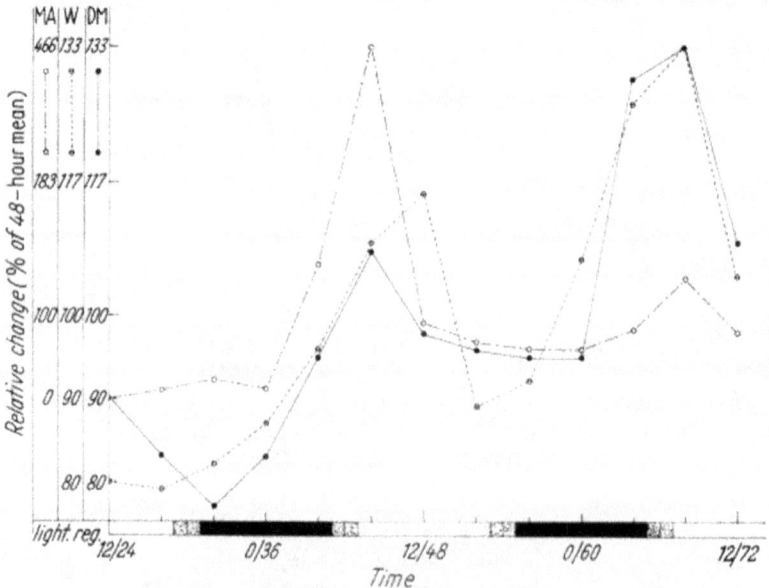

Figure 3.3: Time relations among 24-hour period variables in regenerating mouse liver. MA: mitotic activity. W: water. DM: dry matter. light reg: lighting regimen. Time: time of day/hours post-hepatectomy (see Ref. [5]).

the inherent 24 rhythm persists even after hepatectomy, and the need for rapid replacement of liver parenchyma does not elicit uninterrupted cytoplasmic synthesis.

3.7. The important lesson that I learned

Although my small contribution in the field did not provide the molecular mechanism of liver regeneration, the most important thing that I gained from these experiments was experience in the process of data collection and analysis. The handling of different strains of rodents and understanding their crossing to develop a specific variety of mice strain, and the surgery in these small animals was also invaluable. Another important lesson was learning about experimental design, the statistical power to determine the adequate number of animals per group, and the analysis of data using the right statistical tools. These basic rules were pivotal in my later studies on the pathogenesis of mammary carcinogenesis as well as in the research on environmental carcinogenesis. Echave Llanos was very rigorous about experimental design, and I learned how to do it from him.

Carlos Vilchez, who became a lasting and good friend, was the one who indicated to me that none of the disciples of Echave Llanos had been trained by him, and I was the only one that Echave Llanos personally trained. He explained to me that it was probably because when I entered the institute he had just recovered from a divorce and had a new wife, Rubi Cavourt, who was also working in the Experimental Pathology Laboratory. That new marriage provided him a new outlook and perception of things, and I benefited by starting at this specific moment in his life. In addition, Echave Llanos had recently returned from a sabbatical during which he visited Germany, England, and France, bringing the newest tools available in experimental pathology in those days back to the medical school. Whatever the reason or motivation, he was an extraordinary mentor and teacher for me. I was the youngest of the group, and he was the one who taught me how to do research, from the simple task of planning an experiment to obtaining the conclusions. He taught me the value of statistical power, reproducibility, and quality control. He taught me how to construct scientific tables and figures, and how to make graphics that clearly express data. I absorbed his influence like a thirsty sponge. To this day, I wonder whether he ever realized how much I learned from him and how deeply I have appreciated his mentorship. I still have fresh in my memory the time that I spent by his side at the drawing table, watching how he drew the graphs in China ink and how we also discussed political ideas. He considered himself an atheist and his ideas were toward the left. Although I did not agree with his ideologies, there was a significant and mutual respect in our different ideological positions. One discussion that is engraved in my mind was about the concept of social changes by revolutionary ideas. His statement was something to remember: "*the only people that can do revolutions are those that do not have anything to lose.*" This was probably his position in the continuous disagreements he started having with the authorities of the medical school. In time, he isolated himself from the hostility that he received and he lost the chairmanship of the department, eventually the only thing that tied him to the medical school that he had helped create was the Institute for General and Experimental Pathology. A few years after my departure from the institute in October of 1966, he left Mendoza and dissolved the institute that was so important in my formation as a researcher, as well as for those like R. Piezzi, E. Bade, and A. Badran, who persisted in research.

I have discussed in my previous book [58] that my experience with Echave llanos was the typical example of an *individual exchange*, which I maintained for many years of my scientific apprenticeship. It was during these interactions that I authored my first scientific publications, and where I learned how to present and discuss a paper in a scientific meeting. This type of interaction is extremely valuable, and it is in the scientific apprentice's best interest to find a mentor from whom they can learn and with whom they can work closely with. One of the most important aspects of this formative period for me was that very early on I learned how to handle complex biological processes and even my study of circadian rhythm lost momentum; it wasn't until relatively recently, with the discovery of clock genes [38–42], that the scientific community started to take a second look at this process. In 2003, in collaboration with Irma H. Russo, I acquired funding to study the circadian rhythm of clock genes in the mammary gland of the rat. The importance of the circadian rhythm was further recognized in 2017 with the awarding of the Nobel Prize to the three biologists that contributed to the discovery of the clock genes.

3.8. The clinical training

Although my research work in the institute filled my life, I must also indicate here that I was following the medical curriculum and I learned so much in the study of physiopathology, microbiology, parasitology, and pharmacology that each subject could be a chapter in itself. But I will summarize, saying only that the training that I received in those subjects was so vast and full of laboratory practice supervised by physician scientists that each subject increased my dexterity and learning of new techniques and procedures but most importantly each of those disciplines taught me how the scientific process of discovery worked. I will not go into details about who were the ones that taught us the disciplines of the so-called basic science, but only I will refer to few of the memories collected in my personal journal that give an idea of the caliber of those physician scientists. Of particular relevance in my studies in physiopathology was Prof. Juan Carlos Fasciolo [54]. He was the chairman of the department, and he taught us physiopathology. He was a disciple of Dr. Bernardo Houssay, winner of the Nobel Prize in medicine, and the one that together with another Nobel Prize recipient, Dr. Luis Leloir, structured the scientific research in Argentina, and all of us who were trained in Argentina received the benefit of their efforts. Dr. Fasciolo made his doctoral thesis with Dr. Houssay. He demonstrated that a hypertensive substance was secreted by the ischemic kidney. Fasciolo used the findings of Harry Golblatt, in the United States, who discovered that the mechanism of constriction of the renal artery induced in dogs a permanent hypertension. Fasciolo grafted an ischemic kidney to a normal dog and produced the hypertension, indicating that the effect was produced by a substance secreted by the kidney. Houssay understood the importance of these findings and gathered around Fasciolo other researchers like Muñoz, Taquini, Braun, Menéndez, and Leloir [55]. Leloir and Muñoz were the biochemists; Braun, Menéndez, and Fasciolo the physiologists; and these studies led to the discovery of the angiotensin. In Chicago, Irvine Page had found the same results calling the substance renin, and for many years both names were used in the literature until in 1957 Braun, Menéndez, and Page found a solution to the terminology [56,57]. And from there on the terms used in all the medical texts are angiotensin and angiotensinogen. In 1952, Fasciolo moved to Mendoza, and he was one of the founders of the medical school and organized the department of physiology. He created a cadre of teachers and researchers, among them was his successor Dr. Alberto Binia, who I worked with as a secretary of the Biology Society of Cuyo during the years of 1968–1971. The research environment created by Fasciolo was oozing during my medical school days, and on April 6, 1962, I remember meeting for the first time Dr. Bernardo Houssay, who came to Mendoza in honor of Fasciolo. A small piece of history was gathered together that day.

My last 3 years of clinics started in 1963 and marked a different reality for me. The glamour of the research laboratory ideas and scientific discussion was replaced by patient needs and learning that diseases are not isolated entities, but they are attached to real human beings. The clinical experience and the humanness related to it gave me the dimension of medicine that has been so invaluable in my research career. The human suffering and death in the hospital beds and the fragile health of my mother were a continuum of images and feelings that made me suffer watching the human condition. I wanted to eliminate all of that suffering of our human flesh, and for me to succeed in research on curing diseases my only consolation was that someday all that suffering would be stopped. I was in those days in my early twenties and now I'm 76 years of age, and I still have the same feelings, thoughts, and frustrations. I entered that feeling in my private journal on October 26, 1964, when I wrote: *An old and dirty white sheet separates the man with his rattle of death and the only sounds in the ten bedrooms of the hospital that separate him from all the other still living patients who were in silence awaiting his final moments. I know that in few minutes or maybe a little longer life will disappear and only a corpse will remain. I know that in my Christian belief in immortality but I cannot separate from me the terrible abyss between life and death, health and disease.*

It was also in this period that I wrote an essay that I titled *The Essence of Being a University Student*. It was well received among my peers, and basically I introduced the importance of having an inquisitive mind in our learning process. That essay was the core that later on I developed into my book: *The Handbook for the Apprentice of Biomedical Research: The Tools of Science*, published in 2011 [58].

During those 3 years of clinical sciences in the medical school curriculum, I also made a *tour de force* of studying German. It was ambitious and unrealistic but the place I would train after finishing medical school and the postdoctoral fellowship were also in the back of my mind. In retrospect, I should have concentrated on English only and forgotten about German, but in my own defense of that silly decision it was because Heidelberg was prominent in the scientific environment of those days.

Medical students of the present generation are trained differently, and they will learn how to be physicians not *physician scientists*. Even now the Medical School of the University National of Cuyo in Mendoza is not different than the curriculum of any medical school in the United States. I am a rarity for the new generation where most of the scientists are not physicians and only few of them take the route of science. I am telling my story not because it was better, but because it was different and made me what I am. I was extremely fortunate to be trained by the physician scientists, and although things are not the same now, they existed and were part of my life.

3.9. New perspectives

As I discussed in my previous book [58], "Individual exchanges during the training process must be limited, otherwise they could be detrimental to the scientific apprentice in the sense that he or she may become too dependent on the mentor, ultimately narrowing his or her long-range intellectual growth." When I was at the end of my medical training and needed a new plan of action, I paid Professor Burgos a visit and soon after moved to his institute. Burgos was a different type of mentor than Echave Llanos; he outlined general ideas and let people work from that point forward. He was there when we needed him, but he allowed us the intellectual freedom of our own research interest and that was exactly what I was looking for. My own style of mentorship has in the past followed the individual exchange model based on my experience with Echave Llanos. Lately, my schedule does not allow me the luxury of spending so much time one-on-one with each postdoc, but in order to maintain a close mentor–apprentice relationship, I have adopted Burgos's style. I entrust, however, most technical aspects of the work to the associates who I trust the most to be sure that the methods of transmitting knowledge and skill are similar to the way I would do it. If it were at all possible, I would take the time to work individually with each person, yet by giving my scientific apprentices room to think and grow, I think I have given them something much more valuable [58].

References

[1] Testut, L. and Latarjet, A. *Tratado de Anatomia Humana*, Salvat Editores, S.A. Barcelona. 1959.

[2] Saunders, J. B. de C. M. and O'Malley C. D. *Andreas Vesalius, The Classics olf Medicine Library*, Gryphon Editinons, New York. 1993.

[3] De Robertis, E. D. P., Nowinski, W. W. and Saez, F. A. *Citologia General*, Libreria El Ateneo Editorial, Buenos Aires. Tercera edición. 1957.

[4] Echave-Llanos J. M., Jaffe, I. E., Russo, J. and Bade, E. G. Hipertrofia del riñón en ratones hepatectomizados. *Revista Latinoamericana de Anatomia Patologica* 7: 17–24, 1963.

[5] Russo, J. and Echave-Llanos, J. M. Twenty-four hour rhythm in the mitotic activity and the water and dry matter content of regenerating liver. *Zietschrift fur Zellforschung* 161: 824–828, 1964.

[6] Echave Llanos, J. M. and Russo, J. Action of a homogenate of rat pituitary gland on mouse regenerated liver. *Die Naturwissenchaften* 13: 312–313, 1964.

[7] Echave Llanos, J. M. and Russo, J. Action of pituitary gland homogenates from untreated and hepatectomized rats on hepatic regeneration. *Die Naturwissenchaften* 3: 63–64, 1965.

[8] Needham, A. E. *Regeneration and wound-healing*, Methuen & Co. Ltd, London.1952.

[9] Nye, H. L., Cameron, J. A., Chernoff, E. A. and Stocum, D. L. Regeneration of the urodele limb: a review. *Dev. Dyn.* 226: 280–294, 2003.

[10] Tanaka, E. M. Cell differentiation and cell fate during urodele tail and limb regeneration. *Curr. Opin. Genet. Dev.* 13: 497–501, 2003.

[11] Bosch, T. C. G. Why Polyps Regenerate and We Don't: Towards a Cellular and Molecular Framework for Hydra Regeneration. *Dev. Biol.* 303: 421–433, 2007.

[12] Yu, H., Mohan, S., Masinde, G. L. and Baylink, D. J. Mapping the dominant wound healing and soft tissue regeneration QTL in MRL x CAST. *Mamm. Genome.* 16: 918–924, 2005.

[13] Kawasaki, S. Liver regeneration in recipients and donors after transplantation. *Lancet* 339: 580–581, 1992.

[14] Michalopoulos, G. K. Hepatostat: Liver regeneration and normal liver tissue maintenance. *Hepatology* 65(4): 1384–1392, 2016. doi: 10.1002/hep.28988. (Epub ahead of print).

[15] Brues, A. M., Drury, D. R. and Brues, M. C. A quantitative study of cell growth in regenerating liver. *Arch. Path. Lab. Med.* 22: 658–663, 1936.

[16] Litman, T., Halberg, F., Ellis, S. and Bittner, J. Pituitary growth hormone and mitoses in immature mouse liver. *Endocrinology* 62: 361, 1958.

[17] Di Stefano, H. S. and Diermieir, H. F. Effect of hypophysectomy and growth hormone on ploidy distribution and mitotic activity in rat liver. *Proc. Soc. Exp. Biol.* 92: 590–594, 1956.

[18] Hemingway, J. T. and Carter, D. B. Effects of pituitary hormones and cortisone upon liver regeneration in the hypophysectomized rat. *Nature* 181: 1065–1066, 1958.

[19] Houssay, A. B. *Hipofisis y crecimineto*, El Ateneo, Buenos Aires. 1947.

[20] Swann, M. M. The control of cell division: A Review. II. Special Mechanisms. *Cancer Res.* 18: 1118–1160, 1958.

[21] Ungar, F. and Halberg, F. In vitro exploration of a circadian rhythm in adrenocorticotropic activity of c mouse hypophysis. *Experientia* 19: 158–160, 1963.

[22] Gardner, W. U. Hormonal aspects of experimental tumorigenesis. *Adv. Cancer Res.* 1: 173–232, 1953.

[23] Beltrami, A. P. Evidence that human cardiac myocytes divide after myocardial infarction. *N. Engl. J. Med.* 344: 1750–1757, 2001.

[24] Bergmann, O. Evidence for cardiomyocyte renewal in humans. *Science* 324: 98–102, 2009.

[25] Bhushan, B., Poudel, S., Manley, M. W. Jr, Roy, N. and Apte, U. Inhibition of Glycogen Synthase Kinase 3 Accelerated Liver Regeneration after Acetaminophen-Induced Hepatotoxicity in Mice. *Am. J. Pathol.* 187: 543–552, 2017.

[26] Piran, R., Lee, S. H., Kuss, P., Hao, E., Newlin, R., Millán, J. L. and Levine, F. PAR2 regulates regeneration, transdifferentiation, and death. *Cell Death Dis.* 7: e2452, 2016.

[27] Juskeviciute, E., Dippold, R. P., Antony, A. N., Swarup, A., Vadigepalli, R. and Hoek, J. B. Inhibition of miR-21 rescues liver regeneration after partial hepatectomy in ethanol-fed rats. *Am. J. Physiol. Gastrointest. Liver Physiol.* 311: G794–G806, 2016.

[28] Langiewicz, M., Schlegel, A., Saponara, E., Linecker, M., Borger, P., Graf, R., Humar, B. and Clavien, P. A. Hedgehog pathway mediates early acceleration of liver regeneration induced by a novel two-staged hepatectomy in mice. *J. Hepatol.* 66: 560–570, 2017.

[29] Shang, N., Arteaga, M., Chitsike, L., Wang, F., Viswakarma, N., Breslin, P. and Qiu, W. FAK deletion accelerates liver regeneration after two-thirds partial hepatectomy. *Sci. Rep.* 6: 34316, 2016.

[30] Fu, S. Y. and Gordon, T. The cellular and molecular basis of peripheral nerve regeneration. *Mol. Neurobiol.* 14: 67–116, 1997.

[31] Akimenko, M., Johnson, S. L., Wseterfield, M. and Ekker, M. Differential induction of four msx homeobox genes during fin development and regeneration in zebrafish. *Development* 121: 347–357, 1996.

[32] Gardiner, D. M., Blumberg, B., Komine, Y. and Bryant, S. V. Regulation of HoxA expression in developing and regenerating axolotl limbs. *Development* 121: 1731–1741, 1995.

[33] Torok, M. A., Gardiner, D. M., Shubin, N. H. and Bryant, S. V. Expression of HoxD genes in developing and regenerating axolotl limbs. *Dev. Biol.* 200: 225–233, 1998.

[34] Johnson, C. *Chronobiology: Biological Timekeeping*, Sinauer Associates Inc., Sunderland, MA. 2004, 67–105.

[35] Bass, J. Circadian topology of metabolism. *Nature* 491(7424): 348–356, 2012.

[36] Halberg, F. Some physiological and clinical aspects of 24-hour periodicity. *J. Lancet* 73: 20–32, 1953.

[37] Sharma, V. K. Adaptive significance of circadian clocks. *Chronobiol. Int.* 20: 901–919, 2003.

[38] Goto, M., Mizuno, M., Matsumoto, A., Yang, Z., Jimbo, E. F., Tabata, H., Yamagata, T. and Nagata, K. I. Role of a circadian-relevant gene NR1D1 in

brain development: possible involvement in the pathophysiology of autism spectrum disorders. *Sci. Rep.* 7: 43945, 2017. doi: 10.1038/srep43945.

[39] Singh, D. and Kumar, V. Extra-hypothalamic brain clocks in songbirds: Photoperiodic state dependent clock gene oscillations in night-migratory black headed buntings, Emberiza melanocephala. *J. Photochem Photobiol B.* 169: 13–20, 2017.

[40] Mieda, M., Hasegawa, E., Kessaris, N. and Sakurai, T. Fine-Tuning Circadian Rhythms: The Importance of Bmal1 Expression in the Ventral Forebrain. *Front Neurosci.* 11: 55, 2017.

[41] Shimizu, T., Watanabe, K., Anayama, N. and Miyazaki, K. Effect of lipopolysaccharide on circadian clock genes Per2 and Bmal1 in mouse ovary. *J. Physiol. Sci.* 67(5): 623–628, 2017. doi: 10.1007/s12576-017-0532-1.

[42] Kiessling, S., Beaulieu-Laroche, L., Blum, I. D., Landgraf, D., Welsh, D. K., Storch, K. F., Labrecque, N. and Cermakian, N. Enhancing circadian clock function in cancer cells inhibits tumor growth. *BMC Biol.* 15: 13, 2017.

[43] Kleithman, N. Biological rhythms and cycles. *Physiol. Rev.* 29: 1–30, 1949.

[44] Halberg, F. Physiologic 24-hour rhythms: a determinant of response to environmental agents. *Int. Symposium on Submarine and Space Medicine*, 1958, New London, CT.

[45] Halberg, F. and Howard, R. B. 24-hour periodicity and experimental medicine. *Postgrad. Med.* 24: 349–358, 1958.

[46] Fabry, P. and Hruza, Z. On diurnal rhythmic changes in liver glycogen and protein reserves in fasting rats. *Physiol. bohemoslov.* 5: 142–148, 1958.

[47] Barnum, C. P., Jadetzky, Ch. D. and Halberg, F. Time relations among metabolic and morphologic 24-hour changes in mouse liver. *Amer. J. Phyisol.* 195: 301–310, 1958.

[48] Vasama, R. and Vasama, R. On the diurnal cycle of mitotic activity in the corneal epithelium of mice. *Acta anat. (Basel)* 33: 230–237, 1958.

[49] Halberg, F., Visscher, M. B. and Bittner, J. J. Relation of visual factors to eosinophil rhythm in mice. *Amer. J. Physiol.* 179: 229–235, 1954.

[50] Blumenfeld, C. M. Periodic and rhythmic mitotic activity in the kidney of the albino rat. *Anat. Rec.* 72: 435–443, 1938.

[51] Halberg, F., Peterson, R. E., and Silber, R. H. Phase relations of 24-hour periodicities in blood corticosterone, mitoses in cortical adrenal parenchyma and total body activity. *Endocrinology* 64: 222–230, 1959.

[52] Echave Llanos, J. M. and Piezzi, R. S. Twenty four rhythm in the mitotic activity of normal mammary epithelium on normal and inverted lighting regimens. *J. Physiol. (Lond.)* 165: 437–442, 1963.

[53] Jaffe, J. J. Diurnal mitotic periodicity in regenerating rat liver. *Anat. Rec.* 120: 935–954, 1954.

[54] Fasciolo, S. *Juan Carlos Fasciolo: del hombre al científico*, Editorial de la Universidad Nacional de Cuyo, Mendoza. 2010, 300.

[55] Paladini, A. C. *Leloir: Una mente brillante*, EUDEBA, Buenos Aires. 2010, 256. *Medicina (Buenos Aires)* 70: 396–397, 2010.

[56] Braun, M. E. and Page I. H. Suggested revision of nomenclature — Angiotensin. *Science* 127: 242, 1957.

[57] Braun, M. E., Fasciolo, J. C., Leloir, L. F., Muñoz, J. M. and Taquini, A. C. *Hipertensión arterial nefrógena*, El Ateneo, Buenos Aires. 1943. Traducción al inglés: Renal hypertension. Springfield, III : C.C.Thomas, 1946.

[58] Russo, J. *The Tools of Science: The handbook for the apprentice of biomedical reserach*, World Scientific, Singapore. 2011.

Suggested reading

Edgar, R. S., Green, E. W., Zhao, Y., van Ooijen, G., Olmedo, M., Qin, X., Xu, Y., Pan, M., Valekunja, U. K. Peroxiredoxins are conserved markers of circadian rhythms. *Nature* 485: 459–464, 2012.

Russo, J. *The Training of Cancer Researchers*, World Scientific, Singapore. 2017.

Chapter 4

Irma, the Turning Point

4.1. The portrait

As I write my memoirs in January of 2017, I am looking at a photographic portrait of my wife, Irma (Figure 4.1). She was a beautiful woman with a cryptic smile, and the portrait was intended to capture her strength. Irma was then in her early forties with the assured poise of a woman who has everything. She had passed two medical boards, both surgical and clinical pathology; she was the Principal Investigator (PI) of a research project grant (RO1) from the National Cancer Institute and a Co-PI of another grant that I was holding as a PI; she had given birth to a beautiful girl, Patricia; and she had a loving husband by her side.

Irma and I were working together at the Michigan Cancer Foundation in Detroit, Michigan, but she was also directing two private clinical laboratories, which made her an equal contributor to our annual income. We lived in a beautiful Tudor house on Three Mile Drive in Grosse Pointe Park (Figure 4.2). It was her dream place — she had spotted it even before it was on the market. The photograph shows her as a powerful, beautiful, intelligent woman possessing so much energy and sexual drive that any man would admire and feel proud to be with her. She made me feel complete. All of that was expressed in that portrait.

4.2. How I met Irma

It was 1961, and I was in my second year of medical school when I saw her for the first time. She was entering the main hall of the Central Hospital of the medical school and I was coming out when

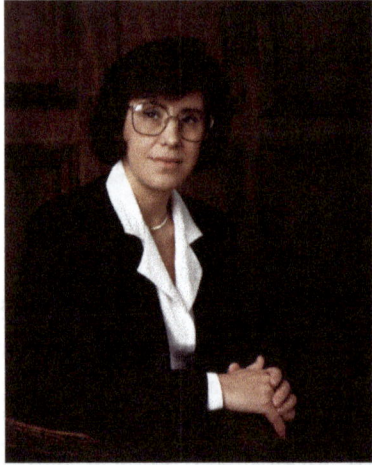

Figure 4.1: Irma in 1985. This photograph was taken by Carl Carmichael in our home in Grosse Pointe Park. Irma is wearing the Donna Karan suit that was her favorite.

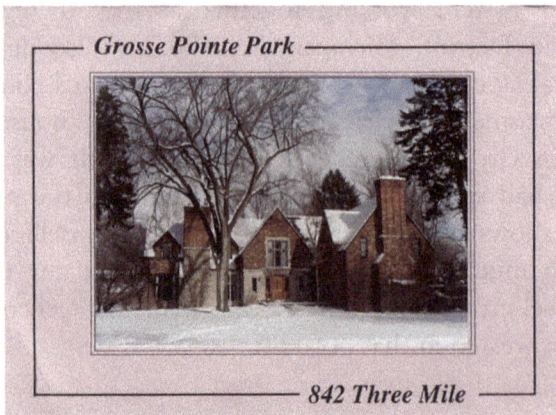

Figure 4.2: Tudor house at the Three Mile drive in Grosse Pointe Park, Michigan.

I saw her. Our eyes met, and she smiled and I smiled, and her image was burned in my retinas forever. She was wearing a short, dark green corduroy coat over a white turtleneck sweater and held a white coat and a book to her chest. She was a first year medical student then, volunteering with Sister Anna to administer medications and shots to the patients of the Central Hospital in her free time. She had the fresh look of a 19-year-old woman, accentuated by a symmetrical face with a small and perfect nose and brown eyes. She had short, dark hair styled in the Grace Kelly fashion of those days. She was the right height and had a beautiful body. But it was her face, her look, her smile, and her sensual lips that were engraved in my memory that day. I did not see her again until 2 years later when I was an Instructor in pathology, and she was one of my students. But still, I did not really talk with her until I met her again on April 26, 1965, the day I started working in the Institute for Histology and Human Development. Ms. Irma Haydee Alvarez, as everybody called her, was in charge of teaching human development, or embryology, to the second year medical students.

At that time, I was an instructor of pathology under Professor Julian Echave Llanos, but I was planning to leave the Department of Experimental Pathology because if I stayed there I would be unable to obtain my postdoctoral fellowship with the CONICET, or National Council for Scientific Research and Technology, an organization founded by Bernardo Houssay, Argentinean and 1947 recipient of the Nobel Prize in Physiology or Medicine. Having this plan in mind, I discussed my options with Professor Mario H. Burgos. He was the Chairman of the department, although he preferred to be called the Director of the Institute of Histology and Embryology. I wanted to be a part of his group to help my application to the CONICET. Professor Burgos was extremely positive and supportive of that move, but he did not have an open position for me at that moment. So I continued to hold the position of Instructor in pathology and at the same time worked *ad honorem* in his department while I waited for something to open up.

In addition to my employment situation, I had a significant academic *tour de force* in front of me. I was finishing the regular classes of the medical school and would soon take exams in six major disciplines, among them two clinics, medical and surgical plus pediatric. Passing those tests would qualify me to start a one-year internship in medicine, surgery, obstetrics and gynecology, and pediatric medicine. In addition to this curriculum, my work in histology and embryology was fundamental in keeping me up to date in the new techniques of cell biology and learning electron microscopy, which was one of the strongest points of the institute. This skill would allow me to be more competitive in my application to the CONICET. To achieve this plan, I must finish all my exams before March 1966 and start my internship that same month. Then I would be able to finish my one-year internship in time to begin the fellowship in the CONICET the following March, otherwise I would need to wait for another year. In addition to that, my plan also included finishing my doctoral work and defending my thesis in 1968. In the middle of this frantic and detailed academic plan, Ms. Irma Haydee Alvarez again appeared in my life.

Working at the institute, the path of Ms. Irma H. Alvarez crossed with mine every day because we were sharing the same laboratory space. In those days, the institute was lodged in a three-story building that used to be one of the most distinguished private residences in Mendoza, near the Boulogne Sur Mer and Emilio Civit Avenues, where the affluent society once lived. Now, most of the affluent people have moved to the suburbs of Mendoza, and the luster of the place is lost, replaced by businesses. But in those days, it was a beautiful place near the majestic doors of the San Martin Park. The permanent building of the medical school was still under construction in the place called the University Center, near the northwest border of the San Martin Park, and later on the institute moved there.

Ms. Alvarez had been working in the institute for the last 4 years, and she was pivotal in teaching developmental biology or medical embryology because not many members of the institute considered this topic fashionable — or so they said, in reality, it was too complicated for most of them. As a consequence, Irma was well respected and they left her alone. Ironically, developmental biology was the most expanding field in biology during the period of 1970–1990. Ms. Alvarez also had a supportive group of female friends who would have done anything for her; she was loved by all of them.

Ms. Alvarez was not from Mendoza; she was born and raised in San Rafael, a city located 230 km south of Mendoza. San Rafael is a beautiful town with sycamore-lined streets, which contribute to the clean and fresh air that is easy to breathe. The southern city has a wonderful dark blue sky, the stars seem to be almost within reach; and interestingly, San Rafael was a hub for many European immigrants other than Spanish and Italian. The town is surrounded by large vineyards where famous wines, including Malbec, were and still are produced. She came to Mendoza to study medicine and was living in a rented apartment in the city, which she shared with Ms. Lula Rodriguez, the sister of Dr. Esteban Rodriguez, who was a young researcher at the institute. She was also a good friend of Susana Bringa, another medical student who worked with her in embryology. The secretary, Ms. Esther Sosa, and the chief histo-technologist, Ms. Matilde Massot, were ardent guardians of Ms. Alvarez. They guarded her from her numerous suitors — medical students and teaching assistants and even a couple of mothers of already established doctors who saw in Ms. Alvarez a desirable candidate for marriage to their sons. Her friends felt that she was such a good catch and that they must filter the right man for her. Certainly, she did not need their protection, but the women had already decided that they must be her chaperones and protectors.

The environment of the institute was completely different from the Department of Experimental Pathology. The latter was silent and metrically designed by Julian Echave Llanos, who kept the department running like a ship. The institute's location on the sixth floor of the Central Hospital gave it the sober and sterile atmosphere of a healthcare facility. But the institute that Mario H. Burgos was directing was a different place altogether. The medical school and the institute also had very different visions on how to do science. Echave Llanos, as we called him, was more from the European school of science, whereas Burgos had trained with Houssay and also at Harvard with Dawn Fawcett and had the typical American approach to science and to the world. Burgos had a large group, and each of the researchers pursued his/her own theme of research, providing a great variety of topics and interests. It was a friendly and highly motivating environment formed by already established researchers and others who were coming from abroad to start their independent careers in the CONICET. There were many fellows who were ready to start their training at the institute or preparing to go abroad. This meant that the institute was full of young budding researchers, and I felt that this was the right environment for me. I was anxious to absorb this new environment, which made me even more conscious of time. The location of the institute near San Martin Park also contributed to this awareness and invited leisurely walks during the siesta break time and early in the morning, the sun giving the sensation of freedom and openness.

San Martin Park is an iconic place, and as Geronimo Sosa described [1], it represents the spirit of those born in Mendoza, or Mendocinos, who were able to transform the desert into green pastures, an oasis in the arid pre-Andean Mountains. The meaning of this can only be appreciated by those who live or that have lived there; they truly understand how difficult it was to make something grow in the arid soil of the area. Originally called the Park of the West, it was the inspiration of Dr. Emilio Civit, the Minister of Hacienda in 1897. The park was designed by Carlos Thays, a French-born naturalized Argentinean. The idea of the park was considered by many as an impossible one to realize. But it was nonetheless built on 1260 acres of desert with an annual precipitation rate of 220 mm a year. It is now an oasis, something that only those from that particular generation, the builders of Argentina, were able to conceive and create. It was with this unfettered frame of mind that Carlos Thays designed the park that contained a rose garden, fountains like the one representing all the continents, and many statues, including the *Horse of Marly*, the *Purity*, *Diane and Endymion*, the *Greeting of the Sun*, and the Spanish *Prado*, to mention a few iconic pieces. There is also an artificial lake large enough for regatta competitions. The park contained 40,000 trees that were brought from over the world. Poplars from Italy, paraisos from India, casuarinas, aromos, and grevilleas of Australia, eucalyptus of Tasmania, palms of Chile and the Canary Islands, the oaks of France, magnolias and elms from the United States. A special system of irrigation was constructed to keep all of this alive.

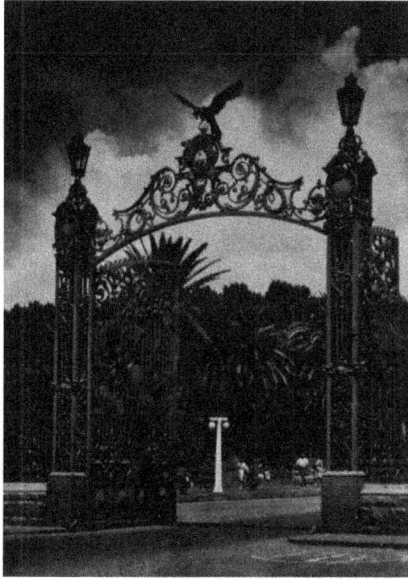

Figure 4.3: Central gate to San Martin Park.

The entrance to the park (Figure 4.3) is a large, ornate gate that opens to the *Horses of Marly* and a large avenue that disappears into the pre-Andean mountains. These gates are the park's trademark. They were built in England by order of the Sultan Abdul-Hamid II, or the Red Sultan, but because he was deposed by the Turkish people before they were completed, the sale was never effected. Thus, in 1909, Dr. Emilio Civit negotiated their purchase for Mendoza's new park with a few modifications. The imperial crown and the crescent moon of Islam were replaced by the condor and Mendoza shield.

My home was to the east of San Martin Park, and the institute on the other side of town, about 3 km away. The parish was called San Jose, and it was part of the Guaymallen district. The name came from an Indian chief who belonged to the Huarpe tribe, the primitive inhabitants of the area. The entrance to Guaymallen was San Jose Parish and a small square holding three large stone statues, each 12 feet tall and serving as the guardians of the few remnants of the Huarpes. I calculated that if I walked from the institute to my home for dinner, I would be able to reach my parents' house almost 30 minutes earlier than if I used the public transportation. Walking on the streets of Mendoza was a great way to reach places because almost everything was within walking distance. Walking was pleasant even in winter and also a good mental and physical exercise.

Ms. Alvarez must also have done the same calculation and reached the same conclusion, although in her case the destination was the university diner. This coincidentally shared logistic proved fortuitous one evening when both of us came out of the institute at the same moment, and we started walking the same path, going east on Emilio Civit Avenue until we reached the Plaza Independence on Chile Street, and from there we took Rivadavia Street, where the university diner was located near San Martin Avenue, Mendoza's main street. It was almost three quarters of the way to my home. In my first walk with her, we started talking, but the time and the distance was too short for us to finish discussing the many topics in which we shared an interest.

During those daily walks, I learned several things about Ms. Alvarez, one of them was that she had been born in San Rafael on February 28, 1942, and was 24 days older than me. She had two sisters, the older one, Martha, and the youngest, Estela, both of whom were studying in Provo, Utah. Her mother, Carmen Maria, was a widower. Irma's father had died when she was 16 years old, and her mother raised three daughters with the support of an extended family, all of them first generation Argentineans of Spanish ancestry. When Irma was 18 years old, she was preparing for her marriage to Rodolfo (Fito) Bianchi, an engineer and the older son of a family that owned many vineyards and wineries. Irma had received a teacher's diploma after graduating from the Normal School in San Rafael and was teaching her first assignment at an elementary school. Apparently Irma and Fito were interested in tinkering with ideas and higher pursuits at the intellectual level. They designed a special system to protect the vine arbors from the icy weather of Mendoza's winter, which can be devastating for those who earn their living from the revenues of the spring harvest. In the middle of these endeavors and preparing for their wedding, they also took a vocational test. The test determined that both of them had an aptitude for the biological sciences. Irma took that so seriously that she ended her engagement to Fito and instead took the examination tests to enter the medical school in Mendoza. The medical school examinations were extremely difficult and constructed to select only 80 of the 700 applicants to the University National of Cuyo Medical School, located in Mendoza. She passed all the tests and started studying medicine in 1961.

I also learned from Irma that wittiness and free thinking were trademarks of her family. One her mother's side, everyone except her Catholic aunt Elena declared themselves atheist. Irma and her sisters were religious by nature, however, and had been searching for a religion from a young age. The three of them found a way to canalize their religious natures in the missionaries of the Church of Jesus Christ of the Latter-day Saints, or Mormons, in San Rafael. Martha embraced that religion as did Estela, although she had a more torturous path. She even married one of the elders in the big Church of Salt Lake City but after several years she ended her marriage and returned to Catholicism. Irma had several conflicts due to the rational basis of that Church, and because she had been baptized as Catholic by one of her aunts from her father's side, she started exploring Catholicism. She was in that search when our walks began.

For me, being a Catholic was extremely important and many of my friends, but not all of them, belonged to the Catholic Movement, also called Catholic Action, and I was a serious practitioner of my faith. My beliefs had been energized in my college years, spurring a serious commitment to Catholicism during my medical school years, including the Ignatius spiritual exercises [2] and retreats under Father Lloret from the Jesuit order. My Catholic upbringing was a part of my being. It was in this circle that I had met many young women, some of them quite attractive and intelligent. I had developed feelings for some of them, but interestingly in every case, I felt the initial joy and pain of love then after a few months, the feeling dissolved into either a good, lasting friendship or simply got lost in the current of time. Probably that happened at that moment because my priority was to be a medical researcher, and everything else, including romantic relationships, was secondary.

When Irma H. Alvarez entered my circle, she awakened in me memories of our first encounter in the hall of the medical school, but I felt, knowing my priorities and romantic history, Ms. Irma H. Alvarez was a candidate to become a good friend, a laboratory partner, and a smart woman with whom I could discuss any topic without embarrassment — at least that is what I thought would happen.

Irma liked philosophy, and I was mesmerized listening her talk about philosophical ideas. She was so logical and witty. She liked Latin and knew volumes about the Gallic War, as it had been her hobby to read about it when she was in college. She remembered all the declinations of the main verbs, and she was very precise, speaking about mitochondrion or mitochondria, never mistaking singular for plural. Before deciding on medical school, she'd wanted to be a missionary in Africa, fighting diseases and helping people improve their living conditions. I told her that those ideas were foreign to me; although I wanted to help people, I was convinced that my way was by doing medical research. She was so transparent and full of care for others. Her passion for tinkering with ideas and concepts was equal to her love of the opera. I confessed to her that I was a dilettante and ignorant in musical knowledge. I was her public, and she used to sing me almost complete partitures of opera in Italian or French. I was impressed by her prodigious mind and talents. I never believed that she was doing this because she wanted to impress me, rather she was only showing what she was, and I started enjoying her company and secretly began to look forward to seeing her each evening when we made our walk together.

Irma and I were so different: she was musical and I was not; she had a caring and loving nature, while I was aggressive and full of energy to struggle against the world, where I felt like Don Quixote, ready to conquer the world; she was calm and patient, whereas I was impatient; she was tolerant of the weaknesses of others, and I was not. Interestingly, those differences probably made us look for more inside the other and were an attracting force between us. We agreed on one important point, to be intransigent in questions of fidelity and love.

At the institute, each member had an assignment, or a theme, for their work, but because I was still in pathology and I was working in liver regeneration, Burgos did not give me an assignment. Irma was in developmental biology, and Burgos assigned her to work on the metrial gland, an organ that Burgos had worked on with George Wislocki when he was at Harvard [3]. In many rodents, the metrial gland is formed during pregnancy with the appearance of large granular cells in the mesometrium at each implantation site. In rats, during the week following implantation, the size of these glandular structures increases rapidly and becomes very prominent during the second week of gestation. The metrial gland acquires the shape of a triangle that makes it easy to dissect from the rest of the placenta. The function of this gland was unknown except that it related to pregnancy because it disappeared after pregnancy, therefore the main question of the research was to find the gland's physiological role. Based on the fact that the gland increased its number of cells during pregnancy, Irma postulated that the gland could secrete oxytocin. To test this hypothesis, she developed a system to keep the uterus of the female rat out of the body in a thermostatic bath with an adequate culture media and connected to an electrode that measured the electrical potential and also the contraction of the uterus. Using this method, she was able to show that the extract of the metrial gland secreted an oxytocin-like substance that helped the uterus to contract and facilitated the delivery of the pups. She postulated that the metrial gland functioned as a relay, allowing each part of the uterus to contract not simultaneously but locally, facilitating the delivery of the pups in a certain order. If the contraction of the uterus was not coordinated for each pup (in general, rats have about ten pups per litter), the process of parturition could be jeopardized; instead the local control allowed each pup to be delivered in a sequential order, according to the position in the uterus. Although Burgos was not happy when people mixed with each other in their assignments, I provided Irma some help with this study, but it was clear to him and to everybody that she was the main driver of all the studies. The experiments needed to be carefully planned, and they were very time-consuming because they required that one group of animals be made pregnant in order to get enough metrial glands, and meanwhile someone must prepare the saline extract to be used, and also the study required another group of female rats to be one handed, these primed with estrogen so that their uteruses would be receptive to the oxytocin effect of the extract. The experiments required significant amounts of samples and confirmations to generate strong statistical significance. I started working with her on this project in May of 1965, and we published our first paper together in 1966 [4].

In August of 1965, I was doing pediatric medicine when I contracted hepatitis B from one of the kids in the ward and was ordered to be in bed for four weeks. Those weeks were an eternity for me because I could not study, go to class, or to the institute. I was very sick. During those weeks, Irma came to visit me several times at home. She captured the heart of my mother, Teresa, and my grandmother Dominga, who was living with us then. I knew what their female intuition drove them to think, but I was quite clear with them that Ms. Irma H. Alvarez was a friend and a colleague who worked with me at the institute.

After my recovery, I was back to my usual routine, and my daily walks with Irma were once again an enjoyable experience. However, my mind was fixed on the objectives ahead of me. I finished the medical courses on Saturday, October 30, 1965. I had been keeping a journal of my life since I was 16 years old, and I wrote in my journal that day: *I feel like I am in an alien land that never has been explored before, in which there is no path, no road in front of me that needs to be crossed — only a deserted plain.* I interpreted the crossing as six examinations, the internship, the postdoctoral fellowship, and the doctoral thesis. Like all dreams, this one is open to interpretation, and apparently I saw what was obvious for me, but I had yet to realize that another path was to choose having Irma in my life.

One of the main contributions of the Catholic Movement to my formation as a person was teaching me discipline. In college, I trained myself to endure 14–16 hours a day of study. My method was to study for 50 minutes and have a nap of 10 minutes, which significantly helped me to retain all the information that I needed to assimilate. I used to study standing up and in a loud voice to avoid falling asleep, mainly for that first hour of the morning. I would wake up at 5 a.m. and study until 6.30 a.m., then go to Mass at the chapel of the

Dominican sisters, and then breakfast, and then more studying until 11 p.m. Later I learned that both Leonardo da Vinci and Thomas Edison used this same method of taking periodical naps while working to increase their intellectual output. Thomas Edison kept a bed in the laboratory to facilitate this, and it was part of the memorabilia on display at his house in Orlando, Florida. Now there are scientific data showing that the initial steps of knowledge acquisition may be completed first during the waking hours, but the post-acquisition process takes longer, extending into sleep [5,6]. I can certainly say the system worked quite well for me.

My reading on the Cistercian monks and their disciplines in the daily hours were later on reinforced by Jesuit retreats [2] and have provided me some kind of mystic contemplative experience in my medical studies. This enjoyment of the solitude and contemplation while absorbing new knowledge made me very hesitant to spend my time with others. It was the total awareness that time was the only possession that I had and that I was the only one who could open or close that treasure chest, which was a part of my worldly existence. *Now I realize that love is time.* When you give your time to others that is the true manifestation of love. It is not the gift of material goods that count; it is only time, and the time that we have as human beings during our stay in this world is the only thing that belongs to us. I remember that Irma used to come to visit me and ask questions regarding the analysis of statistic data from her work on the metrial glands, and she would laugh when my eyes turned to find a watch to check how much time I was wasting on things that were not related to my study. Irma had a better sense of Christian life than I, because *she knew that real love was time.*

In March 5, 1966, I finally succeeded, and I started my medical internship. The same day I resigned my position of Research Teaching Assistant in pathology and gave the keys of my laboratory to Professor Echave Llanos. I had also obtained a paid position as an instructor in histology and medical embryology at the institute. This was the last time that I saw Echave Llanos. I remember that he was sad that I was leaving the Department of Experimental Pathology, but probably because he also knew that his mission in the medical school at the

University National of Cuyo was coming to an end. He'd had a big fight with the conservative management of the university, which clashed with his liberal and leftish position, and he was losing the battle, but he was a good scientist. He left Mendoza 2 years later and took a position as Chairman in the Department of Histology at the University of La Plata in Buenos Aires. Only one of his six disciples moved with him. Ernesto Bade had already returned to his country of birth and obtained a position in Heidelberg; Carlos Vilchez and Irma Safe went into the practice of medicine; Ramon Piezzi and I moved to the institute; and Alfredo Badran, the last to be incorporated in the initial team of six, moved with Echave Llanos to La Plata.

The deserted plain that I saw in front of me when I finished my medical courses started to show a more defined path, and on March 5, 1966, I saw very clearly that it was not a turning back for me. Instead my path to become a physician researcher was taking a new turn with a big difference that I had never expected to happen — I would not be walking alone.

4.3. Our first date

During the early morning of Saturday, April 2, Bernardo Hochman, a good friend from college and also from the university, went to visit a laboratory in the Department of Agrarian Sciences directed by Dr. Palleroni, a scientist who was working in auxins and gibberellins, hormones that control the growth of plants. Bernardo was a good friend and I was also very close to his Jewish–Polish family. They were immigrants, and they were good and tenderhearted people. I had joined their lunches and dinners many a times when I visited his home. There my palate got used to Polish sauces and other Jewish European dishes. Bernardo was a tinkerer, and he became fascinated with new ideas all the time. That was why he was so determined to go to Palleroni's laboratory that day. I already had met Palleroni before, in a regular meeting of the Biology Society of Cuyo, which gathered all the scientists in the region. He was probably one of the most serious of that group, and the hormone-like behavior of the auxins and gibberellins, which behaved as morphogen-like characteristics, was also something that interested me. We met again and we had a very productive intellectual morning.

On our way back, Bernardo asked me if I would like to join him for a party that night, explaining there would also be other guests that I had met a few weeks earlier. He remarked that I could find the same girl that I had danced with before. I told him that I would not be able to accept his invitation because that night I had a date with Ms. Irma H. Alvarez. He was excited about this and wanted to know how I got a date with her, as he felt that she was out of his league. I explained, without telling him too much, that I had met her in the institute and that we had been talking and walking a lot. I was grateful that we reached the center of the city at that moment, and from there we took different paths to our homes. Bernardo was very expansive and had a good heart, and I miss him. He tested my Christianity all the time, and his many theological questions helped me reinforce my knowledge and manage the Marxist dialectic. On the other hand, he was very impulsive, and I remember one day in 1957, when we were in college, he came to my home extremely excited because he had joined the Communist Party. His reason was that if the Soviet Union had been able to launch the first artificial Earth satellite, called Sputnik 1, then they would next conquer Western civilization. Therefore, he had decided to reinforce his leftist ideas by joining the party. Many years later when I was already in the United States, I received the news from my father that Bernardo had moved to Israel to be part of the Yom Kippur War, which began in October 1973. After that, I never heard any more about him. But back on that Saturday in April 1966, Bernardo was the first to know of my date with Irma.

I had been working, talking, and walking with Irma for almost a year before I invited her to have our first date. We decided on dinner and dancing. I picked her up at 9 p.m., the customary time for dinner in Mendoza. She was wearing a tweed, dark gray dress that contoured her body, insinuating her stunning form but not in excess. She had a touch of blush on her cheeks and her eyes were accentuated with slightly blue shadow. To my eyes, she was smashing that night.

Irma had not taken my invitation to dinner and dancing literally and was surprised when we entered the five-star restaurant of the Plaza Hotel, on the corner of Chile and Avenida Sarmiento, in front of the Plaza Independence and to the left of the Independence theatre. The Plaza Hotel is now the Park Hyatt Mendoza Hotel Casino and Spa but it still maintains the nineteenth century Spanish colonial facade. The restaurant used to have a dance floor and live music during the weekends. It was a very high-class place. I do not really remember what we had for dinner that night because in my journal I wrote only that: *I started dancing with her when the orchestra played a song that Irma told me was her favorite.* The song was "Smoke Gets in Your Eyes" by the Platters, a popular group in the 1960s. The lyrics were beautiful and very appropriate:

> *They asked me how I knew*
> *My true love was true*
> *I of course replied*
> *Something here inside cannot be denied*
> *They said someday you'll find all who love are blind*
> *When your heart is on fire*
> *You must realize, smoke gets in your eyes...*

That song has been the hallmark of our life, and every time that we heard it, we danced. Even one time when we were cooking together and Irma recognized that Henry Mancini and his orchestra were playing it on the radio, we stopped what we were doing and danced. Another time we heard it in the elevator of a Brussels hotel, and lucky us, we were alone.

Holding Irma in my arms and dancing with her on that first date was the most wonderful experience of my life. For the first time, I felt that I was meeting a warm and free woman, no guile, no hiding or playing games; this was something different than what I had felt before. I remember that I kissed Irma and I told her that I loved her, and she responded that she loved me too. I asked her if she remembered the first time that we crossed each other in the hall of the Central Hospital, and she said that she never forgot it.

I understood that night that all of my previous feelings of love were nothing compared to what Irma had awakened in me during all those months of working together and sharing our thoughts and dreams, and I was so grateful that she felt the same way. We danced until the orchestra left, and then we walked home, holding hands and treasuring that moment. I left Irma in her apartment and went to my parents' house still intoxicated by the warmest feeling I had ever experienced in my life. We were 24 years old.

I am an old man now and living alone as I write the memoirs of my life, but that moment of my first date with Irma is still as fresh as it was 52 years ago. I also feel that all the other young women before Irma gave me a small flavor of what love really is. I remember the women who came before her, and I thank all of them because through them I understood the feminine dimension of life and how important the impact of each of those brief encounters was; everything together makes the whole of us. Lord Tennyson was right when in his poem *Ulysses* he wrote:

> *I am a part of all that I have met;*
> *Yet all experience is an arch wherethro'*
> *Gleams that untravell' d world...*

That is the value of human relationships and the sanctity of life, because we will never know when we might impact — or be impacted by — someone merely by the fact that we were a part of their life, even for a brief period of time.

4.4. Romance

The day after our date was a Sunday, and we met at the Church of the Jesuits. This was a common place for the Catholics in the university to gather in those days. That night I missed dinner with my parents so that Irma and I could keep talking about our feelings; we decided to keep them a secret, to treasure for a while the marvelous sentiments we shared. We agreed that we would act as usual and continue to behave as good friends and coworkers.

Walking was the most natural thing for us to do, and even now every plaza in Mendoza is a reminder of those days. The Plaza Spain with its beautiful tiles depicting the story of the foundation and colonization of Mendoza; the Plaza San Martin, sober but full of pride and heroism; Plaza Independence with its multiple paths and fountains. In those days, every corner of our city looked precious and beautiful. Even the dust that was and still is the big concern of every inhabitant of Mendoza did not bother us. But our secrecy lasted scarcely two months because Tito Freyre, a classmate of Irma, saw us holding hands when we were on our walks. When he broke the news of our romance, the general reaction was that he was probably imagining things, that I was likely helping Irma to cross some obstacle on the street; the idea we were a couple was impossible for them to accept, and Susana Bringa, one of the Irma's friends, even bet her entire month's salary to other members of the institute that it was not true. Her female friends felt that their intuition and perspicacity had failed when they realized that they had no idea how this had happened without them suspecting a thing, and worst of all, without Irma saying a word to her closest friends, not even confiding in her roommate, Lula Rodriguez, or the protective Esther de Sosa or Matilde Massot.

On the other hand, it was equally difficult to believe that Jose, the serious, the intellectual, the best medical student, and the super Catholic, would be involved in romance. Apparently, they felt I was too busy to be a courtier. Everybody liked to court Irma, she was a woman that many would like to date and marry, one of the most sought after of all the women in the medical school. But even worse than those conjectures was why Jose Russo was looking outside of all the Catholic girls in his circle when nobody was really certain that Irma was Catholic. That was the major puzzle.

When Irma was confronted by her friends at the institute, she confessed it was true that we were in love. With this confirmation given, the following day, Tito Freyre announced in the middle of a class that Irma was in love with Pepe Russo, as I was known in the medical school circle. The immediate ripple effect was that most of the young women of my Catholic circle did not greet Irma for a while, as she was seen as an intruder. But very soon everything returned to normality, and our romance was seen as a beautiful thing. Better still Irma and I were fully accepted into a new circle — one of couples in love or recently married.

4.5. Families and friends

The most important part was how to face our families and our friends and make the many decisions suddenly in front of us. I was part of the group called the Catholic Action, which had played an important role in Argentina as well as in many countries that had been affected by the anti-Catholic actions of the government, for example, Spain, Italy, France, and Belgium — and even Argentina in the time of Peronism [7]. Historically, one of the most violent episodes against the Catholic Action was done in Germany by Adolph Hitler, that famous night of the long knives [8]. But the Catholic Action is not a political entity; it is populated by laypeople interested in improving the society by making known the principles of Catholic faith in everyday life. The Catholic Action in Argentina was separated into groups by age and activities. I was a part of the university group of Catholics. That group integrated all the different disciplines that our university in Mendoza had in those days, including philosophy, economics, arts, social and political sciences, and medicine. It was a great way to meet and get to know people of different disciplines and interests, and of course a great opportunity to mingle and socialize. In Argentina, the Catholic Action is still an active institution [9].

Almost a week after Irma and I declared our sentiments, I had a meeting with a friend of mine, Father Jorge Munoz, who was the spiritual leader of our group at the university. I narrated to him how I met Irma and what had been the result of our date. He was so positive and happy to know of my awakening as I explained to him my concerns about Irma becoming a fully practicing Catholic. As a result, he wanted to meet her, and so Irma did. Father Munoz told me later that I should not worry about her Catholicism because Irma would surprise me. He was so right because she turned out to be a source of wonderful surprises and even an example for my own daily Christian and Catholic life.

After the secrecy of our romance was broken, I told my mother first and then the rest of my family. My mother and grandmother had already met Irma but my father and sister had not, and their first reaction was that I should invite her for dinner. As an Italian family, lunch and dinner were sacred in our home, especially dinner which was a way to solidify events in the family.

The first of Irma's family to know of our romance were Aunt Elena and her husband, Miguel, who encountered us one afternoon in a cafe called El Molino, a regular place for meeting friends and family located in the northern arm of San Martin Avenue.

In the Mendoza of my time, the afternoon was broken up by a tea with croissants or cake or biscuits at 5 p.m. This custom was taken from the English and the pastry from the French and was probably embraced as an additional way to enjoy the company of friends and family. There were four customary breaks in the Mendoza of those days. At 10 a.m. coffee with a biscuit, lunch at around 1 p.m., then the tea at 5 p.m. and dinner at 9 p.m. The normal working day started at 8 a.m. and lunch break in Mendoza lasted from 1 to 4 p.m., and then work in general ended at 8 p.m. with dinner at 9 p.m. Most of the movies and theaters opened at 10 p.m.

After our chance meeting with Elena and Miguel, who in those days lived in San Rafael, Irma was eager to share the news with her mother, Carmen, and her grandmother Marcelina, along with the rest of her family. So on May 24, I traveled to San Rafael and met all the Clan Martinez, as they used to call themselves. Martinez was the maiden name of Carmen, and they were old residents and colonizers of San Rafael; Irma's grandmother Marcelina and her grandfather Julian Martinez had arrived at the end of the nineteenth century, when there was still an indigenous population from the tribe of the Tehuelches scattered in the nascent town. Therefore, the Clan Martinez had a long tradition and knowledge of the town. That night Irma and I had dinner with Elena and Miguel, and it was a real pleasure to know them in their own environment. She was a Realtor and also had a book-binding shop while Miguel was a judge in the Labor Court of the town. They were recently married and had a wonderful relationship between them and with the rest of the family.

Although Miguel passed away few years ago, I am still in contact with Aunt Elena, who is 92.

Carmen, Irma's mother, as well as her aunts and their families were very kind and social and accepted me quite well, but her grandmother Marcelina made clear she'd been expecting a taller and more handsome man for her favorite granddaughter. Later on Irma told me that her grandmother liked tall and handsome men in general, as her husband had been that way. Marcelina loved Irma, and they were always very close; according to Irma, her grandmother had raised her and probably forged in her character the hard work and rigid morality of truthfulness held by the real Castellans who populated Argentina at the end of that century.

Although my first visit to San Rafael was brief, it was rich in beautiful moments, and in a certain way, it brought us one step further in our relationship. More important for me was to see Irma surrounded by her cousins, uncles, aunts, nephews, and nieces; it made me realize even more how sweet and tender a human being she was.

Irma easily integrated in my family circle, and everybody liked her because she was humble and effortlessly adapted to different people, situations, and environments. She conquered all. The same happened with my closest circle of friends, among them the recently married Marcelo and Estela Palero, and all the members of my Catholic group at the university. I had met Marcelo at one of the university camps that we used to have during the summer in Mendoza's mountains. He had recently qualified as a lawyer and hailed from Cordoba, a city east of Mendoza and half the distance to Buenos Aires. He was doing labor laws and had a great heart and dedication to the cause of the poor. Our friendship grew with the years and with Estela the couple became natural members of our circle.

In November of 1967, I met Estela, Irma's sister, who was returning from Utah. She was extremely extroverted and social with an artistic temperament diametrically opposed to Irma's more cerebral personality. Despite those differences, Estela has remained very close to us in the many happy and sad moments of our lives. Irma's older sister, Martha, was still in the USA then, and I met her later on.

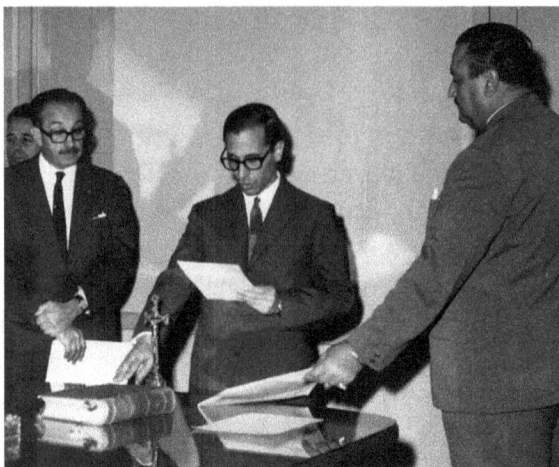

Figure 4.4:   Taking the Hippocratic Oath on March 11, 1967. The Dean of the medical school, Dr. Roger Zaldivar, is to my left.

In March of 1967, I took the Hippocratic Oath (Figure 4.4) and started my postdoctoral fellowship with the CONICET. Our life in those days centered on our work at the institute. Irma was still finishing her last year of medical school and preparing to take her final examinations.

Our friends and fellow members of the institute created a beautiful social circle, and we were very well integrated in it. Every weekend we had a dinner or a social gathering, and when not with those friends we were with my family, who were extremely jealous to share us with anybody else. I visited San Rafael several times and became friendly with Irma's cousins and extended family. Those were joyful days.

4.6. Social environment

An important figure in our circle was Father Jorge Munoz, and at many of our social gatherings his baritone voice sang "Granada," a Spanish song that was very common in those days. He was also the spiritual leader of the group, and I was very sad when he left Mendoza to accept a post in Recife, Brazil, searching for a deeper social engagement. Many years later, I learned that his move to Recife was not an assignment by Mendoza's bishop. Hélder Pessoa Câmara, a

Brazilian Roman Catholic archbishop in Recife, was an advocate of liberation theology, and when Jorge moved to Recife it was to be part of his movement. Câmara played a significant role in drafting the *Pastoral Constitution on the Church in the Modern World* [10] and challenged his brother bishops to live lives of evangelical poverty — without honorific titles, privileges, and worldly ostentation. He taught that "the collegiality of the bishops finds its supreme evangelical realization in jointly serving the two thirds of humanity who live in physical, cultural, and moral misery." However, the problem was not in that message. It was when the members and followers of the liberation theology started behaving as a political and social movement, putting forth the idea that Christ was not the Son of God and Our Savior but rather a political figure, a revolutionary, the subversive of Nazareth, and that is not the message of the Gospel or the Church.

The main topics of discussion in our university circle were social inequality and the poor. The discussion was led by those coming from the economy and philosophy sides of the spectrum as well as from the many students of law and social sciences. Remembering those days, I realized in retrospection that the departure of Jorge Munoz was the tip of the iceberg concerning the reality of what was taking place in the Church as well in the Argentinean society of those days. For us in the medical field, poverty and the misery of hospital life were a part of our training; it was not an intellectual exercise, it was real. When the poor came to our hospitals, we treated them to the best of our abilities, and we did not have time to think about the reasons for their poverty as we were focused on how to solve their medical problems. We as medical doctors were trained in reverse: taught to solve the problem of each human being one at a time, and probably we were not able to see the large societal problem as that was beyond our scope and training. I also was convinced that the big medical problems must be solved by the individual enterprise of medical researchers and that they needed to be very focused on solving one problem at a time. To my mind, there was no other way to see the problem, neither in those days nor now. This concept of the importance of the uniqueness of each person, their individual potential, importance, and sacred value was so rooted in us that any idea or social movement or force that could break the importance of the person as a whole was unacceptable. Probably our friends saw that and left Irma and I out of their inner turmoil.

We were aiming to finish medical school and then start our research enterprise, which probably shielded us from what was really happening. Was it an act of love on their part to keep us separate from the fomentation that some of them were part of? Did our ivory tower insulate us from the rest? I still do not have an answer, only conjecture. What I realized later on was that although other priests replaced Jorge Munoz, the Church was suffering a large and seismic movement produced by the liberation theology and many of the priests we knew left priesthood. Mendoza's seminary lost many seminarians and priests, and later on, the Pope decided to close that seminary and many others in Latin American to stop the spreading infiltration of the left and the famous liberal theology.

We saw priests who were our dear friends, like Munoz, Pujol, Brascelli, and Santoni, carried off by that current of social reforms and eventually leave the Church. It was a slow process but the shake-up started in those days of 1967–1969, and by the time it was finished, we were already in the United States. But in the beginning, Irma and I saw all these intellectual discussions as an interesting exercise, and it never crossed our minds that those ideas would be put in action and finally end in Argentina's dirty war. This initial social fomenting at the intellectual level was nurtured by different sources, not just communism but also the leftist movement that was permeating university life, mainly for those in the humanistic sciences. But then Peronism emerged again as the justicialist doctrine mixed with the ideas of the Cuban revolution, and these were all components of a mixture that moved both bad and good people to want to make social changes. Later on, I found out that our lawyer friend Marcelo Palero had been accused of communism and incarcerated by a military junta. He was so maltreated that he died of a stroke at the age of 40, leaving Estela with six children. Those tremendous forces were there in 1966, but we were not touched by them. Regardless, many people suffered and some died for changes in the Church and in the political movement of Argentina.

The "dirty war" was the name used by Argentina's military government for their fight against state terrorism. There are hundreds of articles that have been written on the subject, which historically took place from 1974 to 1983, but in 1967–1969, the period I am covering in this memoir, I realize now that the ferment was already there. I am not qualified to talk about this subject but in retrospect I feel that the eventual protagonists were around us and some were even our friends and acquaintances, but we did not recognize them nor did they share with us what they were really thinking. For reasons that I cannot explain, those events did not touch our life and we followed our own path.

4.7. Marriage

We were in the 26th month of our relationship when two independent events happened to shake our idyllic time. One was that I was late to pick Irma up for dinner because I was delayed by a female medical student who was very persistent about wanting my personal attention during that year. That particular day I arrived very late and Irma did not like it.

The second event took place at a party with some friends from our Catholic Movement. When the party was starting to lose steam, only about eight of us remained at the insistence of the hostess, a woman I knew from the medical school. A few years back, we'd been very connected and had spent many hours talking, mainly discussing medicine and social issues. But this mutual curiosity had dissolved after a few months, and we never had a formal date or even used any word indicating any special commitment. From my part, our connection was something that dissolved over the course of time. But apparently that was not the case for her, and that night she asked us to listen as she played a song by Luigi Tenco called "Ho Capito che Ti Amo."

The lyrics are like this:

Ho capito che ti amo
quando ho visto che bastava
un tuo ritardo
per sentir svanire in me
l'indifferenza

per temere che tu
non venissi piu...

Although the song was in Italian, Irma's fondness for opera surely allowed her to understand that the song was a clear declaration of love by somebody who was realizing what she had lost and finally understanding it was almost too late to recover it. That evening when Irma was walking to her apartment, I noticed that she was distant, but still I was not fully aware of what she was feeling. The following day, July 26, 1968, she told me that we must have a temporary separation because she was not sure if we should continue our engagement. She left later that day for San Rafael.

The whole world fell to my feet, and I could not understand her reaction. She would not answer my calls, and I felt miserable. I assumed that she'd probably had the same reaction when she'd broken her engagement with Fito Bianchi, but why? Maybe she wanted to pursue something different, like becoming a missionary? Or possibly dedicate herself to serving the needy without the attachment of a family? All those speculations crossed my mind as I pondered a million and one scenarios — none of which was the right one.

Irma came back from San Rafael on August 1, and I saw her in the institute. The re-encounter was tense because she extended her hand instead of offering her cheek for my kiss. We talked for hours and the Gordian knot of the problem emerged. We remembered this moment many times in our marriage, and later we laughed about it, but the message that day was very clear about what she wanted from me. She was categorically certain that she loved me without reservation but she would never share me with anybody else, and she wanted to be sure that she was the only person I loved. This could be interpreted as jealousy, but in Irma it was truthfulness and a commitment to her vision of the future; in short, she was not sure that I was fully ready for her. In that moment, I saw that it would be useless to explain to her that I did not have control over the female medical students' infatuation, and that I had never, in neither thought nor action, done anything to offend our love and commitment, and that the song played at that party was something mean-spirited that I had no control over. Instead of telling her all of that, in that moment I instead told her *that I loved her more than anybody else and that she was and will be the only woman of my life.* That day I told her that we must get married, and she agreed.

I presented my doctoral thesis dissertation in September of 1968, and I passed with honors. I was the 10th physician to complete the doctoral work in the whole history of the medical school, which started in 1950.

In January of 1969, I received the notification that my postdoctoral fellowship in the CONICET was renewed for two additional years, and our marriage was planned for the second month of that year. In January, Irma's older sister, Martha, arrived from Salt Lake City. The surprise was not meeting her but the knowledge that she came to stop our wedding because she felt that Irma was making a mistake by marrying me. Irma later explained to me that her sister's main objection was that I was Catholic and for a Mormon like her that was unacceptable. Martha did not prevail, and in time she accepted me as her brother-in-law.

There were two incidents that saddened those blissful days. One was that I saw my mother crying when I was empting my room at their home, where I had lived for so many years — during elementary school, college, and medical school. I only understood her sadness when my own daughter, Patricia, left home for college. The other sad situation was that my dear grandmother was hospitalized because she developed a strangulated hernia that resulted in removal of a part of her small intestine that was necrotized. She had a long surgery and recovery period. My grandmother Dominga had witnessed our romance since the beginning, and she loved Irma and that feeling was mutual. Before we went on our honeymoon, we visited her in the hospital.

Our marriage took place on February 9, 1969 (Figure 4.5). Our godmother and godfather in our marriage were Irma's mother, Carmen, and my father, Felipe, and Estela and Marcelo Palero. We married in the Church of our parish in San Jose where I grew up, and Father Santoni heard our vows. One of the beautiful meanings of having a Church ceremony is that the priest is the witness of our

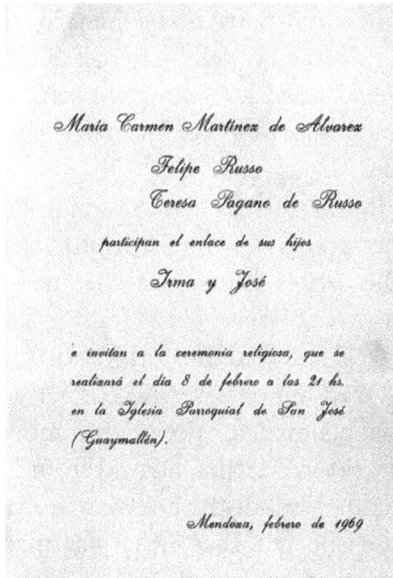

Figure 4.5: Our wedding invitation.

commitment to the Church and the community that surrounds us. At the end, Christian life is a personal and individual choice of love. The Dominican sister's choir sang the "Magnificat" when we left as a couple. It was a small ceremony full of meaning and attended by all the people who loved us. We had reached the marriage and saved our chastity for each other. The "Magnificat" was a song that the Dominican sisters choir sang every day at the 6.30 a.m. mass in the chapel that was two blocks from my home and which had been a part of my routine when I was a college and medical student.

After a 10-day honeymoon in the Ville of Carlos Paz in Cordoba, we moved to an apartment in Mendoza at 1973 Patricias Mendocinas, which we rented from the Salcedos, old friends of my mother's family. We stayed in that place until we came to the United States in 1971.

My father built all the furniture for our new home and some of it is still preserved in the house I lived in Rydal, Pennsylvania, almost 12,000 km from our native Mendoza, but still holding the beautiful memories of those days when I met and married Irma. She was the turning point of my life, and it was impossible to foresee 52 years ago how meeting her would be so important for our work together and my life as a cancer researcher.

References

[1] Sosa, G. *Parque General San Martin*. Edicion Oficial, Adhesion del Gobierno de Mendoza al Sesquicentenario de la Independencia Argentina, Mendoza. 1964.

[2] Martin, J. *The Jesuit Guide to (Almost) Everything*, Harper One, New York. 2010.

[3] Wislocki, G. B., Weiss, L. P., Burgos, M. H. and Ellis, R. A. The cytology, histochemistry and electron microscopy of the granular cells of the metrial gland of the gravid rat. *J. Anat.* 91: 130–140, 1957.

[4] Russo, J. and Alvarez, I. H. Accion ocitocica del homogeneizado de placenta sobre el utero aislado de rata. *Acta Physiol. Lat. Am.* 16: 1–6, 1966.

[5] Rasch, B. and Born, J. About sleep's role in memory. *Physiol. Rev.* 93: 681–786, 2012.

[6] Stickgold, R. Parsing the role of sleep in memory processing. *Curr. Opin. Neurobiol.* 23: 847–853, 2013.

[7] Karush, M. B. Chamosa, O, Editors.

[8] Truman, T. *Catholic Action and Politics*, The Merlin Press, London. 1960.

[9] http://www.accioncatolica.org.ar/

[10] O'Connell, G. "Call Him a Saint?" America. April 27 issue, 2015.

Chapter 5

My Postdoctoral Years in Argentina (1967–1971)

5.1. Postdoctoral fellowship in Argentina from April 1967 to April 1969

When I ended my medical studies, I had a clear idea what steps I needed to follow in my training as a physician scientist. This was possibly due to the existence of the National Scientific and Technical Research Council (CONICET), the main organization in charge of the promotion of science and technology in Argentina. The principal objective of this agency is to boost and implement scientific and technical activities in the country and in all different fields of knowledge. When I finished my medical studies and internship in March of 1967, I followed the structure available to me at that time. If you wanted to be a medical researcher, you must apply for 2 years of postdoctoral fellowship to the CONICET with an optional 2 additional years and after this 4-year training in Argentina, or you could opt for training outside of the country and upon your return you would be qualified to apply to enter the CONICET as a scientific researcher. Of course, not everybody followed that path, but those were the basic steps to pursue.

The CONICET was established in 1958 by a decree of the national government, and its first director was Bernardo A. Houssay, recipient of the Nobel Prize in medicine. In a certain way, it was the perseverance and vision of Dr. Houssay that made this institution a reality. Bernardo Alberto Houssay was born in 1887 and died in 1971. He was the prototype of a physician scientist, and in 1947, Dr. Houssay received the Nobel Prize for Physiology or Medicine for his discovery of the role played by pituitary hormones in regulating the amount of blood sugar (glucose) in animals. As early as 1919, he was appointed the chair of physiology at the University of Buenos Aires Medical School. He not only transformed this department into an outstanding one but made it a first class place in research internationally. Because he had ideas contrary to the political environment of the Argentina of those days, he was deprived of his university posts and forced to re-establish his research activities and staff at the privately funded Instituto de Biología y Medicina Experimental. When Peron was ousted from power in 1955, Dr. Houssay was reinstated at the University of Buenos Aires, where he remained until he died. In 1957, he used all his energy and influence to create the National Scientific and Technical Research Council [1]. In one way or another, every scientist in Argentina owes his training and status to Bernardo A. Houssay. It was only possible for me to follow a path of training and become a cancer researcher because of his efforts and his disciples'.

On April 1, 1967, I started my first year of postdoctoral research fellowship under Dr. Mario H. Burgos at the Institute of Histology and Embryology. I had already been there for 2 years (see Chapters 3 and 4), and it was clear that any study related to cancer was out of the question. As I have indicated in previous chapters, there were many researchers in that department and they were at different levels of training and stages in their careers. Therefore, I assessed my situation and realized that I needed to learn and define a specific area of research. My immediate concern was to choose a theme for my doctoral thesis, but first I needed to integrate myself into the Burgos projects. I was a part of his closest team of researchers working on the project of mitochondrial respiration of the Sertoli cells under the effect of FSH and LH that was supported by a grant of the USA Population Council. The aim was to explain how the interaction of FSH and/or LH with the oxidative pathway of the mitochondria could be involved in the release of the mature spermatozoids or spermiation from the Sertoli cells. The compilation of this research was published in 1972 as a book chapter [2] in which I was honored to be the third author of that publication. One member of the team was Alberto Vitale Calpe, 2 years my senior, who had developed such a great mastery in electron microscopy that he was really first class. Another member of the group was Dr. Fabio Sacerdote, with whom I learned my rudiments of tissue culture; he had been brought to Mendoza to develop this area of research, but he did not meet Burgos's expectations, and also I realized that it was difficult to compete in that field with the resources allocated to this section. Probably for these and other reasons Burgos moved Fabio Sacerdote to work in his group. An important plus of this team was the technical expertise of Daniel Bari, who was in the technical career track of the CONICET. Daniel Bari was a talented person who knew about instrumentation, techniques, and he was the key to learning the use of expensive equipment needed for cell biology, such as ultracentrifuges that allowed us to separate different organelles and cell fractionation, spectrophotometers, and other analytical equipment like polarimeters. Luis Gutierrez was also on this team, and he was the personal electron microscopist of Dr. Burgos and generously taught me the techniques of preparation for electron microcopy studies such as embedding, sectioning, and staining. However, the use of the electron microscope was heavily regulated by the Director of the section, a retired Army engineer. He had very good relations with Vitale Calpe, making it difficult for me as a newcomer to compete with his high level of proficiency. Therefore, I was in a place where electron microscopy was the main feature of the program but I could not touch the instrument as much as I wanted. Therefore, I decided to first work on my basic electron microscopy skills, like sectioning using the Porter Bloom ultra-microtome with glass knives. I mastered how to make them with a glass knife instead of using a diamond knife, which was not provided to me until later on. This technique was vital for doing good electron microscopy in those days; therefore, I worked on mastering them until my window of opportunity opened up, and I was able to use the electron microscope with more freedom. The use of the electron microscope also required a better access to film and the dark room and all the materials needed to make the final prints for studying as well as for publishing. This was basically monopolized on the Burgos Team by Vitale Calpe. The window opened for me when the institute moved to its new building in the medical school, and I volunteered to move first, together with the electron microcopy facility. In the new building, not only did I have my own laboratory but I could use the electron microscope as much as I wanted because there were not many users in the new facility. In fact, it took almost a year to complete the move, making this time a valuable breathing space for acquiring not only skill but also a great dexterity in the whole specialty of electron microscopy. Learning that was extremely important for my postdoctoral fellowship in the USA as well as for my first job as a cancer researcher in Michigan (Chapter 7). I must also acknowledge that the new director, Mr. Helmut Dobeslaw, a German engineer trained by Siemens, was extremely kind and spent time with me allowing me to earn his confidence in my use of this beautiful machine.

While all these changes were taking place, I got to know two excellent biochemists: one was Maria Teresa Inon, a young investigator starting her career in the CONICET who had obtained her degree from the University of La Plata in Buenos Aires, and the other was Dr. Francisco Bertini, a senior investigator in the CONICET who had completed his training at the University of Chicago and was working in lysosomes. Both of them were excellent colleagues and friends, and also good discussants and critical of new ideas. They and Dr. Burgos were the first to know the blueprint of what would become my doctoral thesis. The idea that I presented to Professor Burgos was to study the *localization, function, and regulation of the acid phosphatase in the testis*. Burgos supported the work and from those studies many publications besides my thesis dissertation originated [3–7].

5.2. My doctoral thesis

My thesis work was the foundation for my independent work because, while I was still being mentored by Burgos, the topics as well as the planning of the experiments were my endeavor and gave me the chance to expand my collaboration networks with different members of the institute. Using my training in experimental pathology, I oriented my studies toward something related to cancer, like control of development, differentiation, and mainly to increase my knowledge and skills in biochemistry and cell biology. An additional benefit of this work was also that it gave me my first taste of directing people working under me. I recruited three medical students who were interested in my work, and they became an extremely helpful team. I remember Mr. M. Marchevsky, Mr. C. Cuccia, and Mr. D. Lenouguer coming with me at five o'clock every morning to help with the tissue collection and biochemical testing. Also, there was no competition to use the instruments until almost 10 a.m., meaning that for five hours every weekday we would have the entire institute to ourselves. I started working on my thesis on October 7, 1967, and I made my dissertation on September 18, 1968. During this period of my career, I worked 12–14 hours a day. My dissertation was so scholarly done that I still tremble with the emotion of that day. My thesis tribunal was speechless that I was able to present so many data and give so much foundation for my reasoning that they unanimously gave me the highest grade and congratulations. *I was the 10th medical doctor to graduate in almost 20 years since the medical school had existed.*

I divided my thesis work into three parts: The first part was a description of the localization and distribution of the acid phosphatase in the testis of different species and its biochemical characterization followed by functional changes induced by age, circadian rhythm, and station variations. The second part of the work was the hormonal regulation of the acid phosphatase activity as well as other enzymes in the testis of the mouse. And the third part was the experimental manipulation of different physiological conditions for a better understanding of the role of the acid phosphatase as well as other enzymes in the testis.

5.2.1. *Localization, distribution, and biochemical properties of the acid phosphatase of the testis*

In this first part of the thesis, I described that the histochemical location of the acid phosphatase was in the Sertoli and Leydig cells in

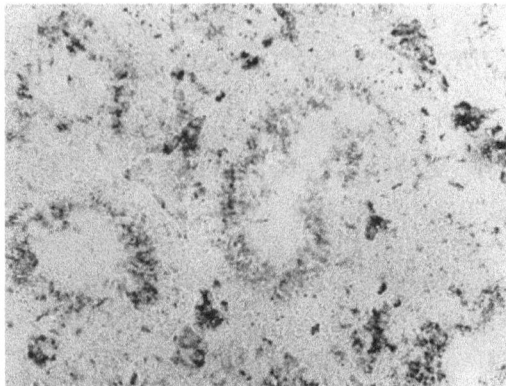

Figure 5.1: Cryostat section of the testis of *Mus musculus* presenting positive reaction in the apical portion of the seminiferous tubule and in the interstitial Leydig cells (100×).

seven species of vertebrates including the *Bufo arenarum Hensel, Lectodactylus chaquensis, Mus musculus, Rattus norvegicus, Misocricetua aureatus, Cavia porcellis, and Felix domesticus.* I am in debt to Mr. Luis Castro who was in charge of the animal facility and made it possible for me to obtain all these species for my work. Figure 5.1 shows the localization of the acid phosphatase in the adult testis of the mouse. The histological distribution of the acid phosphatase in all the species studied clearly indicated that this enzyme must play an important role in spermatogenesis as well as in the spermeation, or release of the sperm, from the Sertoli cells and as well must play a role in the steroid secretion in the Leydig cells.

The acid phosphatase biochemically shows that the optimum activity is at pH 5, and it is thermo-labile, destroyed at a temperature of 60°C. The enzyme is inhibited by formaldehyde and sodium fluoride. The enzymographic study shows that more than one isoenzyme exists for each of the studied species. The subcellular fractionation of testis homogenate showed that the enzyme is localized mostly in the supernatant (65–70%). The activity of the lysosomal fraction is only 20% latent, probably because of the fragility of the testicular lysosomes.

5.2.1.1. *Subcellular localization*

Cellular fractionation procedures have provided information on the localization of acid phosphatase in different fractions of liver, kidney, prostate, and other organs. The richest is the lysosomal fraction, and according to De Duve *et al.* [8], the acid phosphatase, like other hydrolytic enzymes, has an optimum activity at or near pH 5, and it was recovered in a "light mitochondrial" or lysosomal fraction. My work was the first to report the localization of the acid phosphatase in the testis. Using differential centrifugation [7], I obtained different fractions designated N (nuclear), M (mitochondrial), L (lysosomal), P (microsomal), and S (supernatant). Basically, what I found was that 65% of the acid phosphatase of the mouse testis is found in the 105,000 × g supernatant, whereas the lysosomal fraction contains 19%. The fact that the activity of the latter fraction was stimulated by activation indicates that the enzyme was present in the particulate form, meaning in the lysosomes [3].

5.2.1.2. *Role of age*

The localization of the acid phosphatase underwent modifications during the aging of the animal. In the newborn mouse, the enzyme was localized in the Sertoli cell, while at the 15th day of age it also appears in the Leydig cells, accompanied by a very significant increase of the total enzyme activity in the cell homogenate (Figure 5.2) [4].

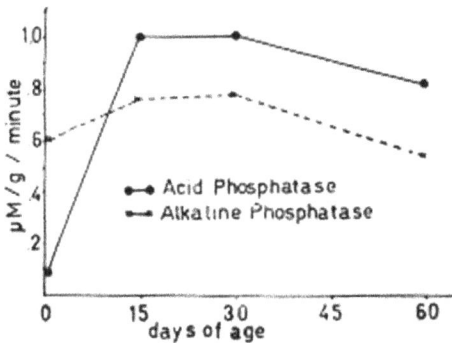

Figure 5.2: Acid and alkaline phosphatase activities expressed in μM/g/minute in testis homogenates at different periods of postnatal development.

5.2.1.3. *Circadian rhythm*

I found that in the mouse testis the expression of acid phosphatase shows a circadian rhythm (Figure 5.3).

Whereas no variation in the content of protein, water, or dry matter was observed during the 24-hour period, there was instead an increase in the activity of the enzyme at midday and a decrease at 8 p.m. followed by another increase at 4 a.m. [5]. The effect of light on the gonad had been reported as early as 1935 by Benoit [9] and demonstrated to be mediated by the hypothalamic–hypophyseal axis [10–12]. *The reporting of a circadian rhythm of the mouse testicular acid phosphatase was a novel observation indicating that the enzymatic activity could be exerted by the pituitary gland through the gonadotropins,* since the blood level of LH is at its highest [13] when the enzymatic activity of acid phosphatase is at its minimum. In later studies done in collaboration with Francisco Bertini and Ramon Piezzi [6], I provided further evidence in favor of a hypothalamic–hypophyseal mechanism

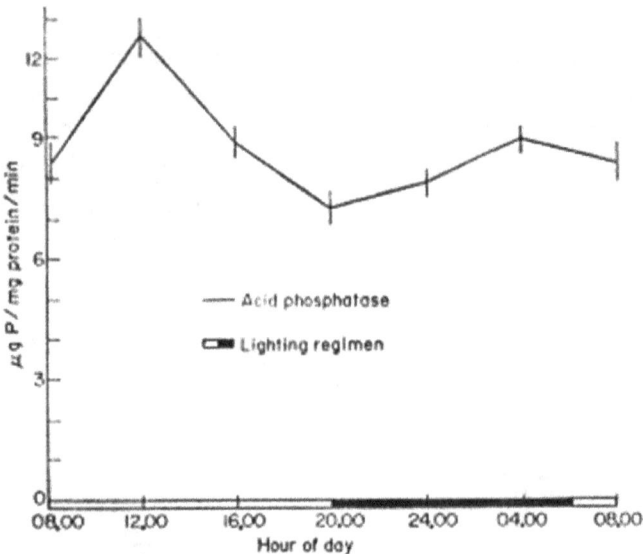

Figure 5.3:   The variations of acid phosphatase activity during a 24-hour period present a circadian rhythm related to the lighting regimen in the animals' habitat.

by the finding that hypophysectomy produces an increase of acid phosphatase in the summer testis of *L. chaquensis*. These events indicated that the acid phosphatase of the testis depends on hormonal variations, mainly LH [14].

5.2.2. *The effect of gonadotropin hormones*

In this part of my studies, I incorporated not only the acid phosphatase but also the Na^+K^+-ATPase, Mg^{++}-ATPase, and respiratory activity. I used the toad as an experimental model based on work done on that species in Argentina. These data were published with Mario Burgos in *General and Comparative Endocrinology* [14].

The effect of gonadotropins upon the toad testis has been studied since 1929 by Houssay and collaborators [15–17] who reported that pituitary extract stimulates the release of spermatozoa and suggested that the target cell of gonadotropin was the Sertoli cell. Further work demonstrated [18] that the increase in water content of the seminiferous tubules was an important factor in sperm release. In an ultra-structural study of the toad testis under gonadotropin stimulation (LH), it was shown that the Sertoli cell cytoplasm was the main target of the luteinizing hormone (LH). I demonstrated that Na^+K^+-dependent ATPase fell to 34%, and the Mg^{++}-dependent ATPase fell to 32% of the controls (Figure 5.4). Also, I found that 30 minutes after injection of HCG, the oxygen consumption decreased to 46% of the control values and was maintained even after 120 minutes post HCG administration [14]. A depression of the acid phosphatase-specific activity, also near 50% of the control activity, occurred in the 30 minute HCG-injected group. This effect was maintained during the first two hours (Figure 5.5).

HCG increased the water content in the toad testis in the order of 50% and the sodium content increased 39%, whereas potassium, instead, appeared to move in the opposite direction decreasing 30% in relation to the control. All these changes were associated with the increase of spermatozoa in the cloacal fluid after HCG administration (Figure 5.5). These data indicated that the inhibition of the sodium

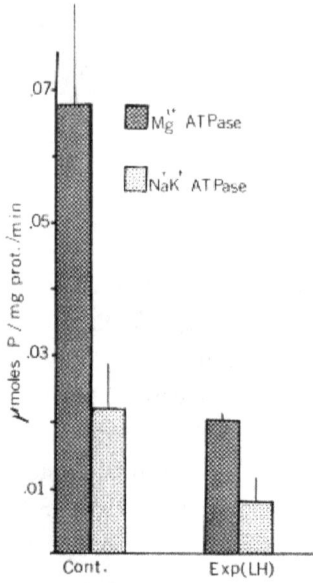

Figure 5.4:   ATPase activity in the testes of control and experimental toads.

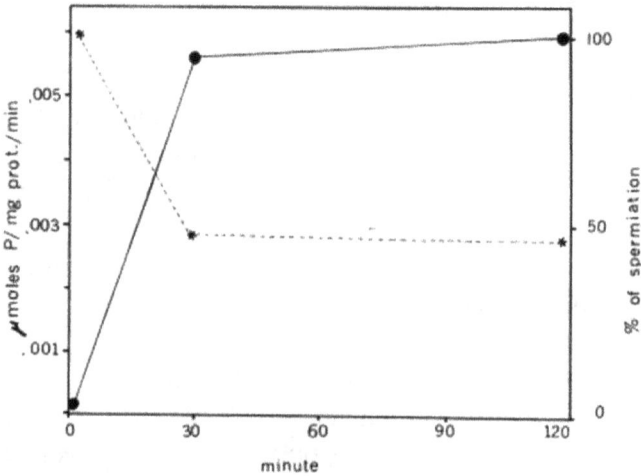

Figure 5.5:   Acid phosphatase activity (broken line) and percentage of spermiation after HCG (solid lines). The acid phosphatase was determined using the method described by Bodansky [41].

pump was the cause of the swelling of the Sertoli cells being the endoplasmic reticulum, the main target at the subcellular level [19]. *I postulated that the marked decrease in* Mg^{++}-ATPase *activity may be caused by a direct effect of the hormone on the mitochondrial ATPase or may be mediated through the respiratory chain, since the oxidation of succinate falls. This was determined using the oxygen consumption in a Warburg apparatus using 0.1M sodium succinate. I also postulated that the diminution of acid phosphatase activity after HCG administration was attributable to a release of acid phosphatase into the excretory ducts during spermiation* [14] (Figure 5.6).

I further supported these data by showing that in the mouse testis HCG depresses acid phosphatase [20]. Moreover, I showed that

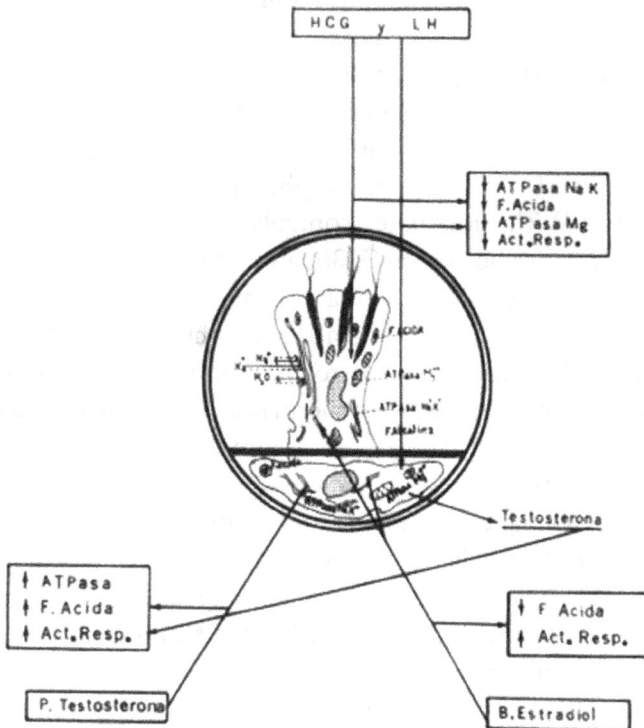

Figure 5.6: Summary of the hormonal control of the enzymatic activity in the testis. Reprinted with permission from Ref. [20].

hypophysectomy increases the specific activity of this enzyme in the testis of *Leptodactyllls chaquensis,* whereas HCG decreases it [6]. Mating produces a decrease of acid phosphatase in mice and hamsters [20], and in the hamster this inhibition of acid phosphatase during copulation was coincidental with the secretion of pituitary LH [13, 15].

5.2.3. *Experimental demonstration of the role of pituitary gland*

5.2.3.1. *Hypophysectomy*

In collaboration with Francisco Bertini and Ramon Piezzi, we published a paper in *Acta Physiologica Latino Americana* [6] showing the role of the pituitary gland in the regulation of the acid phosphatase in the testis of *Leptodactylus chaquensis.* This is an amphibian that undergoes a seasonal cycle of spermatogenesis during which they present remarkable changes of size and variations on the spermatogenic wave. We studied the effect of hypophysectomy during summer when the testes reached the maximum weight and the spermatogenic wave is complete. With adequate controls, the hypophysectomized specimens were sacrificed at 5, 7, 30, and 50 days after the operation. Early changes were observed at 5 and 7 days after the operation when the spermatocytes diminished. On day 30, clusters of spermatozoa were seen closely packed and inserted into Sertoli cells detached from the basal membrane, while the spermatogenic elements were very poorly represented. On day 50, the weight of the testes was reduced to 10% of the controls and a fibrotic process appeared to be installed replacing the normal elements. The acid phosphatase, firstly localized in the Sertoli cells in relation to the clusters of spermatozoa, became related at this latest stage with degenerating cells. The decrease in number of the spermatocytes, observed early after the hypophysectomy, may be a clue to the fact that these cells are differentiated into spermatide without being replaced by differentiating spermatogonia. *One important conclusion of this work was that the acid phosphatase does not disappear with the progressive detachment of spermatozoa from the Sertoli cells, but it remains highly active in the latter and in relation with degenerating cellular elements* [6]. *These observations supported the phagocytic role of Sertoli cells postulated by other researchers* [21,22] *and also indicated the importance of acid phosphatase in cellular degeneration and death, perhaps by a mechanism of autophagy that was clear in the animals sacrificed 50 days after hypophysectomy* [6]. *This concept of autophagy was a new one in those days and only started to be relevant in the literature around 2010.*

5.2.3.2. Comparative effect of mating with the exogenous administration of LH or HCG

In a study that I published with M. H. Burgos, F. Sacerdote, and R. Vitale Calpe [2, 15], we highlighted the comparative effect of LH and mating in the sperm release showing that the gonadotropin hormone LH controls the process of spermiation or sperm release from the Sertoli cells. A physiological stimulus such as mating, by increasing the LH levels, provoked a decrease of the acid phosphatase, Na^+K^+-ATPase, and Mg^{++}-ATPase as the exogenous administration of these hormones does. The LH or HCG depress the Na^+K^+-ATPase inhibiting the transport of sodium that, in the Sertoli cells, induced the swelling of the endoplasmic reticulum and release of the spermatozoa. We postulated that either LH or HCG, or mating might also have an uncoupling role in the oxidative phosphorylation of the testis by depressing the Mg^{++}-ATPase on the oxygen consumption. The effect of the hormone as well as mating in the acid phosphatase indicated that the lysosomes played a role on the degradation and rearrangement of the cytoplasmic components during the profound changes that the Sertoli cells show during spermiation, whereas in the Leydig cells it appeared to be necessary for the maturation and normal metabolism of these cells. These studies pointed to two important differences taking place during the physiological process of mating. One is that during mating the release of spermatozoa, which occurs at the level of the seminiferous tubules, was controlled by luteinizing hormone, or LH. This process has nothing to do with the spermatozoa released during mating from the tail of the epididymis. The spermatozoa mature in the epididymis for almost 14 days and pass from the head to the tail. This number of spermatozoa is ejaculated during mating. At the same time, LH is released in plasma and induces a new release of spermatozoa which travel from the testes to the head of the epididymis [2, 15].

5.2.4. *The lessons learned during my first two years of postdoctoral training, from April 1967 to April 1969*

The finalization of my doctoral thesis and my work on Burgos's team as well as with other members of the Institute of Histology and Embryology was a great period in my formation as a researcher because it gave me significant dexterity in multiple cell biology techniques that added to my experience in experimental pathology and made me feel empowered and, most importantly, I felt that my coworkers had confidence in my work, in my data, and in the way that I was interacting with them. They probably will never know how much I received from each one of them.

Professor Mario H. Burgos, Director of the institute and also my mentor, was a remarkable man, full of energy and enthusiasm, and he provided an exemplary role model of the high standards needed to do scientific research. He emphasized all the time that "research is a vocation and not something that we have to do because we are obliged to do it, we do research because we want to do it and as a consequence we must do it right and honestly."

However, this period was harsh for me economically because I was facing an impending marriage to Irma and at the same time helping my parents; my salary from the fellowship was never enough. Burgos helped me by adding a supplement to my salary using the grant that he had from the Population Council. This support was extremely meaningful to me not only for the monetary help but as a vote of confidence in my work and a sign of his affection toward me.

5.3. My scientific research training in Argentina from April 1969 to December 1971

The start of 1969 was full of excitement because Irma and I had set the date of our marriage date for February 8 and also because I was waiting to hear from the Center for Reproduction and from the CONICET about my further postdoctoral research training.

The fellowship from the Center for Reproduction was a prestigious fellowship, and Burgos not only sponsored my application but he was extremely eager that I have this opportunity. The competition for this fellowship was quite strong because it was open to all the young Latin American scientists, it was very well remunerated, and it also entailed a full training of 2 years in the best equipped and most reputable centers located in Buenos Aires, Uruguay, Chile, and Brazil. I was disappointed when I received the notification that my application was not approved. It was a sour feeling that I was not measuring up with the other applicants. However, I received shortly after the news that the CONICET would continue the support for my third and fourth year of training, before I applied for my training abroad.

We can only evaluate the importance of the events in our lives when they are looked at in retrospect. The negative answer from the Center for Reproduction was the best thing that could have happened to me. That fellowship would have interrupted my budding family life with Irma, her internship in the medical school, and separated me from my parents when I still was very attached to them and had already seen them suffering when I moved out from my home and started a new one with Irma. Besides these consequences, if I were a part of these trainees, it could mark me as a reproductive biologist and separate me from my path to becoming a cancer researcher. With the CONICET's fellowship, instead, I was freer to craft my training and choose the place for my studies abroad. It was undoubtedly a more uncertain path, but it was definitely the best path for me to control what I wanted to be. *Although reproductive biology is a fascinating specialty, it would never measure up to my ambition of being a cancer researcher.* Therefore, in this period of my training, I had several objectives to accomplish: (1) To develop a line of research that provided my own entity. (2) To fill the gaps in my training, which I realized was weak in the biochemistry of proteins, DNA and RNA, biostatistics, and the management of radioactive material that was crucial for performing advanced cellular and molecular studies. (3) To identify the center abroad where I could complete my training, and that would also involve mastering a second language.

5.4. Developing my line of research

The Leydig cell of the testis was not studied at the institute, and so I decided to concentrate on this cell type and orient the studies on two different fronts: first, its differentiation from the fetal period to adulthood, and second, to unveil the response of this cell to gonadotropin hormones, mainly HCG. In this period, I also mentored Dr. Juan C. De Rosas, who recently graduated and was interested in research. We made a good team, and he kept working at the institute when I left in 1971.

The morphological changes observed in the Leydig cell of the testis during the embryonic and fetal periods have been studied in different species, such as the dog, pig, boar, horse, rat, sheep, and man [23], but not in the mouse, and therefore to study this cell from the developmental process could give me an idea of the differentiation process and a way of testing whether my observations and conclusions were in line with data in the literature and also with the confidence that something original would come from these studies. I found that the Leydig cells of the testis arise from cells which cannot be distinguished from fibroblasts. Their scanty cytoplasm increases in amount and becomes more granular, and I described that the differentiation steps could be divided into three phases (Figures 5.7 and 5.8). During phase 1 (days 11–15), the spindle-shaped cell becomes an immature Leydig cell which contains numerous free ribosomes and some polysomes. This phase is characterized by a peak of mitotic activity that decreases as the cell differentiates (Figure 5.9).

I also quantitated the number of prominent cytoplasmic features in the different phases of differentiation (Figure 5.10). The phase 2 (days 16–19) is characterized by a marked development of smooth endoplasmic reticulum and by an equally important decrease in ribosomal population. Mitochondria are increased in number by 100% (Figures 5.10 and 5.11).

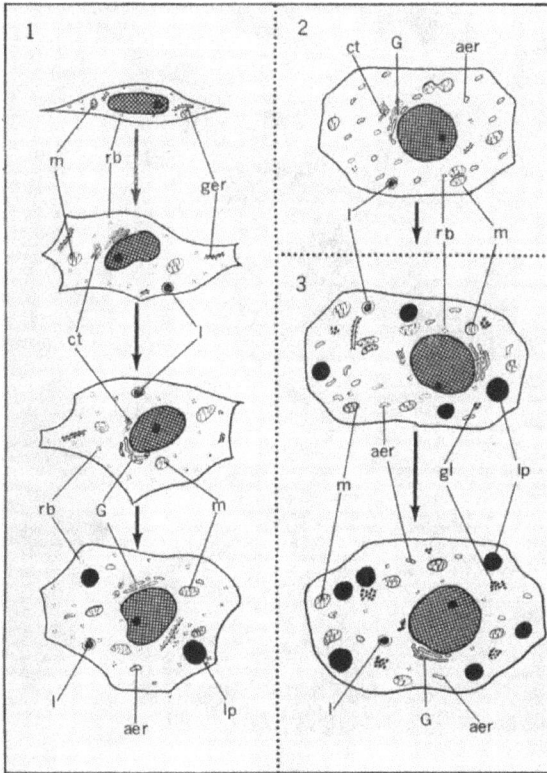

Figure 5.7: Evolution of the Leydig cell in the fetal mouse testis. Leydig cell differentiation is divided into three phases. Phase 1 shows the transformation of the spindle-shaped cell into a primitive fetal Leydig cell (days 11–15). A cell in phase 2 has a rich, smooth endoplasmic reticulum, few free ribosomes, and numerous mitochondria (days 16–19). A cell in phase 3 shows an increase of lipids and glycogen. The other organelles, such as smooth endoplasmic reticulum, are well developed (day 19 to birth); aer, smooth endoplasmic reticulum; ct, centrioles; G, Golgi complex; ger, rough endoplasmic reticulum; gl, glycogen; l, lysosomes; lp, lipids; m, mitochondria; rb, ribosomes.

Phase 3 (day 19 to birth) (Figures 5.12 and 5.13) is characterized by maximal lipid and glycogen content. Close to the time of birth, smooth endoplasmic reticulum decreases in extent and becomes vesicular. The peak in prenatal Leydig cell differentiation as judged by development of the endoplasmic reticulum occurs during phase 2. The

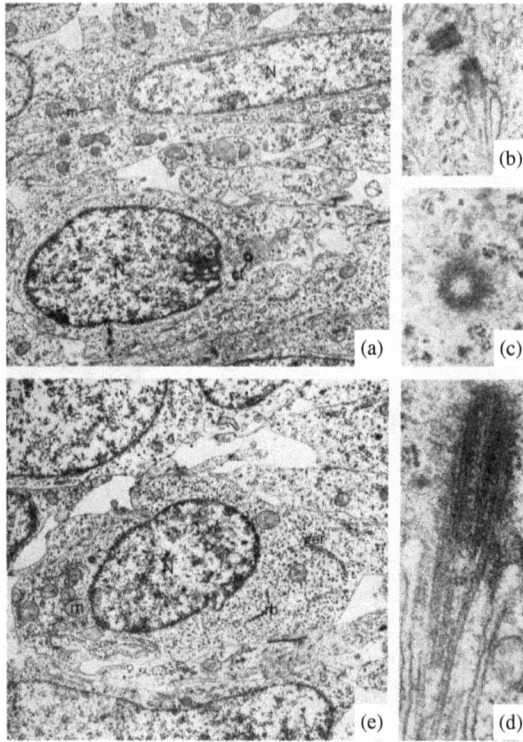

Figure 5.8: (a) Low-power magnification showing spindle cells and intermediate cells (day 12); ct, centrioles; G, Golgi apparatus; m, mitochondria, N, nucleus (×6,100). (b) Pair of centrioles, one of them giving rise to a cilium (×20,000). (c) Cross-section of a centriole. (d) High magnification of a cilium centriole (×82,500). (e) Leydig cell at phase 1 (12 days); ger, rough endoplasmic reticulum; m, mitochondria; N, nucleus; r, ribosomes (×6,900).

originality of this study was the demonstration that the differentiation pattern displayed by the Leydig cells from its spindle morphology characterized by the abundance of ribosomes in phase 1 to the replacement in phases 2 and 3 by the smooth endoplasmic reticulum. The scarcity of endoplasmic reticulum and the richness in ribosomes are common characteristics of embryonic and undifferentiated cells, as has been described previously by other authors [24–26].

Development in the smooth endoplasmic reticulum is an important criterion of specialization of the Leydig cell as an androgen-secreting

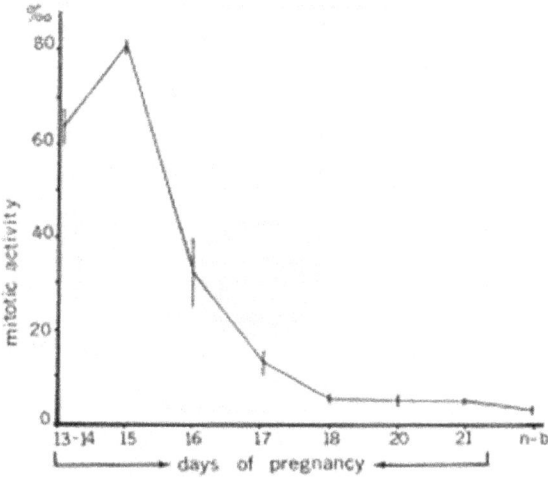

Figure 5.9: Percentage of cells showing mitotic activity. (Mean +/− standard deviation).

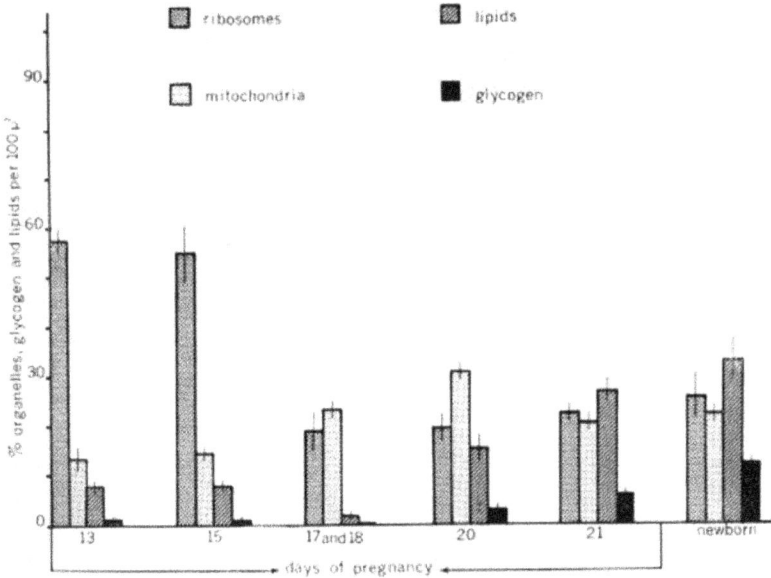

Figure 5.10: Average percentages in occurrence of four cytoplasmic parameters (ribosomes, mitochondria, lipids, and glycogen) as counted in 40 areas of 100 μ^2 each in micrographs at a final magnification of 5,150 times. The results are expressed as the percentage of each parameter in an area of 100 μ^2 with their standard deviations.

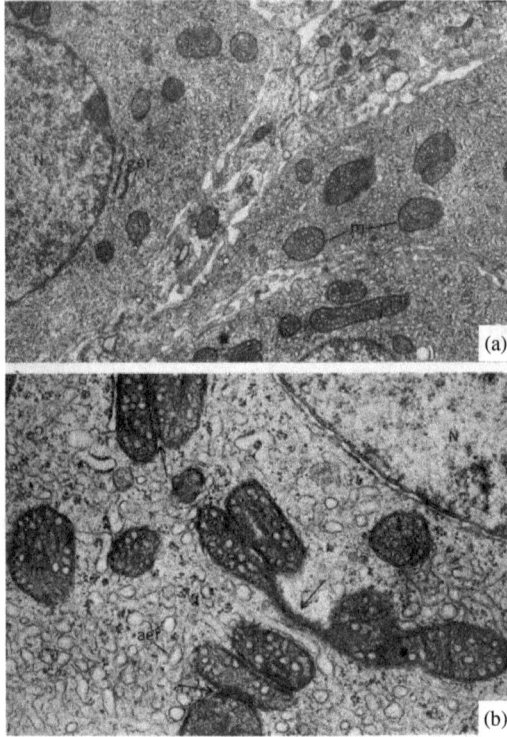

Figure 5.11: (a) The Leydig cell on day 17 has a richly developed smooth endoplasmic reticulum and a considerable number of mitochondria. These cells are poor in lipids and other inclusions; ger, rough endoplasmic reticulum; m, mitochondria; N, nucleus (×9,900). (b) High magnification of the fetal Leydig cell of day 17 (phase 2). Arrows point to the middle constriction of mitochondria with close contact of the external membranes. The rough endoplasmic reticulum (ger) shows signs of continuity with the smooth endoplasmic reticulum (aer). M, mitochondria; N, nucleus (×28,500).

cell; the peak of its growth during phase 2 indicates that the fetal mouse testis secretes androgens [23, 27]. Besides the endoplasmic reticulum the number of mitochondria in phase 2 is twice that of phase 1 and in phase 3 it increases more. The observation that HCG stimulates the division of the mitochondria has a significant relevance since this organelle cannot be generated *de novo*. The mitochondria must replicate their genome and divide it in order to be inherited by

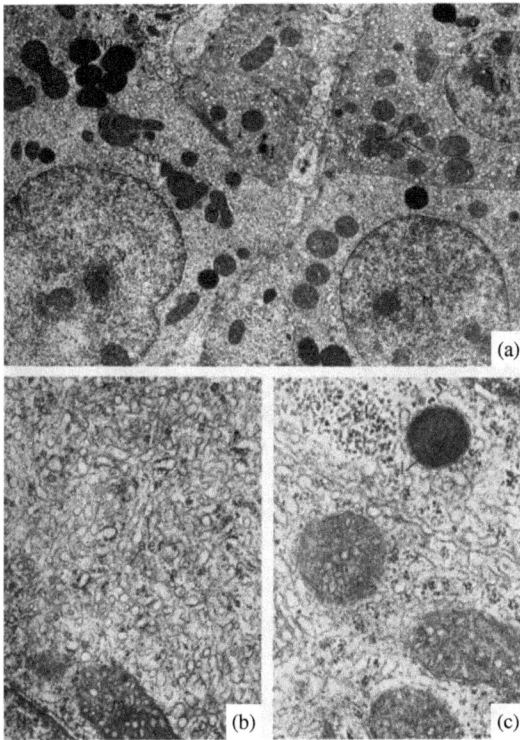

Figure 5.12: (a) Low-power electron micrograph of cell at day 20 (phase 3). The number of mitochondria has increased in relation to phase 2; some are undergoing division (arrow). The lipid droplets are more numerous than in previous phases; l, lysosomes; lp, lipids; m, mitochondria; N, nucleus (×9,800). (b) High magnification of a Leydig cell at day 20. The smooth endoplasmic reticulum is richly developed whereas rough endoplasmic reticulum is scanty; m, mitochondria; N, nucleus (×21,200). (c) High magnification of a cell at day 20 showing glycogen beta particles and other organelles; gl, glycogen; l, lysosomes; m, mitochondria (×24,800).

each daughter cell during mitosis. The division of the mitochondria is a structural challenge that requires the substantial remodeling of membrane morphology. In a paper published in *Nature* in 2016 [39], it was shown that the constriction that lead to mitochondria division is controlled by a dynamin-related protein (Drp1, Dnm1 in yeast) that works in concert with dynamin 2 (Dyn2) to orchestrate sequential constriction events that build up to division. Alteration in mitochondrial

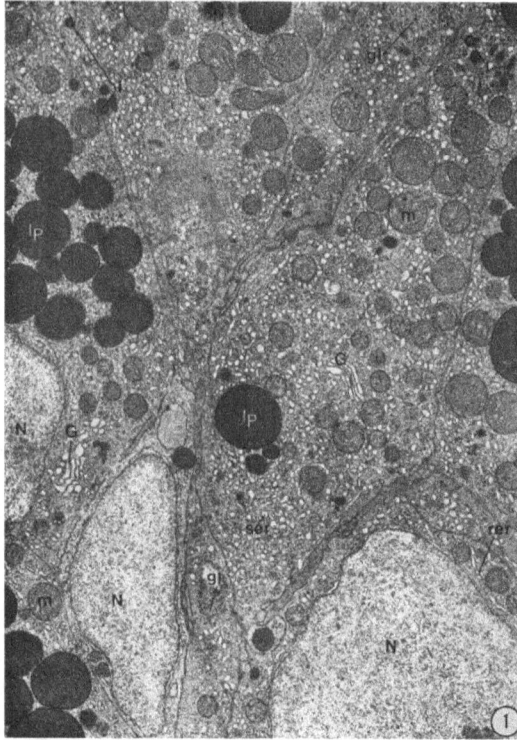

Figure 5.13: Low-power electron micrograph showing a Leydig cell of a newborn mouse containing a poorly developed smooth endoplasmic reticulum (ser) and numerous lipid droplets (lp), glycogen (gl) particles; m, mitochondria; l, lysosomes; G, Golgi complex; rer, rough endoplasmic reticulum; N, nucleus (×7,200).

dynamics may contribute to many neurodegenerative diseases like Charcot–Marie–Tooth disease and centro nuclear myopathy [40]. Another novelty of my work was the observation of the striking increase in lipids and glycogen. My speculation was that an inverse relationship existed between lipids and glycogen content, on the one hand, and Leydig cell differentiation, on the other. For example, there was a decrease in lipids and glycogen during the postnatal development whereas there was an increase in lipids and glycogen between the last intrauterine hours and the first postnatal days, marking a period of regression [28, 29]. An experiment that I started with Dr. Agustin Aoki was the injection of human chorionic gonadotropin into four-day old mice and the ultra-structural study showing disappearance of glycogen and lipids, with concomitant growth of smooth endoplasmic reticulum [30]. This observation was important for my studies but was also my first disappointment in science when Aoki, who was my senior and had already completed his training abroad, published this data without me. The lesson that I learned from this disappointment was to be fair with all my coworkers. Even though I was disappointed, I was not discouraged because my vision as a physician scientist was beyond his narrow scope as a morphologist; for him this was only an observation, conversely, I was interested in a process. In summary, these data suggested that, as in the case of man, gonadotropins also play a role in the postnatal development of the mouse Leydig cell. Although the level of placental gonadotropins was not known for the mouse, the changes in organization of the prenatal Leydig cell, which are similar to those reported for man [27], seem to be a strong indication that gonadotropins control prenatal differentiation of the cell in mouse also.

In summary, Leydig cell differentiation in mouse occurs during two periods, both of which are characterized by conspicuous smooth endoplasmic reticulum. The first peak is prenatal, and the second peak occurs at the 20th–25th day of extra uterine life, i.e., at puberty [28,29].

After birth, I found that there are two stages of Leydig cell development: The first period includes the changes taking place during the first three weeks after birth, whereas the second period comprises the events occurring from the fourth week on.

In the first period, the Leydig cell shows a round or an ovoid nucleus with a loose chromatin, one or two nucleoli, and a few fenestrations in the nuclear envelope. The cytoplasm contains a poorly developed smooth endoplasmic reticulum (Figure 5.14).

After the 10th day, a slight increase in the number of vesicles and tubules of the smooth endoplasmic reticulum is observed (Figures 5.14(a) and 5.14(b)). These tubules start to establish connections between them that give the smooth endoplasmic reticulum a labyrinth appearance (Figure 5.14(b)). Free ribosomes and a few cisternae of the rough endoplasmic reticulum can be found scattered among the smooth endoplasmic reticulum and in the vicinity of the nucleus (Figures 5.14 and 5.15).

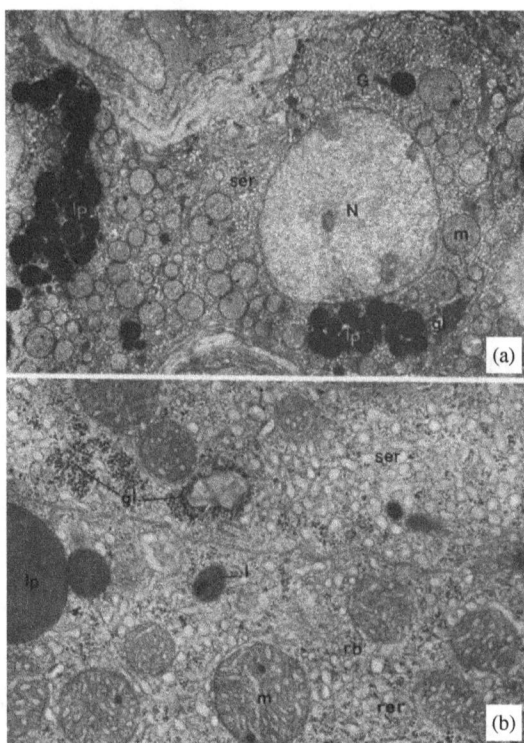

Figure 5.14:   (a) Leydig cell from a 10-day-old mouse; gl, glycogen; G, Golgi complex; lp, lipid droplets; m, mitochondria; N, nucleus; ser, smooth endoplasmic reticulum (×6,500). (b) Leydig cell of a 15-day-old mouse showing a relatively well developed smooth endoplasmic reticulum (ser); ribosomes (rb), and a few cisternae of the rough endoplasmic reticulum (rer) are scattered throughout the cytoplasm. Clusters of glycogen particles (gl) are also found; l, lysosomes; lp, lipid droplets; m, mitochondria (×27,000).

In the Leydig cell of the newborn (Figure 5.15), the glycogen particles, 200–400 A° across, are arranged in numerous clusters. The endoplasmic reticulum, instead, is poorly developed. Figure 5.16, shows that, on the other hand, the mature Leydig cell only contains very moderate numbers, if any, of scattered glycogen particles, isolated or in small clusters, whereas the smooth endoplasmic reticulum is quite richly developed.

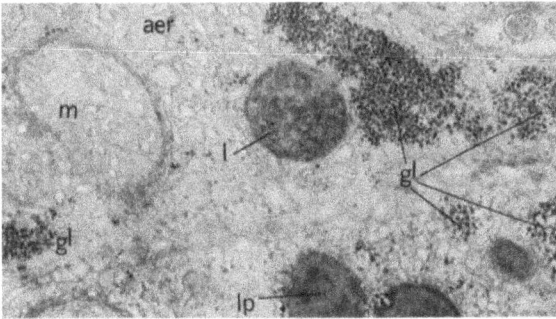

Figure 5.15: Leydig cell of a newborn. The abundance of glycogen clusters is evident; aer, agranular endoplasmic reticulum; gl, glycogen; l, lysosome; lp, lipid; and m, mitochondria (×31,580).

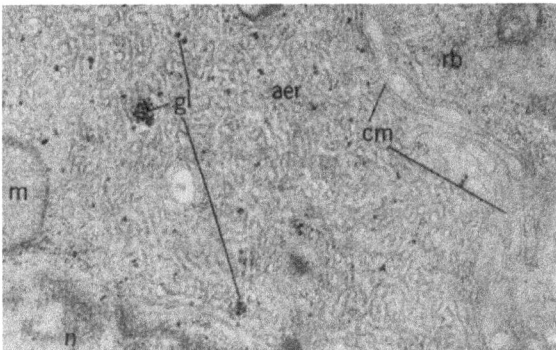

Figure 5.16: The cytoplasm of the mature Leydig cell contains a very rich labyrinthine network of smooth reticulum, whereas little glycogen is scattered in the cytoplas; aer, agranular endoplasmic reticulum; cm, cytoplasmic membrane; gl, glycogen; m, mitochondria; n, nucleus; and rb, ribosomes (×30,000).

The glycogen particles, 200–400 A° across, are arranged in numerous clusters in the testis of the newborn (Figures 5.17(a) and 5.17(b)). This is consistent with the biochemical data, which show high glycogen content in the testis during this period (Figure 5.18) and a decrease in the testis of the adult mice (Figure 5.18).

In the second period of adult life, which starts around the fourth week of life, the smooth endoplasmic reticulum hypertrophies considerably, occupying a large portion of the cytoplasm (Figure 5.19).

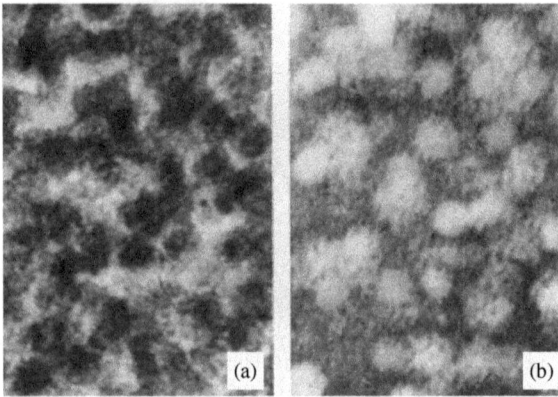

Figure 5.17:   (a) Glycogen particles 200–400 A in diameter (beta type) (×80,000). (b) In negatively stained preparations of isolated particles (beta type), these are similar to those found in situ (×80,000).

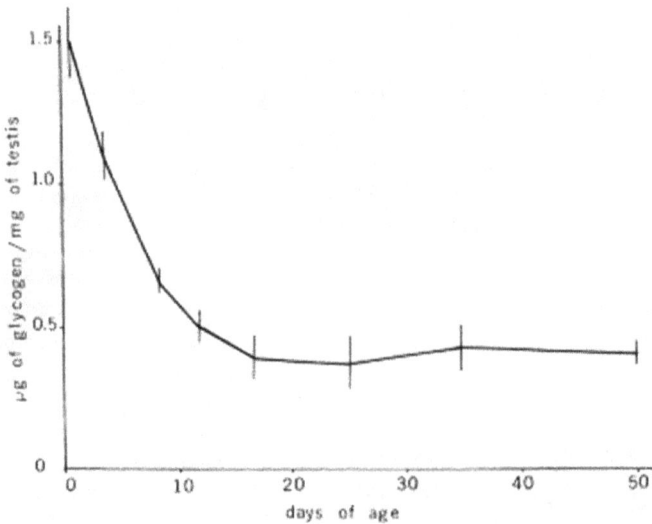

Figure 5.18:   Diagram showing μg of glycogen/mg of testis in the ordinate and postnatal days of age in the abscissa where the change studies are most obvious.

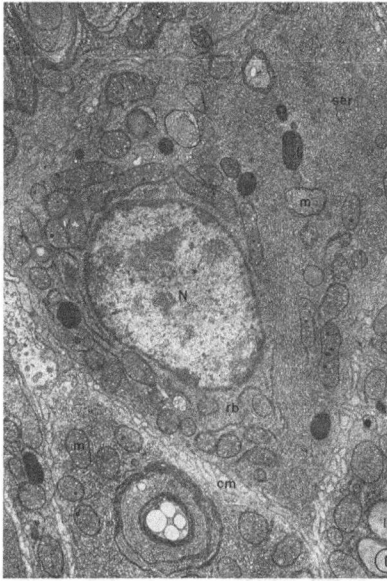

Figure 5.19: Low-power electron micrograph showing a mature Leydig cell of the mouse. This cell is characterized by a rich development of smooth endoplasmic reticulum (ser) and numerous interdigitations with other Leydig cells (cm); m, mitochondria; l, lysosomes; lp, lipid droplets; N, nucleus; rb, ribosomes (×8,400).

Different to the first period of postnatal development at the beginning of the adult life of the mouse, a few ribosomes and polysomes are present in those areas of the cytoplasm devoid of reticula. Mitochondria are generally conglomerated in the proximity of the nucleus, although they may also be found scattered throughout the cytoplasm. The second period is also characterized by the appearance of double-walled tubules, and by a marked decrease in the number of glycogen particles and lipid droplets. Lipid droplets remained as isolated inclusions (Figure 5.19). In the mature Leydig cell, primary lysosomes are also found and frequently observed in close relation to lipid droplets with formation of lipofucsin granules (Figure 5.20).

The relevance of the description of the prenatal and postnatal pattern of Leydig cell development is that it provided me a framework

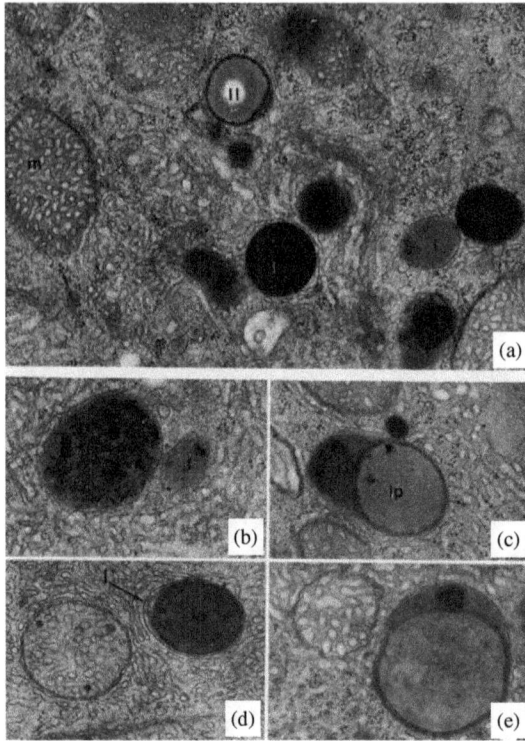

Figure 5.20:   (a) Cytoplasmic portion of a mature Leydig cell showing the presence of lysosomes (l) and "lipo-lysosome" bodies (ll); m, mitochondria (×27,000). (b) Primary lysosome (×34,000). (c) A "lipo-lysosome" body; lp, lipid droplet (× 20,500). (d) Lysosome (l) containing a lipid droplet (lp) (×33,000). (e) Lipofucsin granule (×30,000).

for further experimental work on the role of LH and mainly HCG in the control of the differentiation of these cells that is described in Section 5.5. Of relevance was the finding that, at the end of the fetal period, the cytoplasm of the Leydig cell contains a large number of lipid droplets and glycogen particles, whereas the amount of smooth endoplasmic reticulum decreases, demonstrating a relatively quiescent perinatal period. The first peak of differentiation that takes place during the fetal life is regulated by the chorionic gonadotropin in humans. The fact that HCG can induce differentiation of four-day old mice in 96 hours [30], consisting of a great development of the smooth endoplasmic reticulum and a decrease in the number of lipid droplets and glycogen particles, a phenomenon that in the normal postnatal period takes 20 days, points toward the importance of this hormone in the differentiation of the Leydig cells in the prenatal life. Another relevance of this work is the clear demonstration of the biosynthesis of membranes that is accompanied by depletion of glycogen particles, suggesting that the probable role of glycogen in the differentiation process is to serve as a source of energy and/or as a supplier of materials for the formation of new membranes [29]. Whereas the mitochondria of the Leydig cell contain tubular cristae, which are typical of the mitochondria of steroid-secreting cells, I observed that HCG stimulation in the adult testis indeed has a significant target effect in this organelle that made me postulate that the HCG lipolytic effect is mediated by its action on the mitochondria [31].

5.5. Studies on the hormonal control of Leydig cell differentiation

5.5.1. *Effect on the mitochondria*

In the Leydig cells of the adult mouse testis, the human chorionic gonadotropin exerts significant changes in the mitochondria. These organelles are mostly spherical or ovoid with tubular cristae and one or two grana in the moderately dense matrix. Two daily doses of 100 i.u. of HCG induce a constriction in their middle portion, to the point where they exhibit a filament made up of outer membrane structures linking the two portions of the organelle (Figures 5.21 and 5.22).

The mitochondrial intracristal spaces are markedly widened, and some mitochondria have become doughnut-shaped, some bifurcated, and the others have become considerably elongated (Figures 5.21 and 5.22, arrows). Whereas one dose of 100 i.u. of HCG after 24 hours induced these changes, larger doses (>100 i.u.) of HCG do not add pronounced changes. Interestingly enough, smaller doses, such as 20 and 30 i.u. of HCG do not affect the mitochondria. Administration of 50 i.u. doses twice daily induces mitochondrial changes, but has no effect either on lipid droplets or other organelles. The novelty of these

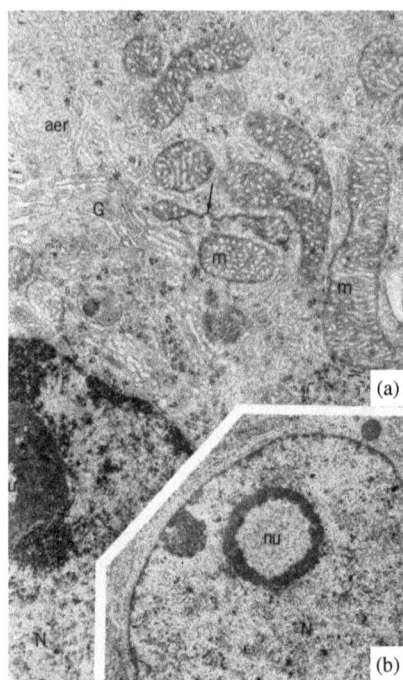

Figure 5.21: (a) The mitochondria (m) exhibit the hormonal effect; they have constrictions (arrow), and are bifurcated. The intracristal spaces are markedly widened. The Golgi complex (G) has developed to a large degree. A portion of the nucleolus (nu) shows the peripheral arrangement of the RNA surrounding a fine-textured nucleolar matrix. N, nucleus; aer, smooth endoplasmic reticulum (×25,000). (b) The nucleolus (nu) of the treated cell exhibits the margination of the RNA. N, nucleus (×9,000).

studies was the observation that mitochondria are the first ones to respond to the effect of HCG [31]. I postulated that the effect in the mitochondria is the first step required for the lipolytic effect of this hormone in order that the steroid synthesis takes place. The HCG may act on lipase stimulation through cyclic AMP requiring ATP and magnesium ions. These observations advanced the hypothesis that the lipolytic effect of HCG demands energy from the mitochondria and mediation of cyclic AMP.

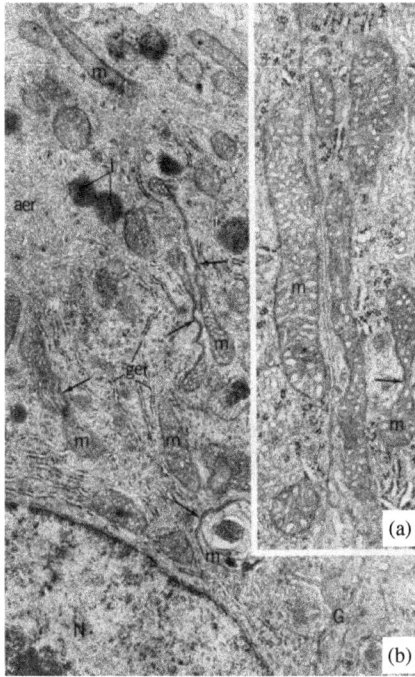

Figure 5.22: (a) The striking, consistent changes undergone by the experimental mitochondria (m) go from constriction (arrow) to doughnut shape (lower arrow). The intracristal spaces are widened; aer, smooth endoplasmic reticulum; G, Golgi complex; ger, rough endoplasmic reticulum; N, nucleus (×15,000). (b) Mitochondria (m) after HOG treatment elongate considerably or become constricted (arrow) (×25,000).

5.5.2. *Effect on the synthesis of cholesterol*

The differentiation of Leydig cells is characterized by the biosynthesis of membranes that is accompanied by depletion of glycogen particles, suggesting that the probable role of glycogen in the differentiation process is to serve as a source of energy and/or as supplier of materials for the formation of new membranes [29]. The HCG accelerates this process of forming new membranes and is associated with a lipolytic effect.

The development of smooth endoplasmic reticulum is accompanied by steroid secretion that uses cholesterol as a basic metabolic substratum. The main role of cholesterol in mammals is to serve as a precursor of steroid hormones and to function as a structural component of the cell membranes. To further analyze the role of HCG in the formation of membrane, meaning smooth endoplasmic reticulum, I used an inhibitor of the cholesterol synthesis called MER-29, or also called triparanol (Figures 5.23 and 5.24). The target of triparanol is 24-dehydrocholesterol-24-reductase [32,33]; inhibition of cholesterol biosynthesis is brought about by preventing the enzymic reduction of the 24, 25 double bond in the side chain, thus causing accumulation of desmosterol. Desmosterol is detectable ultra-structurally by the accumulation of dense, pleomorphic, membrane-limited bodies [34]. These bodies are present in moderate numbers in the normal mature Leydig cell of the mouse testis and in

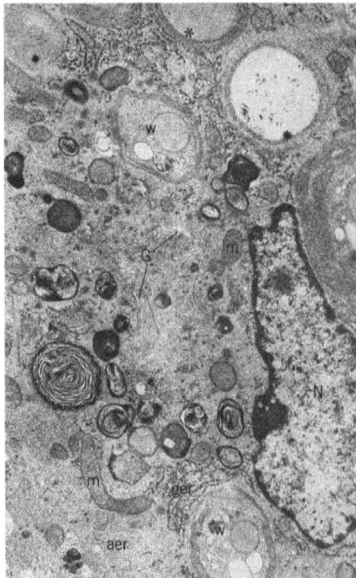

Figure 5.23: Effect of MER-29 alone. The smooth endoplasmic reticulum (aer) shows many whorls (W). Asterisks indicate different stages of the ER whorls surrounding lipid droplets or vacuoles. Dense bodies are quite numerous. The Golgi complex (G) is conspicuous; ger, rough endoplasmic reticulum; lp, lipid droplets; m, mitochondria; N, nucleus (×10,000).

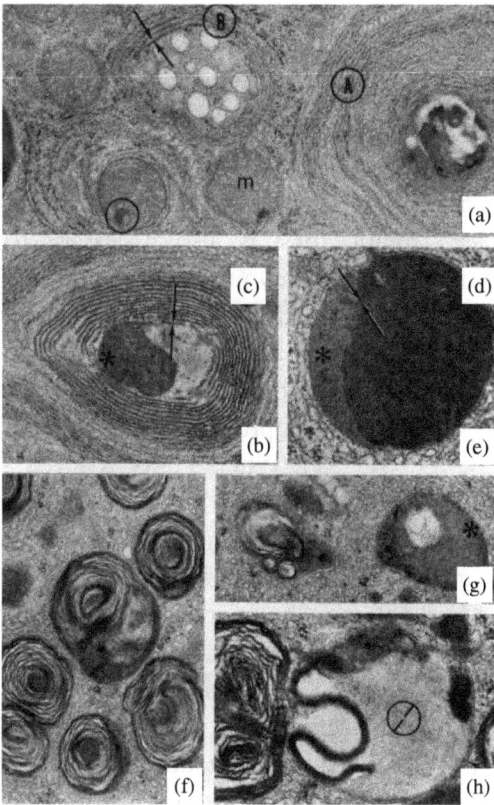

Figure 5.24: (a) Effect of MER-29 alone. Sequence of events leading to dense body formation can be followed from stage A to stage B. Circle encloses one ring-like granum of a mitochondrion (m). Arrows point to a dense body, stage B. Note continuity of the concentric whorls with finely stippled material (×25,000). (b) At stage C, the origin of the dense bodies from the smooth endoplasmic reticulum is confirmed. Finely stippled material (asterisk) is continuous with material filling the lumen of the concentrically arranged smooth membranes (×70,000). (e) Final stage of formation of this type of dense body shows the cap-like arrangement (asterisk) of the material continuous with the whorls. The latter exhibits a well-defined membranous organization (arrows), more closely packed than at stage C (×80,000). (f) Some of the numerous dense bodies after MER-29 alone contain a finely stippled material (asterisk) continuous with myelin-like membranes (×20,000). (g) The finely granular material (asterisk) of the dense body at right is continuous with crescent-shaped lysosomal material (asterisk). Dense body at left contains lysosomal material (small asterisk) continuous with the typical phago-lysosome organization (×20,000). (h) Stippling (asterisk) is in close proximity to the lattice of this dense body. Circle encloses an area of the lattice exhibiting clear-cut periodicity. Note that this dense body has a trilaminar unit membrane (arrow) (×35,000).

the adrenal gland. This indicates that in the adult a moderate accumulation of precursor is a normal finding. In the immature testis, on the other hand, the Leydig cell does not present these bodies, which only appear after administration of triparanol. Accumulation of glycogen and degeneration of some mitochondria are the ultra-structural expression of the effects of triparanol. Cholesterol, a normal component of cell membranes, is also necessary for the normal development of the Leydig cell. On the other hand, HCG induces its differentiation, causing a marked increase of the smooth endoplasmic reticulum. This would seem to be its paramount effect and suggests the triggering of high specialization.

The manner whereby HCG promotes this biosynthesis has been documented [23, 29, 31, 32]. When HCG is given simultaneously with MER-29, the effect of this inhibitor is decreased; when administered after MER-29, instead, the hormone is able to completely overcome the effect of the inhibitor. These results show that HCG is probably a competitor of MER-29; the hormone would trigger the enzyme 24-dehydrocholesterol-24-reductase, thus opening the pathway of desmosterol to cholesterol. This would lead to the construction of membrane systems and therefore of steroid molecules [35, 36].

In the adult Leydig cell, the ultra-structural effects of the hormone are: marked decrease of the dense bodies, lipofuscin granules, and secondary lysosomes (Figure 5.24). In the immature Leydig cell, MER-29 noticeably stimulates the lysosome response, as shown in the figure, whereas HCG causes the desmosterol bodies to disappear and promotes a high metabolization of lipids and glycogen. The end point of the HCG action is the high degree of differentiation attained by this cell at the ninth day of age, as compared with the normal lapse of time, which is 25–40 days.

5.5.3. *Looking at the future*

We only know what is in front of us during our present, and the meaning of what is happening to us only has sense when we see our past. To predict the future is only a guessing game for us mortal beings. It was unimaginable to me that my present line of research and the whole idea of cancer prevention that we started to develop in 1973 were rooted in the studies on the effect of HCG as a differentiating agent of the Leydig cells. The pattern of thinking and research that I developed in this period of my life would be reproduced in my future work. The big difference is that the scope of my work and thinking has been significantly enhanced. However, the basic thinking principles are rooted in those days of my early training in Argentina.

5.6. Filling the gaps of knowledge

The studies of cell differentiation of the Leydig cells made me realize that control of cell differentiation was an important path for understanding cancer. This made me even more aware that I needed not only to know about the basis of the new nascent molecular biology but also that I needed to master all the techniques related to this field. The window of opportunity opened to me in July of 1970, when the Campomar Institute, directed by Dr. Luis Leloir, offered through the University of Buenos Aires and through the CONICET a training in protein synthesis that covered DNA replication, transcription, and translation. The training lasted six months at the Campomar Institute, and it was a great opportunity to fill that important gap in my knowledge. Historically, it was also relevant because in July of that year, Luis Leloir received the Nobel Prize and it was extraordinary to see the event unfolding in front of me recapitulating the history of his first work that led to the Nobel Prize. The investigators at the Campomar Institute were first-class. The lunch meetings and the level of discussion were not easy to follow at the beginning, but in time, I was able to catch up. During the six months that I stayed in Buenos Aires — and Irma joined me during the last four months of our stay — it was a great opportunity to meet many wonderful colleagues, some of whom I continue to correspond with even now. One of them was Dr. Daniel Cardinalli, who was working in the ILAFIR in the pineal gland. Another colleague that I met was Dr. S. Alschule from the

Atomic Energy National Commission that was a very important contact for the course on radioactivity that I developed in 1971 in Mendoza as a secretary of the Cuyo Biology Society.

In July of 1971, I received a fellowship from the American State Organization for a training on regulation of metabolism in mammals, in the laboratory of Dr. Herman Nyemeyer in Santiago, Chile. It was a great exercise during which I met Dr. Gordon Sato, a leader in tissue culture. It was also the first time I used English in my scientific interactions and that made me realize that this would be the language for my communication in the United States.

As secretary of the Society of Biology of Cuyo, I also made a good friendship with Dr. Alberto Binia, who was a professor and later chairman of the Department of Physiopathology, directed at that time by Carlos Fasciolo, and together we organized a course in the use of radioisotopes in laboratory research and another course in biostatistics. These targeted courses helped me to complete the gaps in my knowledge. It was a great experience that allowed me to appreciate and develop a lasting friendship with those budding and already formed scientists in the medical school.

5.7. Planning my training abroad

In January of 1971, I started applying for my postdoctoral fellowship abroad, and I presented my application to CONICET to work in the laboratory of Dr. Howard A. Bern at the University of California in Berkeley. He was well known for his study of breast cancer. The response did not come from Bern but instead from Dr. Dorothy Pitelka, who made her reputation working in the ultra-structure of the mammary gland and was associated with the group studying the RNA virus and mammary cancer. This group had been working since Bittner [37] on developing the specific strain of mice that develop mammary cancer, and the ones that postulated that the hyperplastic alveolar nodules (HAN) are the premalignant lesions of breast cancer in mice. That group was very well known in breast cancer research, and Dr. Pitelka was a well-reputed electron microscopist. Electron microscopy was my main area of expertise, and my recent papers were on that topic, which was probably why Bern asked her to respond to me.

At the same time, I presented my application to the Population Council that was under the Rockefeller Foundation in New York, but I did not choose any mentor and I left in the application a blank space. On May 13, 1971, I received a letter from the Population Council granting me the fellowship and my assigned mentor was Prof. Dr. Charles Metz at the University of Miami in Coral Gables, Florida, at the Institute for Molecular and Cellular Evolution. In that institute, two main laboratories had been concentrated, one directed by Dr. S. Fox that studied the presence of life particles in material coming from space, and the other laboratory was directed by Prof. Charles Metz to study the mechanisms of the immune system and reproduction, an area that was extremely innovative at that time.

Dorothy Pitelka wrote to me several times, and the last time was on August 16 when she asked for my final confirmation of coming to her place. Although going to Berkeley sounded exciting and everybody at the institute, mainly Dr. Esteban Rodriguez, who had returned that year from 3 years of training abroad and who had stayed one year in Berkeley, was extremely excited about the place. However, listening to my own instinct, there was something about the way in which the situation was handled that made me feel uneasy. I had written to Professor Bern, and another person, an associate, wrote back to me about working more in electron microscopy; so I decided not to accept that place and to pursue instead the offer from the Population Council. It is difficult to rationally explain my reaction and choice because the selection was opposite to what I was looking for. However, I visualized that Berkeley would not be the place to develop my career.

Retrospectively that was the right and wisest decision, although it was not a rational one at that time. Why do I say this? Because without accepting the fellowship of the CONICET, I was bound to return to Argentina after 2 years, and my chances to do cancer research were extremely slim to null because there was not a strong group in Argentina to pursue this research, and I would need to go back to continue studying what I had been doing until that moment. The other thing that happened but was impossible to predict was that a few years later Dr. Dorothy Pitelka developed Alzheimer's disease. This would have made my stay in Berkeley an incidental one, without a mentor that could back me in the future. Accepting the Population Council and working with Professor Charles Metz was also an open canvas and working in immune reproduction was an unknown field to me.

Where is the basis to say that it was the wisest decision? First, the Population Council fellowship did not oblige me to return to Argentina. Why I was not bound to return is still not known to me. I do know this situation allowed me to stay in the USA and develop my career in cancer research. A second fortuitous event that was also impossible to predict was that Irma was accepted with open arms by Charles Metz due to her experience in embryology and further training at the University of Buenos Aires under Dr. Armando Pisano in the Experimental Embryology Laboratory while I was doing my training in the Campomar Institute. Metz offered Irma a position to work in *in vitro* fertilization and she received additional training at the University of Pennsylvania under Dr. J. Bedford. Her work in *in vitro* fertilization help her to demonstrate that fertilization of the oocyte could be stopped using an immune mechanism [38].

As soon as we knew that the United States was our destination, we started to improve our English, and it was our priority. This was accompanied by confirming our love and affection to our family and friends. When we departed from Buenos Aires on December 30, 1971, I knew that I would never come back to do research in Argentina. And I knew that I was starting a journey of no return. When I said my last greeting to my dear friend Marcelo Palero, I told him that I would probably never come back to Mendoza. I did not know why I said it, but that was what happened.

References

[1] Young, F. and Foglia, V. G. Bernardo Alberto Houssay 1887–1971. *Biogr. Mem. Fellows R Soc.* 20: 246–270, 1974.

[2] Burgos, M. H., Sacerdote, F. L. and Russo, J. Mechanism of sperm release. Chapter 12, In: Segla, S. J., Crozier, R., Cofman, P., Candleffe, P. C., (eds)

Regulation of Mammalian Reproduction, Charles C. Thomas, Springfield, Illinois. 1972.

[3] Russo, J., Localization, function and regulation of the acid phosphatase in testis. Medical Doctor Degree, Medical School of the National University of Cuyo, Mendoza, Argentina (Doctoral Thesis Dissertation), 1968.

[4] Russo, J. Acid and alkaline phosphatase of the mouse testis at different stages of postnatal development. *Acta Physiol. Lat. Amer.* 17: 302–308, 1967.

[5] Russo, J. Circadian rhythm of acid phosphatase in mouse testis lysosomes. *J. Reprod. Fertil.* 23: 21–24, 1970.

[6] Bertini, F., Russo, J. and Piezzi, R. The effect of hypophysectomy on the histologic acid phosphatase distribution in the testes of Leptodactylus chaquensis. *Acta Physiol. Lat. Amer.* 19: 22–29, 1969.

[7] Russo, J. Subcellular distribution of the acid phosphatase in the mouse testis. *Acta Physiol. Lat. Amer.* 20: 74–76, 1970.

[8] De Duve, Ch., Pressman, B. C., Gianetto, R. Wattiaux, R. and Appelmans, F. Tissue fractionation studies. 6. Intracellular distribution patterns of enzymes in rat-liver tissue. *Biochem. J.* 60: 604–617, 1955.

[9] Benoit, J. Maturite sexuelle et ponte obtenues chez Ia cane domestique par l'eclairement artificicl. *C. r. Seanc. Soc. Bio.* 120: 905–908, 1935.

[10] Assenmacher, I. and Benoit, J. Repercussions de Ia section du tractus porto-tuberal hypophysaire sur Ia gonadostimulation par Ia lumierc chez le canard domestique. *C. r. hebd. Seanc. Acad. Sci.(Paris)* 236: 2002–2006, 1953.

[11] Renaud, D. Influences simultanees de Ia lumiere et d'injections d'hormone gonadotrope sur le developpement testiculaire de colins immatures (Oiseaux Galliformes Odontophorides). *Bull. Soc. Zool. Fr.* 90: 417–422, 1965.

[12] Ferrand, R. Effet de sejour a l'obscurite sur le testicule du verdier (Ligurinus chloris L). *c. r. Seanc. Soc. Biol.* 160: 1715–1718, 1966.

[13] Donoso, A. O. and Santolaya, R. C. Depletion of pituitary LH induced by coitus in the male hamster. *Acta Physiol. Latinoam.* 19: 70–74, 1969.

[14] Russo, J. and Burgos, M. H. Effect on HCG on the enzymic activity of the toad testis. *Gen. Comp. Endocrinol.* 13: 185–188, 1969.

[15] Burgos, M. H., Vitale-Calpe, R. and Russo, J. Effect of LH in seminiferous tubule at the subcellular level. In: Eugenia, R., Geron, X., (eds), *Gonadotropins.* 1968, 213–224.

[16] Houssay, B. A. Hormonal regulation of the sexual function of the male toad. *Acta Physiol. Lat. Amer.* 4: 1–41, 1954.

[17] De Robertis, E. D. P., Burgos, M. H. and Breyter, R. Accion de Ia hipofisis sobre las celulas de Sertoli y el proceso de expulsion de los espermatozoides en los anfibios. *Rev. Soc. Arg. Biol.* 4: 21–25, 1945.

[18] Burgos, M. H. and Mancini, R. E. Expulsion de espermatozoides por accion de las gonadotrofinas en el testiculo de sapo "*in vitro.*" *Rev. Soc. Arg. Biol.* 24: 318–327, 1947.

[19] Burgos, M. H. and Vitale Calpe, R. E. The mechanism of spermiation in the toad. *Am. J. Anat.* 120: 227–252, 1967.

[20] Russo, J. Localizacion, regulacion y funcion de Ia fosfatasa acida testicular. Doctoral Thesis. Fac. de Medicina U.N.C. Mendoza, Argentina.1968.

[21] Carr, I., Clegg, E. J., Meek G. A. Sertoli cells as phagocytes: an electron microscopic study. *J. Anat.* 102: 501–509, 1968.

[22] Cei, J. M. Los fenomenos ciclicos endocrinos sexuales de Ia rana criolla 'L. ocellatus'. *Acta zool lilloana* 6: 283–331, 1948.

[23] Russo, J. and de Rosas, J. C. Differentiation of Leydig cell during the fetal period in mouse testis: Ultrastructural Study. *Am. J. Anat.* 130: 461–480, 1971.

[24] Grasso, J. A., Swift, H. and Ackerman, G. A. Observations on the development of erythrocytes in mammalian fetal liver. *J. Cell Biol.* 14: 235–254, 1962.

[25] Duck-Chong, C., Pollak, J. K. and North, R. J. The relation between the intracellular ribonucleic acid distribution and amino acid incorporation in the liver of the developing chick embryo. *J. Cell Biol.* 20: 25–35, 1964.

[26] Palade, G. E. A small particulate component of the cytoplasm. *J. Biophys. Biochem. Cytol.* 1: 59–68, 1955.

[27] Niemi, M., Ikonen, M. and Hervonen, A. Histochemistry and fine structure of the interstitial tissue in human foetal testis. In: Wolstenholme, G. E. W., O'Connor, M. (eds), *Ciba Foundation Colloquia on Endocrinology of the Testis*, Vol. 16, Little, Brown and Company. 1967, 31–55.

[28] Russo, J. Fine structure of the Leydig cell during postnatal differentiation of the mouse testis. *Anat. Rec.* 170: 343–365, 1971.

[29] Russo, J. Glycogen content during the postnatal differentiation of the Leydig cell in the mouse testis. *Z. Zellforsch.* 104: 14–18, 1970.

[30] Aoki, A. Hormone-induced differentiation of agranular endoplasmic reticulum in the interstitial cells of the mouse testis. *Protoplasma* 66: 263–267, 1968.

[31] Russo, J. and Sacerdote, F. L. Ultrastructural changes induced by HCG in the adult Leydig cell of the mouse testis. *Z. Zellforsch.* 112: 363–370, 1971.

[32] Blohm, T. R., Kariya, T. and Laghlin, M. W. Effects of MER-29, a cholesterol synthesis inhibitor on mammalian tissue lipides. *Arch. Biochem.* 86: 250–263, 1959.

[33] Blohm, T. R. and MacKenzie, R. D. Specific inhibition of cholesterol biosynthesis by a synthetic compound (MER-29). *Arch. Biochem.* 86: 245–249, 1959.

[34] Dietert, S. E. and Scallen, T. J. An ultrastructural and biochemical study of the effects of three inhibitors of cholesterol biosynthesis upon murine adrenal gland and testis — Histochemical evidence for a lysosome response. *J. Cell Biol.* 40: 44–60, 1969.

[35] Russo, J. Combined effect of Triparanol and HCG on the ultrastructure of adult Leydig cell. *Z. Zellforsch.* 113: 249–258, 1971.

[36] Russo, J. Ultrastructural study of the combined effect of MER-29 and HCG on the immature Leydig cell of the mouse testis. *Acta Endocrinol. Panam.* 2: 145–157, 1971.

[37] Bittner, J. J. Some possible effects of nursing on the mammary gland tumor incidence in mice. *Science* 84: 162–164, 1936.

[38] Russo, I. and Metz, C. B. Inhibition of fertilization *in vitro* by treatment of rabbit spermatozoa with univalent antibody. *J. Reprod. Fertil.* 38: 211–215, 1974.

[39] Lee, J. E., Westrate, L. M., Wu, H., Page, C. and Voeltz, G. K. Multiple dynamin family members collaborate to drive mitochondrial division. *Nature* 540: 139–143, 2016.

[40] González-Jamett, A. M., Haro-Acuña, V., Momboisse, F., Caviedes, P., Bevilacqua, J. A. and Cárdenas, A. M. Dynamin-2 in nervous system disorders. *J. Neurochem.* 128: 210–223, 2014.

[41] Bodansky, A. J. *Biol. Chem.* 99: 197–201, 1932.

Chapter 6

My Training in the USA (1972–1973)

6.1. My first impression of the USA

Irma and I arrived in Miami, Florida, on December 30, 1971. Our first night was in the Chateau Blue Hotel in Coral Gables, a beautiful residential area near Miami where we lived for almost 19 months. Our arrival in the USA was full of new and eye-opening experiences that overlapped with the faces of my mother, father, sister, and all the friends we'd bid farewell to in Mendoza. Their faces are still imprinted in my memory because I saw the stoic anguish of my father and the sorrow and pain of my mother seeing me leave, as well as the tears of my sister, who felt the heavy burden of being the only one helping the family. My mind was busy absorbing what my new American life would be and comparing that idea with my time in Mendoza, the place I grew up that has contributed so much to making me the physician scientist that I am. The past, the present, and the future were merging as one reality in my life, and my only wish at that moment was that my coming to this new country made sense and was worthy of leaving my dear Mendoza.

Dr. Charles Metz and Dr. Alberto Seiguer were waiting for us in the Miami airport, and they were extremely generous with their time, providing advice on what and what not to do. Charles Metz had already arranged that the following morning I would meet with the administrator of the Institute for Molecular and Cellular Evolution,

Mr. R. Dockenford, who would help us find an apartment. Mr. Dockenford was extremely friendly and helped us locate our first apartment at 341 Madeira in Coral Gables, just a few miles from the institute. In a matter of days, we realized the difficulties of getting around without a car, and on January 5, Mr. Dockenford helped us finance our first car, a 1971 Ford Pinto. That car helped us move around fast and easily as we had learned that public transportation was almost non-existent in the United States. However, we appreciated the other side of the USA, the dynamic operation of an economy that was built to serve the consumer. The best example was our initial contact with the gas, electricity, and water companies; in just a few hours our needs were met. The utilities companies were extremely efficient in their services and so much different from Argentina where everything was an ordeal. We almost laughed when the phone company not only responded to our request in hours but also asked how many phones and which colors we wanted. The funny part is that in those days in Mendoza getting a phone was a long process, and even then you could get only one phone per household and all of them were black. The other impression that we received was that the people were friendly and in stores the employees were nice and smiled at us. Whatever the reason for this behavior, it was a good feeling. It made us feel welcome. In time, we realized that this friendliness was not fake; it was the spirit of America. It was also part of an inherent graciousness, mainly in the older generation; they were happy to assist you. This welcoming pattern was also found when we moved to Michigan in 1973, but unfortunately we could not find that kindness when we moved to Philadelphia in 1991. In the 1970s, social security was offered to us and obtaining a driver's license was a well-organized and accessible process. In those days, gasoline cost 33 cents a gallon and tips were not customary in restaurants and other service places. We soon appreciated the advantage of credit cards, if you used them judiciously. In less than three months, we felt comfortable moving in our new environment. The glorious weather of Florida was also a contributing factor.

6.2. The Institute for Molecular and Cellular Evolution

The Institute for Molecular and Cellular Evolution was founded by Dr. Henry King Stanford in 1964 as part of his program to increase the research activity of the University of Miami. The institute was a separate set of buildings in Coral Gables, basically in the middle of the residential area. We were almost 3 miles from the main campus and about 10 miles from the medical school, which was in the city of Miami. During our first month, we usually arrived at 8 a.m. and stayed at work until 7 p.m., but very soon we found out that the schedule was not like that, and most of the researchers started at 9 a.m. and by 4 p.m. only the janitors were there. The philosophy was that if you could not accomplish your work in the normal working hours something must be wrong with you. At the beginning, we were reluctant to follow suit, but slowly we learned that the Miami area, and the whole state of Florida, was a place to be discovered. We learned that many extracurricular activities, like concerts and musical festivals as well as art exhibits, took place in the main campus, and all these evening activities were for the residents. We had been married for almost 3 years, and this time in Florida was an extended honeymoon. Once we started our incursions, our Pinto moved us from east to west and from north to south, all over the state in a matter of months. Our first trip was on January 30 to Key West. It was a delightful excursion that was followed by many, many more. In March of that year, I acquired my first 35 mm real photographic camera, a Canon F1, and my photographic enterprise started. There was not so much as a corner that we visited that we did not photograph. Also, we created a darkroom and started developing our own film to become proficient with micro- and macrophotography, meaning that we were discovering all the possibilities that our new space offered to us. It was also in this period that we acquired a Beaulieu 4800 ZMII Super 8 Movie Camera that allowed us to film sperm immobilization, and we even learned how to add a soundtrack. We presented the resulting movie in several meetings, and it was part of my final report to the Population Council. This was our first scientific film and, considering the tools of those days, it was really an excellent one. It was also well received at the Population Council meeting in New York in March of 1973.

Photography and 35 mm slide parties were a typical entertainment in the scientific community of the institute in those days. Every gathering ended by showing beautiful photos and films of volcano eruptions and the processing of rocks from the moon, searching for life particles. I must confess that I admired those beautiful photos and films shown by my Japanese colleagues.

Although Irma did not come with a fellowship, she was hired by Dr. Metz to work in *in vitro* fertilization, and we shared the same laboratory. I adapted what was available to make a functional place for both of us. There were two other couples working in Professor Metz's laboratory; Drs. Amelia and Alberto Seiguer, who were also from Argentina, and we bonded in a long-lasting friendship. The other couple was Carolyn and Robert Conway, graduate students from Virginia. This delightful and highly spirited couple used the laboratory next to us. We had a technical assistant that we knew as Woody who was in charge of taking care of the general maintenance of the laboratories and the rabbits for our experiments. He was also extremely helpful in managing the goats from which we obtained the antibodies for our work. My assignment was to study the mechanism of sperm immobilization.

6.3. The immune system and sperm immobilization

Although it was known that some normal sera contain cytotoxic properties that induce sperm immobilization [1–4] in the presence of complement (C') [1–3,5], the mechanism of immobilization was incompletely understood at the time that my research started. It was known that a correlation existed between sperm immobilization and female infertility [6–9], and the most important part was that the sera of infertile women has a sperm-immobilizing action. It was also known that cell membrane damage was associated with immunological immobilization of sperm. Using this knowledge, I started to search ultra-structurally what was the effect of antibodies against sperm or its parts and the importance of complements in the process of immobilization. I presented my conclusions in a meeting of the American Society of Cell Biology in 1972 [10] and a final publication in 1974 in the *Journal of Biology of Reproduction* [11].

6.3.1. *The procedures*

A visit to a farm in Coral Gables provided me with goats that were immunized either with ejaculated sperm, epididymal sperm, or the semen of vasectomized male rabbits [10,11]. The pre-immune serum or the immune serum was obtained by venipuncture of the jugular vein and from them I purified the immunoglobulins that I used in my experiments [10,11]. The procurement of the sperm or seminal fluid required the use of an artificial vagina that we had covered with the fur of a female rabbit. The male rabbit was first prepared using a female teaser rabbit that we called "Francine." The system was very good and allowed me to obtain the material that I needed for each experiment in our publication, which describes in detail the methodology that I used [11].

6.3.2. *The observations*

The immobilization of the spermatozoa was produced by an immune response against the spermatozoa. The effect was so fast that we filmed the process and documented it in a 25 minute movie that I delivered at a conference in March of 1973 at the Population Council in New York City. The rabbit sperm was immobilized in the first 5 minutes only when mixed with goat antisemen or anti-epididymal spermatozoa antibody plus unheated complement (C'). Immobilization failed to occur when heated (56°C; 30 min), so C′ was substituted for the unheated material. Treatment with goat anti-seminal plasma (immunizing antigen from vasectomized male rabbit) globulin or whole serum plus C′ did not produce sperm immobilization. Sperm immobilization was also observed in the presence of complement using isoimmune serum obtained from female rabbits immunized with rabbit semen. This last data confirmed what was observed in infertile women: that their serum immobilized the sperm of their partners. The effects of antibody plus unheated or heated C′ in terms of the number of affected sperm are given in Figure 6.1. The increase in morphologically altered sperm after exposure to C′ plus anti-whole semen or anti-epididymal sperm antibody was striking; 71.2% and 68.8% of spermatozoa, respectively, showed altered acrosomes. When heated C′ was substituted for active C′ in the sperm–antibody mixtures, the number of altered sperm was

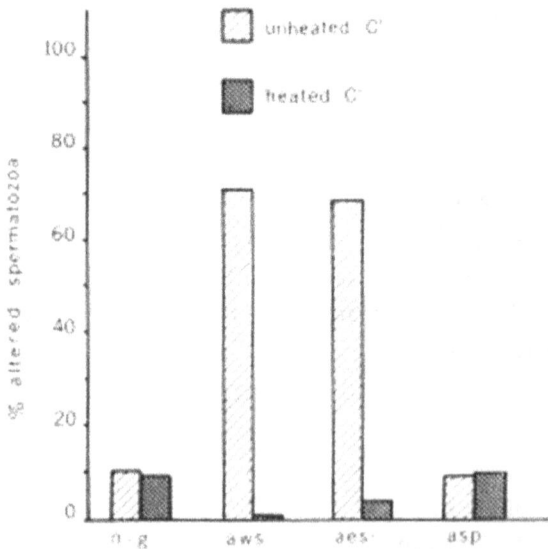

Figure 6.1: Percentages of spermatozoa with altered acrosomes after treatment with normal globulin (n-g), anti-whole semen globulin (aws), anti-epididymal spermatozoa globulin (aes), and anti-seminal plasma globulin (asp). The striking effect of unheated complement (C′) on spermatozoa pretreated with anti-whole semen globulin or anti-epididymal spermatozoa globulin is evident. Percentages are calculated from samples in excess of 300 sperms.

similar to that found in sperm treated with control globulin plus unheated C′ (Figure 6.1).

6.3.3. *Ultra-structural details of cytotoxic action*

I used a new Philips 300 electron microscope that I shared with other researchers who were examining small particulate materials from the moon, searching for signs of life. Most of the scientists working in that project were Japanese, and although I did not know how to speak the language, our non-verbal communication was excellent. I was my own technician, and I needed to process and section my plastic-embedded material as well as develop and print my own photographs. That was probably the most tedious work due to long hours in the dark room. Because I was in a frantic working mood, I produced thousands of photos until I was called by Dr. S. Fox, the other director of the Institute for Molecular and Cellular Evolution, who indicated to me that I was monopolizing the darkroom and the electron microscope. Fortunately, Professor Metz's intervention smoothed the situation, and then I did not have a problem in using those facilities as much as I wanted. It was in this environment that I studied the ultra-structural changes that explained the sperm immobilization induced by an immune response.

Figure 6.2 illustrates the structure of the untreated rabbit sperm head in section at low magnification. The anterior half and equatorial segment of the head (Figures 6.3 and 6.4) show intact cell membrane with a trilaminar unit membrane structure. I have noted that when the rabbit sperm was treated with control goat globulin, head to head clumping frequently occurred. This resulted from the presence of a "natural" agglutinin, and Figures 6.5 and 6.6 show how the sperm heads agglutinated in this manner.

In this normal agglutination process, the integrity of the cell membrane persists (Figure 6.6) in the acrosomal region. The cell membrane of the equatorial and subequatorial regions of the sperm head, the midpiece, and the flagellum all remain intact and indistinguishable from the untreated sperms after exposure to normal or antibody globulin even in the presence of active C′ (Figures 3.6,

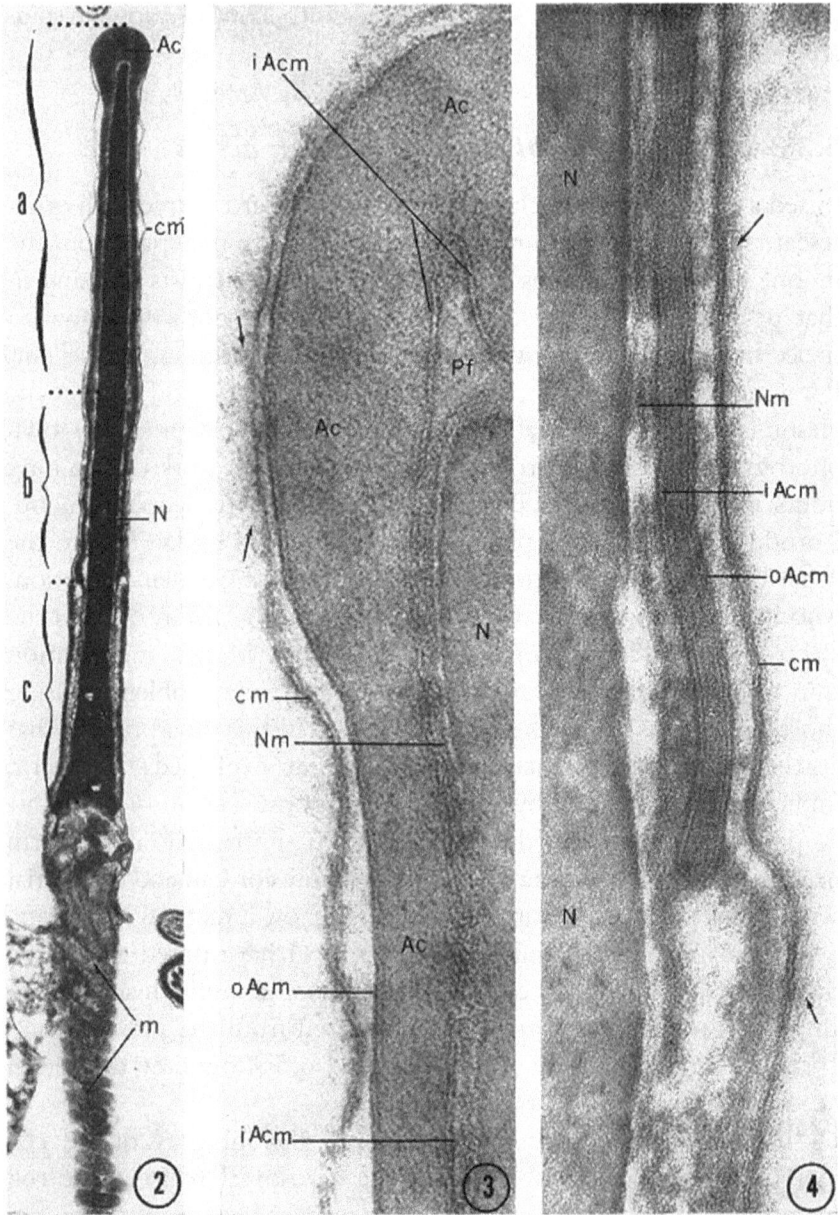

Figure 6.2: Longitudinal section of normal ejaculated spermatozoon. The sperm head is divided into: (a) half anterior portion, (b) equatorial segment, and (c) post-acrosomal segment. The cell membrane (em) envelops the acrosome (Ac) and this surrounds the nucleus (N). The section includes the neck and the midpiece of the spermatozoon with the mitochondrion sheath (m) (×26,200)

3.8–3.11 in Chapter 3), meaning that the sperms treated with goat globulin, either control or antibody globulin, show an amorphous material attached to the cell membrane (Figures 6.3, 6.4, and 6.7). No such material was seen on untreated sperms. This material was especially prominent in antibody-treated sperms (Figures 6.13, 6.18, and 6.20) and may represent antigen–antibody precipitate. It is observed in Figure 6.6 between the heads of spermatozoa believed to be agglutinated head to head.

The same material is observed between the tails of spermatozoa agglutinated tail-to-tail by antibody (Figure. 6.10). In addition to the amorphous surface material, vesicles 50–80 nm in diameter are found external to the sperms after control or, more frequently, antibody globulin treatment (Figures 6.7, 6.11, 6.16, and 6.18).

These vesicles are bounded by a trilaminar membrane-like structure. They are not dependent upon C′, either heated or unheated. Some of the vesicles may be products of antigen–antibody interaction. They could be formed from fragments of cell or acrosomal membranes or remnants of cytoplasmic droplets. The really conspicuous changes in sperm ultra-structure occur after treatment with anti-whole semen or anti-epididymal sperm antibody with active, unheated C′ (Figure 6.21). This series of changes does not result when heated C′ is substituted in the test systems (Figure 6.11). The changes include a swelling of the spermatozoon in the form of

---

Figure 6.3:   (Figure on facing page) High magnification of the anterior portion of the sperm head pretreated with normal goat globulin. The nucleus (N) is enveloped by the nuclear membrane (Nm), and external to this is the inner acrosomal membrane (iAcm). At the apex of the cell, the inner acrosomal membrane and the nuclear membrane form the subacrosomal space or perforatorium (pf). The outer acrosomal membrane (oAcm) and the cell membrane (em) are also shown. The membranes have the trilaminar unit membrane structure. This spermatozoon shows a fine granular material attached to the cell membrane (arrows). This material appears when the cells are treated with normal (control) or antisperm goat globulin without the addition of complement (×200,000).

Figure 6.4:   Longitudinal section at the equatorial and post-acrosomal portion of the spermatozoon. The trilaminar structure of the nuclear membrane (Nm) is visible. The inner (iAcm) and outer (oAcm) acrosomal membranes are joined at the bottom of the equatorial segment..

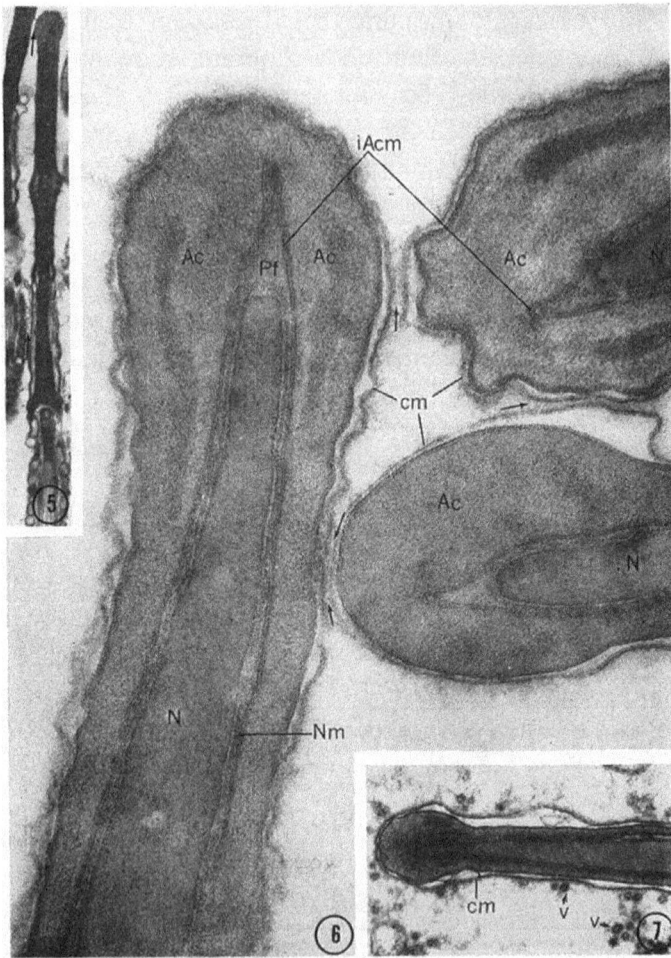

Figure 6.5: Low magnification of the sperm treated with normal (control) gamma globulin plus heated complement. The arrows show the apparent point of agglutination between the spermatozoa (×7,600).

Figure 6.6: Longitudinal section of sperms treated with control gamma globulin plus unheated complement. Head-to-head agglutination is shown; a fine granular material (arrows) is found between the cell membranes (cm) of the spermatozoa. The trilaminar membrane structure is preserved in all the membranes, Nm, nuclear membrane; iAcm, inner acrosomic membrane; oAcm, outer acrosomic membrane; Ac, acrosome; N, nucleus, and pf, perforatorium (×110,000).

Figure 6.7: Section of sperm treated with normal goat serum. Fine granular material is attached to the cell membrane. The vesicles (v) attached to the membrane in clusters are observed more frequently with whole serum than globulin treatment (×30,000).

increased space between the cell membrane and the outer acrosomal membrane (Figures 6.16, 6.17, and 6.21), rupture of the cell membrane, usually in the region of the acrosomal apex (Figure 6.21), followed by coiling of the cell membrane posterior to the level of the equatorial segment, and finally complete detachment of the cell membrane anterior to the equatorial segment (Figures 6.12, 6.13, and 6.21). Additional striking changes occur in the outer acrosomal membrane. These consist of regularly spaced 60–200 nm holes through which acrosomal material apparently exudes (Figures 6.12, 6.14–6.18, and 6.21). In extreme cases, the cell membrane in the acrosomal region, the outer acrosomal membrane, and the acrosomal contents all disappear and only the inner acrosomal membrane persists (Figure 6.19). All of these changes occur only in the region of the sperm head anterior to the equatorial segment (Figures 6.16–6.18). In the equatorial segment and more posterior, the cell membrane and the acrosomal membrane retain their normal relationships and trilaminar structure (Figures 6.13, 6.16, 6.18, and 6.20). It should be emphasized that the cell membrane and the outer acrosomal membrane both retain their normal trilaminar structure except at the points of rupture. Attempts to demonstrate 10 nm "holes" in the sperm cell membrane comparable to those reported [13,14] in ghosts of immunologically lysed sheep erythrocytes were unsuccessful. Such holes were not seen in sections of immobilized spermatozoa or ghosts of immunologically lysed erythrocytes. Negatively stained erythrocyte ghosts showed the characteristic holes. However, attempts to demonstrate comparable holes by negative staining in membranes isolated from antibody and complement-treated sperm were unsuccessful [11].

6.4. The relevance of my work

I was able to demonstrate that sperm immobilization by antiserum is a specific, complement (C′)-dependent, sperm–antibody reaction. This was confirmed by the fact that the anti-seminal plasma serum failed to affect sperm motility in the presence of C′. The sperm immobilization resulted from interaction of intrinsic sperm antigens

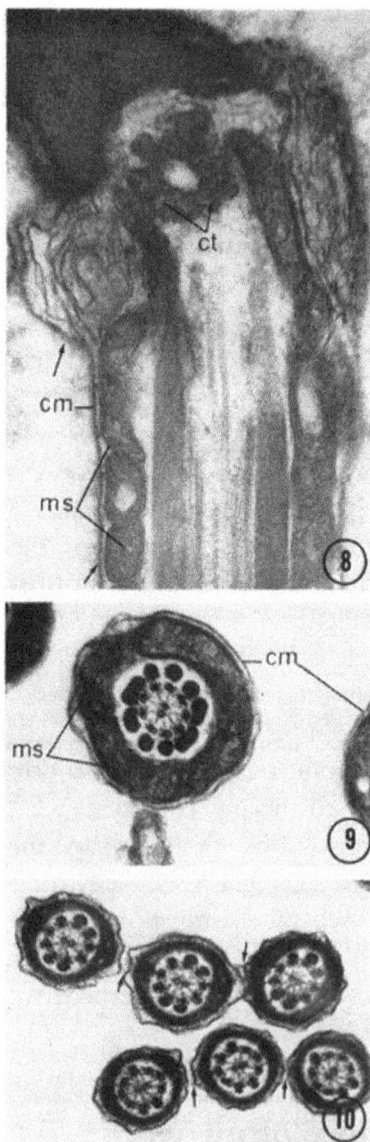

Figure 6.8: Longitudinal section of the neck and midpiece of sperm treated with anti-epididymal sperm globulin plus heated complement. The centriolar apparatus (ct) and the mitochondrial sheath (ms) are well preserved. The cell membrane (cm) is intact; the arrow indicates the fine material attached to it. The same conditions are observed when unheated complement is used (×50,200).

with antibody and C′. The "immobilization antigens" may be related to sperm "antifertility antigens," as has been suggested by Menge and Protzman [12]. They had showed that antisperm, but not antiseminal plasma antibodies, inhibit the capacity of rabbit sperms to produce conception after intravaginal artificial insemination. My work clearly demonstrated that the immunologically immobilized sperms showed alterations at the level of the sperm head, more specifically in the anterior half of the acrosome. In my studies, the continuity and trilaminar fine structure of the treated sperm cell membrane does not show a marked overall change. The alterations resulting from antibody–C′ treatment involve relatively massive swelling followed by membrane rupture, especially at the acrosomal apex. These changes in the cell membrane are reflected in comparable changes in the subjacent outer acrosomal membrane resulting in holes through which the acrosomal contents can escape. These holes were up to 200 nm in diameter, and were far larger than the 10 nm holes produced in erythrocyte membranes in the course of immunological hemolysis [13,14]. My speculation was that the mechanisms of cell membrane damage have common features in the two cases, at least to the extent that antibody and C′ components are involved in both. I postulated that the visible effects on the membranes in the sperm acrosomal region were preceded by subtle changes that I could not distinguish in the time frame of my studies. The liability of the cell and outer acrosomal membranes in the anterior sperm head region suggest membrane-bound antigens specific to the region. This was supported by the literature of those days indicating the localization of sperm surface antigens in that region [15–20]. The fact that the visible effects, though massive individually, are relatively small in

---

Figure 6.9:   (Figure on facing page) Cross-section of a sperm midpiece treated with anti-whole semen globulin plus unheated complement. The integrity of the mitochondrial sheath (ms) and the preservation of the membrane structure are shown (×40,160).

Figure 6.10:   Cross-section of tails apparently agglutinated with anti-whole semen globulin plus heated complement. The arrows indicate the fine material that links the sperms (×38,000).

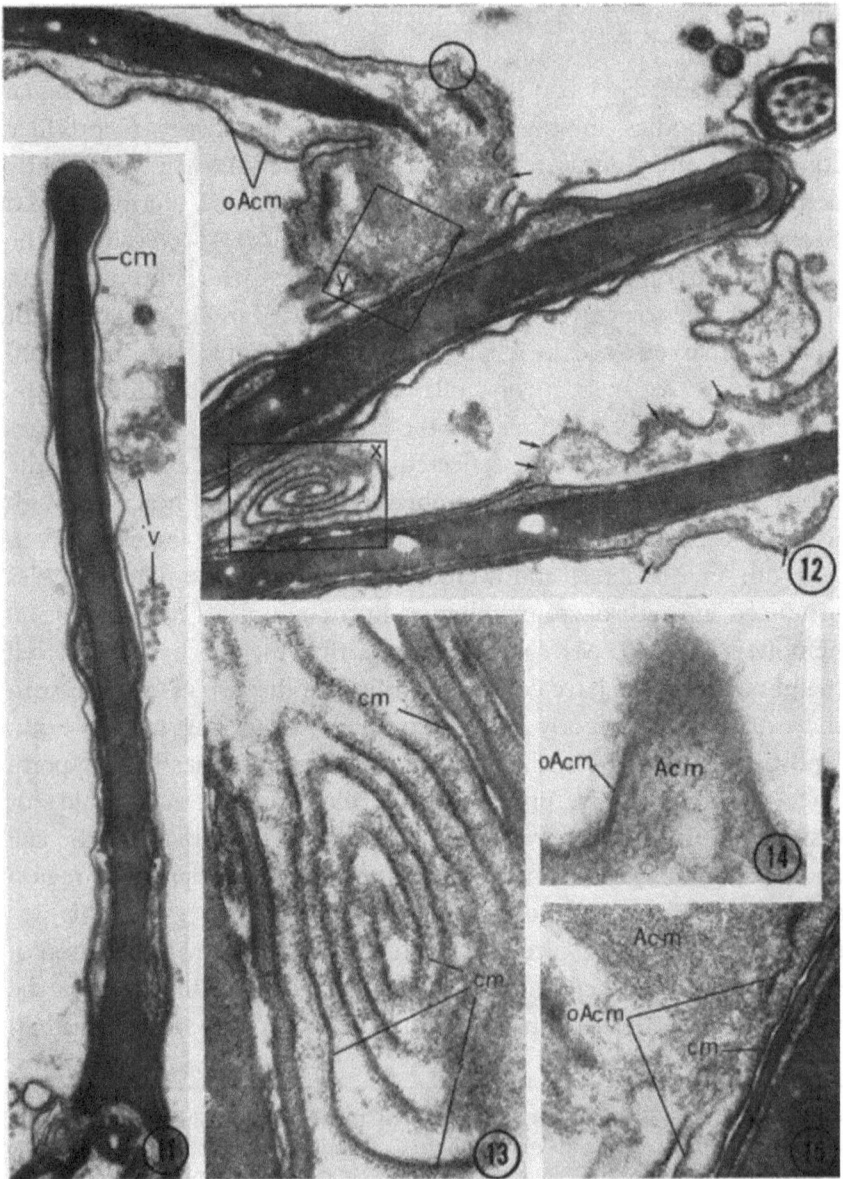

Fig. 11–15. See page 301 for legends.

Figure 6.11: Longitudinal section of sperm treated with anti-epididymal sperm globulin plus heated complement. The integrity of the cell membrane (cm) and vesicles (v) attached to it is retained (×20,000).

number suggested to me that the antigenic material was in clusters or "colonies" of antigens rather than a uniform pattern of individual antigenic sites on the acrosomal membrane. The other relevant observation was that the principal alterations were seen where the acrosomal material was concentrated. Therefore, a modest increase in permeability of the cell and outer acrosomal membranes could result in hydration and consequent swelling of the acrosomal contents with a variety of hydrolytic enzymes which could contribute to the membrane. My studies have shown damage not only to the cell membrane but also the subjacent outer acrosomal membrane, indicating that the C′ action resulted in greater permeability for both membranes. My explanation was that the initial antigen–antibody–C′ interaction at the cell membrane surface would result in a local permeability increase, especially at the sperm apex, permitting passage of additional C′ and antibody to the outer acrosomal membrane. Here a second antigen–antibody–C′ reaction would result in permeability increase of the outer acrosomal membrane. Hydration

---

Figure 6.12: (Figure on facing page) Sperm treated with anti-epididymal sperm globulin plus unheated complement. The cell membrane of one of the cells is missing (left upper corner). The cell membrane of the sperm in the lower portion of the picture is coiled back to the level of the equatorial segment (rectangle X). The outer acrosomal membrane (oAcm) has holes of different sizes (arrows), and the acrosomal material is loose and partly lost. The rectangle Y is at high magnification in Figure 6.15. The circle shows a hole with expulsion of the acrosomal material (×34,000).

Figure 6.13: High magnification of the rectangle X from Figure 6.12. The integrity of the trilaminar cell membrane structure is observed; however, the membrane has coiled. The equatorial segment of the acrosome is comparable to controls (×100,000).

Figure 6.14: High magnification of the hole in the oAcm indicated by the circle of Figure 6.12. The hole formed by rupture of the outer acrosomal membrane (oAcm), liberates acrosomal material (Acm). The trilaminar structure of the membrane is preserved (×100,000).

Figure 6.15: High magnification of the area in the upper (y) rectangle of Figure 6.12. The outer acrosomal membrane (oAcm) shows trilaminar structure; membrane continuity is interrupted by holes produced by the treatment. The acrosomal material is apparently diffusing out (×60,000).

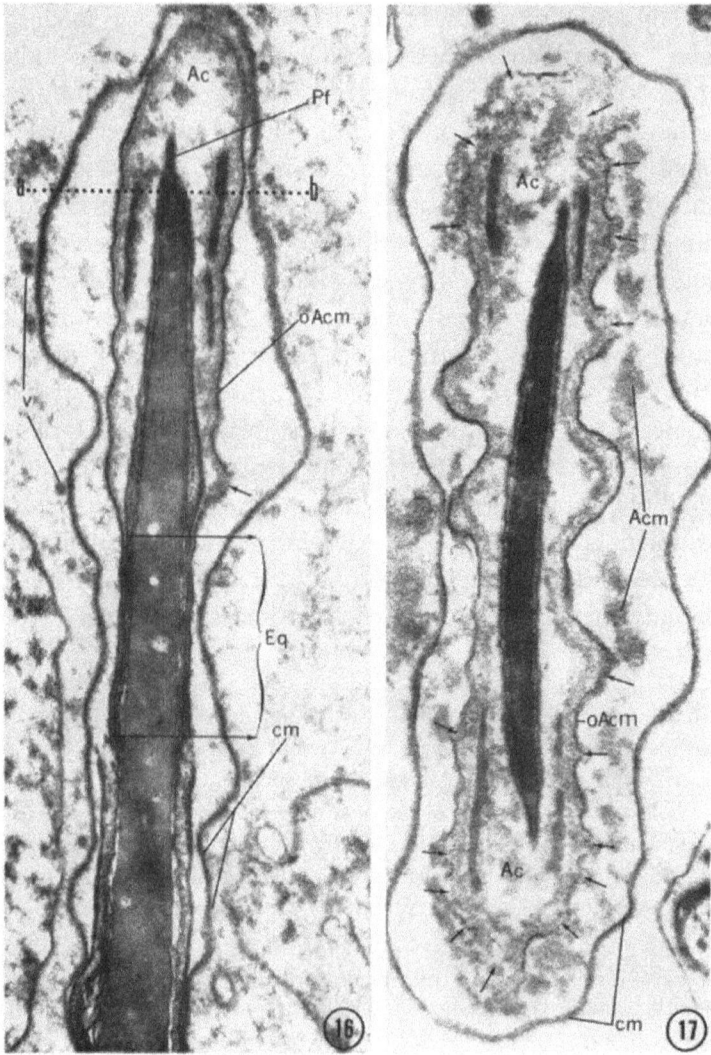

Figure 6.16: Longitudinal section of sperm treated with anti-whole semen globulin plus complement (unheated). The striking changes observed here are the swelling of the acrosomal material and the loosening of the outer acrosomal membrane (oAcm) in the anterior region. The equatorial segment of the acrosome is not modified. The perforatorium (pf) is now separated from the acrosomal material. The arrow indicates a hole in the oAcm. Fine granular material and vesicles (v) are attached to the cell membrane surface. The dotted line (a–b) is at the level of the cross-section shown in Figure 6.17 (×38,700).

and swelling of the acrosomal contents would then follow. Interestingly, the inner acrosomal membrane was not damaged, suggesting that at least the "inner" surface of the acrosomal membrane lacks the requisite antigens. The fact that the cell membrane and outer acrosomal membrane do not appear to undergo membrane fusion after rupture could indicate that the immunological immobilization was associated with true cell membrane holes providing continuity between the sperm cytoplasm and the external environment. This condition contrasted sharply with the normal acrosomal reaction where membrane fusion between the cell membrane and outer acrosomal membrane maintains membrane continuity in spite of the fact that both membranes (mammals) are lost in the process as has been shown by data published in those days [21–23].

My final conclusion was that the physiological mechanism of sperm immobilization is most readily visualized as destruction of the cell membrane permeability barrier followed by depolarization of the membrane and the loss of motility is attributed to creation of a break or hole in the cell membrane.

These observations were followed by a second publication with C. Metz and B. Dunbar in 1975 [24] in which the sperm immobilization was studied using immunofluorescence and scanning electron microscopy. We observed that the rabbit sperm fluoresced relatively uniformly following treatment with goat or rabbit anti-rabbit semen globulin alone or in combination with heated complement. However, following an immobilizing treatment, namely fluorescein conjugated goat or rabbit anti-rabbit semen globulin plus active C′, the sperm fluoresced minimally in the acrosomal region but brightly in the post-acrosomal area. This appearance corresponds to the position of the cell membrane of the sperm head, following the rolling back of the cell membrane that we saw under the electron

Figure 6.17: (Figure on facing page) Cross-section at level of dotted line (a–b) of spermatozoon in Figure 6.16. Conspicuous holes (arrows) are seen in the outer acrosomal membrane with loss of acrosomal material (Acm) into the space between the cell membrane and the outer acrosomal membrane (oAcm) (×42,000).

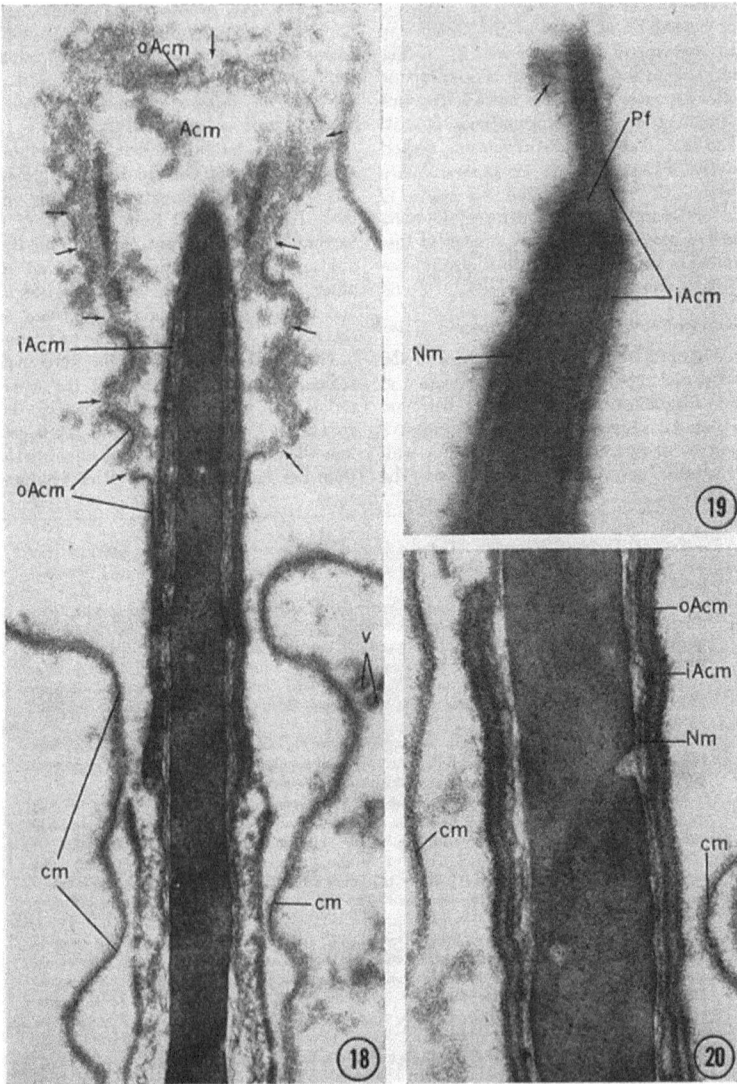

Figure 6.18: Longitudinal section of sperm treated with anti-whole semen globulin plus unheated complement. Lesions in the outer acrosomal membrane (oAcm) are shown in the anterior portion of the head. These include "holes," fragments of membrane and loss of acrosomal material (Acm). The arrows indicate holes, between them pieces of oAcm with the trilaminar structure are observed. The cell membrane (cm) is now separated from the rest of the cell and some vesicles (v) are attached to it. In spite of the damage to the outer acrosomal membrane, the inner acrosomal membrane (iAcm) and the equatorial segment of the acrosome are intact (×54,600).

microscope [11] (Figure 6.21(d)). Comparable posterior fluorescence was observed by indirect immuno-fluorescence. This posterior fluorescent pattern may be diagnostic for immunologically immobilized rabbit sperm. Membrane damage associated with immunological immobilization was also seen with SEM. This appeared as an accumulation of material interpreted as rolling back of the cell membrane from the acrosomal apex.

6.5. Looking forward

My work on sperm immobilization was finished in nine months. This was much earlier than the 24 months that Professor Metz expected and so, in August of 1972, I started to feel anxious about my next step. Although my Population Council's fellowship was not renewed until the end of December of 1973, I felt that I needed to start looking for a place where I could do cancer research. I wrote more than 40 letters based on the advertisements of open positions in *Science* and by January of 1973, I had narrowed my search to four possible places: the Baltimore Cancer Institute, University of Alabama, University of Tampa, and the Michigan Cancer Foundation (MCF) in Detroit with Dr. Marvin Rich. I met Dr. Rich in the Miami Winter Cancer Symposium in February of 1973, and the Michigan Cancer Foundation was the first place that I was invited to visit. I went in March 21 of that year. My presentation was around the work that I had done on the differentiation of the Leydig cells and the role of

---

Figure 6.19: (Figure on facing page) Sperm treated with anti-whole semen globulin plus unheated complement. The cell membrane and the outer acrosomal membrane have disappeared and only the inner acrosomal membrane (iAcm), including that covering the perforatorium (pf), remains. The arrow shows acrosomal material (Acm) attached to membrane (×128,250).

Figure 6.20: Equatorial segment of sperm treated with anti-whole semen and unheated complement. The trilaminar structure of the nuclear membrane (Nm), inner acrosomal membrane (iAcm), and outer acrosomal membrane (oAcm) is intact. The cell membrane (cm) is preserved, but it is detached from this portion of the cell (×102,000).

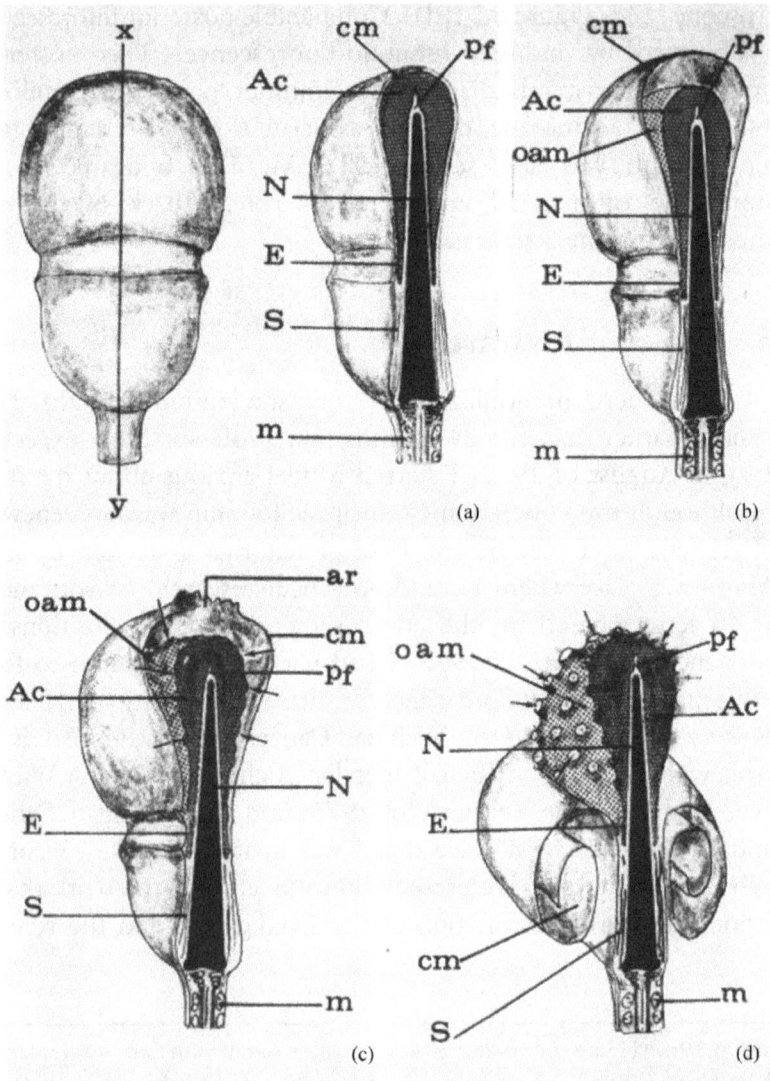

Figures 6.21:   Presumed sequences of acrosomal changes after antibody complement immobilization of sperm. (a) Normal, unaltered sperm. Stereoscopic representation of the normal sperm surface (left). The line x–y is the level of the sagittal sections (right and (b)–(d)); Pf, perforatorium; S, subequatorial segment. Note continuous unbroken cell membrane over the acrosomal region. (b) Early changes in treated sperm. The anterior half of the sperm head is swollen by separation of the cell membrane (cm) from the outer acrosomal membrane (oAcm). Other symbols as in (a).

hCG in the process. The talk was very well received and one of the comments was why I was looking to work in the cancer process when I had done such original work in the Leydig cells?

After visiting all the other places, I had a better idea how to compare the facilities but I did not see too many possibilities to grow as a cancer research scientist except at the MCF. It took several months before the offer was completed but in July of 1973 the final contract was signed, and I started to work there at the end of the summer of 1973 (see Chapter 7).

In the middle of this search, several events took place in my life. In December of 1972, when Irma and I were celebrating Christmas and New Year's with her sister Estela and her family, I visited the University of Utah Medical Center. The facility was impressive in appearance but it was not an attractive place for me. However, I met Dr. Alberto Baldi, who was working in the center, and who I had known during my stay in the Campomar Institute. Alberto Baldi was also orienting himself to work in cancer, and it was good to talk with him and compare possibilities. He was planning to return to Argentina in July of 1973, and he was extremely positive about his return.

In February of 1973, I received a letter from Dr. Alfredo Barbieri, the Director of the Institute of Biology at the University of Tucuman in Argentina, and he offered me the position of Head of electron microscopy facilities in the university. I discussed the pros and cons with Professor Mario Burgos when I saw him in New York — he was doing his sabbatical at Rockefeller University at the same time that I presented my work to the Population Council. We stayed in New York for several days and had a beautiful experience discovering the city. Burgos was enthusiastic about the position in Tucuman, and he encouraged me to take it. However, just a few months later, in

Figure 6.21: (Figure on facing page) (c) Intermediate stage in sperm alteration. Swelling increases, the cell membrane has ruptured at the sperm head apex (ar), holes appear in the outer acrosomal membrane, and the acrosomal contents are less dense. (d) Advanced stage in sperm head damage. The cell membrane has detached from the anterior half of the sperm head and coiled back exposing the outer acrosomal membrane to the equatorial segment. Many holes (arrows) appear in the outer acrosomal membrane.

May of 1973, Dr. Barbieri advised me not to return to Argentina because Tucuman was the center of the guerrilla warfare at the beginning of the tumultuous years that Argentina suffered, ending in the Dirty War (See Chapter 4).

6.6. Reflections on my training in the USA

In retrospect, my formal training in the USA lasted around 19 months and more than acquiring special technical skills at the scientific level, it was basically a learning experience in living abroad and a healthy transition toward my first position as a cancer researcher. Electron microscopy was the line of continuity between my training in Argentina, my fellowship in Florida, and my first position as a cancer researcher at the Michigan Cancer Foundation (see Chapter 7). It was the only key that I had to establish my presence in the scientific world until I could demonstrate that electron microscopy was just one of the many tools that I possessed — until I was able to demonstrate the profile of a cancer researcher that I believed I had.

The record of my scientific production clearly shows what I said above; however, in these memoirs I need to register other facts that took place during those 19 months of my training in Florida that were more fundamental in my life. The arrival to the USA changed my perspective and image of myself as if the mirror in front of me showed someone I did not recognize. I was the best student in college and medical school, I was an outstanding candidate to become a physician scientist. I was more than a physician, I was a medical doctor and a PhD, due to my doctoral thesis dissertation. I had accumulated a profound knowledge of many different fields, and I felt good about my science as well as my knowledge. I was an educated scholar who could discuss even complex subjects besides medicine, such as philosophy, religion, and general sciences.

Although I was the same person, my image in the mirror was reflecting a different person in my new environment. In the new academic environment, I was unable to keep a high level of interaction due to my limited English vocabulary, and even my simplest ideas were difficult to transmit; English was my main barrier, and I could not display the reasoning and argumentative skills that I had developed through the years. My foreign accent was an additional problem when I was speaking to my peers. I was not a physician or a medical doctor; I was a foreign graduate without the privilege to prescribe even the most rudimentary medication, and unable to discuss medical cases because I was short of the tools, the words I needed to do that. I saw others advance in front of me displaying primitive ideas, but I was unable to react because I felt that my English was inadequate. Having lost the fluency and ease of communicating in my native tongue, I felt crippled. The situation was even worse when I saw the abysmal economic imbalance between what I believed my rank and knowledge deserved and what I received. I was naked, terrified, and paralyzed to feel that I was a speck in a great scientific world. However, it was easy for me to recognize that the scientific environment of this country was unique and that I wanted to belong here. I realized my frustration and anger must be transformed into a positive attitude, canalizing my energies to overcome my deficiencies. I had experimented with those feelings before in my early youth, therefore these feelings were not new to me and it would take years of training and education until I would be able to transform those disadvantages into real assets.

These inner changes in my life are likely the most important things I experienced in those 19 months of my USA training. I realized that probably the most important experience of my training abroad was this self-discovery of my own reality, and that is probably the scariest feeling anyone can experience, and also the main reason why many of my colleagues never wanted to leave their country; they preferred to avoid seeing themselves reflected in the mirror of the world. It is a painful reality but probably the most important one that we need to suffer to evaluate our own capabilities.

References

[1] Chang, M. C. The effects of serum on spermatozoa. *J. Gen. Physiol.* 30: 321–335, 1947.

[2] Walsh, L. S. N. Natural auto and homoio spermotoxins in guinea pig serum. *J. Immunol.* 10: 803–809, 1925.

[3] Spooner, R. L. Cytolytic activity of the serum of normal male guinea pigs against their own testicular cells. *Nature (London)* 202: 915–916, 1964.

[4] Yanagimachi, R. In vitro capacitation of golden hamster spermatozoa by homologous and heterologous blood sera. *Biol. Reprod.* 3: 147–153, 1970.

[5] Baun, J., Baughton, B., Mongar, J. L. and Shild, H. O. Autosensitization by sperm in guinea pigs. *Immunology* 4: 95–110, 1961.

[6] Ashitaka, I., Isojima, S. and Ukita, H. Mechanism of experimental sterility induced in guinea pigs by injection of homologous testis and sperm. II Relationship between sterility and a sperm-immobilizing antibody. *Fert. Steril.* 15: 213–221, 1964.

[7] Isojima, S., Li, T. S. and Ashitaka, Y. Immunologic analysis of sperm-immobilizing factor found in sera of women with unexplained sterility. *Amer. J. Obstet. Gynecol.* 101: 667–683, 1968.

[8] Isojima, S. Relationship between antibodies to spermatozoa and sterility in females. *Int. Planned Parenthood Fed. for Immunology and Reproduction*, 1969, London, 267–279.

[9] Isojima, S., Tsuchiya, K., Koyama, K., Tanaka. C., Naka, O. and Adachi, H. Further studies on sperm immobilizing antibody found in sera of unexplained cases of sterility in women. *Amer. J. Obstet. Gynecol.* 112: 199–207, 1972.

[10] Russo, J. and Metz, C. B. Ultrastructural changes in immunologically immobilized rabbit sperm. *J. Cell Biol.* 55, 223a, 1972.

[11] Russo, J. and Metz, C. B. The ultrastructural lesions induced by antibody and complement in rabbit spermatozoa. *Biol. Reprod.* 10: 293–308, 1974.

[12] Menge, A. C. and Protzman, W. P. Origin of antigens in rabbit semen which induce antifertility antibodies. *J. Reprod. Fert.* 13: 31–40, 1967.

[13] Humphrey, J. H. and Dourmashkin, R. R. The lesions in cell membranes caused by complement. *Advan. Immunol.* 11: 75–114, 1969.

[14] Polley, M. J. Ultrastructural studies of Clq and of complement membranes interactions. In: Amos, B. (ed), *Progress in Immunology*, Academic Press, New York. 1971, 597–608.

[15] Henle, W., Henle, G. and Chambers, L. S. Studies on the antigenic structure of some mammalian spermatozoa. *J. Exp. Med.* 68: 335–352, 1938.

[16] Kohler, K. and Metz, C. B. Antigens of the sea urchin sperm surface. *Biol. Bull.* 118: 96–110, 1960.

[17] Srivastava, P. N., Adams, C. E. and Hartree, E. F. Enzymic action of acrosomal preparations on the rabbit ovum in vitro. *J. Reprod. Fert.* 10: 61–67, 1965.

[18] Menge, A. C. Antiserum inhibition of rabbit spermatozoal adherence to ova. *Proc. Soc. Exp. Biol. Med.* 138: 98–102, 1971.

[19] Edelman, G. M. and Millette, C. F. Molecular probes of spermatozoan structures. *Proc. Nat. Acad. Sci. USA* 68: 2436–2440, 1971.

[20] Nicolson, G. L. and Yanagimachi, R. Terminal saccharides on sperm plasma membranes: Identification by specific agglutinins. *Science* 117: 276–279, 1972.

[21] Colwin, L. H. and Colwin, A. L. Membrane fusion in relation to sperm-egg association. In: Metz, C. B., Monroy, A., (eds), *Fertilization, Comparative Morphology Biochemistry and Immunology*, Vol. 1, Academic Press, New York. 1967.

[22] Barros, C., Bedford, J. M., Franklin, L. E. and Austin, C. R. Membrane vesiculation as a feature of the mammalian acrosome reaction. *J. Cell Biol.* 34: C1–C5, 1967.

[23] Franklin, L. E., Barros, C. and Fussell, E. N. The acrosomal region and the acrosome reaction in sperm of the golden hamster. *Biol. Reprod.* 3: 180–200, 1970.

[24] Russo, J., Metz, C. B. and Dunbar, B. S. Membrane damage to immunologically immobilized rabbit spermatozoa visualized by immunofluorescence and scanning electron microscopy. *Biol. Reprod.* 13: 136–141, 1975.

Chapter 7

The Breast Cancer Virus and the Viral Team (1973–1976)

7.1. My first position as a cancer researcher

On a cloudy day in the last month of summer, Irma and I drove our Ford Pinto from our new home in Ann Arbor, Michigan, to 110 East Warren Avenue in Detroit, where a five-story brick building named the Michigan Cancer Foundation, or the Meyer L. Prentis Cancer Center, was located (Figure 7.1). With only 92 researchers, the Michigan Cancer Foundation (MCF) was small in comparison to other cancer centers in the country, but it had a fascinating backstory. According to Dollie Cole [1], in 1941, Columbia University's Crocker Laboratory for cancer research was closing, and they needed to dispose a colony of inbred rats that were maintained by Drs. Maynie R. Curtis and Wilhelmina Dunning. The colony, worth about 2,000 dollars, was finally housed in the basement of a non-descript Detroit building originally designed as a repair shop for trucks. The newly refurbished building and the experimental rat colony constituted the main assets of the newly incorporated Detroit Institute of Cancer Research. It was from this humble beginning that the MCF was born, and by the time that I joined them in that first week of September 1973, the Meyer L. Prentis Cancer Center, named after a former treasurer of General Motors and led by Dr. Michael Brennan, was a freestanding cancer research institution.

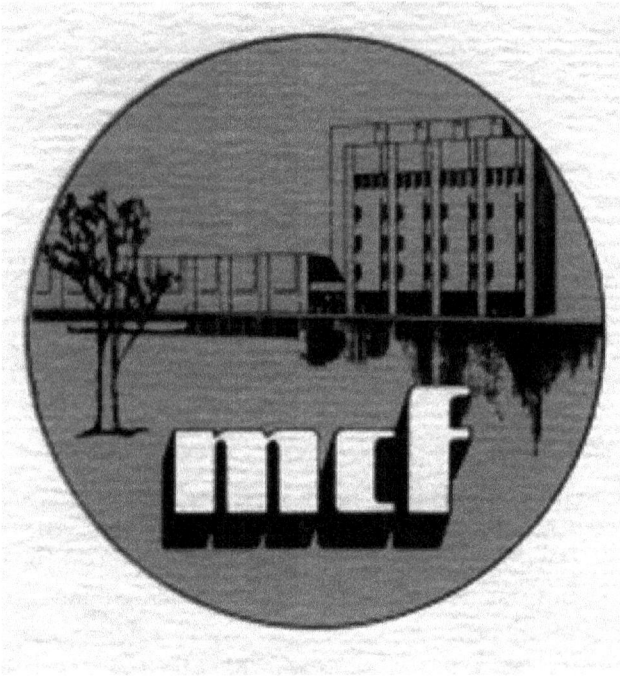

Figure 7.1: Drawing of the MCF in 1973. The structure on the left is the remnant of the Detroit Institute for Cancer Research that was merged with the newer five-story Meyer L. Prentis Cancer Center building.

The first floor of the building was devoted to public service facilities — patient services, public health education, volunteer activities, and the detection clinic. The second floor was a remnant of the old Detroit Institute for Cancer Research and lacked any windows, looking from the outside like a solid, impenetrable brick wall (Figure 7.1). The first and second floors were joined to the new Prentis building; the other four floors had their windows facing all the cardinal points of midtown Detroit. The state-of-the-art facility was dedicated to cancer research and an impressive mark in the city's skyline.

I remember the lobby being warm, and a smiling receptionist led us to the second floor where the Scientific Director, Dr. Marvin Rich, was expecting us. It was difficult to conceive in that moment that this first day of my first job as a cancer researcher in the USA was probably the most important one of my life, and it made sense of so many decisions that had come before — why I emigrated from Argentina, why I studied medicine, and why I chose experimental pathology as my first research training in the Experimental Pathology Department at the University National of Cuyo under Dr. Echave Llanos in my native Mendoza (see Chapter 3). After all, for as long as I could remember, I had dreamed of doing cancer research.

The MCF was part of the medical center where Wayne State University Medical School had its stronghold. The medical center was expanding in the middle of a run-down neighborhood, and the main street was called "the Lady Warren Avenue" by some of the neighbors. The name came because for years it had been the red-light district, and during my first years at that institution it was not unusual to see ladies of the night walking on that street, plying their trade. The most paradoxical aspect of this human situation was that this subreal life was taking place in the middle of a neighborhood boasting the beautiful art museum that held Diego de Rivera's mural, the Engineering Society with its wonderful modern architectural design, the new Harper University Hospital, and the new medical school building. The old women's hospital building was a remnant of what medical care was like before this urbanization spirit took root. All the power of modernization and improvement contrasted tremendously with the surrounding decaying decadency of the place, with its run-down houses that spoke of a better past and playgrounds overgrown by weeds, the free spaces used as garbage dumps. All of these contradictions were beyond my initial understanding — comprehension came later on, when I learned the struggles of the city and the reality of the blue-collar workers linked to a car industry that was remodeling itself in the face of competition from European and Japanese cars. This shifting dynamic was affecting the American autoworkers trapped in their old neighborhoods and being driven away by a city that wanted to revive itself and modernize and catch up with the rest of the country. It took me a few of the almost 19 years that I lived in Michigan before I started to appreciate this and learned to not only understand but also love the humanness and the history of Detroit.

I arrived at the MCF as the chief of the experimental pathology laboratory; later I became a member and Chairman of the foundation's Department of Pathology, as well as becoming a clinical Associate Professor of pathology at Wayne State University Medical School. At the same time, my closest associate, Dr. Irma H. Russo, and I created a small section in the department that we named the Breast Cancer Research Laboratory, with a focus on studying the pathogenesis and prevention of breast cancer (see Chapter 8). Upon my arrival at the MCF (as it was then known, in 1991, the name was changed to the Karmanos Cancer Center, and it became a part of Wayne State University), my main function as a cancer researcher was to be a part of a team that was progressing full speed in the isolation of a putative virus that could be responsible for the etiology and pathogenesis of breast cancer. Working with this team of exemplary scientists, such as Marvin Rich, Michael Brennan, Charles McGrath, Philip Furmanski, Herbert Soule, Ramadandra Das, and Justin McCormick (Figure 7.2), was a

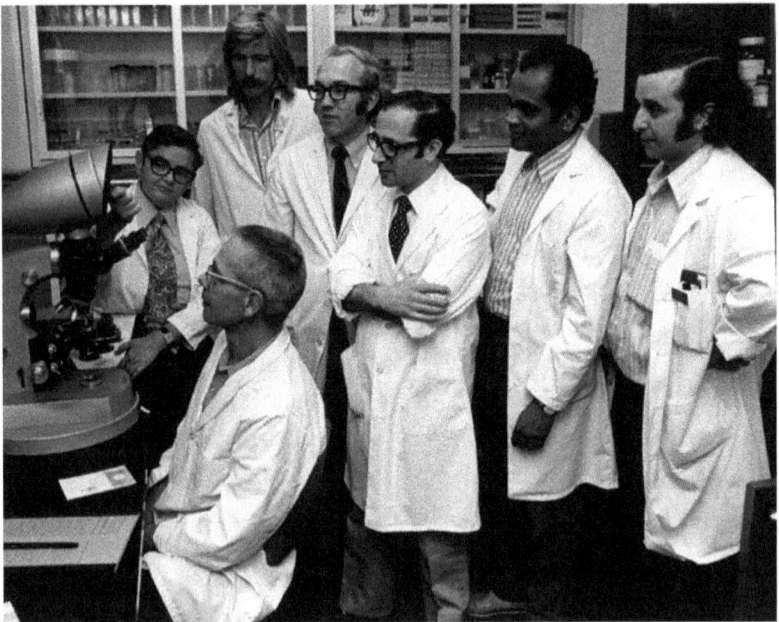

Figure 7.2:   From left to right, Herbert Soule, Marvin A. Rich, Charles McGrath, Justin McCormick, Jose Russo, Ramadandra Das, and Philip Furmanski. (The Experimental Pathology Laboratory was located on the second floor of the Prentis Building.)

wonderful experience. All of them shared so much of their experience with me; they cannot imagine how much I learned from them. To be surrounded by and collaborate with scientists who acted and thought differently was a wonderful experience for a young scientist like me.

7.2. How I learned to direct and organize a cancer research laboratory

My new role as a research scientist at the MCF was completely different than the one where I used to work, and it was not until around November 1973 that I introduced "the work logistic" into my daily jargon. Even though I do not have formal military training, there were certain terms that had stuck with me from my reading about the Gallic war. Therefore, I developed a logistic plan to assess my weakness and strategies, and define my goals. The immediate challenge was to adapt to my new position as a cancer researcher. I needed to quickly learn how to work with a team of researchers that I called the "viral team"; they were already well on their way in the search for a viral particle that could be the etiological factor of one of the most deadly diseases known to man, breast cancer. But it was like trying to catch a train already leaving the station. Whatever I had done up to that moment was only what my brain and hands had allowed me to do — funding had never been my domain. In the past, I'd needed to be the technician, the scientist that analyzed the data, the one that wrote the paper, and the whole research enterprise of my scientific world had been constrained by what I could do and what I knew how to do. In my limited perception, I was "my own boss." Until I arrived at MCF, obtaining the funds for doing research had not been my personal concern; the funds were there because the Director of the department or institute had shared their resources or because I was, after all, a pre- or a postdoctoral researcher. However, as a cancer researcher and also as a member of a team I needed to quickly learn what the others were doing, what I could contribute, how the funds were obtained, and who was behind them — and all this assimilation needed to be done incredibly fast because in those days the intellectual pressure to find the virus was tremendous. It was a national obsession to find a virus that would finally cure breast cancer. In other words, as great as it was to work in a team, my whole being reacted to the realization that the pace or tempo was not established by me but rather the leader of the team, the rest of its members, and the funding institution that was behind the project; in this case, the USA National Cancer Institute (NCI). It was not only the MCF that was on this task but several important laboratories around the world were also working on the same thing. I met most of them in April 1974 at my first meeting of the American Association for Cancer Research, and again at the international meeting in Pisa, Italy, held in October of the same year (Figure 7.3).

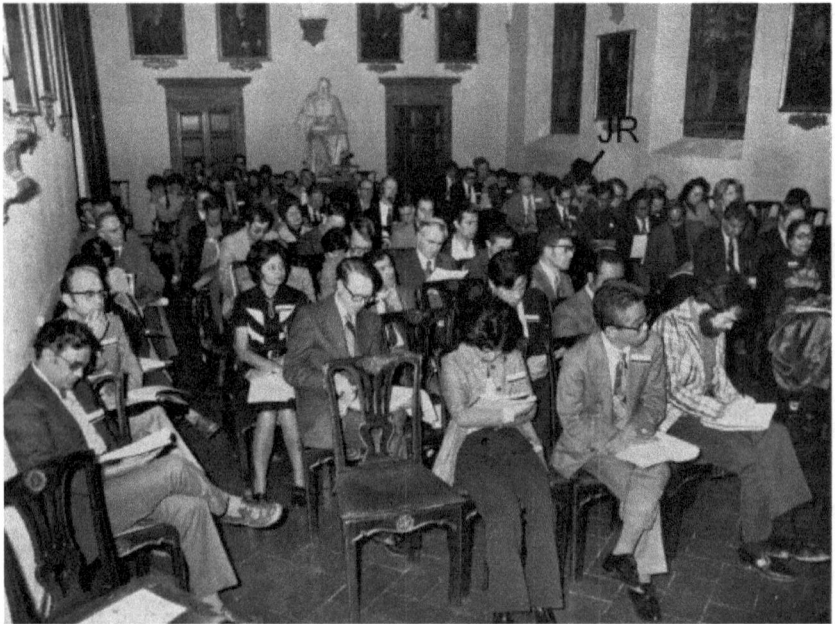

Figure 7.3: Photo of the ninth meeting on Mammary Cancer in Experimental Animals and Man, held in the historical lecture hall of the University of Pisa's Sapienza Building, October 1974. At the back, the memorial sculpture of Galileo Galilei who taught in that same conference room. In this meeting, only 87 participants were admitted, from the United States, the Netherlands, Italy, England, Denmark, Japan, France, Israel, Tunisia, and one each from the German Democratic Republic and Poland.

The first lesson that I learned working on a research team was the importance of deadlines and the establishment of achievable landmarks in the research project. The second thing was the realization that I was immersed in a situation where I felt like the rabbit in the Lewis Carroll story, running all the time in order to try to keep myself in place. This created in me an ambiguous reaction: exhilaration at being in the middle of the action, but also a visceral reaction and anxiety that seeded doubt. I started to wonder if this path was the one that I should follow; in other words, I was not convinced that the pursuit of a virus as the causative agent of breast cancer was not too narrow to be true, but even more than this intellectual challenge, *I felt that I wanted to be more independent.* In my self-searching I admit that the constraint of working on the viral team was the strongest influence on my feelings. An additional factor was that my return to Argentina to take a Professorship at the University of Tucuman was no longer an option due to the guerrillas that were starting to pull apart my native country (see Chapter 6). Therefore, I was in a position to achieve my goal of doing cancer research even though I felt the constraints of the viral team. Realistically, I had no way to return to Argentina until the political situation, later called the Dirty War, cleared. However, despite all these doubts, I realized that it would be premature to change my course and the most important issue was for me to honestly assess my situation. First was my recognition that although I have training in biochemistry and molecular biology (Chapter 4), my way of thinking was rooted in experimental pathology and cell biology, and I had expended many years making electron microscopy my first area of expertise, meaning that I was able not only to interpret the ultra-structure of a cell but also that I had the dexterity of an electron microscopist from the beginning to the end of the process, as I discussed in Chapter 4. More important, because of that expertise, I was hired as an experimental pathologist and electron microscopist. Therefore, I went to the root of my uneasiness, because something continued to niggle at me. I was technically the chief of the experimental pathology laboratory but I had to work within the already existing electron microscopy laboratory that was directed by Dr. William Arnold, and I needed to work with him and his technician

Mr. Ronald Bradley. The difficulty came with the sad realization that my rhythm was too fast for those who were already there. This created significant tensions during my first three months at the foundation. To their eyes I was like a bull in a china shop, disturbing their established rhythm with my accelerated pace. In retrospect, I understand how they felt, but back then I understood that the aim of the viral team, and thus my personal function, was to demonstrate whether or not there was a real viral particle in the breast cells. Therefore, the only way to resolve the situation was to have both Arnold and Bradley under my direct supervision, rather than as collaborators. This could only be achieved annexing the electron microscopy laboratory to my own laboratory, creating a unified unit under my direction. If I accomplished that I would have a broader base of operation as well as a more productive work environment. Marvin Rich understood this conflict and based on the low productivity and slow response of William Arnold, he decided that the electron microscopy laboratory should also be under my direction, and this was achieved before the end of that year. The small victory of broadening my operations made me more conscious that my best alternative was to be humble and to become a team player, learning from the other members of the viral team as much as I could, because the reality was that I had a lot to learn at that specific time of my life, so that is what I did.

7.2.1. *My relationship with the viral team*

Unfortunately, not all the members of the viral team were so easy to deal with (Figure 7.2). Charles McGrath had published in *Nature* and other important journals, and he was the "prima donna" of the group with the attitude that he would get the Nobel Prize for his discoveries while the other team members were only fillers. It should not be doubted that his assumption was partly right, and if the virus was demonstrated it would provide massive recognition for him as the second most important member of the team, after Marvin Rich. McGrath and I had few verbal encounters, so finally I spoke to him very frankly, making him understand that at that time in my life I was not his competitor and that the only thing that I wanted was to be sure that the viral particle was there. In time, I recognized that he also wanted to spread his wings and that he was unconventional for the standard of those days. In a certain way, he felt that the cage of the MCF was too small for him. In addition to our professional differences, there were also big contrasts between us personally: my small physical stature contrasted with his towering six and a half feet; I was monogamous and married to a lovely woman who was faithful to me, while he was divorced and with a tumultuous romantic life at that moment; I was very conservative, and he was liberal with all the mentality of a Berkeley trainee. Importantly, when we clarified our differences, it was more palatable to work with him, however after a few years he left the MCF.

Phillip Furmanski was the complete opposite of Charles McGrath; he had a pleasant, friendly, and informal appearance and personality that made him easy to reach and talk to. He was generous and always ready to teach what he knew; Phillip was a good person and an extremely important member of the team who provided great stability in the tumultuous situation triggered by McGrath. Phillip was a good friend of Marvin's; he was the silent partner that kept the group together.

With Justin McCormick, I developed a close friendship spurred by our trip to Pisa, where we discovered that we have similar tastes for religious art. During our stay, we visited many places near Pisa, journeying to Florence, Assisi, Rome, and the Vatican. Justin has been a lasting friend, and we kept in touch after he moved to Michigan State University in the early 1980s and even after I left the MCF in 1991.

The relationship that I developed with Herbert Soule was a different one; I was hungry to know the way that he had accomplished the isolation of MCF-7 cells, and he provided me a firsthand account of his adventures with the cells, from the specific moment that Michael Brennan gave him the three liters of pleural effusion through how he developed the cells until Brennan came to the lab and asked Soule to throw away the cells because of possible viral contamination. Of course, Herbert never destroyed the cells; he kept going, resulting in his great contribution to cancer research. He gave me, for my own collection, the original slides showing the cancer cells in the pleural effusion, and the primary tumor of Sister Malone. He also gave me the slides showing the MCF-7 cells in their 800 days in culture. He shared with me his early notes when he started culturing the MCF-7 cells. Herbert was a natural for culturing cells and although he was a heavy smoker and on many occasions he interrupted the work to have a cigarette, he never contaminated his cultures. He was a simple man and he liked the work that he was doing. His records were meticulous and he personally took care to maintain the cells alive. My affection for Herbert spurred me to rescue him in 1990 by incorporating him into my payroll when the MCF was suffering severe economic constraints and they were planning to dismiss him.

7.2.2. *Establishing a logistic plan*

The other aspect that I immediately saw in the experimental pathology laboratory was that, while I was well equipped to do morphological work, I lacked the facilities to do tissue cultures and molecular biology studies. I could not incorporate any of those facilities into my hiring package because the viral team already provided that expertise. To acquire those facilities would be more difficult than simply annexing the 2,000 square feet of laboratory space used by Electron Microscopy, which did eventually happen. But I still needed to optimize this situation and so waited until I could reconfigure the experimental pathology laboratory, making it possible to go from cell biology to exquisite molecular studies (see Chapter 10) by acquiring the equipment and tools for performing tissue culture and molecular biology. According to my logistic plan, it was something that I eventually needed to do, but in the meantime I would work with the others to obtain tissue cultures and molecular studies. That was the best course of action during my first 3 years at the MCF.

As chief of the laboratory, I forced myself to avoid the pitfall of micromanagement, and as a consequence my success would depend on hiring adequate technical associates to help me develop the research work. As discussed above, I knew that I could not diversify the resources of my laboratory more than I already had, therefore, the course of action that I found most plausible was to increase the critical mass of people working under my direction. That would help me develop research projects that had enough preliminary data to compete for extramural funds.

The increase in the size of my workforce would also give me enough time and breathing space for analyzing, elaboration of data, and creating new lines of research. I saw that this path was fundamental for my long-term success. Eventually, I was able to secure not only a position for Irma as a research scientist but with the addition of William Arnold, I had two research scientists and three technicians, namely Ronald Bradley, Peter Wells, and Joseph Saby, plus a photographer, Peter Kaspar, who helped us to process the increasing number of photographs that we generated every day in our search for the virus. Two additional people from Wayne State University, William Isenberg and an undergraduate student named David Salomon, joined us in the spring of 1974. This was the configuration of the experimental pathology laboratory at that time (Figure 7.4).

A positive aspect of this new paradigm in my life was that I also had in front of me the *breathing space to start a new line of research*, which could be completely different from the one that the viral team was doing. The caveat for this was that I must obtain extramural support to perform these activities, and this was one of the simplest metrics to measure my success as a scientist. All of these new frontiers in front of me, or in the logistic plans I called "fighting fronts," were not easy to digest at once because I was dealing with colleagues who had graduated and trained in the USA and that gave them a significant advantage over me. They spoke and wrote fluent English, they had done postdoctoral training with important investigators who were at that moment in leadership positions, and they already (at my own age of 31) had grants from the NCI, meaning that basically I was in a tennis match holding a baseball bat. I was a newcomer from the most remote country on the American continent, and during my first five months at the MCF there were moments I felt inadequate to the task of facing all these challenges and self-doubts. My only reassurance was that I had two important weapons on my side. One was that I had

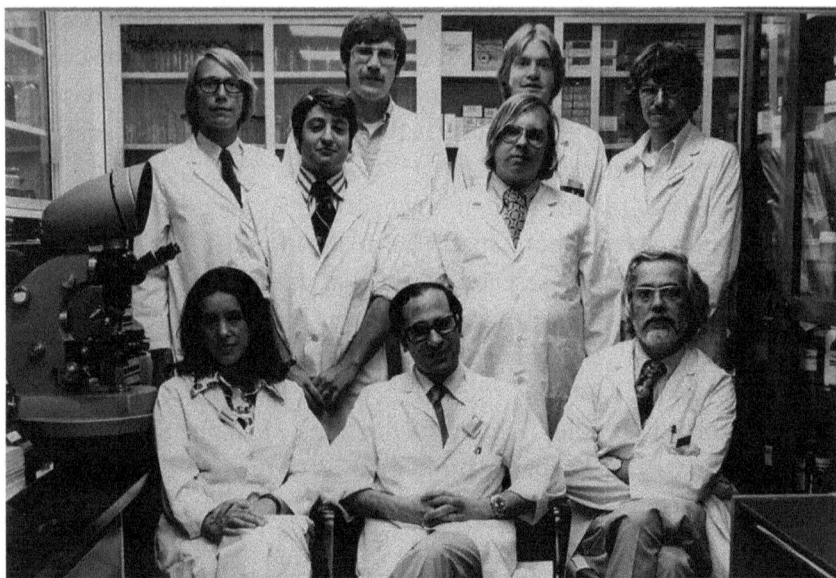

Figure 7.4: The experimental pathology laboratory team in the spring of 1974. From left to right: in the front row, Dr. Irma H. Russo, Dr. Jose Russo, Dr. William Arnold. In the second row: Joseph Saby, David Salomon, Peter Wells, Ronald Bradley, William Isenberg, and Peter Kaspar.

developed an active plan that motivated me to keep going, and the second was that I had the energy to work long hours and the ability to motivate people. In retrospect, I was right and the plan worked and allowed me to achieve the status of an independent research scientist in this country.

My logistic plan was simple. With the resources that I had, I divided my research approaches into three different paths. One was continuing to work with the viral team and ensure that Dr. William Arnold, Ronald Bradley, and Peter Kaspar were involved full-time in the search for the virus. The second group (which I called the experimental group) was formed by Peter Wells and Joseph Saby to work on understanding the process of cell transformation, tumorigenesis, and assimilating the emerging new technologies, such as immuno-cytochemistry at the light and electron microscopy level. Both of these projects were funded by the budget from the viral team.

The third group, funded by institutional funds, was the one that formed the Breast Cancer Research Laboratory (BCRL) with Irma H. Russo, William Isenberg, and Joseph Saby. The undergraduate student was also added to this group. In my logistic plan, the BCRL and the data gathered in the experimental group would give us the basis for constructing an independent research team. This was an excellent plan that brought us to the present time. Dividing the resources in this way allowed me to be not only productive on the viral team but also gave me the chance to develop new lines of research and update the technical landscape that was emerging in those days.

7.2.3. *Knowing to know*

I have learned, or probably inherited from my mother, the ability to listen, and I also developed the patience and stamina to be attentive to what other people say and do. These invaluable qualities allowed me to realize that I needed to know not just the members of the viral team, but also other members of the institution who were my seniors not only in age but in experience, and to learn from them how they had succeeded. Therefore, I started talking and listening to them. I found not only some excellent human beings but also outstanding research scientists with vast and varied experiences who, through their work and example, taught me how to make my plan of action a reality. Among those inspiring people was Dr. Samuel Albert, a Canadian physician who was in charge of biometry at the foundation and had developed a significant outreach program in metropolitan Detroit for collecting human breast milk to be used as a source in searching for the viral particle. The other scientist was Dr. Samuel Horowitz, a biologist-biophysicist working in the water and ion transport in frog ovocytes, a man with a sharp mind and successful grant record. Dr. Jerome Horwitz was a chemist who developed the AZT drug that was later used for AIDS treatment. Dr. Charles King was a chemist working in chemical carcinogenesis with whom I developed a great affinity due to our common work in that field, and Samuel Brooks was a chemistry professor at Wayne State University working in estrogen receptors. I must also recognize that Marvin Rich and his wife, Ruth, turned out to be good friends who helped Irma and I understand many social nuances of the American scientific community. By including us in their group of friends and acquaintances, Marvin and Ruth gave us the opportunity to meet many top researchers of that time, like Francesco Squartini, Hiafa Keydar, Craig Jordan, Russel Hilf, Pietro Gullino, Peter Bentvelzen, Ethiene Lafargues, Sol Spigelman, Michael Gallo, Roberto Ceriani, Diana Lopez, Daniel Medina, Nikki Agnatis, and Leon Dmochowski, to mention just a few. Some of them also became very good friends. Altogether, I developed a great affection for those senior members at the MCF because they offered me a friendship that taught and helped me understand clearly what I needed to succeed as an independent cancer researcher.

Undoubtedly this assessment and the development of a logistic plan was the smartest way to initiate and continue my cancer research career. But I would be extremely remiss if I did not recognize that Irma, my wife, companion, friend, and colleague, was a continuous source of wisdom and strength as I visualized the path to follow. It was her charm, good nature, and wittiness that allowed us to be easily admitted into the social and scientific environment. When I was in doubt, her reply was always, "*Jose, do you have something else better to do?*" The implication of that question was that she would be at my side in any new path we decided to take (see Chapter 4).

7.3. How I was involved in the search for a breast cancer virus

Marvin Rich was a national figure in virus cancer research who directed the MCF in its search for a breast cancer virus, however, later he became the leader of the viral team. When I met Marvin Rich at the Miami Winter Symposium in March 1973, he showed interest in my background in experimental pathology and electron microscopy, and he was the one who initiated my hiring at the MCF. I was employed that same year to be the chief of the experimental pathology laboratory and, as such, to also be part of his group. The aim of the scientific team was based on the knowledge that viruses induced breast cancer in experimental animals and that retroviruses were found in the milk of women who had a particularly high incidence of breast cancer. These findings were initiated to solve a basic problem in breast cancer control — the identification of that portion of the population at high risk of breast cancer. Dr. Samuel Albert, the Director of biometry at the MCF, established an extensive human milk collection network which covered the entire metropolitan Detroit area and was aimed at determining if the presence of a characteristic virus in milk could be indicative of a woman's risk of developing breast cancer. This study was ultimately not successful due to the intrinsic problems in analyzing these viruses in a medium that contains so many enzymes that destroy any type of RNA particle. This originated the idea that viruses could grow in normal or cancer cell cultures, and if this were the case then a vaccine aimed at breast cancer prevention in high-risk women could be developed. It was at this time that I arrived at the MCF, and the immediate task of the project was to search in human breast cells at the ultra-structural level for the presence of a retrovirus. Searching for the retrovirus in the breast cells required the use of an electron microscope, a tool that allowed us to see the internal structure of the cell. I was quite familiar with the electron microscope because of my training in ultra-structural cell biology with Burgos back in Mendoza (see Chapter 3 and Figure 7.5).

The quest for the retrovirus was part of a larger project funded by the NCI within the Virus Cancer Program. The thinking was that if a virus could be identified in this established human breast epithelial tumor cell line, it would link to the viral etiology of breast cancer.

7.3.1. *The viral hypothesis of cancer*

The idea that cancer could be caused by a virus was pioneered by Peyton Rous around 1910. He found a tumor in the back of a Plymouth Rock hen diagnosed as spindle cell sarcoma, but the interesting part of the story is that he could transplant the cells from

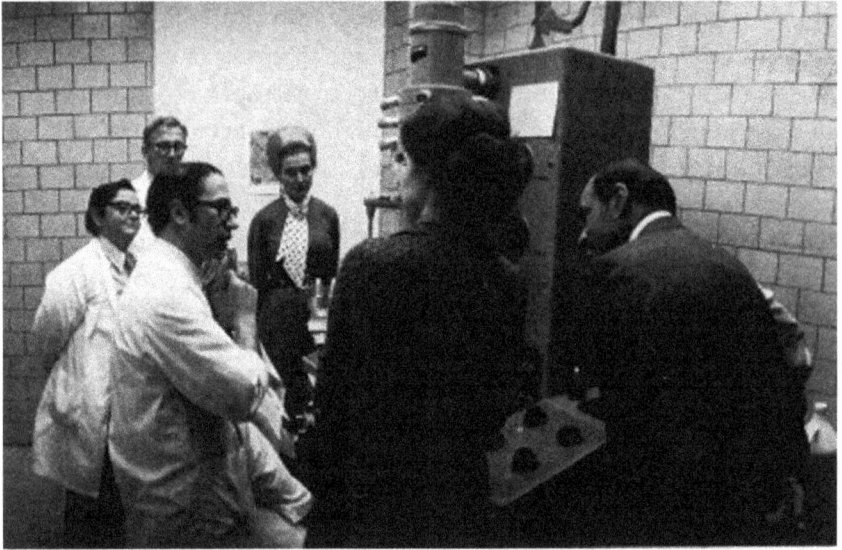

Figure 7.5:   The photo shows the electron microscope that was used to search for viral particles. From left to right: Dr. Jose Russo, Dr. Marvin Rich, Dr. Michael Brennan, Dollie Cole, Marvin A Frenkel and Julie Nixon Eisenhower. The Hitachi microscope was capable of magnifying an image 150,000 times.

one hen to another and the tumor was exactly the same. But his critical experiment was to obtain a filtrated extract of the tumor that did not contain spindle cancer cells and when injected into another hen reproduced the same type of tumor over and over again. The biological material that can pass through a filter is a virus now known as the Rous sarcoma virus (RSV). The discovery of the RSV was followed by the discovery of the Shope papillomavirus in 1935, the leukemia-causing virus in mice in 1940, and the Burkit lymphoma virus in 1958. The relevance of these discoveries was the idea that if viruses were the etiological cause of cancer, then the development of a vaccine could stop an infectious disease. This idea was blowing the minds of the cancer research community during the period from 1950 to 1980, and the viral hypothesis took prevalence in the thoughts of cancer researchers during that time. Excitement about the project also came from Howard Martin Temin, Renato Dulbecco, and David

Baltimore's seminal discovery of reverse transcriptase, for which they shared the Nobel Prize in Physiology or Medicine in 1975. Reverse transcriptase explained how tumor viruses act on the genetic material of the cell and introduced a revolutionary concept that contradicted the "central dogma" of molecular biology that genetic information flows exclusively from DNA to RNA to protein. Certain tumor viruses carry the enzymatic ability to reverse the flow of information from RNA back to DNA, using reverse transcriptase. Reverse transcriptase is the central enzyme in several widespread human diseases, most notably HIV, the virus that causes AIDS.

From 1973 to 1976, I was immersed in the viral etiology of cancer as I was suddenly embedded in the world of American science. I saw how scientists like Michael Gallo, Fred Rausher, Sol Spiegelman, the members of the viral team, and others were presenting evidence and new possibilities for and against the viral hypothesis. Another great moment in science came with the signing of the 1974 Cancer Act, which significantly increased the NCI's appropriations. Suddenly what had once been only a dream, due to financial constraints, was made reality and the sky was the limit. This was a contagious feeling that also got me; it was an exciting time to be a cancer researcher. It was in that period that *Julie Nixon Eisenhower* (Figure 7.5) visited our laboratory as part of the diffusion of the recently signed Cancer Act by then President Richard Nixon. She was a delightful woman who endured my explanation on how we used the electron microscope to search for the virus.

7.3.2. *The viral etiology of breast cancer*

The concept that a virus could be the etiological cause of breast cancer came from experimental data in mice and the discovery that similar virus particles were present in human milk, human mammary epithelial cells, and cell lines derived from human breast cancers. The etiologic role of viruses in the mammary tumors of mice was first demonstrated by John Bittner in 1936 [2]. The classic studies of Bittner established that mammary cancers in mice could be caused by a virus which in turn could be transmitted through nursing milk.

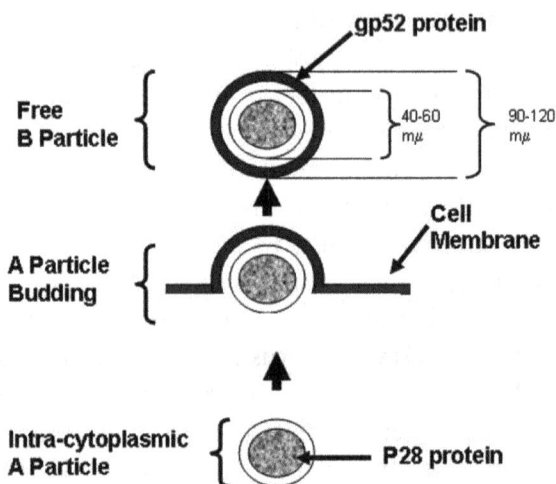

Figure 7.6:   Evolution of the MuMTV from a particle synthesized in the cell and transported to the apical portion of the cell membrane via the Golgi apparatus. The cell membrane (thick solid line) that surrounds the *A particle* reacts against a gp52 protein. After the budding, the *B particle* is free and can infect other cells. The core of the virus (gray in the photo) contains a 70S RNA with reverse transcriptase properties.

These viruses are classified as type B oncornaviruses (Figure 7.6). Their genetic information is coded by 70S RNA. They possess reverse transcriptase (RNA-dependent DNA polymerase) enzymes and biophysical properties similar to those of the other oncornaviruses known to induce neoplasia in several host species. Murine mammary tumor virus, or MuMTV, is an endogenous virus of mice — meaning that the nucleic acid information for MuMTV is contained in the genome of every cell of the host.

It is known that there are at least two routes of natural transmission for the mouse mammary tumor virus: by way of the milk and by vertical transmission through viral genomic information integrated into, and transmitted by, the germ cells. This basic knowledge leads to the speculation that, due to the difference in incidence of the breast cancer population, looking for the presence of a virus in the milk of those women was a viable and credible task which could provide the answer to not only the etiology of breast cancer but also explain the differences in incidence according to race and geographic location [3, 4]. For example, the Parsi community of Bombay was particularly suitable for these studies. The Parsi migrated from Persia to India in the seventh century and as a consequence of their strict prohibition against intermarriage constitute a population that has been inbred for almost 1,500 years. The incidence of breast cancer in Parsi women is somewhat less than that in European women but it is three times higher than in the non-Parsi, Hindu population of Bombay [3, 4]. Virus particles with the characteristics of known animal oncornaviruses were observed in the milk of these women. These particles were morphologically similar to MuMTV. However, the tools which have been available for the detection and quantification of oncornaviruses have proved less than satisfactory when applied to the routine, large-scale testing of complex body fluids. In 1973, three avenues of approach were available for the detection of these viruses: morphological, biochemical, and immunological.

Several electron microscopic studies have described the distribution of virus-like particles in negatively stained preparations of human milk [3, 4]. Unfortunately, exposure to human milk could destroy the morphological integrity of exogenously added MuMTV [5], and furthermore human milk contains membranous vesicles and casein micelles which could be easily mistaken for oncornaviruses in negatively stained preparations. This was the reason the negatively staining technique was abandoned in favor of electron microscopic studies, introducing instead the use of thin sectioning of material embedded in epoxy material and stained with heavy metals like uranium and lead for better contrast. The use of thin sectioning techniques for the electron microscope, in addition to differential centrifugation techniques for the isolation and quantification of these viruses — helped by the discovery of reverse transcriptase and its specific association with RNA tumor viruses [6–8] — provided a more reliable technology in the search for a viral particle.

The first initiative of the MCF, in association with other organizations under the sponsorship of the NCI, was to collect the milk of nursing women in the metropolitan Detroit area. Unfortunately, it was found that human milk contains factors that would obviate the reliable detection of reverse transcriptase [9], and one such inhibitor was ribonuclease, which can mask the activity of more than 108 virus particles per milliliter. These studies were followed by using a particular radioimmunoassay for virus antigens but a crucial step was the isolation of virus proteins of viral cores [10], specifically isolating proteins which were associated with the oncornavirus-like particle in human milk. This protein was present in reverse transcriptase positive milks, and absent in negative milks. Its distribution in density gradients of core preparations coincided with the core-containing bands and their reverse transcriptase activity. However, detection in the milk was found not to be the best approach for isolating and purifying the virus. It was thought likely that the virus-like particles found in human milk originated from the normal, milk secreting, epithelial cells of the breast, and that these cells might be better indicators of the virological status of the human host than the milk itself. The importance of this reasoning was that these cells could serve not only as a potential virus source, but also as a substrate for infectivity studies.

7.4. The search for a virus in normal breast epithelial cells

The discovery that milk was not the best source from which to identify the putative virus led to the idea that culturing normal breast epithelial cells would be another source to identify the pro or viral particles. We were not the first ones to culture breast epithelial cells and others [11–13] had already published some material using breast tissue as a source for culturing breast epithelial cells. Therefore, since human milk was known to contain such cells, members of the viral team attempted to use this fluid as a source for initiating cultures of mammary epithelial cells. It was found that the cells in the milk of actively lactating donors were present in very low concentration (generally fewer than 104 cells per sample), and that most of the cells were damaged and would not grow. Phillip Furmanski used sequential samples of milk from single donors and observed that a peak in the cell concentration of milks occurred just after the onset of weaning, when the volume of secreted breast fluid was drastically reduced. These cells, when placed in culture with the addition of autologous serum, develop into monolayers of growing epithelial cells [14]. The important step was to demonstrate that these cells grown in culture were real epithelial cells and for that purpose we studied them under the electron microscope. Working with Phillip Furmanski, we used breast fluid obtained from human donors after weaning. The cells collected were diluted in a culture medium and grown *in vitro* using the serum from the same woman. After a couple of weeks, they formed monolayers in the culture (Figure 7.7(a)).

It was important to demonstrate that those cells were epithelial and that when we studied them under the electron microscope we needed to be sure that we were able to maintain the morphology of

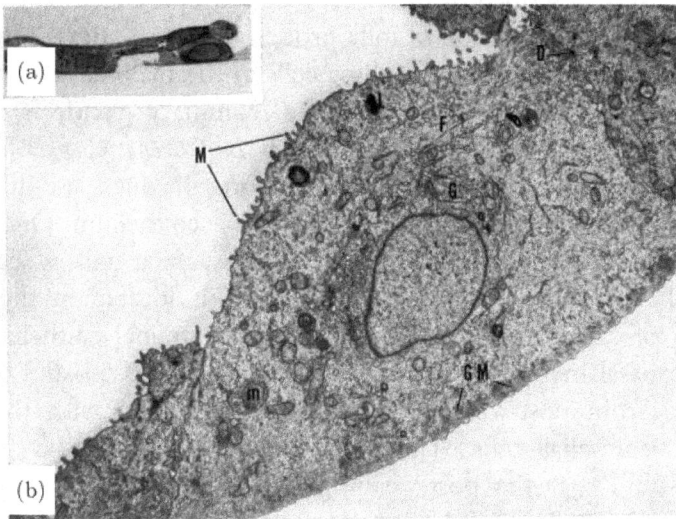

Figure 7.7: (a) One micron section of human epithelial cells from post-weaning fluid in culture, magnification ×850. (b) Human breast epithelial cells from post-weaning fluid after two weeks in culture. Noted are microvilli (M), desmosomes (D), mitochondria (m), filaments (F), Golgi apparatus (G), lysosome (L), granular material in the basal portion cell (GM) (×7,500). Reprinted with permission from Ref. [15].

the cells. We fixed them in the culture flask and detached the full monolayer using propylene oxide, which dissolves the plastic beneath the cells without altering their structure [15] (Figure 7.7(a)). This technical detail of detaching the cells from the plastic using propylene oxide was a significant technical advantage over the usual way of scraping the cells from the flask using a rubber policeman, or scraper. The technique that we developed allowed us to see the cell to cell interaction without interrupting their normal pattern of growth (Figures 7.7(a) and 7.7(b)).

These cultured cells isolated from post-weaning human breast fluids were truly epithelial. They were characterized by having an extensive system of cell junctions, cellular polarity, surface differentiation, and secretory activity, all features of mammary epithelium. We found a finely granular material in the Golgi vesicles, very similar to that in the Golgi vesicles of the lactating mammary gland in mice described by other authors [16,17], which represented the synthesis and secretion of milk protein (Figures 7.8(a)–7.8(c)).

The topographic origin of these cells in the mammary gland was of great interest for our studies. The mammary gland, as I have described in my 2004 book *Molecular Basis of Breast Cancer* [18], is a secretory organ covered by epithelium along the ducts and ductules. Two types of cells are found in the glandular epithelium. One is the epithelial cell that surrounds the lumen into which milk is secreted. The other is the myoepithelial cell, which is located in the basal portion of ducts and ductules, between the luminal epithelial layer and the basal membrane. The ultra-structural characteristics of cells cultured from post-weaning fluids were consistent with those of luminal epithelial cells. Therefore, a main contribution was to demonstrate that the post-weaning fluids contain a much higher concentration of epithelial cells, which retain the capacity to grow in short-term cultures, as has been shown by Phillip Furmanski *et al.* [14]. The cells were detached from the ductal lining during the involution of the breast at the end of lactation, and, more important, they were viable cells that could grow optimally in a culture medium with autologous serum. One of the inherent problems that emerged

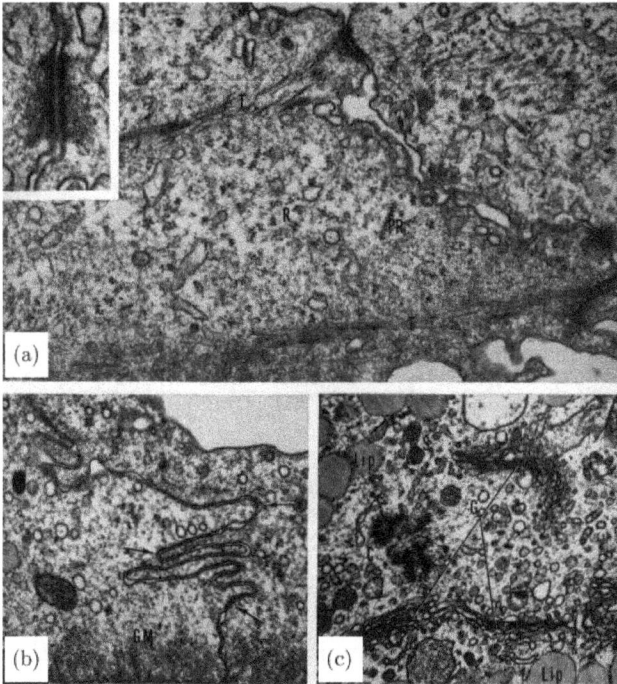

Figure 7.8: (a) Two cells joined by desmosomes in the apical and basal poles of the cells. Numerous tonofilaments (T) are present, some confluent, forming tonofibrils ending in the terminal web of the desmosomes. Free ribosomes (R) and polyribosomes (PR) are in the cytoplasm, (×34,500). The upper inset shows a desmosome (×60,000). (b) Cytoplasmic interdigitations (arrows) between the epithelial cells from the post-weaning fluid. The granular material (GM) is apparently attached to the cell membrane (×18,200). (c) Golgi apparatus (G) and vesicles with secretory material (S) surrounding the centrioles (C). Upper left corner and lower right corner, lipid droplets (Lip) (×18,200). Reprinted with permission from Ref. [15].

from the study of these cells was that after several passages (less than 10), they were not growing any longer and during this small span of time, we were unable to detect at the ultra-structural level any pre-viral or viral particle. The failure to show viral particles in the normal breast epithelial cells obtained from the post-weaning fluid was not a deterrent for us, and we pursued the next phase, which was to seek the virus in a cancer cell line.

7.5. The viral team's quest for a human breast cancer virus

The demonstration by the Sol Spiegelman group [19] that nucleotide sequences homologous to the viruses known to cause cancer in mice were expressed in the messenger RNA fraction of malignant human breast cancers awakened interest in the search for a viral etiology of human breast cancer, and the objective of the viral team was to look not in the human milk or in normal human breast epithelial cells but in a human breast cancer cell line that was originated in the MCF and called the MCF-7 cells [20].

7.5.1. *The first human breast cancer cell line*

MCF-7 is a breast cancer cell line isolated from a 69-year-old Caucasian woman. Dr. Michael Brennan, president of the MCF at the time, was treating the patient, who also happened to be a nun. She had what appeared to be a tumor mass in her right breast, and the tissue removed was not confirmatory of cancer. Five years later, however, after noticing a lump/discoloration, a second operation revealed a malignant adenocarcinoma. Over the next 3 years, local recurrences were treated with radiotherapy and hormonotherapy. In the process of removing the chest wall nodules, a pleural effusion was discovered (Figures 7.9(a) and 7.9(b)).

The cluster of neoplastic cells found in the pleural fluid was strikingly similar to those of neoplastic cells growing in the primary tumor. MCF-7 was the first stable human breast cancer cell to be isolated; it was maintained by Herbert Soule for almost 30 years [20]. In the last 45 years, this cell line has generated more than 26,000 papers. This abundant literature clearly shows the importance of this cell line and to discuss the content of those articles is beyond the scope of this chapter and this book, but it is important to describe here some basic biology of this cell line, first in tribute to the memory of my dear colleague Herbert Soule (Figure 7.2) and second to revise important experiments done in the author's laboratory that paved the way for further development and use of this cell line.

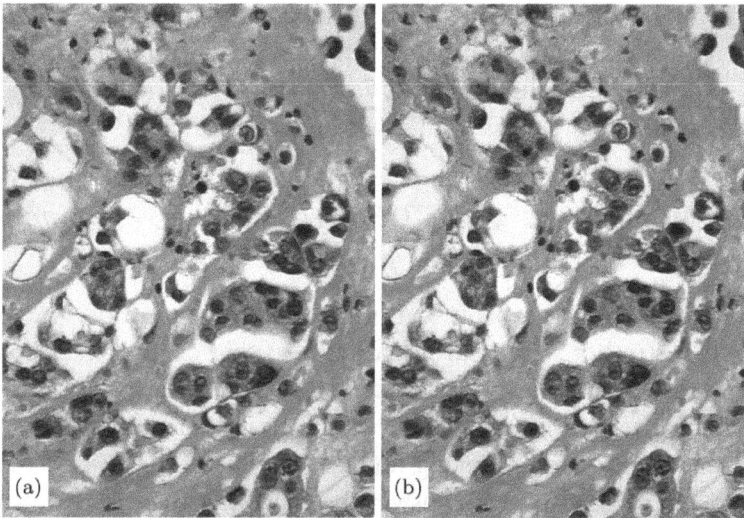

Figure 7.9: Histologic section of pleural effusion clot, from which MCF-7 were originated. Stained with H&E (×200).

Since its initial description [20], MCF-7 has been verified to be from humans both biochemically and cytologically [21]. The demonstration of human alpha-lactalbumin [22] and estrogen receptor protein [23, 24] in these cells supports its origin in the human breast tissue. This cell line contains receptor proteins specific for estrogen, (ER) androgen, glucocorticoids, and progesterone [24]. The high concentration of these receptors in MCF-7 has made the use of this cell line the primary source for the isolation of the ER protein and the developing of antibodies that are used now in the clinic for detecting the presence of estrogen receptors in the paraffin-embedded tissue of breast cancer.

The behavior of MCF-7 cells, as observed morphologically when grown in collagen-coated sponges [25] and in athymic mice [26, 27], indicates the value of the cell line in understanding biological aspects of malignancy at the cellular level. In this chapter of my memoirs, I will dedicate Section 7.6 to describe how I faced MCF-7 cells as a target for a viral search and in Section 7.7, I will narrate the history of the 734B particle as a putative breast cancer virus. Suffice it to say that in my perspective as an experimental pathologist the search for the virus was important in itself and the demonstration (or not) at the ultra-structural level that the virus 734B was there could have a clear indication that a virus was implicated in breast cancer.

7.5.2. *My encounter with MCF-7 cells for understanding basic bio-pathological questions*

In retrospect, I must explain that in that specific period of time from 1973 to 1976 there were burning questions that needed to be solved if we were to focus all our attention on MCF-7, a breast cancer cell line, in the search of a viral particle. Therefore, among my priorities at that moment, besides looking for the presence of the 734B putative virus in MCF-7 cells, was to answer the following questions: Was this cell a bonafide luminal epithelial cell and not a myoepithelial one? Was MCF-7 able to reproduce the original tumor pattern when cultured in a tridimensional matrix mimicking the structures from which the cells were originated in the pleural effusion? Were the MCF-7 cells forming a provirus or viral structure that could be detected using immuno-cytochemical methods? The detection of complex proteins that were enameled in a fashion similar to the oncornavirus observed in the mouse model would be of great value even if the cells were not forming the full budding viral particle as shown in Figure 7.6.

7.5.2.1. *Are MCF-7 cells luminal?*

MCF-7 was initially described by light microscopy [20] as being comprised of polyhedral epithelial cells and confirmed by scanning electron microscopy (Figures 7.10(a) and 7.10(b)). In confluent cultures or in those seeded at a high cell density, cells tended to be compact or laterally compressed, but usually retained contact with the substratum. Cultures less than seven days post seeding and those not grown to confluence contained cells that were low, cuboidal in nature. The pattern of growth — small patches before getting into confluence — was the very characteristic of the MCF-7 cells, and we captured them using the scanning electron microscope depicted in

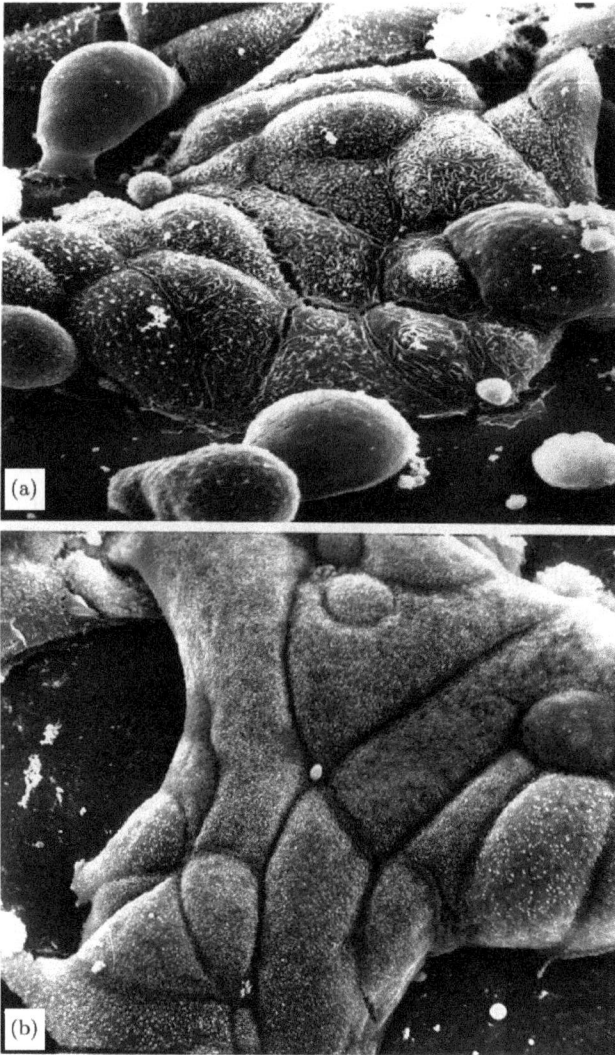

Figure 7.10: Scanning electron micrograph of MCF-7 cells growing in plastic surface (×400).

Figure 7.10. We have described in more detail a comparative morphological pattern of different human breast cell lines *in vitro* in our book *Techniques and Methodological Approaches in Breast Cancer Research*, published by Springer in 2014 [66].

Using the same cells but prepared for thin sectioning after being embedded in plastic, we were able to study them under the electron microscope. The cells maintained the epithelial pattern with separation of tissue and lumen by an interface of contiguous cell margins tightly bound together by occluded junctions (Figure 7.11). This polarity was also observed in breast cells and tumor cultures derived from other mammals [28, 29], but this was the first time that the MCF-7 was scrutinized for ultra-structural observations. The cells were characterized by the presence of microvilli, which increase the luminal surface area, and by the accumulation of secretory vesicles at the free apical cell margins, as depicted in Figure 7.11. We observed differences among individual cells that were entirely consistent with the malignant origins of the cell line [25]. The combination of desmosomes, tonofilaments, and intracytoplasmic lumina, which are the markers used for identifying breast cells in culture [30], were all observed in MCF-7 cells, but seldom were all three markers present in the same cell (Figure 7.11(b)). Desmosomes were infrequent among cells of young, growing cultures which were joined together largely by tight junctions. Microfilaments, likewise, were plentiful in most cells but were bundled into tonofilaments, primarily in cells of long established cultures. Intracellular lumina were extremely rare among our samples but occurred fairly often under certain experimental conditions, such as when inoculated into athymic mice [27]. Two of these characteristics, intracellular lumina and tonofilaments, have been proposed as indicators of malignancy [31], mainly since they are found in carcinoma *in situ* and more frequently in invasive carcinoma [31]. Derivation of the basement membrane from epithelial cells has been described in animals and in cell culture [32]. Although the presence of the basement membrane has not been fully demonstrated in the normal human breast epithelium in the culture, it may be significant that this lamella is lacking in the flask and collagen-coated sponge cultures of MCF-7 [33]. MCF-7 cells have a secretory potential, although it is largely inactive and unregulated. Typical indications of secretory activity were the aggregation of a few vesicles and granules just beneath the plasma membrane at the free surface and a concomitant moderate elaboration of endoplasmic reticulum and Golgi apparatus (Figures 7.11(c) and 7.11(d)). However, a few cells bore large accumulations of membrane-bound material filling the distal

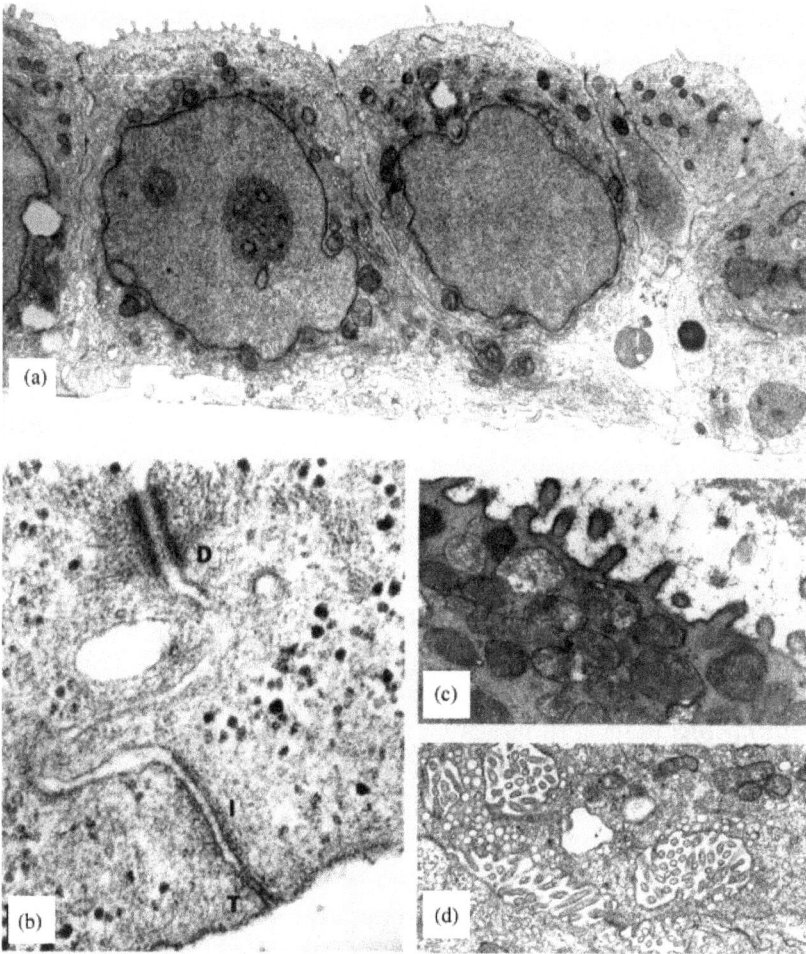

Figure 7.11: (a) Transversal section of MCF-7 cell monolayer (×4,000). (b) Attachment between two cells with a tight junction (T), intermediate junctions (I) and a desmosome (D), (×81,000). (c) Secretory vesicles clustered beneath the plasma membrane (×60,000). (d) Microvilli on a lumen between cells (×50,000). All sections were stained with lead citrate and uranyl acetate.

part of the cytoplasm, with similar structures appearing outside the plasma membrane. Thus, in any given culture, the level of secretory activity varies from cell to cell. In this feature, MCF-7 resembles mammary malignancies and certain previously described dysplasias [31, 34] more closely than normal breast epithelial cells [31, 35–37].

MCF-7 was a cell line with certain ultra-structural characteristics, which allowed it to be distinguished from other human breast cell cultures [30, 35, 38, 39]. It was also morphologically distinct from mammary cultures of other species [40, 41].

7.5.2.2. *Is MCF-7 able to reproduce the original tumor pattern when cultured in a tridimensional matrix?*

Various *in vitro* methods have been used to determine and characterize the malignant potential of tumor cells [42–48]. MCF-7 cells cultured in semisolid media, like agar methocel, formed colonies and when seeded in a collagen matrix they formed ball structures or solid masses of cells indistinguishable from those formed by primary breast cancer cells *in vitro*. We decided to use collagen-coated cellulose sponges for testing the three-dimensional expression of tumor morphology and for the investigations of its cellular inter-relations.

This system has been used in the study of various cells including HeLa, rodent ascites hepatoma, and explants of chick embryonic heart and liver [48]. Different tumors have been tested by the same method, including a mouse mammary carcinoma, a human cervical squamous cell carcinoma, and human explants grew and reproduced the organized structure of the original tumor. With Ronald Bradley (Figure 7.4), we studied the morphologic pattern exhibited by the MCF-7 cells growing in the collagen-coated cellulose sponge, and it was beautifully found that they developed a similar pattern found in both the antecedent primary tumor and the pleural metastasis from which this cell line was derived (Figure 7.12).

The primary breast tumor was a scirrhous carcinoma presenting islands of atypical epithelial cells with large nuclei, prominent nucleoli, and mitoses. In some areas, the cells were fairly close, forming clusters of 6–10 cells per level of section separated by connective tissue. In other areas, the clusters were larger and showed pseudo lumina, which were formed by necrosis of the central cells and determined the formation of duct-like structures.

The metastatic cells obtained from the pleural effusion material (Figure 7.9) were arranged in clusters and duct-like structures. Isolated

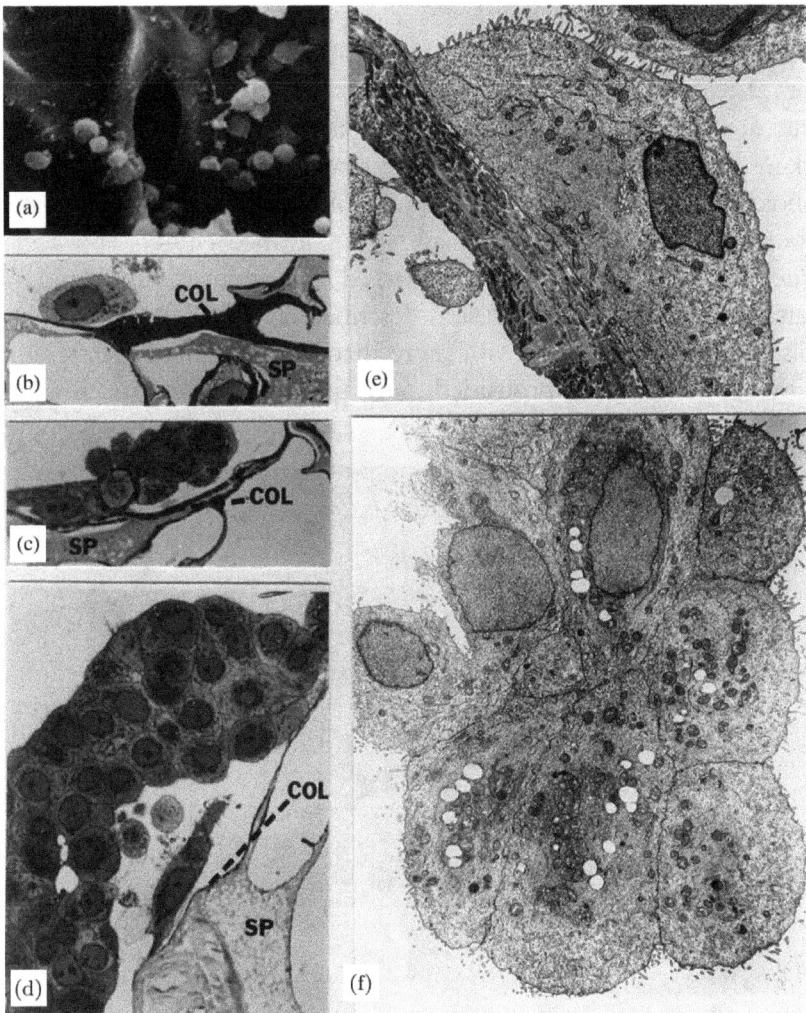

Figure 7.12: (a) Scanning electron micrograph of MCF-7 cells attached to the collagen-coated sponge (×400). (b) A single MCF-7 cell attached to the collagen (COL), SP sponge (toluidine blue) (×600). (c) A single cell attached to the collagen-coated cellulose sponge (×4,000). (d) Small cluster of MCF-7 cells partially attached to the collagen coat (COL), SP sponge (toluidine blue) (×600). (e) Large cluster of MCF-7 cells protruding into the sponge (SP) cavity. The collagen (COL) is seen as a thin, darkly stained layer (toluidine blue) (×600). (f) A vertical section through a cluster of cells similar to that described in 7.12(e) (×2,000). Panels (a)–(f) were reproduced with permission from Ref. [67].

cells were trapped in the fibrin clot, together with erythrocytes, granulocytes, and lymphocytes. The number of cells in a cluster varied from 2 to 50 per level of section. Some clusters showed a lumen-like structure (left by degenerated cells), while in other instances, nuclear pyknosis was observed. The duct-like structure appeared layered with cuboidal or flat epithelial cells. The cells cultured in the collagen-coated sponge did not grow in monolayers, but formed clusters and acinar structures with the same pattern observed in the primary tumor and the material from the pleural effusion described above (Figure 7.13). The cells formed large clusters with more than a hundred cells per level of section. The clusters protruded into the sponge interstices as an

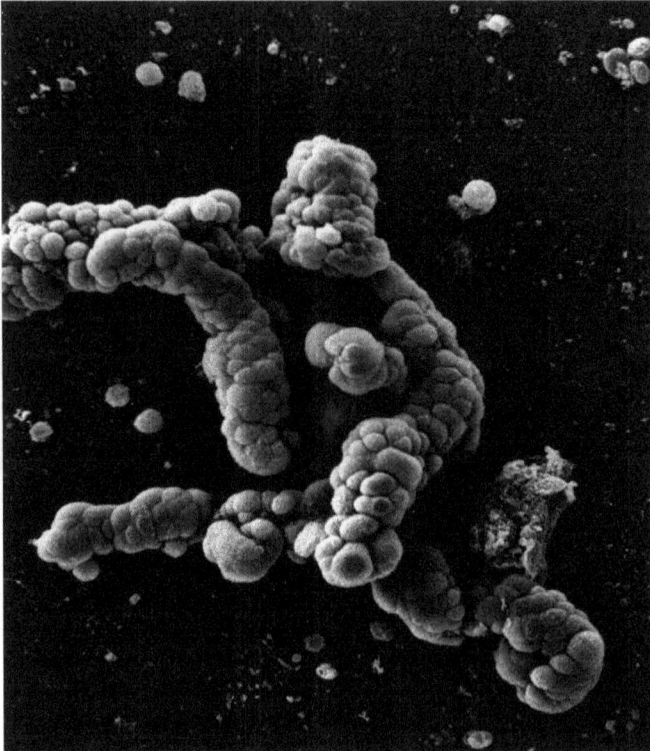

Figure 7.13: Scanning electron microscopy of cells recovered from the supernatant medium by centrifugation on a Millipore filter showing long arrays of densely packed, small round cells, with sharply defined cell limits (×2,000).

organoid structure that remained attached to the collagen coat by only a few cells. Like the original tumor, the clusters formed lumen-like structures via a degeneration of the central cells of the mass; liquid and cell detritus accumulated in the lumina. Lumen formation was at random; some large clusters did not show lumen, whereas others formed lumen eccentrically. Electron microscopic observations revealed that the cells surrounding a lumen in its early formation did not possess microvilli, but appeared in later development and were oriented toward the lumen [25]. The cells grown on sponge presented the same moderate degree of atypia seen in the tumor from which they were derived, but they presented more mitotic figures and fewer pyknotic cells. Similar structure was observed in free-floating cells recovered from the culture medium (cells which apparently became detached from the collagen coating) (Figures 7.13 and 7.14). *The most remarkable finding was that the morphogenesis memory of these cells is unaltered by long passage in vitro.* This had previously been demonstrated for mouse mammary carcinoma cells [49] but never before in human breast cancer cells.

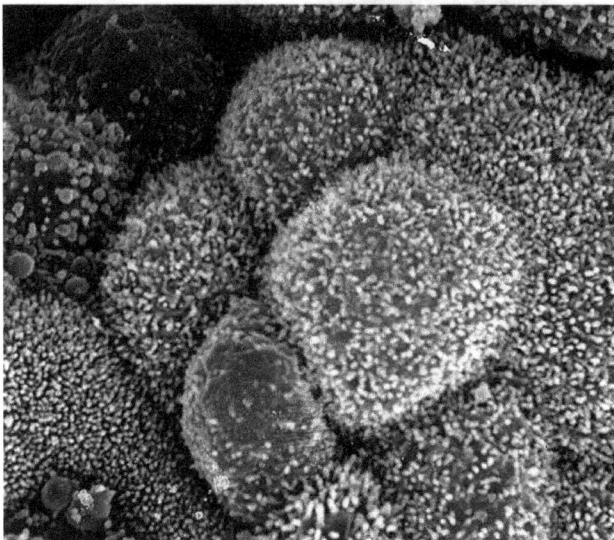

Figure 7.14: Higher magnification of the surface of the cell as shown in Figure 7.13. Covered by uniform type of microvilli all over the surface, but microvilli differ widely from cell to cell, (×20,000). Reproduced with permission from Ref. [67].

7.5.2.3. *Are MCF-7 cells forming a provirus or viral structure that could be detected using immuno-cytochemical methods?*

Because the breast cancer cells were also producing secretory material, it was easy to get confused by proviral or viral particles, making the search more arduous.

Basically, the molecular studies indicated that the amount of viral production would be very low, therefore the search for a vital particle that resembled the oncornavirus depicted in Figure 7.5 was a real task. Structures like the one shown in Figures 7.15–7.17 were commonly observed in our material and none of them were real provirus or viral particles.

In our quest to identify viral particles in human breast epithelial cells, we devised several strategies; one of them was to use

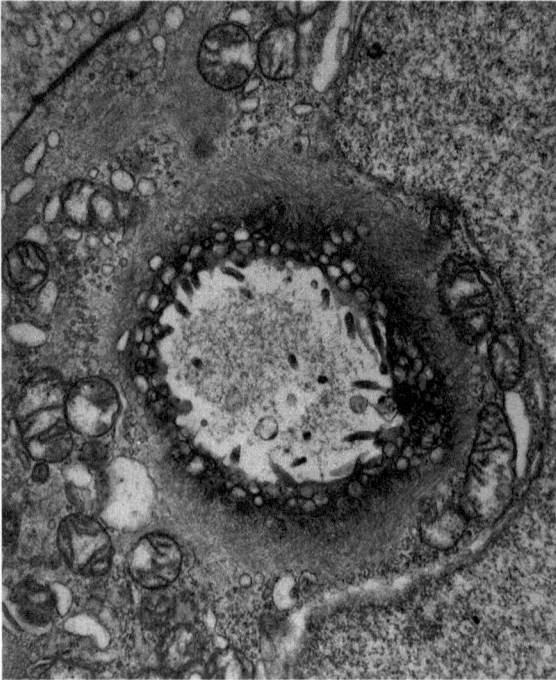

Figure 7.15: Cross-section of a pseudo lumina of MCF-7 cells growing in a heterologous host showing the formation of microvilli and secretory material.

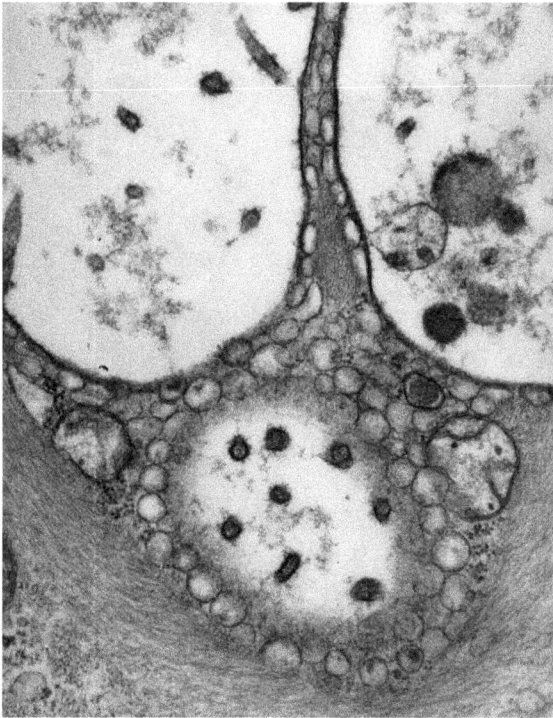

Figure 7.16: Luminal spaces formed in MCF-7 cells showing cross-section of microvilli that look like bound membrane particles.

immune-localization of pre-particles that could indicate that the cell could produce a viral particle. In 1975, working with William Arnold and Herbert Soule, we utilized murine mammary tumor cells obtained from a primary culture of spontaneous adenocarcinoma in BALB/c x C3H mouse and the human cancer cells MCF-8, a stable of cells derived from a hormone-induced tumor cell line developed previously by Herbert Soule that were supposed to contain the oncornavirus [50]. Using these two cell lines, we decided to utilize the technique recently described by Sternberger [51, 52], which consisted of visualizing a cellular protein that works as the antigen, using an antibody against the protein that was coupled to a peroxidase–anti-peroxidase complex which could be visualized as a dark complex under the microscope (Figure 7.18).

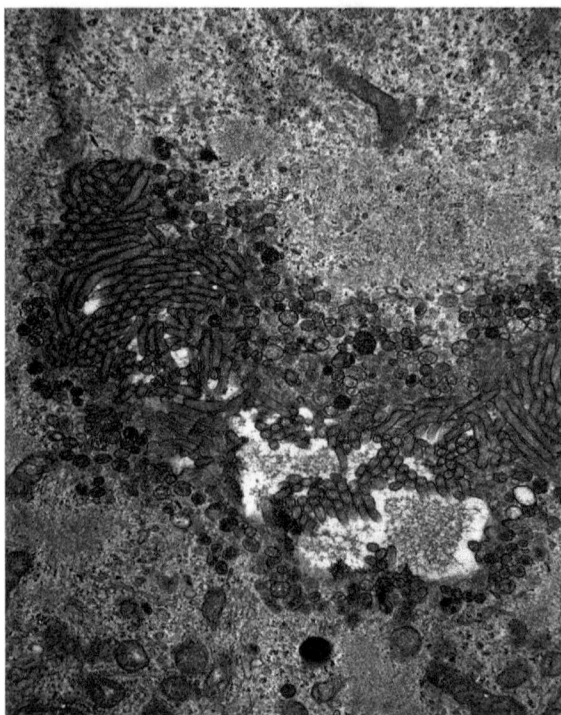

Figure 7.17: Cross-section of an intercellular lumina of MCF-7 cells growing in a heterologous host showing the formation of microvilli and secretory material.

As depicted in Figure 7.18, the reaction was limited to a single layer of PAP molecules which may lie so close together as to render an area nearly electron opaque (Figure 7.18(a)). Preparations revealed considerable structural detail within budding MuMTV particles (Figures 7.18(b) and 7.18(c)). The PAP complex was detecting the gp52 protein that was the external coat of the virus (see also Figure 7.6). Most MCF-8 cells were unreactive and free of PAP particles; of the reactive cells, there was no morphological evidence indicating that these cells produced the proviral proteins or the whole viral particle. No budding virions were seen in MCF-8 cells. Although masterfully done, the technique was a step forward in our abilities to detect viral particles using these new methodologies but it was negative in those cells that were supposed to carry the 734b particle. This negative result forced us to speculate that the PAP complex was too coarse and maybe what was

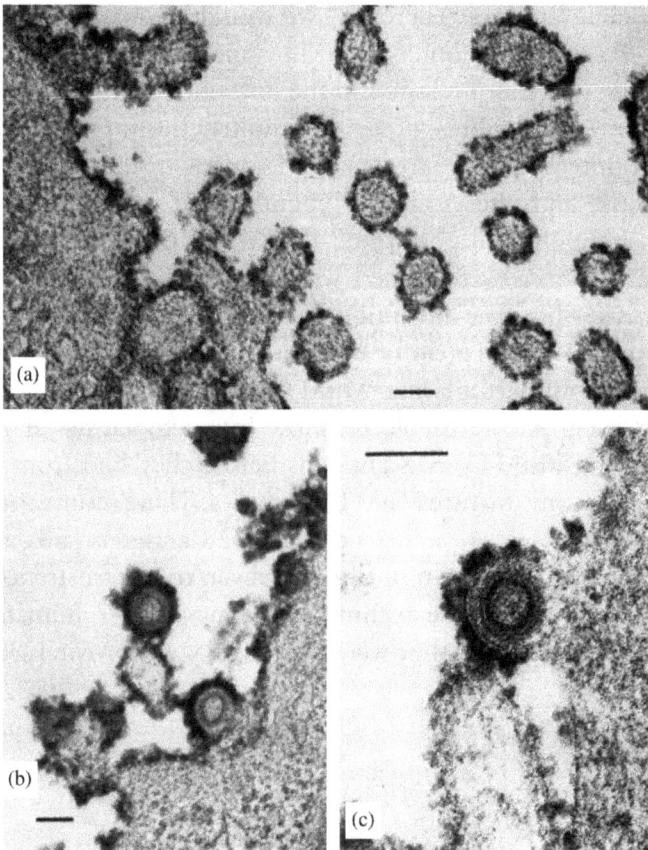

Figure 7.18: (a) Round dense anti-peroxidase molecular complexes pinpoint the position of anti-MuMTV antibodies that recognize the gp52 protein. The reaction is confined to the external plasma membrane surface and surrounds the microvilli of the murine primary tumor cells (MTPC). (Scale 0,1 micrometer). (b) PA complexes cluster tightly over the surface of MuMTV virions budding from a MTPC cell. (c) Concentric layers of PAP, envelope, outer and inner shells, and lucent center in a MuMTV particle in MTPC cell.

needed was to use a finer marker, significantly smaller than the PAP complex (8–12 nm) which could help us detect small proviral complexes. Using this mind frame in collaboration with Dr. Ray Weigand, who had replaced Dr. William Arnold, we decided to use ferritin as a marker. It was more than 10 times smaller than the PAP complex. This method allowed us simultaneous observation of viral ultra-structure and detection of the labelling product. Therefore, we would be able to demonstrate the intracellular localization of a MuMTV antigen.

Both the viral morphology and the immune-ferritin label (labelled MuMTV antigen) could be observed simultaneously. For this purpose, we used a primary culture from a spontaneous mammary tumor of a C3H mouse, and after fixation we embedded in Araldite, a softer plastic than Epon, and performed the typical 600 Å thick sections. These thin sections were etched with hydrogen peroxide to expose the protein for binding the antibody contained in the rabbit antisera against purified p28 protein of the MuMTV (Figure 7.6) which was located in the intracytoplasmic MuMTV, or *particle A*. As illustrated in Figure 7.19, we were able to show intracytoplasmic *A particles* containing the MuMTV p28 antigens before they bud from the cell surface and become mature MuMTV particles. These results confirmed that intracytoplasmic *A particles* contain p28 antigens [53] and that we were able to detect them *in situ*. However, to our frustration when we applied this innovative technique to our MCF-7 human breast epithelial cancer cell line, they were negative for any proviral sequence.

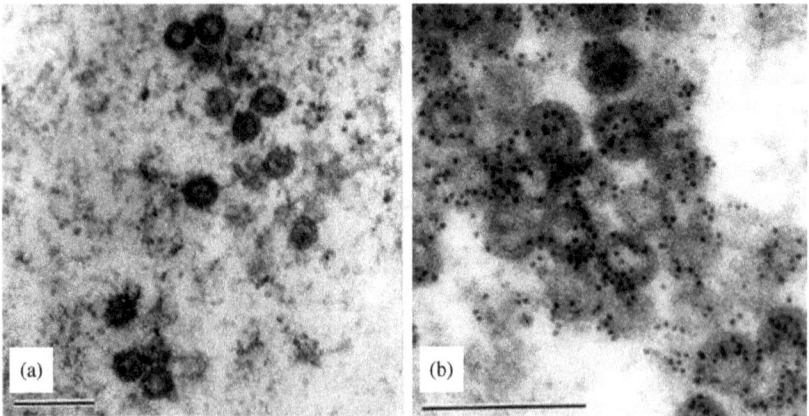

Figure 7.19: These are sections of MuMTV-producing cells that contain intracytoplasmic *A particles*. The complete immune ferritin labeling procedure was performed on each grid. (a) Buffer containing 1% normal goat serum was substituted for the primary antisera and no labelling is observed. (b) The complete reaction procedure shows heavy labelling of the intracytoplasmic *A particles* with little ferritin over adjacent areas of the cell. (Bar equals 0.2 um in all cells.)

7.5.2.4. *Are MCF-7 cells tumorigenic?*

Peter Wells and Joseph Saby, both recent college graduates who joined the experimental pathology laboratory at the MCF in 1973, were our first technical assistants. Peter and Joseph proved invaluable in their help with growing the MCF-7 cells in athymic mice, which resulted in a full demonstration that MCF-7 cells were tumorigenic. Athymic mice are a special strain of BALBC mice born without the thymus, making them immunosuppressed, and therefore able to tolerate exogenous tissues like neoplastic cells. Keeping that particular type of animal alive in those days was not an easy task; Joseph's and Peter's ingenuity and perseverance in designing and constructing a special rack that maintained the cages in a sterile environment kept the mice alive long enough to finish our experiments. It was their sense of purpose that made demonstrating the importance of the hormonal milieu in the growing of MCF-7 cells in athymic mice possible [35].

It was well known at that time that an important criterion of malignancy was the ability of transformed cells to grow in an adequate hetero-transplantation system [54]. Immunologically depressed athymic mice (*nu/nu*) [55–58] have the striking capability of discriminating between normal and neoplastic cells. Normal cells do not induce tumors [57], whereas malignant cells do. MCF-7 cells, cultured as previously described [25], were removed from the culture vessel by trypsinization, suspended in phosphate buffer saline (PBS), and transplanted in 21-day old Balb/c (*nu/nu*) mice into the mammary gland fat pad which was cleared according to the method of DeOme [59]. It is important to emphasize that we learned to clear the fat pad of these small animals which were extremely delicate in constitution and got sick easily due to their immune deficiency. After many trials and rehearsals, we were sure that the technique was in place, and we injected the cells in the fat pad that did not contain any remnant of the mammary gland of the animal to be sure that we had a site of implantation that would support the growth of the cancer cells. The first experiment demonstrated that MCF-7 cells were unable to grow in either female or male athymic mice. These negative results were unexpected, and we repeated the experiment three times to be sure that we were doing everything right and that the number of cells that we injected were adequate, but still the results were negative. We made a detailed gross examination of the area of cell inoculation, and the histological study revealed a complete absence of the inoculated cells; only disorganization of the fat and some fibrosis were observed.

After this failure, it occurred to us that this type of mouse was hormone insufficient and that the levels of estrogen were lower than in the normal strain of mice. This plus the knowledge that MCF-7 cells were estrogen receptors positive led us to use supplementation of the hormonal milieu of these special hosts. We repeated the experiment again and only those mice that had received a transplant of pituitary glands or ovaries from syngeneic mice induced the growth of MCF-7. We noted that 9 of the 11 (82%) inoculated female mice that received pituitary grafts developed palpable tumors within 12–18 days after inoculation. The tumors adhered to the skin and underlying muscle. No macroscopic metastatic growths were observed. Also, 8 of the 13 (61.5%) inoculated female mice that received ovary grafts developed palpable tumors within 12–18 days. Tumors were attached to the skin and underlying muscles; no metastatic growths were observed. The tumors were small oblong masses of 1.5–2.5 mm at their largest diameter. They adhered to the dermis of the skin and to the muscle of the abdominal wall. The tumors were firm, of a rubbery consistency, and presented resistance to sectioning. *We had demonstrated for the first time that MCF-7 was a tumorigenic cell line that required the hormonal milieu for growing in the heterologous host. This was the best model of breast cancer ever designed to study the hormone dependence of human breast cancer.* We also demonstrated that the histological patterns of the 17 tumors studied were identical. The tumors were composed of nests of cells arranged in either clusters or single or double-row strands (Figure 7.20). The inoculated epithelial cells were surrounded by a dense stroma formed by collagen fibers and fibroblasts. Blood vessels were scarce in the central portion of the tumor and more abundant in the periphery and in areas of invasion. The cells presented a considerable degree of pleomorphism and atypia as is depicted in Figure 7.20.

The intense fibrous reaction observed at the inoculation site and in the dermis was not observed around cells invading skeletal muscle (Figure 7.19). Mitoses were frequently observed in areas of invasion.

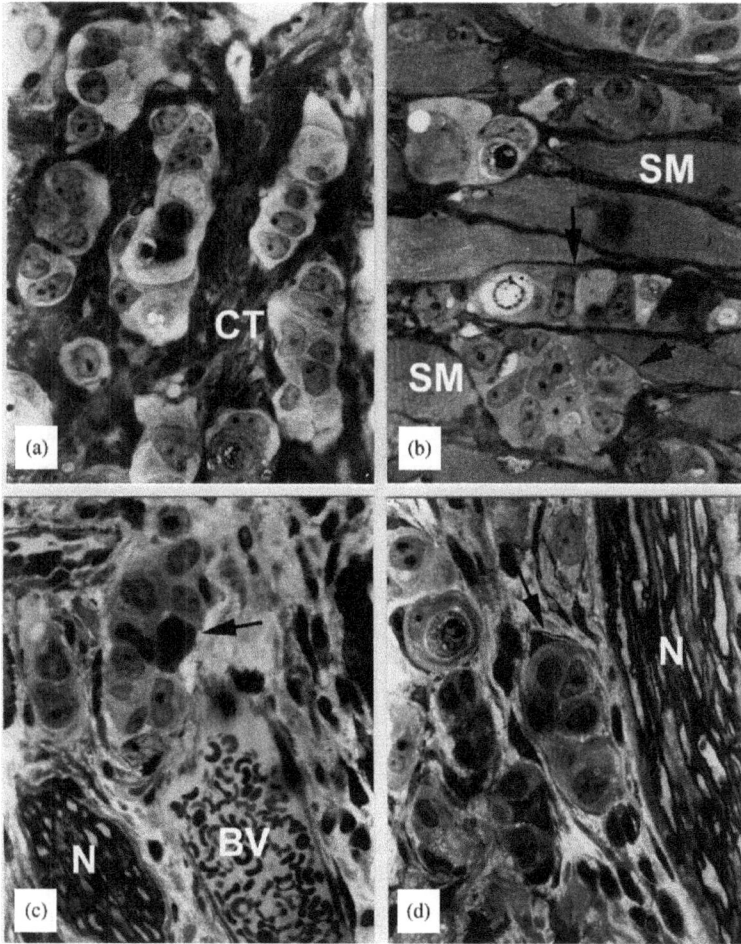

Figure 7.20: (a) Clusters and strands of MCF-7 cells surrounded by a dense stromal reaction in a nude mouse tumor. CT is connective tissue. (b) Strands (long arrow) and clusters (short arrow) of MCF-7 cells among muscle fibers. SM is skeletal muscle. (c) Cluster (arrow) of MCF-7 cells between the adventitia of a blood vessel (BV) and a nerve (N). (d) Cluster of MCF-7 cells (arrow) apposed to the perineurium; N is nerve. All photographs from 1 um sections of plastic embedded material stained with toluidine blue (×240).

No metastases were found in any of the tissues studied; however, clusters of cells attached to the adventitia of blood vessels or adjacent to the perineurium were observed in the periphery of the tumor. The tumors observed in mice isografted with pituitary glands or ovaries were indistinguishable. The successful hetero-transplantation of human tumors [58, 60] and cultured human malignant cells [55, 56] into nude mice has proven to be an excellent model for the study of neoplastic tissue and an effective diagnostic tool for differentiating malignant from benign cells [57]. The growth of MCF-7 cells as tumors in nude mice might be predicted by the malignant nature of the tumor of origin and by the demonstration of several transformation markers. However, MCF-7 cells did not form tumors in all inoculated mice but only in those receiving pituitary or ovarian grafts, thus suggesting a hormone dependency for *in vivo* growth. The fact that more tumors were observed in mice receiving pituitary grafts (82%) than in those receiving ovarian grafts (61.5%) suggested that some pituitary hormone could be involved in the development of these tumors. The inoculation of MCF-7 cells into nude mice induces tumors morphologically similar to the tumor of origin. This property of malignant cells has been described for other cell lines maintained for almost 100 passages *in vitro* [57] and transplanted into nude mice, and for human tumors transplanted into the anterior chamber of the guinea pig eye [61]. MCF-7 cells developed a histological pattern in the nude mice similar to that observed in the tumor of origin. The tumor of origin was an infiltrative ductal carcinoma with productive fibrosis (commonly called scirrhous carcinoma). This same pattern of epithelial cells surrounded by a dense stroma is observed in the mouse, suggesting that it is the neoplastic epithelial cell that elicits a stromal response in the host. This observation was also supported by results obtained in an experimental model developed by us for the study of scirrhous carcinoma [62].

7.5.2.5. *Is the tumorigenic capacity regulated under a specific hormonal milieu?*

The absence of tumors in untreated animals could be explained by an inadequate hormonal milieu for the growth of MCF-7 cells. The fact that the original tumor from which MCF-7 cells were derived was responsive to hormones and that MCF-7 cells still retained specific high-affinity estradiol and progesterone receptors after more than

160 passages in culture supports this explanation. In 1976, the utilization of hormonal supplementation in the growth of MCF-7 cells [27, 63] suggested replacing the isografts by hormone pellets [64]. We found out that the use of castrated male, estrogen supplemented, was also suitable for the growth of MCF-7 cells. The removal of the uterus and supplementation with estradiol either as pellets or Silastic tube containing 5 mg of 17-beta-estradiol in female mice is also a standard procedure presently used in many laboratories around the world. We have described these studies in detail in our book [18].

7.6. The 734B putative human viral particle

After studying the normal human breast epithelial cells, the viral team concluded that we were unable to identify a particle with all of the characteristics of the known oncornaviruses [21]. The 734B putative breast cancer virus shares no identity with mammalian leukemia viruses and has a density of 1.17 gms/cc, contains a true reverse transcriptase, and 70S RNA. Particle synthesis was, however, slightly restricted, with only transient, low-level virus production observed in routine cell culture passages of MCF-7 cells. To define the biological role of this agent, it was necessary to confirm its species of origin. Such determinations were based on the fact that endogenous oncornaviruses of any species were coded by the DNA genome of the native species. Unrelated species do not carry the same coding sequence in their DNA, and consequently, one could expect the viral genome (or a DNA copy of it) to hybridize with the DNA of the species of origin but not with the DNA of unrelated species. The viral team's results suggested that at least some 734B sequences were coded by the DNA genome of human cells and not by non-human cells, and suggested, therefore that 734B was a human endogenous virus. In the mouse mammary cancer system, virus is found in milk, cultured cells derived from tumor, and breast tumors. The question posed by the viral team was: Might we expect the same in man? And the real answer was elusive — at least as was shown in the two articles that we wrote [65, 66].

7.7. Do MCF cells that express the putative 734B viral particle by molecular studies have a morphological equivalent?

For almost 3 years, we took more than 50,000 photographs of putative particles that could resemble a retrovirus (Figure 7.6), but ultimately our studies were unable to isolate the virus or to demonstrate a causal relationship between the retrovirus and cancer, nor were we able to develop a vaccine. There are still researchers working in this area who maintain that a large proportion of human breast cancers may be associated with the human mammary tumor virus (HMTV). This human virus is nearly identical to the MuMTV that is implicated in breast cancer in mice. That is the meaning of the word *research*, to look and look again, or to search again and again.

7.8. The end of the viral team

Although the virus was not demonstrated morphologically in the cells that we studied, we cannot rule out that some sequences of the virus were there and a causative of breast cancer yet could not be detected at our resolution levels. Probably that will be the task of another group of researchers better equipped than we were more than 30 years ago.

My experience in the viral studies of cancer produced much significant work, and for my part, it was important to recognize that I was increasingly skeptic about the role of a viral etiology in breast cancer after listening to hundreds of lectures and spending hundreds of hours in meetings organized by the NCI and the virus program. I felt that something was missing, and every single day the complexity of the data and the interpretations to justify how a virus might induce breast cancer became more convoluted and difficult to follow. Therefore, my logistic plans to find other paths led me to follow the somatic mutation and the role of chemical carcinogens in the cancer etiology. But I will address this topic in other chapters. However, the importance of this period of my career as a cancer researcher, from 1973 to the end of 1976, was extremely rich in experiences at the personal, intellectual, and career levels, and allowed me to answer issues that were not properly addressed at that specific time in the history of breast cancer. Was an MCF-7 cell a breast cancer cell? What did it look like? Did the cell reproduce in culture the same original tumor pattern? Did the cell produce tumors in animals? How was the growth of these cells controlled *in vivo*? I answered these questions, and in addition this period was pivotal for starting my independent career as a cancer researcher. I am sure, in retrospect, that the development of a logistic plan was extremely important to determine a path to follow. I do not know if everything would be different if I had not been part of the viral team but I am certainly glad that I was part of that enterprise.

References

[1] Cole, D. Dolly Cole in breast cancer. Saturday Evening Post, June/July, 1974, 246.

[2] Bittner, J. J. Some possible effects of nursing on the mammary gland tumor incidence in mice. *Science* 84: 162, 1936.

[3] Moore, D. H., Charney, J., Kramarski, B., Lasfargues, E. Y., Sarkar, N. H., Brennan, M. H., Burrows, H.N., Sirsat, S. M., Paymaster J. C. and Valdya, A. B. Search for a human breast cancer virus. *Nature* 229: 611, 1971.

[4] Feller, W. F. and Chopra, H. C. Virus-like particles in human milk. *Cancer* 28: 1425, 1971.

[5] Sarkar, N. H., Charney, J., Dion, A. S. and Moore, D. H. Effect of human milk on the mouse mammary tumor virus. *Cancer Res.* 33: 626, 1973.

[6] Baltimore, D. RNA-dependent DNA polymerase in virions of RNA tumour viruses. *Nature* 226: 1209, 1970.

[7] Temin, H. and Mizutanl, S. RNA-dependent DNA polymerase in virions of Rous sarcoma virus. *Nature* 226: 1211, 1971.

[8] Schlom, J., Spiegelman, S. and Moore, D. H. RNA-dependent DNA polymerase activity in virus-like particles isolated from human milk. *Nature* 231: 97, 1971.

[9] McCormlck, J. J., Larson, L. J. and Rich, M. A. RNase inhibition of reverse transcriptase activity in human milk. *Nature* 251: 737, 1974.

[10]   Feldman, S. P., Schlom, J. and Spiegelman, S. Further evidence for oncornaviruses in human milk: the production of cores. *Proc. Nat. Acad. Sci. (USA)* 70: 7973, 1976.

[11]   Buehring, G. C. Culture of Human mammary epithelial cell. Keeping abreast with a new method. *J. Natl. Cancer Inst.* 49: 1433–1434, 1972.

[12]   Feller, W. F., Stewart, S. E. and Kantor, J. Primary tissue culture explants of human breast cancer. *J. Natl. Cancer Inst.* 48: 1117–1120, 1972.

[13]   Lasfargues E. Y., Coutinho, W. G. and Moore D. H. Pitfalls in the isolation of a human breast carcinoma virus in tissue culture. *J. Natl. Cancer Inst.* 48: 1101–1105, 1972.

[14]   Furmanski, P., Longley, C., Fouchey, D., Rich, R. and Rich, M. A. *J. Natl. Cancer Inst.* 52: 975–977, 1974.

[15]   Russo, J., Furmanski, P. and Rich, M. A. An ultrastructural study of normal human mammary epithelial cells in culture. *Am. J. Anat.* 142: 221–231, 1975.

[16]   Bargmann, W. and Welsh, U. On the ultrastructure of the mammary gland. In: Reynolds, M., Foley, S. J., (eds.), *Lactogenesis, the initiation of milk secretion and parturition*, University of Pennsylvania Press, Philadelphia, Pennsylvania. 1969, 443–452, 1969.

[17]   Wellings, S. R. Ultrastructural basis of Lactogenesis. In: Reynolds, M., Foley, S. J., (eds.), *Lactogenesis, the initiation of milk secretion and parturition*, University of Pennsylvania Press, Philadelphia, Pennsylvania. 1969, 5–25.

[18]   Russo, J. and Russo, I. H. *Biological and Molecular Basis of Breast Cancer*, Springer-Verlag, Heidelberg, Germany. 2004.

[19]   Axel, R., Gulati, S. and Spiegelman, S. Particles containing RNA-instructed DNA polymerase and virus-related RNA in human breast cancers. *Proc. Natl. Acad. Sci. (USA)* 69: 3133–3137, 1972.

[20]   Soule, H. D., Vazquez, J., Long, A., Albert, S. and Brennan, M. A human cell line from a pleural effusion derived from a breast carcinoma. *J. Natl. Cancer Inst.* 51: 1409–1416, 1973.

[21]   McGrath, C., Grant, P. M., Soule, H.D., Glancy, T. and Rich, M. A. Replication of oncornavirus-like particle in human breast carcinoma cell line, MCF-7. *Nature* 252: 247–250, 1974.

[22]   Rose, H. N. and McGrath, C. a-Lactalbumin production in human mammary carcinoma. *Science* 190: 673–675, 1975.

[23]   Brooks, S. C., Locke, E. R. and Soule, H. D. Estrogen receptor in a human cell line (MCF-7) from breast carcinoma. *J. Biol. Chern.* 248: 6251–6253, 1973.

[24]   Horwitz, K. B., Costlow, M. E. and McGuire, W. L. MCF-7: A human breast cancer cell line with estrogen, androgen, progesterone and glucocorticoid receptors. *Steroids* 26: 785–795, 1975.

[25] Russo, J., Soule, H. D., McGrath, C. and Rich, M. A. Re-expression of the original tumor pattern by a human breast. Carcinoma cell line (MCF-7) in sponge cultures. *J. Natl. Cancer Inst.* 56: 279–282, 1976.

[26] Russo, J., Brennan, M. J. and Rich, M. A. Induction of tumor growth by inoculation of a human breast cancer cell line MCF-7 into ovary or pituitary grafted nude mice. *Proc. Amer. Cancer Soc.* 17: 116a, 1976.

[27] Russo, J., McGrath, C. M., Russo, I. H. and Rich, M. A. Tumoral growth of a human breast cancer cell line (MCF-7) in athymic mice. In: Nieburgs, H.E., (ed), 3rd *Int. Symp. on Detection and Prevention of Cancer*, 1976, 617–626, New York, NY.

[28] Arnold, W. J., Soule, H. D. and Russo, J. Fine structure of a human mammary carcinoma cell line, MCF-7. *In Vitro* 10: 356, 1975.

[29] Pickett, P. B., Pitelka, D. R., Hamamoto, S. T. and Misfeldt, D. S. Occluding junctions and cell behavior in primary clusters of normal and neoplastic mammary gland cells. *J. Cell Biol.* 66: 316–332, 1975.

[30] Buehring, G. C. and Hackett, A. J. Human breast tumor cell lines: Identity evaluation by ultrastructure. *J. Natl. Cancer Inst.* 53: 621–629, 1974.

[31] Ozzello, L. Ultrastructure of the human mammary gland. In: Summers, S. C. (ed), *Pathology Annual*, Appleton-Century-Crofts, NewYork. 1971, 1–59.

[32] Pierce, G. B. and Nakane, P. K. Basement membranes: Synthesis and deposition in response to cellular injury. *Lab. Inv.* 21: 27–41, 1969.

[33] Russo, J., Bradley, R. and Soule, H. D. Ultrastructural study of human mammary carcinoma cells (MCF-7) grown in collagen-coated sponge. *Proc. Electron Microsc. Soc. Amer.* 392–393, 1975.

[34] Murad, T. M. Ultrastructure of ductular carcinoma of the breast (*in situ* and infiltrating lobular carcinoma). *Cancer* 27: 18–28, 1971.

[35] Russo, J., Furmanski, P., Bradley, R., Wells, P. and Rich, M. Differentiation of normal mammary epithelial cells in culture: An ultrastructural study. *Amer. J. Anat.*145: 57–78, 1976.

[36] Tannenbaum, M., Weiss, M. and Marx, A. J. Ultrastructure of the human mammary ductule. *Cancer* 23: 958–978, 1969.

[37] Fanger, H. and Ree, H. J. Cyclic changes of human mammary gland epithelium in relation to the menstrual cycle — An ultrastructural study. *Cancer* 14: 574–585, 1974.

[38] Young, R. K., Cailleau, R., Mackay, B. and Reeves, W. J. Establishment of epithelial cell line MDA-IIB-157 from metastatic pleural effusion of human breast carcinoma. *In Vitro* 9: 239–245, 1974.

[39] Cailleau, R., Young, R., Olive, M. and Reeves, W. J. Breast tumor cell lines from pleural effusions. *J. Natl. Cancer Inst.* 53: 661–674, 1974.

[40] Pitelka, D. R., Hammamoto, S. T., Duafala, J. G. and Nemanic, M. K. Cell contacts in the mouse mammary gland. I Normal gland in postnatal development and the secretory cycle. *J. Cell Biol.* 56: 797–818, 1973.

[41] Arnold, W. J., Soule, H. D. and Russo, J. Fine structure of a murine mammary carcinoma cell line. *In Vitro* 12: 57–64, 1976.

[42] Archer, F. L. Normal and neoplastic human tissue in organ culture. *Arch. Pathol.* 85: 62–69, 1968.

[43] Matoska, J. and Siracky, J. Histology and ultrastructure of human breast cancer in organ culture. *Neoplasma* 21: 685–696, 1974.

[44] Tchao, R., Easty, G. C. and Ambrose, E. J. Effect of chemotherapeutic agents and hormones on organ culture of human tumors. *Eur. J. Cancer* 4: 39–45, 1968.

[45] Wellings, S. R. and Jentoff, V. L. Organ culture of normal, dysplastic, and neoplastic human mammary tissues. *J. Natl. Cancer Inst.* 49: 329–338, 1972.

[46] Mareel, L. M., Varaet, L. and De Ridder, L. A. Possibility of distinction between normal and neoplastic cells through transplantation into chick blastoderms. *J. Natl. Cancer Inst.* 51: 809–815, 1973.

[47] Mareel, L. M., *et al.* Possibility of distinction between malignant and nonmalignant cells by transplantation into chick blastoderms: Further evidence from animal and human biopsy specimens. *J. Natl. Cancer Inst.* 53: 1351–1358, 1974.

[48] Leighton, J., *et al.* Collagen-coated cellulose sponge: Three dimensional matrix for tissue culture of Walker tumor 256. *Science* 155:1259–1261, 1967.

[49] Sandford, K. K., Dunn, T. B. and Westfall, B. B. Sarcomatous change and maintenance of differentiation in long-term cultures of mouse mammary carcinoma. *J. Natl. Cancer Inst.* 26: 1139–1183, 1961.

[50] Soule, H. D., Moloney, T., Vasquez, J. and Long A. *Proc. Am. Assoc. Cancer Res.*14: 90, 1973.

[51] Sternberger, L. A., Hardy, P. H., Cuculis, J. J. and Meyer, H.G. The unlabeled antibody enzyme method of immunohistochemistry: preparation and properties of soluble antigen–antibody complex (horseradish peroxidase-antihorseradish peroxidase) and its use in identification of spirochetes. *J. Histochem. Cytochem.*18: 315, 1970.

[52] Sternberger, L. A. *Immunocytochemistry*, Prentice Hall, Englewood Cliffs, NJ. 1974.

[53] Smith, G. H. and Lee, B. K. Mouse mammary tumor virus polypeptide precursors in intracytoplasmic A particles. *J. Natl. Cancer Inst.* 55: 493, 1975.

[54] Sanford, K. K. Biologic Manifestation of Oncogenesis in Vitro: A critique. *J. Natl. Cancer Inst.* 53: 1481–1485, 1974.

[55] Giovanella, B. C., Stehlin, J. S. and Williams, L. J. Jr. Development of Invasive Tumors in the "Nude" Mouse after Injection of Cultured Human Melanoma Cells. *J. Natl. Cancer Inst.* 48: 1531–1533, 1972.

[56] Giovanella, B. C. and Stehlin, J. S. Heterotransplantation of Human Malignant Tumors in "Nude" Thymusless Mice. I. Breeding and Maintenance of "Nude" Mice. *J. Natl. Cancer Inst.* 51: 615–619, 1973.

[57] Giovanella, B. C., Stehlin, J. S. and Williams, L. J. Jr. Heterotransplantation of Human Malignant Tumors in "Nude" Thymusless Mice. II. Malignant Tumors Induced by Injection of Cell Cultures Derived from Human Solid Tumors. *J. Natl. Cancer Inst.* 52: 921–930, 1974.

[58] Povlsen, C. O., Fialkow, P. J. and Klein, E. Growth and Antigenic Properties of a Biopsy-Derived Burkitt's Lymphoma in Thymusless (Nude) Mice. *Intl. J. Cancer* 11: 30–39, 1973.

[59] DeOme, K. B., Faulkin, J. l. T. Jr., Bern, H. A. and Blair, P. B. Development of Mammary Tumors from Hyperplastic Alveolar Nodules Transplanted into Gland-Free Mammary Fat Pads of Female C3H Mice. *Cancer Res.* 19: 350–359, 1959.

[60] Rygaard, J. and Povlsen, C. O. Heterotransplantation of a Human Malignant Tumor to "Nude" Mice. *Acta Pathol. Microbial. Scand.* 77: 758–760, 1969.

[61] Greene, H. S. N. The Significance of the Heterologous Transplantability of Human Cancer. *Cancer* 5: 24–44, 1952.

[62] Russo, J. and McGrath, C. M. Scirrhous Carcinoma in the Mouse: A Model for Human Mammary Carcinoma. Excerpta Medica, Amsterdam, 488, 1975.

[63] Russo, J., Brennan, M. J. and Rich, M. A. Induction of tumor growth by inoculation of a human breast cancer cell (MCF-7) into ovary or pituitary grafted nude mice. *Proc. Am. Assoc. Cancer Res.* 17: 464, 1976.

[64] Shafie, S. M. and Giartham, F. H. Role of hormones in the growth and regression of human breast cancer cells (MCF-7) transplanted into athymic mice. *J. Natl. Cancer Inst.* 67: 51–56, 1981.

[65] Rich, M. A., Furmanski, P., McGrath C. M., Mc Cormick, J., Russo, J. and Soule, H. The etiology of Breast Cancer. In: Menon, K. M. J., Reel, J. R., (eds), *Steroid Hormone Action and Cancer*, Plenum Press, New York. 15–27, 1976.

[66] McGrath, C. M., Furmanski, P., Russo, J., McCormick, J. J. and Rich M. A. 734B: a candidate human breast cancer virus. In: Freedman, H., (ed), *Tumor virus infection and Immunity*, Chapter 4. 63–87, 1976.

[67] Russo, J., Bradley, R. H., McGrath, C. M. and Russo, I. H. Scanning and transmission electron microscopy study of a human breast carcinoma cell line (MCF-7) cultured in collagen-coated cellulose sponge. *Cancer Res.* 35: 2004–2014, 1977.

Chapter 8

The Breast Cancer
Research Laboratory (BCRL)
(Defining the Aims 1973–1978)

8.1. The creation of the Breast Cancer Research
Laboratory (BCRL)

We moved from Florida to Ann Arbor, Michigan, late in the summer of
1973 and made our new home in an apartment right on a branch of the
Huron River. We took long walks along the river, enjoying and loving
that beautiful pastoral place. It was during those walks that we started
to question ourselves and what we wanted to do in cancer research.
What would be our imprint? Our signature? Our legacy? It was there
that the idea of a laboratory dedicated entirely to breast cancer research
was born. Our stay in Ann Arbor lasted less than a year, ending when
Irma discovered Grosse Pointe, a place we found more appealing and
closer to Detroit. Our daily commute from Ann Arbor to Detroit in the
morning and then back in the evening was a treacherous drive, mainly
because winters in Michigan seem to be longer than anywhere else. Our
move to Grosse Pointe was triggered when a couple of scientists that
worked at the Michigan Cancer Foundation had a fatal accident on the
I-95 — the only road that we used for our daily commute. The reason
was a solid one, so we moved to Grosse Pointe Farms and rented a
house on Mapleton Avenue for three years until we bought our first
home on Audubon Street in Grosse Pointe Park. Both places were near
Lake Saint Clair, and we used to walk for hours along the shore of the

lake, admiring dream homes interrupted by the red brick Church of Saint Paul facing the lake where our daughter, Patricia, was baptized in 1980. The main topic of conversation was our research work and how we would merge the resources for constructing and expanding in the MCF with an independent research team or the Breast Cancer Research laboratory (BCRL).

The BCRL grew slowly as an entity, together with my new responsibilities as Chief of the experimental pathology laboratory from 1973–1978. In this initial phase, we established and clarified our aims, and that will be the subject of this chapter of my memoirs. The period that began after 1978 and lasted until 1991 was a special one because it was the time that we expanded our wings, and it coincided with the revalidation of our medical degrees and our taking the specialty board in pathology, plus I was promoted from member to Chairman of the Michigan Cancer Foundation's Department of Pathology, as well as being a clinical Associate Professor of Pathology at Wayne State University Medical School. This was also the period when we felt that we needed a larger "pond" to swim in. We wanted to be on the peak of the mountain. This was accomplished by expanding the BCRL, not only in personnel and grant support but also by developing its own entity as a research laboratory. Physically, the laboratory was housed at the Michigan Cancer Foundation until 1991 when we moved to Philadelphia and I became a Chairman of the Department of Pathology in the Medical Division at Fox Chase Cancer Center. Almost the entire membership of the original BCRL made the move to Philadelphia (see Chapter 10), and even though the BCRL was part of the Pathology Department at Fox Chase, we continued expanding our lines of research until eventually we were established as a separate entity in 1994. After Irma's death on June 25, 2013, the BCRL was renamed *The Irma H. Russo, MD, Breast Cancer Research Laboratory of the FCCC-Temple-Health* in her honor.

8.2. Defining our line of cancer research

Our line of cancer research began when we decided to start using a single experimental model for studying mammary carcinogenesis using the basic model developed by Charles Huggins in 1960 [1], consisting of the intragastric administration of 7,12-dimethylbenz-(a)-anthracene (DMBA) to young virgin Sprague Dawley rats. In that model, the mammary gland's susceptibility to developing neoplasms has made this organ a unique target for testing the carcinogenic potential of specific chemicals. Several carcinogens, which induce mammary tumors in both mice and rats, have been extensively studied in both species, and we have described them in our book *Molecular Basis of Breast Cancer* [2] as well as in a review that I wrote in 2016 [3]. Tumors induced by administration of chemical carcinogens constitute useful tools for dissecting the multistep process of carcinogenesis, which involves initiation, promotion, and progression, and served as a baseline for testing the carcinogenic potential of chemicals in risk assessment [3, 4]. The knowledge that we generated from these studies was possible thanks to three grants that we received during the early period of our research; these grants contributed significantly to our understanding and further development of our work. We received two grant awards from the NCI for studying the basis of mammary gland susceptibility to carcinogenesis and a third grant from the American Cancer Society to study DNA repair and mammary gland carcinogenesis.

8.3. Finding the target of carcinogenesis

We were the first ones to point out the importance of the differentiation status of the target organ as a determinant of the susceptibility to carcinogenesis [4]. The selection of the DMBA tumor model for our studies was based on the criterion that the model must mimic the human disease, meaning that we were able to ascertain the influence of host factors such as ovarian, pituitary, and placental hormones, among others, as well as overall reproductive events because these factors, in turn, influence the development and degree of mammary gland differentiation [5–8], which are subject to a multiplicity of endocrine stimulatory and inhibitory influences from embryogenesis onward [5]. In 1975, we presented our first set of data at the meeting of the American Society for Cancer Research in

San Diego, California, describing the pathogenesis of a rat mammary carcinoma induced by DMBA [9], and from these studies we were able to establish *a biological law that the carcinogenic potential of a given chemical is in great part modulated by the biological conditions of the target organ, which determines its susceptibility to neoplastic transformation* [1, 10]. In the rat, this requires that a carcinogen act on the stem cells of a specific compartment of the mammary gland, the terminal end bud (TEB), which gives origin to the mammary tree as well as the carcinogenic process. The TEB of the rat mammary gland is the equivalent of the terminal ductal lobular unit, or Lobule type 1 in the human breast, and both are undifferentiated structures and the site where the stem cells are nested [10]. When the TEB differentiates into alveolar buds (ABs) and lobules, they lose the susceptibility to neoplastic transformation, which explains why the window of susceptibility in the rat is around 45–55 days of age.

After that age, the number of TEBs decreases and becomes less susceptible to developing cancer (Figures 8.1 and 8.2). The

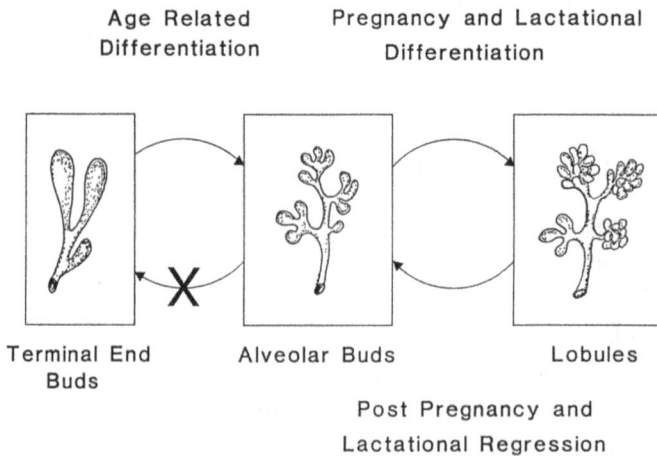

Age Related Differentiation

Pregnancy and Lactational Differentiation

Terminal End Buds

Alveolar Buds

Lobules

Post Pregnancy and Lactational Regression

Figure 8.1: Terminal end buds, alveolar buds, and lobules. Arrows indicate differentiation of terminal end buds into alveolar buds and lobular structures. After weaning, neither alveolar buds nor lobules regress to terminal end buds. Reprinted with permission from Ref. [8].

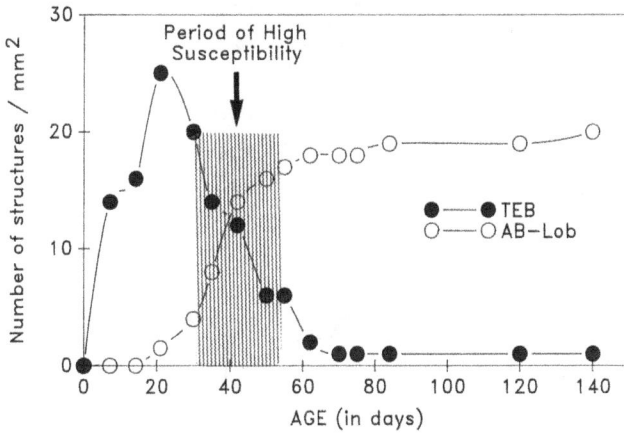

Figure 8.2: Histogram representing the number of structures /mm² (ordinate) of the rat mammary gland in relation to age (abscissa). Hatched area, period of highest susceptibility of the mammary gland to neoplastic transformation by chemical carcinogens. Reprinted with permission from Ref. [8].

importance of this observation is that it mimics what was observed in the human breast, where most of the cancer starts in the ductal structures; in 1990, we published a paper establishing the similarities between rat and human mammary glands [11]. These studies have been seminal in developing the concept of the window of susceptibility to mammary carcinogenesis and environmental exposure that is the basis of several programs initiated by the National Institute of Environmental Health Sciences and the National Cancer Institute, such as the UO1-ESO26130 that is supporting our present research.

Altogether, this seminal work opened the gateway to developing new concepts in the understanding of the susceptibility of the mammary gland to carcinogenesis, concepts such as the role of differentiation and rate of cell proliferation of the mammary gland at the time of exposure to a given chemical carcinogen on its binding, DNA repair, and tumor incidence, that have influenced the way in which the study of mammary cancer is pursued by researchers worldwide [6, 7, 10, 11] (Figure 8.3).

272   *Memoirs of a Cancer Researcher*

Structure	DNA-LI	T_C	Cell cycle	GF_5	^{3}H-DMBA	Lesions
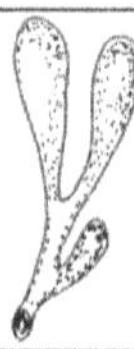 TEB	34%	11.65 h	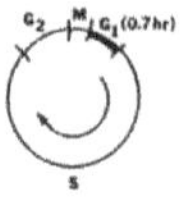	0.55	6.8±2.8	Carcinoma
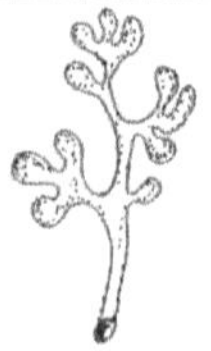 AB	4%	28.18 h	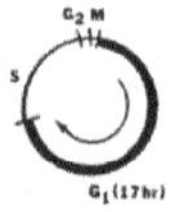	0.13	1.3±0.8	Cysts HAN Adenomas Fibro-Ad.
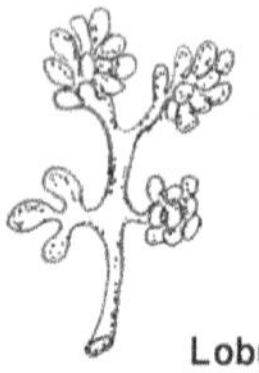 Lobule	0.1%	49.63 h	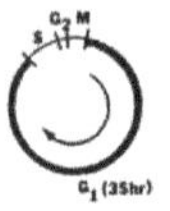	0.0049	0.9±0.5	None

Figure 8.3: Correlation between type of structure, terminal end bud (TEB), alveolar bud (AB), and lobule with their rate of ^{3}H-thymidine incorporation, or DNA-labeling index (DNA·LI), length of the cell cycle in hours (Tc) cell cycle, and growth fraction (GF5), or rate of ^{3}H·thymidine incorporation after five days of continuous infusion. Nuclear uptake of ^{3}H-DMBA, detected by autoradiography and expressed as the number of grains/nucleus, is directly proportional to the DNA-LI and GF5 and inversely proportional to the T_c of each specific structure. The development of carcinomas also correlated with high DNA-LI, T_c, and DMBA binding, whereas benign lesions or the absence of neoplasms were inversely related. Reprinted with permission from Ref. [8].

8.4 The terminal end bud (TEB)

Mammary cancer is the result of the interaction of a carcinogen with the target organ, the mammary gland. This target, however, is extremely complex, since the mammary gland does not respond to the carcinogen as a whole, rather only specific structures within the gland are affected by a given genotoxic agent. The incidence of DMBA-induced tumors reaches 100% when the carcinogen is administered to rats aged 30–55 days, but the highest number of tumors per animal is observed when the carcinogen is given to animals between the ages of 40 and 46 days, coincident with the period in which the mammary gland exhibits a high density of highly proliferating TEBs (Figure 8.2). We attributed this high susceptibility to the specific characteristics of the mammary gland prevailing during that period of life. Administration of DMBA to virgin rats induces the largest number of transformed foci when TEBs are decreasing in number due to their differentiation into ABs (Figure 8.2). These structures, instead of differentiating into ABs, become progressively larger due to epithelial proliferation, with multilayering, secondary lumen formation, and early papillary projections to the widened lumen. At this stage, transformed TEBs are called intraductal proliferations (IDPs) (Figures 8.4 and 8.5).

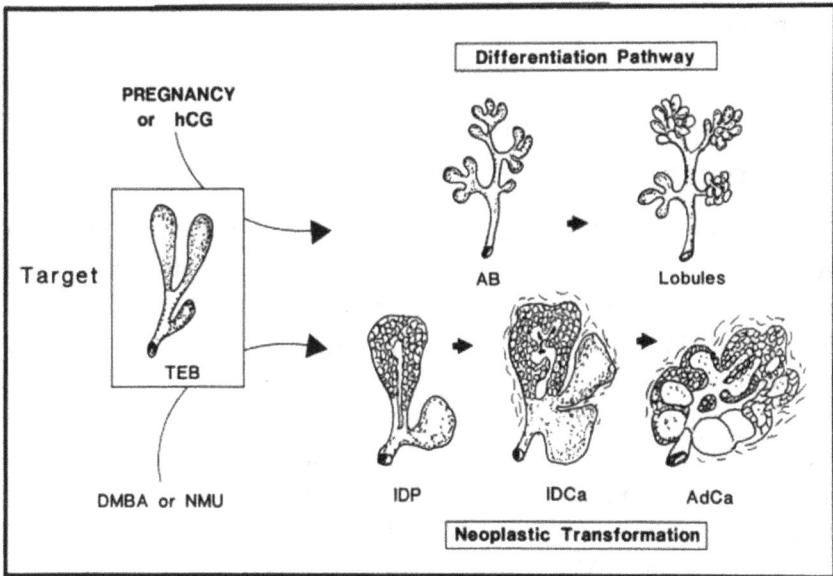

Figure 8.4: Pathogenesis of chemically induced rat mammary tumors. The undifferentiated terminal end bud (TEB) affected by the carcinogen progresses to intraductal proliferation (IDP), and in situ ductal carcinoma (IDCa) that exhibits various histopathological types. Further tumor growth and coalescence of neighboring lesions originate invasive adenocarcinomas (AdCa), which might become metastatic. Figure 8.5: (a) Whole mount of a TEB (toluidine blue) (X 4). (b) Histological section of a TEB (H&E) (X 10). (c) High magnification of b, (X 40). (d) Whole mount of an IDP, in the rat mammary gland. This lesion is observed 21–41 days post-DMBA administration.

Their confluence leads to the formation of micro-tumors that histologically are classified as adenocarcinomas, first intraductal, which progress to invasive, developing various patterns such as cribriform, comedo, or papillary types [1, 12].

The proliferation starts in the TEBs and expands to the ductal structures. (e) Histological section of d with moderate desmoplastic reaction in the stroma (H&E) (X 4). (f) Whole mount of a carcinoma *in situ* stained with toluidine blue, x 4. (g) Histological section of carcinoma *in situ* showing early papillary patterns and intense desmoplastic reaction in the stroma (H&E) (X 10). (h) Whole mount of an intraductal carcinoma, cribriform pattern stained with toluidine blue (X 4). (i) Histological section of g showing epithelial clusters surrounded by intense desmoplastic reaction and lymphocyte infiltration (H&E) (X 10).

8.5. The progression of terminal end bud to cancer

Even though TEB differentiation into AB is inhibited by carcinogen treatment, not all the TEBs present in the mammary gland at the time of DMBA administration progress to IDPs. Some of them still differentiate into Abs, but their number is always lower than that of the control animals. Occasional lobular development is observed, although it is negligible. Some TEBs become smaller with an atrophic appearance, at this stage they are called terminal ducts (TDs). TDs are also susceptible to neoplastic transformation and are the main target of carcinogens in older animals [6, 7]. Those TEBs that were already differentiated into ABs and early lobular structures before DMBA administration do not develop carcinomas. Most of them either remain unmodified or undergo dilatation of the lumen, giving rise to hyperplastic lesions, such as AB hyperplasia (Figure 8.5). Others exhibit epithelial proliferation, forming tubular adenomas, and give rise to cystic dilatations, or fibroadenomas (Figure 8.5). When DMBA is inoculated into older virgin females, ranging in age from 180 to

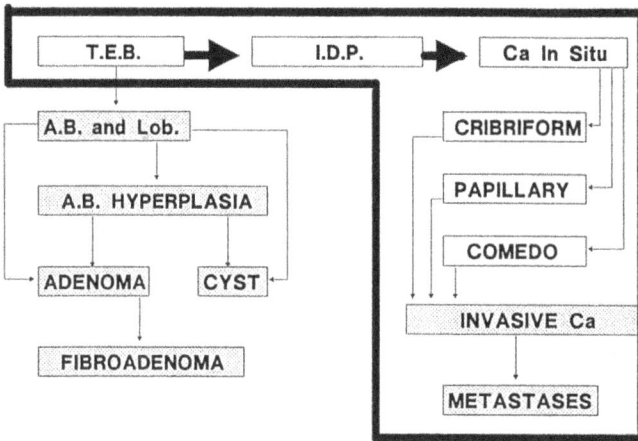

Figure 8.5: Chart representing two different pathogenetic pathways for benign and malignant lesions. Malignant lesions originate from TEB and appear earlier than benign lesions originated from AB. The earliest lesion detected after DMBA administration is the IDP.

330 days, they develop tubular adenomas. These lesions develop predominantly in the abdominal glands, where a higher incidence of tumors is observed in older animals. The observation that mammary carcinomas arise from undifferentiated structures of the gland, namely TEBs and TDs, and that the number of adenocarcinomas is directly related to the number of these structures in the mammary gland (Figure 8.6), whereas benign lesions such as adenomas, cysts, and fibroadenomas (Figure 8.5) arise from structures that were more differentiated at the time of carcinogen administration, *indicates that the carcinogen requires an adequate structural target, and the type of lesion induced is dependent upon the area of the mammary gland that the carcinogen affects.*

Thus, the more differentiated the structure at the time of carcinogen administration the more benign and organized is the lesion that develops. This in turn is related to the number of cells in growth fraction, or proliferating, and the amount of binding of the carcinogen to the different structures of the mammary gland (Figure 8.3).

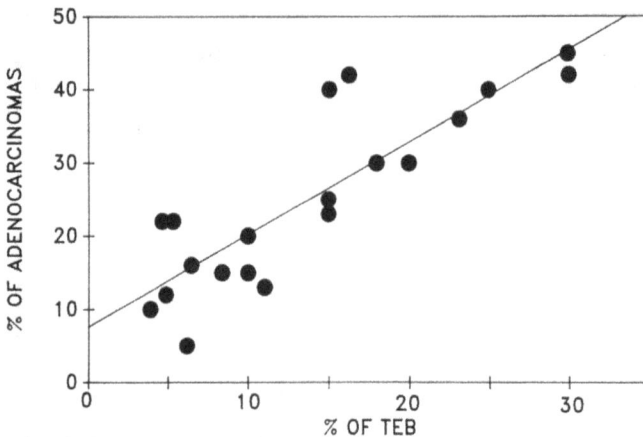

Figure 8.6: Regression curve showing the high correlation (cc, 0.87; p = 0.001) between percentage of adenocarcinomas and percentage of TEBs.

8.6. Cell kinetics and mammary carcinogenesis

Our seminal contribution, that the target of the carcinogen was in the TEB and that the type of lesion depends on the degree of differentiation of the different structure present in the mammary gland at the time of the carcinogenic insult, was also supported by our cell kinetic studies published in *Cancer Research* in 1980 [13]. In every tissue, normal or abnormal, cell composition consists of a balance of three different cell populations: cycling cells, resting cells (cells in G_0), and dying cells (cell loss). In the cell mammary gland, these three cell populations can be identified through the study of the cycle and determination of the growth fraction and the rate of cell loss (Figure 8.3).

The growth fraction refers to the fraction of cycling cells, while the rate of cell loss refers to the fraction of cells that die or migrate to other tissues. Both cell cycle time and the growth fraction determine the number of cells produced per unit of time, and the rate of cell loss determines the number of cells lost per unit of time. The growth of normal cells involves the net increase in cell number resulting from more cells being born than dying. In the differentiated tissue or in the adult tissue, in which growth has ceased, the number of cells produced per unit of time is equal to the number of cells that die. The higher susceptibility of the TEB to neoplastic transformation is attributed to the fact that this structure is composed of an actively proliferating epithelium, as determined by the mitotic index (MI), DNA-LI, T_c, and growth fraction (GF5) (Figures 8.7 and 8.8). Both the MI and DNA-LI are very high at the tip of TEBs, decreasing progressively

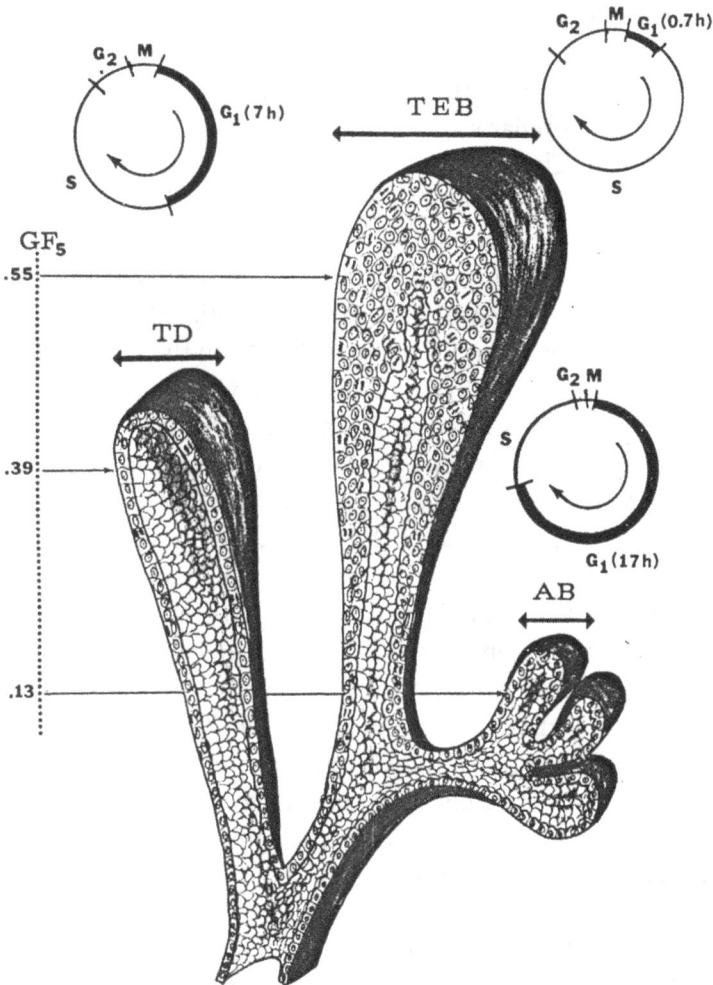

Figure 8.7: Schematic representation of terminal structures in the mammary gland of young virgin rats. The diagram of the cell cycle partitioned into its phases represents the relative length of each phase for each one of the three structures shown. Reprinted with permission from Ref. [13].

toward the ductal or proximal portion of the gland and even further in ABs and lobules (Figures 8.7 and 8.8). TEBs are also characterized by having the highest growth fraction, which progressively diminishes in the more differentiated ABs and lobules (Figure 8.7). By using these cell kinetic parameters, we have calculated the rate of cell loss in each one of the compartments of the mammary tree. Interestingly enough, the TEB is not only the structure with the highest proliferative ratio, but also with the lowest percentage of cell loss in comparison with other parenchymal structures. The rate of cell loss is very high in the lobular structures present in the mammary gland of parous rats. This clearly indicates that the TEB of the young virgin female is the truly proliferating structure of the gland that reaches a steady state only after acquiring full differentiation.

The differences in proliferative activity and growth fraction observed between TEBs and the more differentiated structures of the mammary gland are also reflected in variations in the length of the cell cycle or T_c (Figure 8.7). T_c in TEBs of young virgin rats has an average length of 11 h, increasing to 20.81 h and 28.18 h in TDs and ABs, respectively. Further mammary gland differentiation as a consequence of aging and pregnancy results in an even longer T_c, mainly due to a lengthening of the G_1 phase of the cell cycle (Figure 8.8) [13]. The length of T_c also varies according to the cell type and the specific compartment in which each given cell type is located in.

The shortest T_c is observed in intermediate cells located in TEBs, whereas it lengthens when the same cell type is located in ABs or lobules. These variations in the length of T_c are due mainly to differences in the length of the G_1 phase of the cell cycle, whereas all the other phases remain constant. Intermediate-type cells located in TEBs have a T_c lasting 13 h. When the same cell type is located in more differentiated structures, such as ABs, it exhibits a lengthened T_c, lasting 34 h. *These differences in cell kinetic parameters among the different cell types could explain the higher susceptibility of the intermediate cell of the TEBs to be affected by the carcinogen, which causes further expansion of the proliferative compartment of the intermediate cells and depression in the dark cell population after initiation of the carcinogenic stimulus* [14, 15].

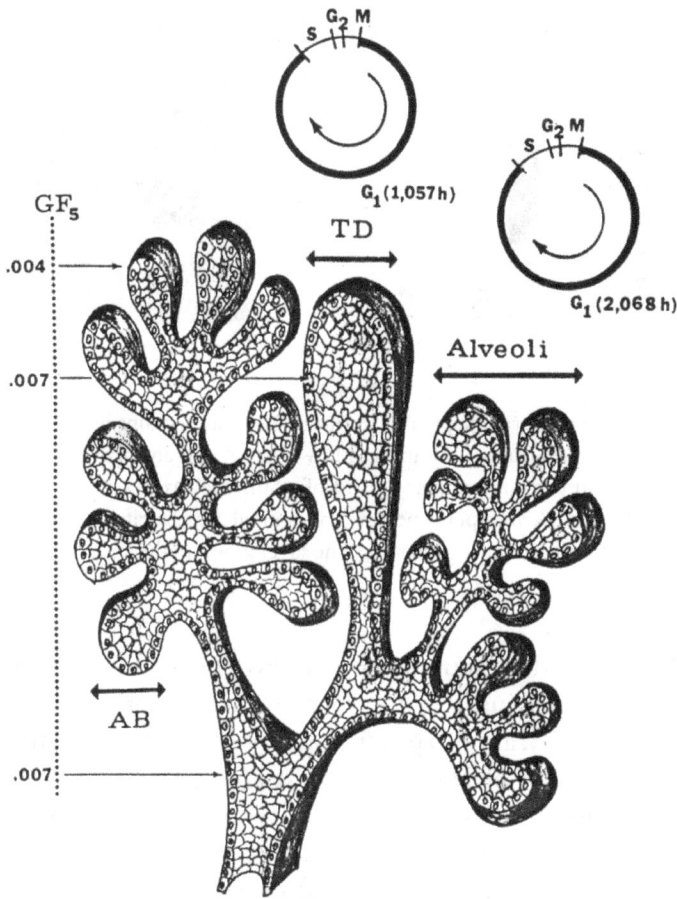

Figure 8.8: Schematic representation of terminal structures in the mammary gland of parous rats. The diagram of the cell cycle shows the relative length of the various phases of the cycle for each structure. Reprinted with permission from Ref. [13].

With Lee K. Tay, in 1981, we published our findings [16, 17] that the mammary epithelial cells metabolize DMBA to polar metabolites with the formation of epoxides that cause DNA damage. When dissociated mammary epithelial cells of young virgin and of parous animals, which basically represent the cells of the TEBs and of the lobules, respectively, are grown *in vitro*, they exhibit different rates of formation of polar metabolites.

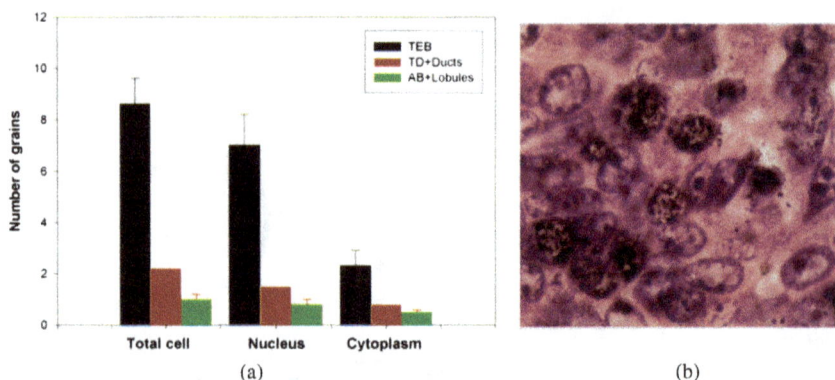

Figure 8.9: (a) Histogram depicting the number of silver grains in the terminal end buds (TEBs), terminal ducts, and ducts (TD + Ducts), and alveolar buds and lobules (AB + Lobules), in the rat mammary gland of a Sprague Dawley rat inoculated with 1 µCi of [^{3}H]-DMBA intraperitoneally. The animal was sacrificed 24 h later and processed for autoradiography studies. (b) The silver grains in the TEB. Counterstained with H&E (×40).

TEB cells produce more polar and less phenolic metabolites than lobular cells, indicating that the former, in addition to their higher proliferative activity, are also producing more epoxides, as is manifested by a higher binding of DMBA to DNA [2, 5, 16, 17] (Figure 8.9). Autoradiography studies performed *in vivo* confirm the observation that the greatest uptake of [^{3}H] DMBA occurs in the nucleus of epithelial cells of TEBs, and the lowest in ABs and lobules, indicating that the highest DMBA–DNA binding is associated with the structure of the gland with the highest replicative properties [2, 5]. The ability of the cells to remove DMBA adducts from the DNA is an indication of their capability to repair the damage. TEB cells remove adducts formed less efficiently than lobular cells. This is attributed to the shorter G_1 phase of T_c and not to a lack of reparative enzymes [10, 16, 17]. *Our studies allowed us to conclude for the first time that the differentiation of the mammary gland modifies the following: 1) glandular structure; 2) cell kinetic characteristics of the mammary epithelium, decreasing the growth fraction and lengthening the cell cycle, mainly the G_1 phase; 3) decreasing formation of polar metabolites and increasing phenolic metabolites; and 4) decreasing binding of the* *carcinogen. All the parameters listed above affect the susceptibility of the mammary gland to carcinogenesis, and so should be taken into account when assessing chemicals for cancer risk.*

8.7. Developing the concept of stem cell and the role of the stroma in mammary carcinogenesis

Our studies also provided strong evidence that in the rat mammary gland there are four different cell types designated as dark, intermediate, light, and myoepithelial and pointing to the intermediate cell type as the stem cell that populates mammary tumors. We published these observations [2, 5, 14, 15], and although not frequently acknowledged, our work in the identification of the cell of origin in mammary carcinogenesis was pioneering work, and I consider that historical reviewers will be able to trace those contributions because they were seminal works in the field of mammary gland stem cells [14, 15].

In this memoir, I also want to emphasize our pioneering contribution on the role of the stroma and inflammatory process in the emergence of the neoplastic lesions. These data have been ignored in the literature although they were described in detail in our book published by Springer in 2004 [2] and in a previous publication in 1996 [5] and even earlier in 1989 [18]. *We were the first ones to identify the role of inflammatory cells in the emergence of ductal hyperplasia and ductal carcinoma in situ.* We have shown that the TEB damaged by the carcinogen evolves to IDP, and this in turn to carcinoma *in situ* (CIS) (Figures 8.3–8.5). IDPs are morphologically distinguishable from TEBs by their size, which is more than twice that of the TEB, and by the homogenous cell composition, which consists preponderantly of intermediate cells (Table 8.1). As it is depicted in Figure 8.10, the induction of IDPs is by no means a rare event. Within 3 weeks of DMBA administration, there are between 10 and 20 IDPs per mammary gland, and this number increases with time, such that by 6–10 weeks after treatment there are approximately 30 lesions per gland, and around 200 per animal. Although IDPs occur

Table 8.1:   Differential diagnosis of TEB, lDP, and carcinoma *in situ* (CIS)

Tissue components	TEB	IDP	CIS
Basement membrane	Present	Present	Present
Periductal stroma	Normal	Moderate desmoplastic reaction	Marked desmoplastic reaction
Inflammatory reaction	Absent	Moderate	Marked
Luminal border	Smooth	Serrated	Irregular
Secondary luminae	Absent	Absent	Present in cribriform pattern
Micropapillae	Absent	Some	May be prominent
Epithelium	Heterogeneous, three cell types	Predominance of one cell type	Predominance of one cell type
Mitoses	Numerous	Numerous	Numerous

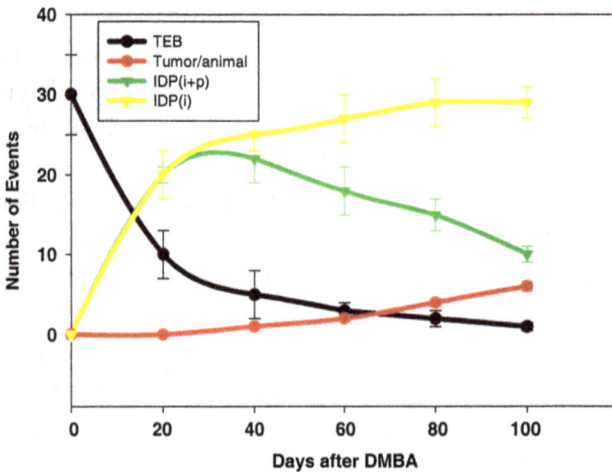

Figure 8.10:   Emergence of pre-neoplastic lesions lDP(i), lDP(i+p), and carcinomas (tumor/animal) as the number of TEBs decreases with time in the mammary gland at different periods after DMBA administration.

in large numbers following DMBA administration, the likelihood of any one IDP progressing to carcinoma in the intact mammary gland is lower than that, since the maximal tumorigenic response rarely goes beyond 5–6 adenocarcinomas per animal (Figure 8.10).

This is attributed to the fact that there are two different types of IDPs. The one that we call "initiated" IDP, [IDP(i)], increase in numbers steadily with a concomitant decrease in the numbers of TEBS; they reach a plateau by 60 days post-DMBA (Figure 8.10). The IDP(i) is characterized by a diameter larger than that of the TEB and is composed of a greater number of epithelial cells. *They do not elicit a response* in the surrounding stroma and remain unchanged during the whole post-carcinogen observation period. A second type of IDP, which we call "initiated and promoted", [IDP (i+p)], arises at the same time and reaches the same level as IDP (i); by 20–30 days post DMBA, they are also characterized by having a larger diameter and a greater cell number than TEBs. *They elicit a marked stromal reaction, consisting of collagen deposition and infiltration by mast cells and lymphocytes.*

IDPs(i+p) progress to CIS and to invasive carcinoma. The fact that not all the IDPs progress to carcinoma indicates that although both IDPs(i) and (i+p) are pre-neoplastic lesions, there are factors that regulate the progression of initiated cells, which affect IDPs(i) and IDPs(i+p) differently. We have been able to identify a host response elicited by the initiated cells that might play a role in this mechanism of progression of the initiated cells: IDP(i), which does not elicit stromal reaction and fails to progress to CIS, and IDP(i+p), which is surrounded by numerous mast cells and lymphocytes and originates malignant lesions (Figure 8.11). The number of mast cells around the IDP(i+p) is three times higher than in TEBs and IDP(i) (Figure 8.11). This IDP(i+p) increase in mast cells is accompanied by an increase in lymphocytes, fibroblasts, collagen fibers, and proteoglycans. Mast cells that are found in different parts of the body are also in the mammary gland. In their cytoplasm, the mast cells contain numerous granules measuring up to $0.8–1.1\mu m$ in diameter

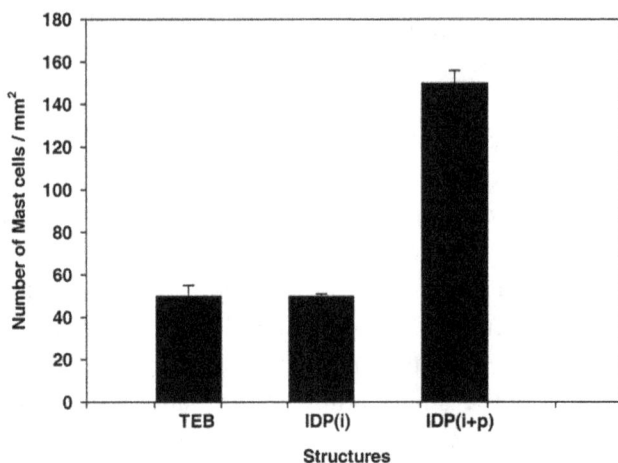

Figure 8.11:   Distribution of mast cells in TEB, IDP(i), and lDP(i+p).

which stain metachromatically with toluidine blue or Alcian blue (Figure 8.12). Mast cells have membrane receptors to IgE, which participate in immediate and delayed-type hypersensitivity. (*This phenomenon is difficult to visualize using hematoxylin for staining the mammary gland; instead using toluidine blue produces this metachromatic response, making it possible to observe the mast cells.* When an antigen combines with IgE and binds the cell receptor, the cell degranulates releasing histamine and heparin. Heparin is a heparan sulfate that has been shown to stimulate cell proliferation [19]. It has been shown that transplanted tumors in the chick embryo may increase by 40-fold the number of mast cells around the tumor implant before new capillaries arise [20]. Mast cell lysates or mast cell-conditioned medium stimulate locomotion of capillary endothelial cells *in vitro* [21, 22], an effect that is attributed to heparin. It has been postulated that heparin or fragments of heparin on the surface of endothelial cells may selectively bind endothelial cell mitogens that are also angiogenic [19]. Interestingly enough, there are several growth factors that have great affinity for heparin [23, 24]. It has also been shown that heparin-coated tumor cells exhibit altered transplantation and cytotoxicity reaction [25, 26], presumably due to blockage of cell surface antigens by heparin. Thus heparan sulfate

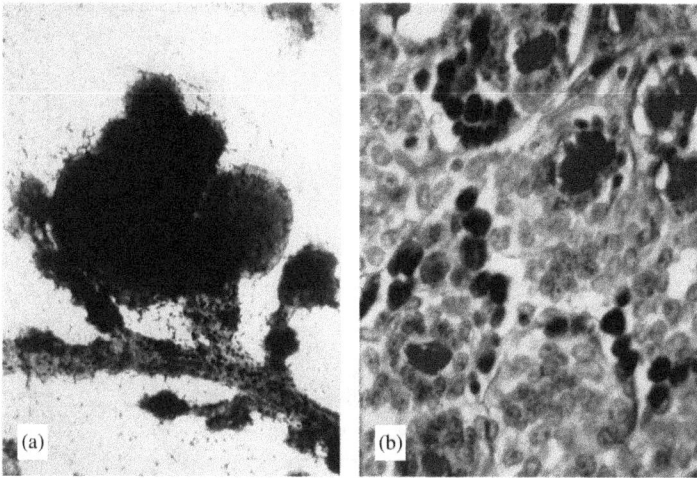

Figure 8.12: (a) Whole mount of adenocarcinoma showing the mast cells surrounding the tumor, stained with toluidine blue (×10). (b) Histological section of the tumor depicted stained with PAS–Alcian blue (×4).

proteoglycans may also be deposited in an annulus around the tumor and may modulate the immunoreactivity or accessibility of the enclosed cells. An early change that we observed during the process of transformation was the synthesis of a large amount of proteoglycans by IDP(i+p), which is evidenced by the deposition of an electron-dense material on the cell surface of the epithelial cells and by an increased reactivity with Alcian blue, pH 2.7, and PAS [2, 5, 18]. We demonstrated that this is accompanied by an increase in uptake of ^{3}H-fucose and ^{3}H-glucosamine (Figure 8.13). The number of cells taking up these precursors is almost three times the number found in TEBs and IDPs(i). *All these data clearly indicated to us that the initiated cells that are progressing to malignancy are secreting proteoglycans, which accumulate in the stroma.*

Furthermore, we postulated that these proteoglycans were either influencing the response of the host by eliciting a higher mobilization of mast cells and inhibiting the cytotoxic effect of lymphocytes or by inducing angiogenesis, desmoplasia, and cell proliferation. Some of these proteoglycans, such as heparan sulfate, were acting as receptors

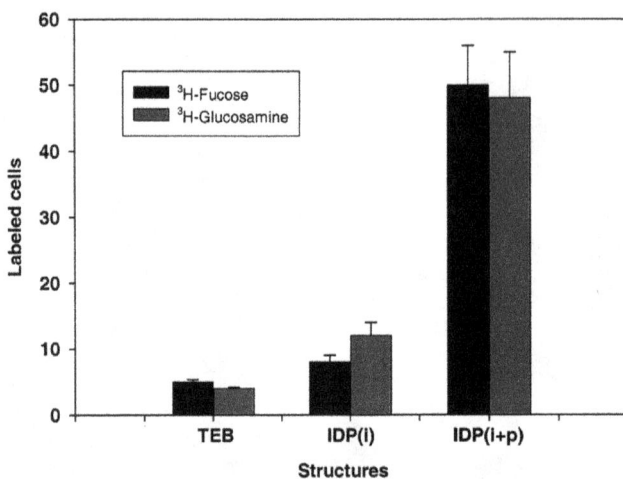

Figure 8.13: Histogram showing the percentage of cells labeled with ^{3}H-fucose and ^{3}H-glucosamine in TEB, IDP(i), and IDP(i+p).

for growth factors, which in turn initiate an autocrine response. Proteoglycans occur on the plasma membranes of mammalian cells and in the extracellular matrix [27–29]. They are neutral glycoproteins, stained by PAS, which are negative with Alcian blue pH 2.7 and contain fucose residues, and acid mucopolysaccharides, which react positively with Alcian blue pH 2.7 and negatively with PAS. Neoplastic transformation of cells dramatically alters proteoglycan synthesis both in the tumor and in the surrounding tissues [30]. This was thought to stimulate tumorigenic growth by decreasing the adhesion of transformed cells to the extracellular matrix [30]. We speculated that the production of proteoglycans allows the IDP to progress to CIS by stimulation of cell proliferation and by interference with an immune reaction toward the cells. Of these newly synthesized proteoglycans, both those that incorporate ^{3}H-D-glucosamine and stain with Alcian blue pH 2.7 and those that uptake ^{3}H-fucose and stain with PAS may act like epiglycanin [2, 5, 18], a high molecular weight sialo-glycoprotein present in mouse mammary carcinoma (Ta3) cells, which is thought to mask histocompatibility antigens. These, in turn, can prevent the generation and penetration of cytolytic lymphocytes [25].

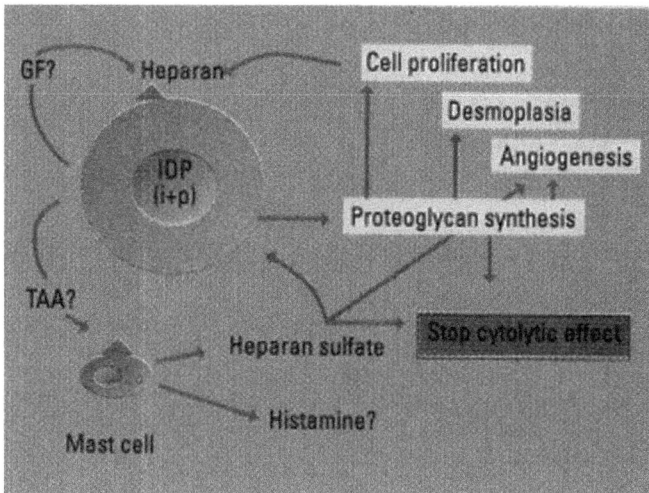

Figure 8.14: The transformed epithelial cells composing the intraductal proliferation (IDP) initiated and promoted (i+p) interact with stromal elements, attracting mast cells and stimulating local regulatory factors that result in increased synthesis of proteoglycans, which in turn affect cell proliferation, desmoplasia, and angiogenesis. GF, growth factor; TAA, tumor-associated antigens. Reprinted with permission from Ref. [5].

In Figure 8.14, I summarize what I interpreted on the interaction between the initiated cells and the stroma [5].

8.8. Impact and relevance of our studies in rat mammary carcinogenesis

Our studies provided a new look to the pathogenesis of breast cancer. Until our studies were published, the concept of pathogenesis of mammary cancer was overpopulated with data originated in mice and based on the viral theory postulating that the hyperplastic alveolar nodules developed after pregnancy were the ones that originated in adenocarcinomas (see Chapter 7). The mouse model of breast cancer did not match with the observations in humans, and we introduced not only a histological basis for understanding breast cancer but also provided a model that mimicked the human disease and provided a mechanistic basis for the susceptibility of the mammary tissue to carcinogenesis.

After our first presentation at the American Cancer Society meeting in 1975 [1], invitations to present our data grew every year, and we consistently presented our work in the yearly meetings of the American Association for Cancer Research (AACR) as invited or plenary speaker. Our first international platform to present these data was the Second Ibero Latinoamerican Congress of Cell Biology in *Mendoza, Argentina* (1978); followed by the Workshop on Chemical Carcinogen–Hormone Interaction in Transformation of Mammary Epithelial Cells *In Vitro*, in *Bethesda, Maryland* (1981); at the University of *Buenos Aires, Argentina* (1981); at the XI Triannual World Congress of Pathology, in *Jerusalem, Israel* (1981); at the Second International Conference on Carcinogenic and Mutagenic N-Substituted Aryl Compounds, in *Hot Springs, Arkansas* (1982); at Michigan State University, in *East Lansing, Michigan* (1982); at the Brookhaven National Laboratory Associated Universities, in *New York* (1983); at the Second International Symposium of the Society of Toxicologic Pathologists, in *Arlington, Virginia* (1983); at the Ludwig Institute for Cancer Research, in *Toronto, Canada* (1984); at the International Symposium of the Argentinean Foundation for Endocrinology in *Buenos Aires, Argentina* (1984); at the Gordon Conference on Mammary Gland Biology, *Colby-Sawyer College, New Hampshire* (1985); at the Institute of Pathobiology, in *Aspen, Colorado* (1985); at the Gordon Conference Hormonal Carcinogenesis, in *New Hampton, New Hampshire* (1985); at the Lakes Regional Discussion Group of the Society of Toxicologic Pathology, in *Ann Arbor, Michigan* (1985); at the Mastology Society, in *Mendoza, Argentina* (1986); at the Fifth Meeting of Society of Pathology of Ecuador in *Quito, Ecuador* (1986); at St. Mary University, in *San Antonio, Texas* (1986); at Wayne State University in *Detroit, Michigan* (1986); at the Institute Adolfo Lutz and University of *Sao Paulo, Brazil* (1986); at the University of Puerto Rico, in *San Juan, Puerto Rico* (1986); at the International Life Sciences Institute (ILSI), in *Hannover, West Germany* (1987); at the International Congress on Progress in Oncology, *Mendoza, Argentina* (1987); at the Liga Argentina de Lucha Contra el Cancer, in *Buenos Aires, Argentina* (1987); at the Boundaries Between Promotion and Progression During Carcinogenesis, in *Cleveland, Ohio* (1988); at the Japanese Cancer Association, in *Nagoya, Japan* (1988); at the Allegheny Singer Research Institute, in *Pittsburgh, Pennsylvania* (1988); at the Hospital Italiano, in *Mendoza, Argentina* (1988); at the Laboratory of Reproduction and Lactancy, in *Mendoza, Argentina* (1988); at the International Association for Breast Cancer Research, *Tel Aviv, Israel* (1989); at the Eppley Institute for Cancer Research in Cancer and Allied Research, in *Omaha, Nebraska* (1989); at the International Life Sciences Institute, in *Nara, Japan* (1989); at the International Life Science Institute, in *Baltimore, Maryland* (1989); at the Fifteenth International Cancer Congress Union International against Cancer, in *Buenos Aires, Argentina* (1990); at the Center for Reproduction and Lactation (LARLAC), in *Mendoza, Argentina* (1990); at the Eleventh Annual Meeting of the American College of Toxicology, in *Orlando, Florida* (1990); at the Smith Kline Beecham Animal Health, in *West Chester, Pennsylvania* (1991); at Harvard School of Public Health, Harvard University, in *Boston, Massachusetts* (1992); at the Symposia in Oncology, in *Pisa, Italy* (1992); at the Albert Einstein Medical Center, in *Philadelphia, Pennsylvania* (1993); at the Gordon Research Conference, *Salve Regina* University, in *Rhode Island* (1993); at the First Ibero-American Congress of Pathology, *Santiago de Compostela, Spain* (1993); at the International Symposium on Molecular Mechanisms of Radiation and Chemical Carcinogen-Induced Cell Transformation, *Mackinac Island, Michigan* (1993); at the Karolinska Institute, *Stockholm, Sweden* (1994); at Schering, *Berlin, Germany* (1994); at the Ninth International Conference on Carcinogenesis and Risk Assessment in *Austin, Texas* (1995); at the Workshop on Stem Cells and Carcinogenesis, in *Oahu, Hawaii*. (1995); at the Working Group on Hormone Related Cancer of the European Cancer Prevention Organization, in *Elbigenalp, Austria* (1996); at the National Institute of Environmental Health Sciences, in *Raleigh, North Carolina* (1996); at the Basic and Clinical Aspects of Breast Cancer, in *Keystone, Colorado* (1997); at the Toxicology seminar series at Texas A&M University, in *Dallas, Texas*

(1997); at the NIEHS workshop on characterizing the Effects of Endocrine Disrupters on Human Health and Environmental Exposure Levels, in *Raleigh, North Carolina* (1998); at the NCI Workshop on Comparative Pathology of Animal Models for Mammary Cancer, *Annapolis, Maryland* (1999); at the VI Congreso Venezolano de Mastologia, *Margarita Island, Venezuela* (1999); at SHARE, *New York* (1999); at the Think Tank 10, in *St. Maarten, Netherlands Antilles* (2000); at the International Academy of Pathology in the Symposium Comparative Pathology of Carcinogenesis, in *Nagoya, Japan* (2000); at the Maurer Foundation, in *Long Island, New York* (2005); at the Breast Cancer Environment Research Centers in the Kellogg Conference Center, in *Lansing, Michigan* (2005); at the National Health and Environmental Effects Research Laboratory, Reproductive Toxicology Division, in *Oakland, California* (2009).

Of all these scientific meetings, the one organized by the International Life Sciences Institute (ILSI) helped us to establish our classification of the rat mammary tumors as a standard for risk assessment evaluation and, more important, a long-lasting friendship with researchers around the world. We generated numerous publications with them [6, 7, 11, 12], and we were also asked to do a complete review of our work, published in *Environment Health Perspectives* in 1996 [5], and the cover of the journal featured the IDP originated in the TEB structures (Figure 11.2).

In 2014, the Society of Toxicology Pathology also invited me to write a special review article on "the significance of rat mammary tumors for human risk assessment" [3].

From July 16–17, 2017 we organized a workshop on the techniques and methodology for preparation and analysis of rat mammary gland whole mounts sponsored by the National Cancer Institute and the National Institute for Environmental Health Sciences that took place in our laboratories at the FCCC in Philadelphia. In this workshop, our criteria for evaluating the differentiation of the rat mammary gland and its evaluation as a surrogate maker of environmental action were accepted. In the compendium of the workshop [31], we published step by step the dissection of the mammary gland and the process to follow for the staining and preparation of the whole mounts with a description of the morphological analyses and quantitation of their structures. The idea behind this workshop was not only to unify the breast cancer researchers on how to study the mammary gland but also for the National Toxicology Program to adopt the study of the whole mounts for evaluating chemical substances. *The work that we initiated with Irma 42 years ago is still relevant.*

8.9. On how we developed a new paradigm in breast cancer prevention

Irma and I created the BCRL to question how breast cancer was initiated and developed, and we acquired a significant amount of data as explained in the previous sections, but at the same time we also asked *the opposite question: Why do certain women never develop breast cancer?* The only answer that we found was from epidemiological observations showing a direct association of breast cancer risk with nulliparity and of protection conferred by an early first full-term pregnancy [32–38]. Although the epidemiology was strong, it was not an explanation or a mechanism by which pregnancy protects the breast against cancer. We thought in 1974 that this *was* a window of opportunity that nature offered us for learning how a physiological event produces in 25% of parous women a complete protection against cancer. We used this basic concept as a blueprint to develop a new paradigm in breast cancer prevention [39–48]. From this initial idea, we were able to *unveil the biological principle underlying the protection conferred by an early first full-term pregnancy and by demonstrating experimentally that it induces in the breast the expression of a specific signature that results from the completion of a cycle of this organ's differentiation, driven by the reproductive process. It took almost 30 years before we were able to publish what was a signature specific for pregnancy that could be responsible for its protective effect* [49–55]. More important, *we have been able to harness this biological principle* by demonstrating in an experimental model that a short treatment with human chorionic gonadotropin (hCG), a placental hormone secreted during pregnancy, induces the same genomic signature as pregnancy, inhibiting not only the initiation but also the progression of mammary carcinomas, stopping the development of early lesions, such as IDPs, and CIS. These observations indicate that hCG administered for a very short period of time has significant potential as a chemopreventive agent, protecting the normal cell from becoming malignant [39–48]. *This new biological concept also implies that when the genomic signature of protection or refractoriness to carcinogenesis is acquired, hormonal treatment with hCG is no longer required. This is a novel concept that contraposes the current knowledge that a chemopreventive agent needs to be given for a long period to suppress a metabolic pathway or abrogate the function of an organ* [56, 57]. Therefore, in these memoirs, I will describe how we developed this knowledge, ending in Chapter 14 on what I believe will be my legacy.

8.10. The role of pregnancy

It was late in the afternoon one spring day in 1976 when Irma came to my office and showed me the TEB (Figure 13.2) that we saw in the virgin rats but were no longer present in the animals that had been going through pregnancy and lactation and that have been regressed over 21 days. *The TEBs had disappeared from the mammary glands of animals that had been going through the process of full pregnancy followed or not by lactation. We presented those data the following year at the meeting of the AACR [58] and published the full paper in 1978 [4].* That initial observation by Irma gave us the first hint that the protective effect of pregnancy was the elimination of the TEBs that were the target of the carcinogenic insult. We postulated that the differentiation of the mammary gland through pregnancy was responsible for the protective effect, and this was one of the aims of our NCI grant CA 27026. The changes induced by pregnancy alone or by pregnancy and lactation induced complete differentiation of all TEBs to lobules, which show active secretionary activity during lactation [see Ref. 2]. Those glands that have regressed to a pre-gestational condition, such as occurs after several weeks of weaning, do not appear extremely different in morphology from the glands of

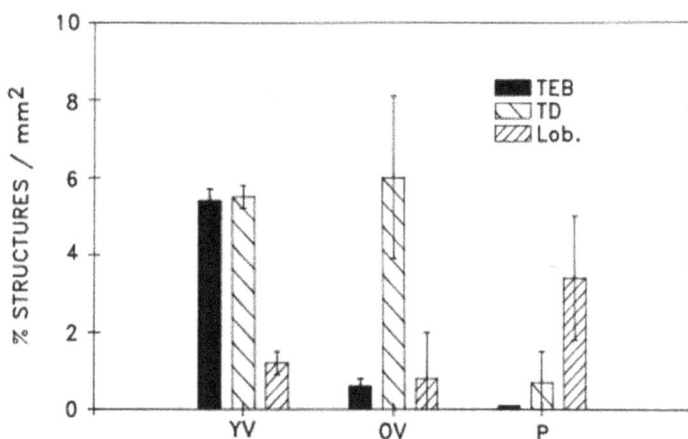

Figure 8.15: Number of structures/mm$_2$ (ordinate) in young virgin (YV; 55 days of age), old virgin (OV; 180 days of age), and parous (P; 180 days of age) animals. TEB, terminal end buds; TD, terminal duct; Lob., lobule. Reprinted with permission from Ref. [8].

virgin animals except for the absence of TEBs, fewer TDs, and more ABs and lobules (Figure 8.15) [4, 59].

These structures, however, show a marked diminution of growth fraction (GF) and a lengthening of the T_c. Very few TDs show active DNA synthesis, having only occasional cells labeled with [^{3}H] thymidine. The DNA-LI of ABs, which is 7.9% and 10.9% in young (55-day-old) and old (180-day-old) virgin rats, respectively, diminishes to 0.3% in parous rats (Figures 8.8 and 8.9). Parous rat mammary epithelial cells also have a lower binding of DMBA to DNA and a more efficient DNA repair (Figure 8.16) [4, 16, 17, 59]. In addition to tumor incidence, tumor type correlates with the degree of differentiation of the mammary gland at the time of exposure to the carcinogen. All of the tumors developed by young virgin rats are carcinomas of ductal origin. Both young and old virgin rats present a higher incidence of hyperplastic alveolar nodules, adenomas, and cysts than multiparous rats [10, 60]. Fibroadenomas, on the other hand, are twice as frequent in multiparous rats as in age-matched old virgin rats (Figure 8.17) [60]. Importantly, in order for pregnancy to be

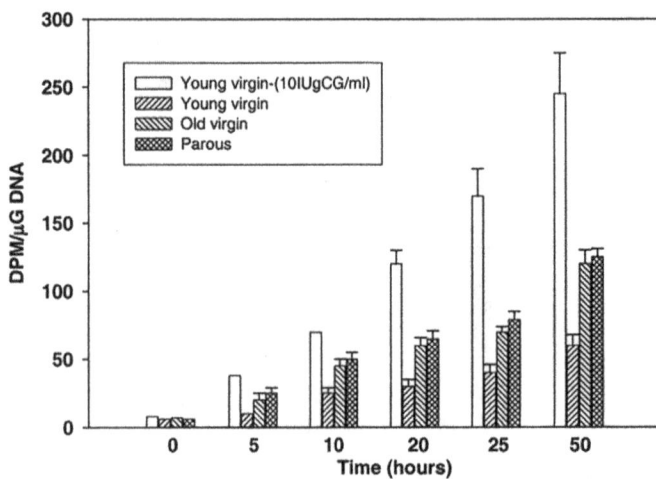

Figure 8.16: DNA excision repair in rat mammary epithelial cells treated with 0.1 mg of DMBA/mL of medium, expressed as disintegrations per minute per μg DNA (ordinate).

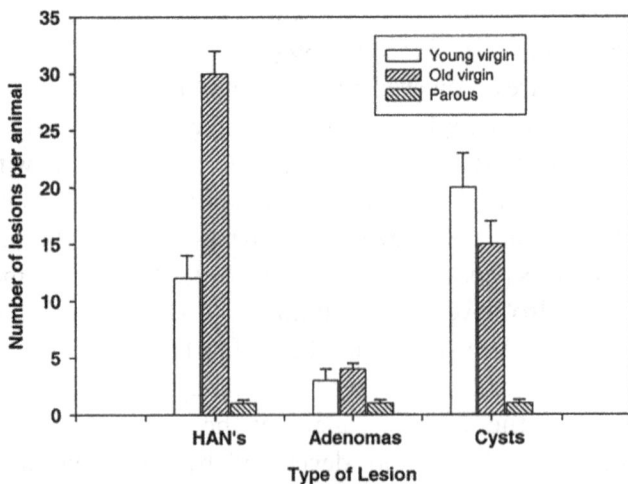

Figure 8.17: Histogram depicting the type of lesions identified in the mammary glands of virgin and parous rats. HANs, hyperplastic alveolar nodules.

protective it must be complete, because pregnancy interruption in these animals is not associated with protection, and the animals developed the same number of tumors and malignant lesions as those virgin controls [61].

8.11. Mimicking pregnancy

It was obvious to us that the pregnancy protection was a hint on how to pursue further. The fact that pregnancy before carcinogen administration seems to be the only truly protective factor in chemically induced mammary gland carcinogenesis suggested to us that placental hormones could play an important role in mammary growth and development during pregnancy and that, on the other hand, the hormonal changes of pregnancy accelerate DMBA-induced mammary tumor growth when mating occurs after carcinogen administration, indicating to us that *the most important event in determining the role that placental hormones plays in either preventing initiation or in promoting tumor growth is the sequence in which they reach the mammary gland. The first experiment that we performed was* DMBA administration at 21 days after the termination of hCG inoculation in doses of 1, 5, 10, or 100 IU/day for 21 days, starting when the rats were at 50 days old, markedly reducing the incidence of tumors from 42.0% in control to 14.0%, 12.5%, 12.5%, and 0%, respectively, in animals treated with the above listed doses. The role of hCG was specific because treatment of 50-day-old rats with 0.5 mg/day of placental lactogen alone or in combination with 1 IU of hCG for 21 days before DMBA administration significantly increases the incidence of carcinomas with regard to control animals. Like pregnancy, hCG induces a greater differentiation of the gland, resulting in a greater number of ABs and lobules, with a consequently decreased number of TEBs and TDs. These changes are accompanied by a decreased DNA-LI [39–48, 62]. Instead, placental lactogen administration, either alone or in combination with hCG, fails to stimulate gland differentiation, and glands from animals thus treated have more TEBs and TDs and fewer ABs and lobules than do glands of control animals.

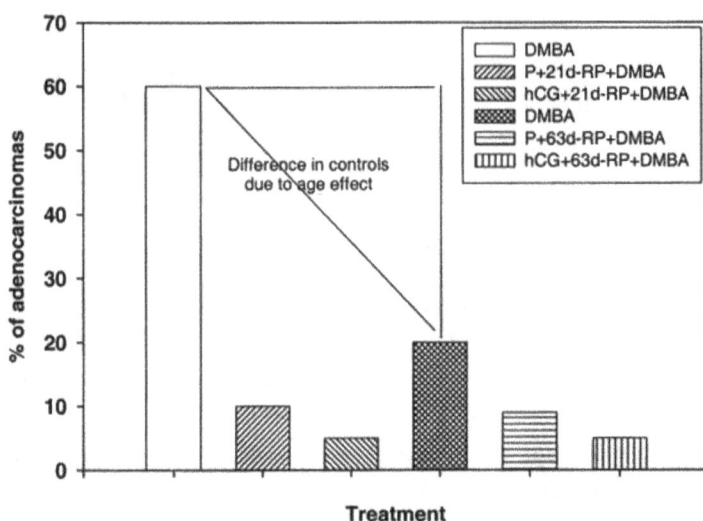

Figure 8.18: Adenocarcinoma incidence (ordinate): percentage of animals developing mammary adenocarcinomas. DMBA, 7, 12-dimethylbenz(a)anthracene; P, pregnancy; RP, resting period post-pregnancy; hCG, human chorionic gonadotropin.

The DNA-LI in all of these terminal structures is similar or slightly higher than that of control animals [62]. Of great importance from these studies was the demonstration that the reduction in cancer incidence is permanent, as demonstrated by the similar degree of reduction when DMBA was administered after a delay of 21, 42, or 63 days after termination of hCG treatment (Figure 8.18).

8.12. Contraceptive hormones in cancer prevention

The use of hCG was a new idea and also very attractive for those who had an open mind but not for the majority of our peers. Therefore, we decided to do more experiments to demonstrate that hCG was really the way to prevent breast cancer. Irma and I obtained another NCI grant to study the effect of contraceptives as preventive agents based on the knowledge that their use does not result in increased breast cancer risk [63].

For this purpose, we administered to nulliparous females of young age hormone combination norethynodrel–mestranol, and of the progestagenic agent medroxyprogesterone acetate (MPA). These studies led to several important discoveries. These two agents differ in their mechanism of action; norethynodrel has a weak progestagenic activity and is considered to be atypical since it induces perinuclear vacuolization of endometrial epithelium, an effect similar to that of estrone [64], and in addition it is administered in conjunction with the estrogenic compound mestranol. MPA is an acetoxyprogesterone derivative more potent than progesterone [64] that significantly reduces estradiol receptor levels in human endometrium [65] and cervical epithelium [66]; however, when both agents are administered at the same dose used for contraception, they induce a degree of mammary gland development which suffices to reduce cancer incidence by more than 85%. However, maximal protection is achieved only when the hormones are administered to young but sexually mature animals ranging in age from 55 to 65 days old (Figure 8.19) [67, 68]. We call this period the "protection window" which overlaps with the

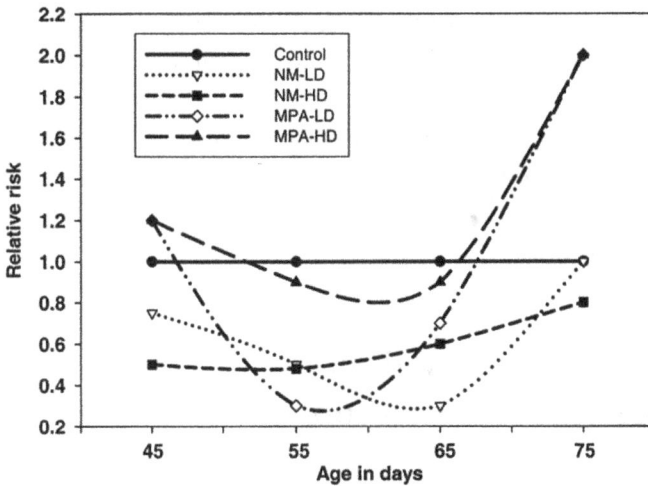

Figure 8.19: Comparative curve of the risk to develop mammary cancer in DMBA-treated animals that have been treated with norethynodrel–mestranol (NM) or medroxyprogesterone acetate (MPA) at low (LD) or high doses (HD).

"risk window" since the same age range represents the peak of susceptibility to neoplastic transformation [9, 10]. Treatment at a younger age, but after puberty and after 65 days of age, either diminishes the protective effect of the combination contraceptive or increases the risk of breast cancer development when the progestagenic contraceptive is used (Figure 8.19) [67, 68]. The selective susceptibility of the mammary gland's TEBs to respond with either differentiation under hormonal stimuli, or transformation under a carcinogenic stimulus, at that specific age indicates that both systems act on the same target and probably utilize the same receptors. Of greater concern was the effect of MPA, which, when administered to post-pubertal females or to old virgin females, stimulates the TEBs of the young animals or reactivates the quiescent TDs of old animals, thus expanding the "risk window" for carcinogenesis. These observations were confirmed by data demonstrating that prolonged treatment with progestagens results in development of mammary nodules [69, 70] and malignant neoplasms [69–71]. Epidemiological observations concur with these findings, as directly proportional to the number of TEBs that are at their peak of cell proliferation [4, 62, 72–75]. Stimulation of the development and differentiation of the gland, resulting in profuse lobular development and depression of DNA synthesis, such as it occurs during pregnancy, or after completion of a 21-day treatment of virgin rats with hCG, reduce the susceptibility of the mammary epithelium to be transformed by the carcinogen. The reduction in cancer incidence is permanent, as demonstrated by the similar degree of reduction when DMBA is administered after a delay of 21, 42, or 63 days after termination of hCG treatment.

8.13. The cellular and molecular mechanism of cancer prevention

We had been able to demonstrate experimentally that pregnancy induces mammary cancer prevention and that the same effect can be obtained by hormonal manipulation and narrowing down to hCG as the hormone that was more efficient in inducing gland differentiation and therefore a complete abrogation of the carcinogenic effect of the polycyclic hydrocarbon DMBA. The next step was to provide the cellular and molecular mechanisms that explain this protection. This was a great challenge for us as experimental pathologists.

In 1982, William McGuire, then editor of the *Journal Breast Cancer Research and Treatment,* invited us to write a review article of our work [10]. At that specific time of our studies we concluded that the protective effect of pregnancy was due to the induction of mammary gland differentiation, inhibition of cell proliferation, increase in the DNA repair capabilities of the mammary epithelium, decrease in the binding of the carcinogen to the DNA, and activation of genes controlling programmed cell death (PCD) [42–48]. The activation of these genes by hCG is of great relevance because PCD is a physiological and phylogenetically conserved form of active cell death (or apoptosis) that has been associated with specific phases of development that control cell proliferation and differentiation [46]. In those days, we also thought that inhibin could be the mediator of the process, and we published several papers supporting this contention [see References 9 and 10] until we realized that not all the pieces of the puzzle fit together, and we pursued identifying other genes that could also be involved in the process. At that time Dr. Pramod Srivastava joined our laboratory. Pramod turned out to be a talented molecular biologist who conducted solid work not only on inhibin but also other transcription factor and genes that later on we confirmed using more advanced techniques like cDNA arrays and sequencing [72]. Even early on, we were able to identify that PCD or apoptosis could be an important mechanism involved in protection. Treatment with hCG induced an increase in the apoptotic index, which reached its maximum when the animals were 85 days old, and it remained elevated at the same level even after cessation of the hormonal treatment (Figure 8.20).

Administration of hCG after DMBA induced a steady increase in the apoptotic index, which reached a peak by the time the animals were 105 days old, but its value decreased sharply after the discontinuation of the hormonal treatment (Figure 8.20). The

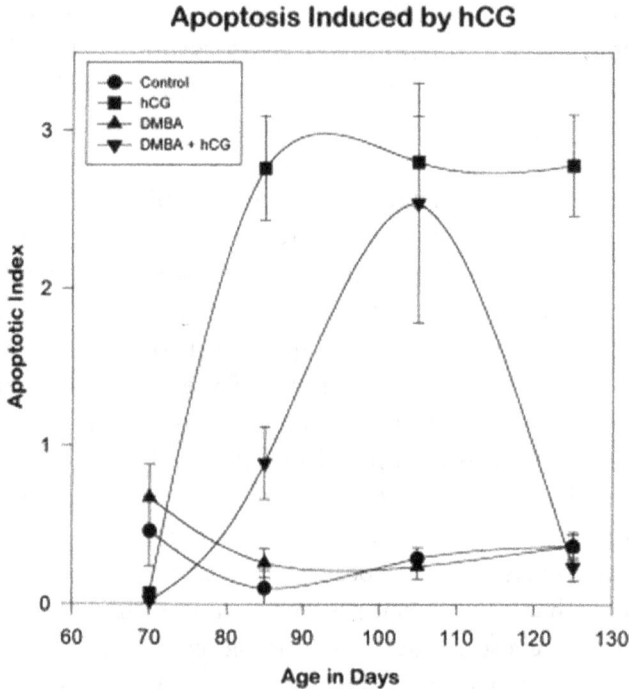

Figure 8.20:   Detection of apoptotic cells in non-tumoral mammary glands of four groups of rats (Control, hCG, DMBA, and DMBA+hCG). Results are expressed as the number of immunocytochemically positive cells per total number of cells counted, and expressed as a percentage, or apoptotic index (ordinate). Rats were sacrificed at 70, 85, 105, and 125 days of age (abscissa). Bars represent the mean ± standard deviation of 5 animals counted per group and per time point. Reprinted with permission from Ref. [3].

apoptotic index of DMBA-induced mammary carcinomas was markedly lower than that of the non-tumoral mammary gland of the animals in the same group. HCG treatment resulted in a marked increase in the apoptotic index of mammary adenocarcinomas with respect to the values found in the tumors of the DMBA group, and it was also higher than in the non-tumoral mammary gland of the same group of animals (Figure 8.20), meaning that the treatment of virgin rats with hCG, in which the mammary carcinogenic process had been initiated with the chemical carcinogen DMBA, induces PCD.

Therefore, the data clearly showed us that the use of agents that induce apoptosis, like hCG, may constitute a useful approach for the prevention and therapy of breast cancer. However, one challenging question was to demonstrate that the effect of hCG was due to the hormone and not an indirect consequence of changes in the ovary, meaning the real question was whether the hCG or the hormones of the ovaries were responsible for the protective effect that we saw.

For this purpose, we performed ovariectomy after DMBA administration (group 3) (Table 8.2) and compared these animals with intact animals in group 1 or animals that were challenged with DMBA. As expected, the tumor incidence and the number of tumors per animal were significantly reduced by ovarian ablation as well as by hCG (groups 2 and 4). Estrogen supplementation in the ovariectomized animals reestablished the tumor incidence and number of tumors per animals (group 5); however, in those supplemented animals hCG significantly reduced the number of tumors per animal as well as the incidence (group 6). These data clearly indicated that hCG has a direct effect on the mammary gland, independent of the ovarian function. This also suggests that hCG could be a tumor-static agent in postmenopausal women, even in the presence of hormone replacement therapy as we show later on [76]. We further pursue the demonstration that hCG has a direct effect on the mammary epithelial cells by treating human breast epithelial cells (HBECs) with hCG (Figure 8.21).

Table 8.2: Experimental protocol to determine the direct effect of hCG in the rat mammary gland

Effect of ovariectomy and HCG treatment in DMBA-induced mammary carinogenesis

Group	An.	An. w T/An	%	Tumors	Tumors/An.
1 DMBA	18	18/18	100	60	3.30
2 DMBA + hCG	20	9/20	45	20	1.00
3 O.V. + DMBA	18	1/18	6	4	0.22
4 O.V. + DMBA + hCG	20	0/20	0	0	0.00
5 O.V. + DMBA + E.P.	18	6/18	33	8	0.44
6 O.V. + DMBA E.P. + hCG	20	2/20	10	2	0.10

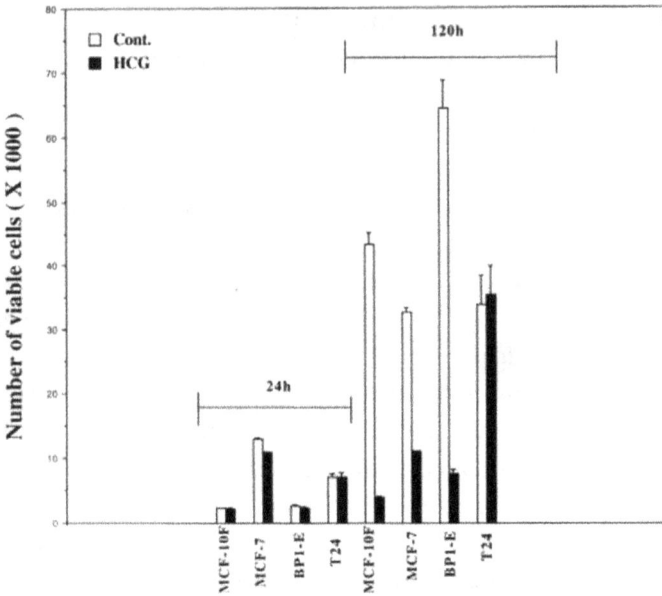

Figure 8.21:   Effect of hCG treatment on cell growth. MCF-1 OF, BPI-E, and T24 cells were treated daily with 100 IU/mL hCG and harvested at 24 and 120 h for cell growth determination by WST-colorimetric assay. Control cells were treated with vehicle only. Values represent the mean number of viable cells (×1,000) ± SD. Reprinted with permission from Ref. [78].

Our studies *in vitro* allowed us to better manipulate the experimental conditions and to show not only the direct effect of the hCG but also understand the molecular mechanism of its action. We showed that hCG inhibits the proliferative activity of the cells and induces activation of apoptotic genes. Inhibition of cell growth was observed only in HBEC, whereas the urothelial cells T24 were not affected by this treatment (Figure 8.21). We tested the human breast epithelial cell lines [77, 78] and showed that hCG induced activation of the apoptotic genes TRPM2, ICE, TGF-b, p53, bax, and p21WAFI/CIPI (Figure 8.22). We also tested in two other cell lines, the BP1-E cells, derived from BP-transformed MCF-l0F cells were also growth-inhibited; however, the pattern of gene activation differed from that exhibited by the parent cells. BP1-E cells exhibited

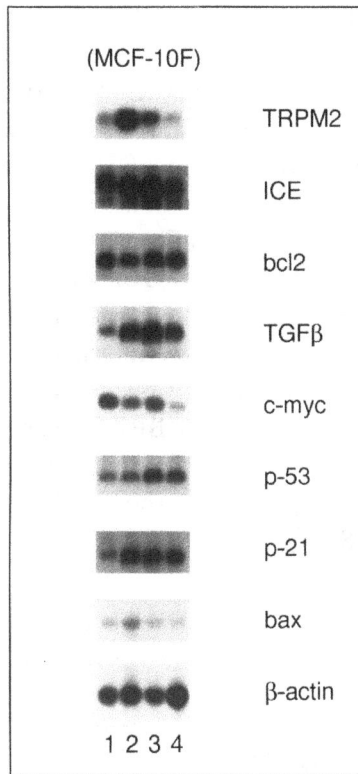

Figure 8.22: Northern blot analysis of TRPM2, ICE, bcl2, TGF-β, c-myc, p53, bax, and p21 gene expressions in MCF-10F cells. Polyadenylated RNA was isolated from cells treated daily with 100 IU/mL hCG and harvested at 24 and 120 h. Lanes 1 and 2 represent control cells treated with vehicle solution for 24 and 120 h, while Lanes 3 and 4 represent cells treated with hCG for 24 and 120 h, respectively. β-actin was used for detecting the amount of RNA loaded in each lane. Reprinted with permission from Ref. [78].

activation of only ICE, bax, and p21 WAFI/CIPI, and significantly down-regulated bcl2, but did not modify TGF-p, p53 or *cmyc* expression. The urothelial cells did not show activation of any of the apoptotic genes. The lack of activation of the genes that control PCD in these latter cells coincides with the selectivity of hCG in the inhibition of *in vitro* cell proliferation, which was observed only in HBECs but not in T24 cells [78].

This specificity of action was attributed to a receptor-mediated effect of hCG on HBECs. We had discussed these data extensively in the manuscripts that we published with Pramod Srivastava in 1998 [77, 78]. The evidence that we had at that time was that the induction of apoptosis was mediated by both p53 and *c-myc*, which are the major players in the context of growth arrest and apoptosis. Basically, we found that hCG treatment significantly induced the expression of p53 and p21 WAFI/CrPr in MCF-10F cells, an observation that suggested that the cell growth arrest was mediated by the tumor suppressor p53 through its downstream target gene p21 WAFI/CIPI [77, 78]. The observation that p53 was significantly activated by hCG treatment in MCF-10F, but not in BP1-E cells, led us to postulate that the activation of apoptotic genes might have occurred through those two different pathways for the inhibition of *in vitro* cell proliferation (Figure 8.23).

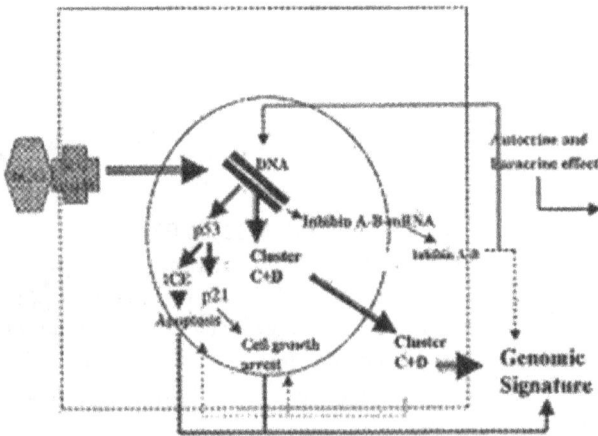

Figure 8.23: Postulated model of hCG-induced cell cycle arrest and apoptosis in human breast epithelial cells. In the presence of hCG for 24 h, breast epithelial cells bind the hormone to a putative membrane receptor. This triggers a cascade of programmed cell death gene activation through the cAMP/PKA pathway, as well as through activation of TGF-β. hCG treatment activates (upregulates)TRPM2, ICE, TGF-β, p53, and p21 in MCF-1 OF cells; in BP1-E cells, it activates TRPM2, ICE, p21, and bax, but does not activate TGF-β, c-myc, or p53, leading us to postulate that p21 and bax activation in these cells proceeds through an alternative pathway, i.e., TF/ DF (broken arrow). Reprinted with permission from Ref. [78].

Our observations suggested that in MCF-10F cells hCG arrested the progression of the cell cycle by inducing (probably through its receptor) the CAMPPKA and p53, as well as the TGF-β pathways, for acting on their target gene p21 WAFI/CIPI, proceeding then toward cell cycle arrest and apoptosis (Figure 8.23).

8.14. Connecting the dots

Many of the data that I presented in this chapter were published as late as 1998, but I have described them here because they were the product of the line of research that we conceived during the period 1973–1978. Those were the years that allowed me to develop the blueprint that gave me the opportunity to carve my independence as a cancer researcher. It is extremely important that I also emphasize that it was the close partnership with Irma that made developing this line of research possible. *It was in this period that Irma and I worked closer together than in any other time of our life.*

We grew together in this new scientific environment, and the need to face so many uncertainties, including mastering the English language, made us spend hours face-to-face analyzing the data and writing the results and discussing each single word for its meaning and repercussion. Irma was brilliant at crafting the right sentence, and she rewrote, and rewrote the sentence until it sounded perfect, whereas I was consumed by ensuring that the data were presented properly and that the ideas were accompanied by the right illustration, table, or figure. Irma and I had the best partnership imaginable. It was difficult for anybody to compete with both of us, and even harder to enter in our circle. Our discussion across the table was about ideas and how to understand and express them. When in later years we were uncertain about how to face our research, our memories and professional path came back to this period of our life because we knew that this was the way. Those years definitely unified us in purpose, and our love for each other was consolidated and matured. In those years, the need to have a child was also growing on us, and so it was in this period that we really took a serious look at our future in the United States. It is important to emphasize that many different events took place during that period that also made the love between Irma and I grow. Irma underwent breast and thyroid surgery, but the result was that it was a benign processes in both cases, but this scared us enough in our sense of mortality. In 1975, we visited Argentina, and although reencountering family and all the friends who had been our circle when we left Argentina was revitalizing and memorable, the country did not look prosperous and a cloud of uncertainty was permeating all the layers of society. My parents made their first visit to Michigan; they were expecting the big surprise of a grandchild, and I know that they were disappointed — it was not until 1980 that my only daughter was born.

It was also at the end of 1975 that we realized that the USA was the country in which we must pursue our dreams. The Argentina of our youth did not exist anymore, and we found that although effectively the nexus was not lost, we had acquired a new dimension in our research and lifestyle and we could not turn back the clock, but we also realized that being foreigners was not a plus, and our chances of fulfilling our expectations and dreams in the USA would require a significant effort on our part. We palpated firsthand the real situation of us as foreigners in the US, and we realized that at least we should take a proactive attitude or our situation would not get better. Irma took the first step and became an approved Foreign Medical Graduate in January of 1976, starting a residency in pathology at Wayne State University in July of that year. I followed her steps three years later, but by then she was taking the initiative to be a board-certified pathologist. Also, we decided to acquire our first home in February of 1976, and we finally bought one at 1226 Audubon Street in Grosse Pointe Park. It was in that house that Patricia was born in 1980.

The period of 1973–1978 was the one in which we saw the scientific environment with a more objective perspective, and we were able to see the main parameters that could decide our future. Publications and grants were the two main tickets to our success, and we pursued these venues with extreme effort and energy. But there was something that bothered us: the fact that we were not recognized as medical doctors. We were simple researchers but not attached to any famous laboratory group in the USA. We were, in a certain way, out of the pack. The only solution was to make ourselves visible for our own merits, and so we decided to validate our medical degrees, obtain a medical certification or license to practice medicine, and pursue a specialization that made us board certified as a way to be trained in this country. When Irma started the residency in pathology in 1976, she was able to spend few hours a day in the laboratory and most of the evening working on our grants and publications. Our orientation to pathology was a natural one based on our training, and by the end of 1978, Irma was completing the last year of her residency program, and had passed the FLEX examination that allowed her to practice medicine in this country. My situation was more difficult because I wanted to continue minding the BCRL and I had also started a new project that was called "The Brown Book," a major research project replacing the "viral group" that had already been phased out. The Brown Book's aim was to validate in paraffin-embedded tissue prognostic factors that could be used for predicting survival. This project was supported by the NCI, and my role was to manage the pathology core and provide support by coordinating a pathology core formed by four representative pathologists of the main hospitals of the Metropolitan Detroit. This put me in direct contact with the best breast tumor pathologist, an opportunity that I used to negotiate my US training in pathology. I had already become an approved Foreign Medical Graduate in March of 1978 and started to negotiate how I could be the BCRL and the experimental pathology laboratory director at the MCF, and at the same time validate my training in pathology to get my board certification. This ambitious plan and the independence we gained by the new grants from the NCI and the American Cancer Society triggered tension with our superiors, mainly Marvin Rich, and the situation reached a point of significant tension, further aggravated by the mismanagement he was accused of that finally ended in his dismissal of the MCF. Although I was not in his close circle and did not know the details, I felt the tension that the situation had created around us. We considered moving on, and we looked at the Mayo Clinic, Michigan State University, and Northwestern University in Chicago. The problem was that the new place must accept both of us and must also help us finish our board certifications in pathology and in addition provide laboratory space for continuing our research that was already funded by the NCI and the American Cancer Society. Our moving out of the MCF never materialized, and we stayed in Michigan for many more years, solidifying our position at the intellectual level and reasserting our line of research, and at the same time we learned to stay separate from the political turmoil at the MCF in that period and pursue our own path.

References

[1] Russo, I., Saby, J. and Russo, J. Pathogenesis of a rat mammary carcinoma induced by DMBA. *Proc. Am. Assoc. for Cancer Res.* 16: 654, 1975.

[2] Russo, J. and Russo, I. H. *Biological and Molecular Basis of Breast Cancer*, Springer-Verlag, Heidelberg. 2004.

[3] Russo, J. Significance of rat mammary tumors for human risk assessment. *Toxicol Pathol.* 43: 145–70, 2015.

[4] Russo, I. H. and Russo, J. Developmental stage of the rat mammary gland as determinant of its susceptibility to 7,12-dimethylbenz (a) anthracene. *J. Natl. Cancer Inst.* 61: 1439–1449, 1978.

[5] Russo, I. H. and Russo, J. Mammary gland neoplasia in long-term rodent studies. *Environ. Health Perspect.* 104: 938–967, 1996.

[6] Russo, I. H., Tewari, M. and Russo, J. Morphology and development of rat mammary gland. In: Jones, T. C., Mohr, U., Hunt, R. D., (eds), *Integument and Mammary Gland of Laboratory Animals*, Springer-Verlag, Berlin. 1989, 233–252.

[7] Russo, I. H., Medado J. and Russo, J. Endocrine influences on mammary structure and development. In: Jones, T. C, Mohr, U., Hunt, R. D., (eds), *Integument and Mammary Gland of Laboratory Animals*, Springer-Verlag, Berlin. 1989, 252–266.

[8] Russo, J. and Russo, I. H. Toward a physiological approach to breast cancer prevention. *Cancer. Epidemiol. Biomarkers Prev.* 3: 353–364, 1994.

[9] Russo, J., Saby, J., Isenberg, W. and Russo, I. H. Pathogenesis of mammary carcinoma induced in rats by 7,12-dimethylbenz (a) anthracene. *J. Natl. Cancer Inst.* 59: 435–445, 1977.

[10] Russo, J., Tay, L. K. and Russo, I. H. Differentiation of the mammary gland and susceptibility to carcinogenesis. *Breast Cancer Res. Treat.* 2: 5–37, 1982.

[11] Russo, J., Gusterson, B. A., Rogers, A. E., Russo, I. H., Wellings, S. R. and van Zwieten, M. J. Comparative study of human and rat mammary tumorigenesis. *Lab. Invest.* 62: 1–32, 1990.

[12] Russo, J., Russo, I. H., van Zwieten, M. J., Rogers A. E. and Gusterson, B. Classification of neoplastic and non-neoplastic lesions of the rat mammary gland. In: Jones, T. C., Mohr, U., Hunt, R. D., (eds), *Integument and Mammary Glands of Laboratory Animals*, Springer-Verlag, Berlin. 1989, 275–304.

[13] Russo, J. and Russo, I. H. Influence of differentiation and cell kinetics on the susceptibility of the rat mammary gland to carcinogenesis. *Cancer Res.* 40: 2677–2687, 1980.

[14] Russo, I. H., Ireland, W. and Russo, J. Ultrastructural description of three different epithelial cell types in rat mammary gland. *Proc. Electron Microsc. Soc. Am.* 34: 146–147, 1976.

[15] Russo, J., Tait, L. and Russo, I. H. Susceptibility of the mammary gland to carcinogenesis III. The cell of origin of mammary carcinoma. *Am. J. Pathol.* 113: 50–66, 1983.

[16] Tay, L. K. and Russo, J. Formation and removal of 7,12-dimethylbenz (a) anthracene nucleic acid adducts in rat mammary epithelial cells with different susceptibility to carcinogenesis. *Carcinogenesis* 2: 1327–1333, 1981.

[17] Tay, L. K. and Russo, J. 7,12-dimethylbenz (a) anthracene (DMBA) induced DNA binding and repair synthesis in susceptible and non-susceptible mammary epithelial cells in culture. *J. Natl. Cancer Inst.* 67: 155–161, 1981.

[18] Russo, J. and Russo, I. H. Boundaries in mammary carcinogenesis, In: Sudilovsky, O., Pitot, H. C., Liotta, L. A., (eds.),*The Boundaries Between Promotion and Progression During Carcinogenesis*, Plenum Publishing Corp., New York. 1989, 43–50.

[19] Folkman, J. How is blood vessel growth regulated in normal and neoplastic tissue? *Cancer Res.* 46: 467–473, 1986.

[20] Kessler, D. A., Langer, R. S., Pless, N. A. and Folkman, J. Mast cells and tumor angiogenesis. *Int. J. Cancer.* 18: 703–709, 1976.

[21] Zetter, B. R. Migration of capillary endothelial cells is stimulated by tumour-derived factors. *Nature* 285: 41–43, 1980.

[22] Azizkhan, R. G., Azizkhan, J. C., Zetter, B. R. and Folkman, J. Mast cell heparin stimulates migration of capillary endothelial cells in vitro. *Exp. Med.* 152: 931–944, 1980.

[23] Gospardorowicz, D. Cheng, J. Lui, G. M. Baird, A. and Bohlent, P. Isolation of brain fibroblast growth factor by heparin-sepharose affinity chromatography: identify with pituitary fibroblast growth factor. *Proc. Natl. Acad. Sci. U.S.A.* 81: 6963–6967, 1984.

[24] Lobb R. R. and Fett, J. N. Purification of two distinct growth factors from bovine neural tissue by heparin affinity chromatography. *Biochemistry* 23: 6295–6299, 1984.

[25] Lippman, M. Transplantation and cytotoxicity changes induced by acid mucopolysaccharides. *Nature* 219: 33–36, 1968.

[26] McBride W. M. and Bard, J. B. L. Hyaluronidase-sensitive halos around adherent cells. *J. Exp. Med.* 149: 507–515, 1979.

[27] Ito, I. Radioactive labeling of the surface coat on enteric microvilli. *Anat. Res.* 151: 489a, 1965.

[28] Bekesi J. G. and Winzler, R. J. The metabolism of plasma glycoproteins: Studies on the incorporation of L-fucose-1-14C into tissue and serum in the normal rat. *J. Biol. Chem.* 242: 3873–3879, 1967.

[29] Bossmann, H. B. Hagopian, A. and Eylar, E. H. Cellular membranes: The biosynthesis of glycoprotein and glycolipids in the HeLa cell membranes. *Arch. Biochem.* 130: 573–533, 1969.

[30] Esko, J. D., Rostand, S. and Weinke, J. L. Tumor formation dependent on proteoglycan biosynthesis. *Science* 241: 1092–1096, 1988.

[31] Salovich, D., Santucci-Pereira, J. and Russo, J. Techniques and methodology for preparation and analysis of rat mammary gland whole mounts. Workshop on the *Techniques and Methodology for Preparation and Analysis of Rat Mammary Gland Whole Mounts* sponsored by the National Cancer Institute and the National Institute for Environmental Health Sciences, July 16–17, 2017, Philadelphia, PA.

[32] Trapido, E. J. Age at first birth, parity and breast cancer risk *Cancer* 51: 946–948, 1983.

[33] MacMahon, B., Cole, P. and Lin, T. M. Age at first birth and breast cancer risk. *Bull. World Health Organ* 43: 209, 1970.

[34] Chie, W. C., Hsieh, C., Newcomb, P. A., Longnecker, M. P., Mittendorf, R., Greenberg, E. R., Clapp, R. W., Burke, K. P., Titus-Ernstoff, L., Trentham-Dietz, A. and MacMahon, B. Age at any full-term pregnancy and breast cancer risk. *Am. J. Epidemiol.* 151: 715–722, 2000.

[35] Holmberg, E., Holm, L. E., Lundell, M., Mattsson, A., Wallgren, A. and Karlsson, P. Excess breast cancer risk and the role of parity, age at first childbirth and exposure to radiation in infancy. *Br. J. Cancer* 85: 362–366, 2001.

[36] Vessey, M. D., McPherson, K., Roberts, M. M., Neil, A. and Jones, L. Fertility and the risk of breast cancer. *Br. J. Cancer* 52: 625–628, 1985.

[37] Kelsey, J. L. and Horn-Ross, P. L. Breast Cancer: Magnitude of the problem and descriptive epidemiology. *Epidemiol. Rev.* 15: 7–16, 1993.

[38] Lambe, M., Hsieh, C. C., Chan, H. W., Ekbom, A., Trichopoulos, D. and Adami, H. O. Parity, age at first and last birth, and risk of breast cancer: A population-based study in Sweden. *Breast Cancer Res. Treat.* 38: 305–311, 1996.

[39] Russo, I. H. and Russo, J. Chorionic gonadotropin: A tumoristatic and preventive agent in breast cancer. In: Teicher, B. A. (ed.), *Drug Resistance in Oncology*, Marcel Dekker, Inc., New York. 1993, 537–560.

[40] Russo, I. H., Koszalka, M. and Russo, J. Human chorionic gonadotropin and rat mammary cancer prevention. *J. Natl. Cancer Inst.* 82: 1286–1289, 1990.

[41] Russo, I. H., Koszalka, M. and Russo, J. Effect of human chorionic gonadotropin on mammary gland differentiation and carcinogenesis. *Carcinogenesis* 11: 1849–1855, 1990.

[42] Russo, I. H. and Russo, J. Role of hCG and inhibin in breast cancer. *Int. J. Oncol.* 4: 297–306, 1994.

[43] Srivastava, P., Russo, J. and Russo, I. H. Chorionic gonadotropin inhibits rat mammary carcinogenesis through activation of programmed cell death. *Carcinogenesis* 18: 1799–1808, 1998.

[44] Mgbonyebi, O. P., Tahin, Q., Russo, J. and Russo, I. H. Serum levels of chorionic gonadotropin in treated female rats during the progression of D MBA-induced tumorigenesis. *Proc. Am. Assoc. Cancer Res.* 37: 1564a, 1996.

[45] Tahin, Q., Mgbonyebi, O. P., Russo, J. and Russo, I. H. Influence of hormonal changes induced by the placental hormone chorionic gonadotropin on the progression of mammary tumorigenesis. *Proc. Am. Assoc. Cancer Res.* 37: 1622a, 1996.

[46] Russo, J and Russo, I. H. Human chorionic gonadotropin in breast cancer prevention In: Ethier, S. P (ed.), *Endocrine Oncology*, Humana Press Inc., New Jersey. 2000, 121–136.

[47] Alvarado, M. E., Alvarado, N. E., Russo, J. and Russo, I. H. Human chorionic gonadotropin inhibits proliferation and induces expression of inhibin in human breast epithelial cells in vitro. *In Vitro Cell. Dev. Biol. Anim.* 30A: 4–8, 1994.

[48] Alvarado, M. V., Russo, J. and Russo, I. H. Immunolocalization of inhibin in the mammary gland of rats treated with hCG. *J. Histochem. Cytochem.* 41: 29–34, 1993.

[49] Russo, J., Balogh, G. A. and Russo IH. Full term pregnancy induces a specific genomic signature in the human breast. *Cancer Epidemiol. Biomarkers Prevent.* 16: 1–16, 2008.

[50] Belitskaya-Lévy, I., Zeleniuch-Jacquotte, A., Russo, J., Russo, I. H., Bordas, P., Ahman, J., Afanasyeva, Y., Johansson, R., Lenner, P., Li, X., Lopez de Cicco, R., Peri, S., Ross, E., Russo, P. A., Santucci-Pereira, J., Sheriff, F. S., Slifker, M., Hallmans, G., Toniolo, P. and Arslan, A. A. Characterization of a genomic signature of pregnancy in the breast. *Cancer Prev. Res.* 4: 1457–1464, 2011.

[51] Peri, S. López de Cicco, R., Santucci-Pereira, J., Slifker, M., Ross, E. A., Russo, I. H., Russo, P. A., Arslan, A. A., Belitskaya-Lévy, I., Zeleniuch-Jacquotte, A., Bordas, P., Lenner, P., Åhman, J., Afanasyeva, Y., Johansson, R., Sheriff, F., Hallmans, G., Toniolo, P. and Russo, J. Defining the genomic signature of the parous breast. *BMC Med. Genomics* 5: 46, 2012.

[52] Russo, J., Santucci-Pereira, J., López de Cicco, R., Sheriff, F., Russo, P. A., Peri, S., Slifker, M., Ross, E. A., Mello, M. L. S. Vidal, B. C., Belitskaya-Lévy, I., Arslan, A., Zeleniuch-Jacquotte, A., Bordas, P., Lenner, P., Ahman, J., Afanasyeva, Y., Hallmans, G., Toniolo, P. and Russo, I. H. Pregnancy-induced chromatin remodeling in the breast of postmenopausal women. *Int. J. Cancer* 131: 1059–1070, 2012.

[53] Russo, J., Santucci-Pereira, J. and Russo, I. H. The genomic signature of breast cancer prevention. *Genes* 5(1): 65–83, 2014.

[54] Barton, M., Santucci-Pereira, J. and Russo, J. Molecular pathways involved in pregnancy-induced prevention against breast cancer. *Front. Endocrinol. (Lausanne).* 10(5): 213, 2014. doi: 10.3389/fendo.2014.00213. eCollection 2014.

[55] Russo, J., Santucci-Pereira, J. and Barton, M. Molecular pathways involved in pregnancy-induced prevention against breast cancer. *Front. Endocrinol.* section Cellular Endocrinology 5: 215, 2014.

[56] King, M. C., Wieand, S., Hale, K., Lee, M., Walsh, T., Owens, K., Tait, J., Ford, L., Dunn, B. K., Costantino, J., Wickerham, L., Wolmark, N. and Fisher, B. Tamoxifen and breast cancer incidence among women with inherited mutations in BRCA1 and BRCA2: National Surgical Adjuvant Breast and Bowel Project (NSABP-Pl) Breast Cancer Prevention Trial. *JAMA* 286: 2251–2256, 2001.

[57] Narod, S. A., Brunet, J. S., Ghadirian, P., Robson, M., Heimdal, K., Neuhausen, S. L., Stoppa-Lyonnet, D., Lerman, C., Pasini, B., de los Rios, P., Weber, B. and Lynch, H. Tamoxifen and risk of contralateral breast cancer in BRCA1 and BRCA2 mutation carriers: a case-control study. Hereditary Breast Cancer Clinical Study Group. *Lancet* 356: 1876–1881, 2000.

[58] Russo, J., Russo, I. H., Ireland, M. and Saby, J. Increase resistance of multiparous rat mammary gland to neoplastic transformation by 7,12-DMBA. *Proc. Am. Assoc. Cancer Res.* 18: 140, 1977.

[59] Russo, J. and Russo, I. H. DNA-labeling index and structure of the rat mammary gland as determinants of its susceptibility to carcinogenesis. *J. Natl. Cancer Inst.* 61: 1451, 1978.

[60] Russo, I. H and Russo, J. Atlas and histologic classification of tumors of the rat mammary gland. *J. Mammary Gland Biol. Neoplasia.* 5: 187–200, 2000.

[61] Russo, J. and Russo, I. H. Susceptibility of the mammary gland to carcinogenesis. II. Pregnancy interruption as a risk factor in tumor incidence. *Am J. Pathol.* 100: 497–512, 1980.

[62] Russo, J. Basis of cellular autonomy in susceptibility to carcinogenesis. *Toxicol. Pathol.* 11: 149–155, 1983.

[63] The Centers for Disease Control Cancer and Steroid Hormone Study. Long term oral contraceptives use and the risk of breast cancer. *JAMA* 249: 1591, 1983.

[64] Edgren, R. A. The biology of steroidal contraceptives. In: Lednicer, D. (ed.), *Contraception: Chemical Control of Fertility*, Marcel Dekker, New York. 1969, 23.

[65] Gurpide, E., Tseng, L. and Gusberg, S. B. Estrogen metabolism in normal and neoplastic endometrium. *Am. J. Obstet. Gynecol.* 129: 809, 1977.

[66] Rail, H. H., Soto-Ferreira, J. and Janssens, K. Y. Effect of medroxyprogesterone acetate contraception on cytoplasmic estrogen receptor content of the human cervix uteri. *Int. J. Fertil.* 23: 41, 1978.

[67] Russo, I. H., Gimotty, P., Dupuis, M. and Russo, J. Effect of medroxyprogesterone acetate on the response of the rat mammary gland to carcinogenesis. *Br. J. Cancer* 59: 210–216, 1989.

[68] Russo, I. H. and Russo, J. Hormone prevention of mammary carcinogenesis by norethynodrel-mestranol. *Breast Cancer Res. Treat.* 14: 43–56, 1989.

[69] Coleman, M. E., Murchison, T. E. and Frank, D. Mammary nodules in dogs receiving Depo-Provera and progesterone: an interim progress report. *Toxicol. Appl. Pharmacol.* 37: 213a, 1976.

[70] Wazeter, F. X., Geil, R. G., Cookson, K. M., Berliner, V. R. and Lamar, J. K. Seven years progress report on long term oral contraceptive studies in female dogs and monkeys. *Toxicol. Appl. Pharmacol.* 37: 208a, 1976.

[71] Finkel, M. J. and Berliner, V. R. The extrapolation of experimental findings (animal to man): the dilemma of the systemically administered contraceptives. *Bull. Soc. Pharmacol. Environ. Pathol.* 4: 13, 1973.

[72] Russo, J. and Russo, I. H. *Role of the Trasncriptome In Breast Cancer Prevention*, Springer, New York. 2012.

[73] Russo, I. H., Pokorzynski, T. and Russo, J. Contraceptives as hormone-preventive agents in mammary carcinogenesis. *Proc. Am. Assoc. Cancer Res.* 27: 912a, 1986.

[74] Russo, I. H., Al-Rayess, M. and Russo, J. Role of contraceptive agents in breast cancer prevention at the *Proceedings of the Biennial International Breast Cancer Research Conference*, March 24–28, 1985, London, UK, p. 87.

[75] Russo, I. H., Al-Rayess, M. and Sabharwal, S. Effect of contraceptive agents on mammary gland structure and susceptibility to carcinogenesis. *Proc. Am. Assoc. Cancer Res.* 26: 460a, 1985.

[76] Janssens, J. P., Russo, J., Russo, I. H., Michiels, L., Donders, G., Verjans, M., Riphagen, I., Van den Bossche, T., Deleu, M. and Sieprath, P. Human chorionic gonadotropin (hCG) and prevention of breast cancer. *Mol. Cell. Endocrinol.* 269: 93–98, 2007.

[77] Srivastava, P., Silva, I. D., Russo, J., Mgbonyebi, O. P. and Russo, I. H. Identification of genes differentially expressed in breast carcinoma cells treated with chorionic gonadotropin. *Int. J. Oncol.* 13: 465–469, 1998.

[78] Srivastava, P., Russo, J., Mgbonyebi, O. P. and Russo, I. H. Growth inhibition and activation of apoptotic gene expression by human chorionic gonadotropin in human breast epithelial cells. *Anticancer Res.* 18: 4003–4010, 1998.

Chapter 9
The Breast Cancer
Research Laboratory — Part 1
(Expanding the Wings 1979–1991)

9.1. Expanding the wings

The period of my life from 1979 to 1991 was 13 remarkable years full
of uncertainties, challenges, and mainly awakening to my surrounding
environment, and perhaps the best way to describe this period of my
life is that this was when I was expanding my wings and starting my
solo flight.

Our line of research had been delineated, and the fact that I had
received federal and other funding to carry on our original ideas was
a clear demonstration that I had initiated my walk on a new path of
scientific discovery. However, that was not enough. Irma was the first
to understand that unless we were medical board certified in a
specialty, we would not completely reach the level of authority and
economic independence that we sought. That was her intuitive line of
thinking, which pushed her to take the foreign medical examination,
the FLEX, and then the board certification in pathology. In my case,
it took a few more years before I was finally ready to spread my wings
in these uncharted territories. This chapter is a narration of what
happened in those years of my life.

9.2. Brown Book Project and my training as a surgical pathologist

In June of 1978, the Michigan Cancer Foundation (MCF) was funded by the National Cancer Institute (NCI) to study the use of prognostic markers in breast cancer based on a project conceived earlier by Dr. Michael Brennan and named the *Breast Cancer Prognostic Study*. Because the draft of the application was published for internal circulation in a book format with a brown cover, the project was also known as the *Brown Book Project*. The total study consisted of 646 primary breast cancer patients collected from 12 different hospitals in the metropolitan Detroit area. The participation of these hospitals allowed expeditious handling of breast biopsies and mastectomy specimens. The project was well conceived because the primary breast tumors were obtained and handled under sterile conditions. Each tumor was sliced into ten or more slabs, depending upon the size of the tumor. Three alternate sections were fixed in 10% neutral buffered formalin and processed for histologic evaluation. One of the sections was frozen at −70°C for steroid receptor assay, and the remaining sections were placed in the chilled culture medium and processed for various experimental protocols from which numerous papers were published with my participation on them [1–14]. My role in that project was the management of the pathology core in which all the paraffin blocks of primary breast cancer processed from the different hospitals of the Detroit metropolitan area were collected and coordinated by the pathology panel that was formed by Dr. Gerald Fine from the *Departments of Anatomic Pathology of Henry Ford Hospital;* Dr. Mujtaba Hussain, *from Sinai Hospital;* Dr. Herbert I. Krickstein, *from St. John Hospital in Detroit;* Drs. Thomas O. Robbins and Barbara Rosenberg *from the William Beaumont Hospital, Royal Oak.* My function in the pathology panel was to coordinate and provide a histopathological diagnosis of the tumor using the accepted classification common in those days [15] and evaluate each tumor with regard to histological grade (HG), mitotic grade (MG), and nuclear grade (NG) by each panelist. Tumors were graded according to the criteria established by Bloom and Richardson [16] and Black [17, 18], and we also added other pathological parameters like size, lymph nodes status, blood vessel invasion, necrosis, and inflammatory infiltration. I published the results of this work in the *American Journal of Clinical Pathology* in 1987 [10]. The organization of the pathology panel immediately put me in contact with practical surgical pathologists who were outstanding microscopists and from whom I learned significantly. My role in the Brown Book was a natural one because I was the Chief of experimental pathology and therefore the most logical to understand what the objective of the project was. In addition, the work fitted quite well with my plans to start a residency in pathology and become a board certified pathologist. At this time in my narrative, it is important to emphasize that my search for a place to do my formal training in surgical pathology and obtain my board certification had started at the beginning of 1978, and from that search I selected four places: Ann Arbor, Wayne State University, Northwestern University, and St. John Hospital; the last two were interested in offering a residency program that would allow me to keep my grants and research laboratories and give me the training that would be recognized by the College of American Pathologists, allowing me to get the board certification. Prof. Dante Scarpelli, the Chair of the Department of Pathology at Northwestern University was very eager that I move to his department, mainly because of my grants, but they wanted my training to be for 6 years, and the facilities that they could provide me were meager in comparison to what I already had at the MCF in Detroit. Instead, St. John Hospital offered me a package of 27 hours a week for 3.9 years without salary from their part but I could maintain my position as Chief of experimental pathology at the MCF without any change in my salary and privileges as a member of that institution. In the end, I realized that this was the best option because it also meant that Irma could finish her last year of residency at Wayne State University without the need to move and sell our home, and more important, I would be able to commute from my home, the hospital, and the MCF more easily because all of them were relatively short driving distances. The negotiation between Dr. Herbert I. Krickstein, the Chief of the Department of Pathology, and Dr. James

Humes, the Medical Director at St. John Hospital, with Dr. Michael Brennan, the President, and Marvin Rich, the Scientific Director of the MCF, took several months but finally was approved and on January 15, 1979, I was admitted in the residency program of St. John Hospital. I worked in the hospital from 8 a.m. to 1 p.m. from Monday to Saturday, and in the afternoon from 1.30 to 7 p.m. in the laboratory at the MCF.

St. John Hospital was a new experience altogether. I was in the lower scale of all the physicians on the medical staff. I was only a resident in the Department of Pathology of a well-recognized and well-run hospital in Detroit. The Director was Dr. James Humes, a prominent pathologist who was on the team that performed the autopsy of President John F. Kennedy. He was a massive man, seven feet tall, with an impressive figure that imposed by his size alone, but also he had a great personality and was a gentle and caring man. He participated in the everyday slide conference and personally ran a monthly pathology slide seminar that agglutinated all the hospitals of the metropolitan and surrounding areas. He was a natural leader. The other pathologists in the department included Dr. H. I. Krickstein, Dr. A. Giraldo, Dr. I. Lawson, and F. Lander, all were well seasoned and some had experience in scientific research; those that did not had a respectful appreciation for it. I felt welcome in the group. The learning process was arduous, and what was most difficult for me to accept was that I was only a resident and so I needed to follow instructions and orders of the work to do. This was not good for my ego, however, very soon I called the attention of the medical staff for my well-prepared case presentations and seminars. That in itself gave me a significant edge over all the other residents and also the medical staff. My research experience and academic background made me fitter and more than compensated for my deficiencies and ignorance about the specialty and medicine in particular. My first year was rough, but I became comfortable after taking my FLEX examination on June 13, 1980, and slowly I conquered my ignorance and started to really feel like a Medical Doctor. Lasting memories and friendships like the one that I developed with Francisco Martinez are still active and alive after 37 years.

My daughter, Patricia, was born on September 11, 1980, and my journal entry on my 39th birthday reads:

Patricia is already six and a half months old. She is beautiful and has plenty of energy. She has learned to recognize us, to play and even to get from us whatever she wants. Patricia Alexandra walks already with my help and has acquired a tremendous ability for moving herself from one place to another with the help of a walker. She has touched my heart and I love her very deeply. I see in her all our genes and potentialities. I recognize Irma and myself in her. She was the perfect example of gene distribution. My heart is jumping in joy when I see her or think about her. She is so radiant and full of vitality that she is a refreshing spring in my taxing days. We have been blessed with her and we are thankful to God for giving her to us, for taking care and educating her.

In April of 1981, Marvin Rich resigned as Scientific Director and Vice President of the MCF after an open power struggle with Dr. Michael Brennan, who took over his presidency. Rich moved to Colorado taking with him valuable people like Philip Furmanski and many other young investigators. Those times were turbulent in the sense that each day brought new conjectures about his successor until Dr. Gloria Heppner was designated as the new Scientific Director. In the meantime, Irma passed her board and started working as a pathologist at Harper Hospital, and although we still kept our research, she could no longer devote 100% to our research projects; however, her input was as important as ever, and our work and reputation kept growing. There were long hours each day because after finishing her work in the hospital at 4 p.m., she came to the Breast Cancer Research Laboratory (BCRL), and we went home together late in the evening. Thanks to her mother, Carmen, who moved in with us and took care of Patricia, we dedicated most of our time to our work.

In the spring of 1982, I started to develop serious gastric problems, and I was diagnosed clinically with a gastric cancer, or linitis plastic, test after test was confirming the diagnosis until Dr. Paul

Rizzo, a surgeon at St. John Hospital, decided to make an exploratory laparotomy. In my June journal entry, I wrote:

Almost four months have passed since my surgery. Only a large scar from my sternum to my pubis remains. The nightmare is over but the fear is still with me. The lesion resulted to be benign and the diagnosis was a chronic gastritis. I remember waking up from the anesthesia and Irma saying that it was a benign process. Irma's courage in this ordeal came afterward, but I know how she has been suffering, helping me and being with me through the whole process. Love and compassion were seeping from every single pore of her skin. Her presence and touch made my ordeal less painful. Irma's suffering in this process cannot be understated; she has been hearing terrible things at Harper Hospital when they discussed my case, giving me only few weeks to live because the diagnosis was a linitis plastic or carcinoma that had taken the whole wall of the stomach. The only one who gave her comfort was an old pathologist at Harper, Dr. Rafmaninoff. He told her that many times this process that looks so bad in a radiological image results to be benign. We cried together and our love and care for each other seemed to have erased all the difficulties of the previous weeks and months. Even Patty perceived that something was wrong with me and she asked if Daddy was sick.

In the middle of my recovery, Dr. John Batsakis, the Chairman of the Department of Pathology at the MD Anderson, was interested in recruiting me for his staff. The offer was tempting, more so because Irma had decided to stop working at Harper Hospital and return to work full-time in the BCRL. That made the offer of the opening a new perspective for both of us. This opportunity was also encouraged by the instability that the MCF was experiencing at that time. However, moving to MD Anderson meant that our collaboration must be finished because they could not have us in the same department due to a nepotism law that was in place at that time at the MD Anderson. Therefore, she would have to relocate into another institution. Although we had even taken the medical license board to practice in Texas, we realized *at the end that our unity as a research team was more valuable than anything else.* MD Anderson would no doubt be an important step forward for my career, with a six-digit salary, but the separation of us as a team was a high price to pay, so we decided to stay and keep fighting in Michigan.

We are part of what we have met says Tennyson in his poem *Ulysses,* and on June 22, 1982, I wrote the following in my journal:

> *Argentina was bitten by England in the fight over the Falkland Islands or Malvinas. I was dying and bitten with every Argentinean who died or was bitten in the fight to keep the Malvinas as part of Argentina. This was a reflection of what Argentina wants to be and to show that can fly like an eagle, but at the end showed that she has only the wings of a Cornish hen. This was a painful war and defeat to see.*

9.3. The pathology reference laboratory

In the late summer of 1982, I finished my residency in pathology and passed the board in November of that year. I was named Chairman of the Department of Pathology at the MCF, and I was assigned a secretary, a budget of department funds, and a private parking space as the perks of being a chair. The residency was paying off and was also associated with a significant increase in salary and status at the organization that had seen me crawling. Now I was in a position that I could really apply not only innovative approaches but also take part in the future decisions of the institution.

The USA economic situation in 1982 and the following years created a low point for grant acquisition, and we were encouraged to be innovative in generating more revenues to keeping our research alive. One of the approaches that we took with Irma was to create a Pathology Reference Laboratory (PRL) inside of the BCRL. The PRL offered electron microscopy and immunocytochemistry in tumor diagnosis, detection of estrogen and progesterone receptors in primary tumors, and toxicologic analysis. The PRL was created with the purpose of generating a permanent resource of funds to keep our research alive. The initiative was well received in the MCF and other researchers like Sam Brooks and Charles McGrath joined the initiative by performing estrogen and progesterone receptors determination, and Dr. Jerome Horwitz, a reputed chemist who discovered AZT, offered his invaluable expertise in mass spectrometry for detecting and confirming drugs in the samples for the toxicologic analysis. Many publications [19–33], and among them my first four books, resulted from that enterprise [34–37]. The PRL allowed me to maintain the histology and immunocytochemistry laboratory at the BCRL, and most important, the electron microscopy section that had two electron microscopes, a scanning electron microscope, several ultra-microtomes, ancillary equipment, and a full dark room. With the revenues, we also were able to maintain three senior technicians and a driver that made the sample collections for the toxicology services. Irma acted as the Director of the clinical services, and I was in charge of the diagnostic microscopy.

In order to make us visible in the community, we organized several tutorials and workshops in tumor diagnosis, emphasizing the use of electron microscopy (Figure 9.1) and immunocytochemistry. The latter was an emerging field imposing over the use of electron microscopy in later years.

During the preparation of our first workshop on the use of electron microscopy in 1983, I received the sad news that on August 19 of that year Marcelo Palero had died. He was a great friend and a godfather of our marriage, together with his wife, Estela (see Chapter 5). The only thing that I have from him now is a small obituary from *Los Andes*, a local paper in Mendoza.

The tutorials and workshops were a success on all fronts. They allowed me to develop a significant profile of academic authority in the community, and nationally, it was an excellent networking system to interact and befriend the most distinguished researchers and pathologists that were the pioneers in these areas and also created a great source of revenues that was easily appreciated by the upper echelon of the MCF (Figures 9.3 and 9.4).

To hammer my visibility, I decided to publish my first book on immunocytochemistry in tumor diagnosis in 1985 [34], spurred by the workshop on this subject that took place in Detroit in 1984 (Figure 9.2). The book was published by Martinus Nijhoff, which was

ELECTRON MICROSCOPY
WORKSHOP

Electron Microscopy in Tumor Diagnosis

October 6th and 7th, 1983

Engineering Society of Detroit
Detroit, Michigan

Organized by

Pathology Reference Laboratory
Michigan Cancer Foundation

Co-sponsored by
Michigan State Medical Society

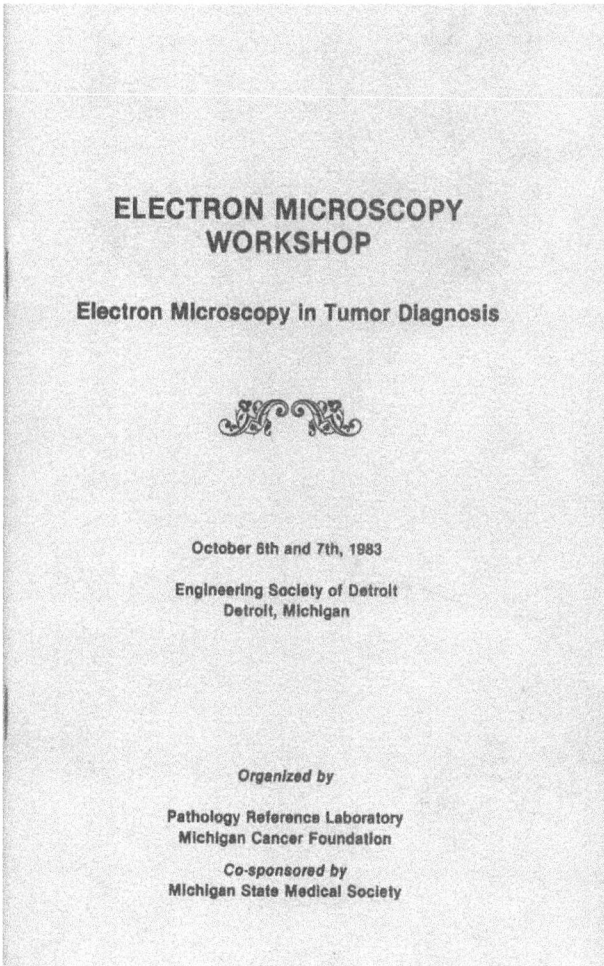

Figure 9.1: Facsimile of the program of the electron microscopy workshop in tumor diagnosis. Engineering Society of Detroit. Detroit, MI, 1983.

part of the Kluwer Academic Publishers Group in Boston. Now it is a part of Springer, and the book can still be obtained through this publisher. The importance of this book is that it summarized the work of great pioneers in immunocytochemistry. This technique was emerging, and the pathologists that were a part of this workshop were pushing the field forward. Immunocytochemistry was still in the

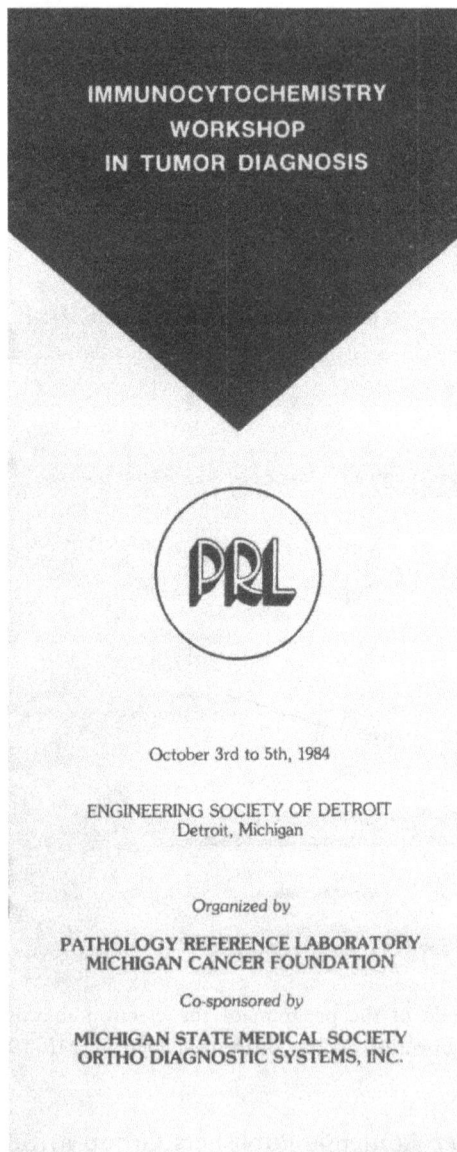

IMMUNOCYTOCHEMISTRY
WORKSHOP
IN TUMOR DIAGNOSIS

PRL

October 3rd to 5th, 1984

ENGINEERING SOCIETY OF DETROIT
Detroit, Michigan

Organized by

PATHOLOGY REFERENCE LABORATORY
MICHIGAN CANCER FOUNDATION

Co-sponsored by

MICHIGAN STATE MEDICAL SOCIETY
ORTHO DIAGNOSTIC SYSTEMS, INC.

Figure 9.2: Facsimile of the program *Immunocytochemistry Workshop in Tumor Diagnosis*, Engineering Society of Detroit, Detroit, MI, 1984.

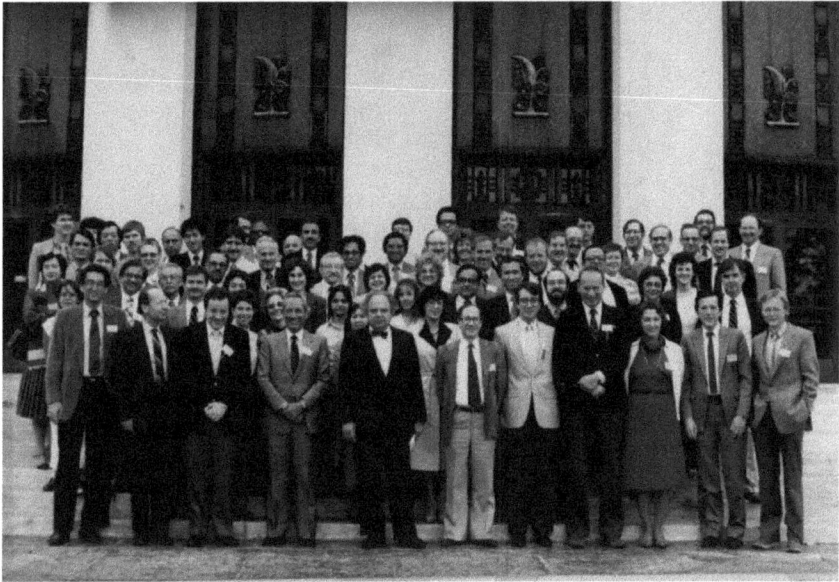

Figure 9.3: Participants in the tutorial and workshop on the use of immunocytochemistry and electron microscopy in tumor diagnosis, Engineering Society of Detroit, Detroit, MI, 1985.

process of being standardized, and it was not as precise as today but the book is a testimony of how in 1984 this methodology was in diagnostic pathology. Main contributors to the book were L.A. Sternberger, N.H. Sternbeger, H. Battifora, E.S. Jaffe, R.A. Tubbs, V.E. Gould, K. Kovacs, M.L. and A.J. de Bold, G.L. Green, C. Cordon-Cardo, R.E. Scully, F.K. Mostofi and I.A. Sesterhenn, D.R. Ciocca, R.L. Ceriani, A.R. Morales, M. Nadji, and J.T. Thornthwaite (Figure 9.2).

Empowered by this book, I also decided to publish three volumes on the electron microscopy in tumor diagnosis [35–37]. The publication of the first volume of this book was more difficult for me because none of the publishers were interested in it as they did not see high rewards; instead, they saw electron microscopy as a dying tool in clinical diagnosis. This was a new experience for me so I sought the help of Dr. Sheldon C. Sommers, a good friend of Michael

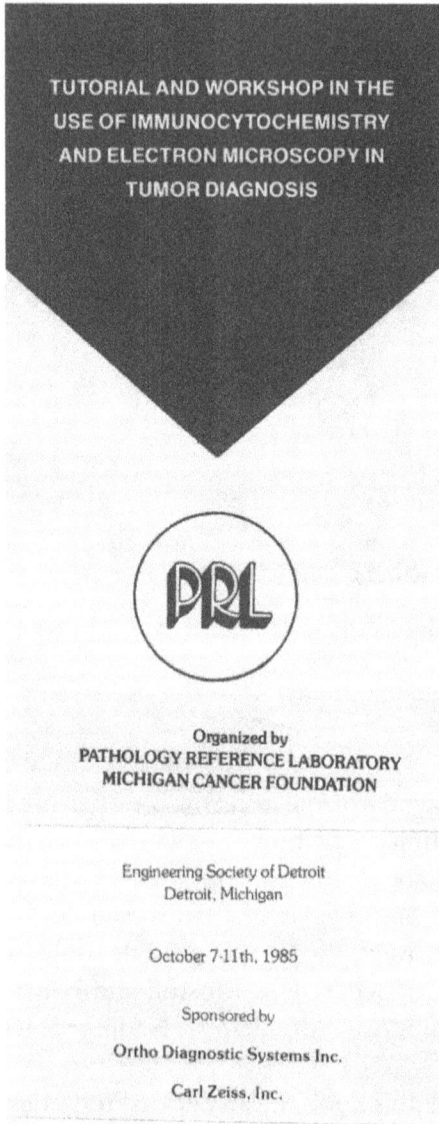

TUTORIAL AND WORKSHOP IN THE
USE OF IMMUNOCYTOCHEMISTRY
AND ELECTRON MICROSCOPY IN
TUMOR DIAGNOSIS

PRL

Organized by
PATHOLOGY REFERENCE LABORATORY
MICHIGAN CANCER FOUNDATION

Engineering Society of Detroit
Detroit, Michigan

October 7-11th, 1985

Sponsored by

Ortho Diagnostic Systems Inc.

Carl Zeiss, Inc.

Figure 9.4:   Facsimile of the program for the *Tutorial and Workshop in the use of Immunocytochemistry and Electron Microscopy in Tumor Diagnosis*, Engineering Society of Detroit, Detroit, MI, 1985.

Brennan and also a pathologist, by asking him to be my co-editor in the three books. He accepted gladly for Volume 1, in which he also contributed to the first chapter, but he did not want to be in the second and third volumes because he argued that was not his area of expertise; however, I insisted and told him that it was my honor to put him as a co-editor. Dr. Sommers put me in touch with a publisher, Field, Rich and Associates of New York, and he published our three volumes (Volume 1 in 1986, Volume 2 in 1988, and Volume 3 in 1990) at no cost to me. And this was the first time that I received royalties from publishing books.

More important than the royalties was the interaction with great electron microscopists like Bruce McKay, from MD Anderson; Cecilia Fenoglio Preiser, who at that time was at the University of New Mexico; Richard Sibley from Stanford University in California; Keith Porter from the University of Maryland; Ronald De Lellis from the New England Medical Center in Boston; Eva Horvath from the University of Toronto; Robert Erlandson from Cornell University; Antonio Campos from the University of Granada in Spain; Vincent Johannessen from the Norwegian Radium Hospital in Oslo; and M. Immaculada Herrera from the National Center of Microbiology in Madrid, Spain (Figure 9.3). The only one who did not contribute in the books was Feroze Gadhiali, who had copyrighted his work in his previous books [38, 39]. However, he was a speaker at all the workshops in electron microscopy that I organized. The three volumes on tumor diagnosis were a good state-of-the-art on how to use this technique on the main types of tumors found in the human pathology [35–37].

The last conference that I organized under the PRL in the MCF was on the *Diagnosis and Management of Breast Cancer* in November 22, 1989 (Figure 9.5).

We kept the PRL open until the end of April 1991, almost two months before we moved to the Fox Chase Cancer Center in Philadelphia. The PRL was a very valuable experience in managing a diagnostic laboratory and, more important, taught me how to create my own environment using the resources that were available around me. Nobody in the Detroit metro area had the initiative of generating

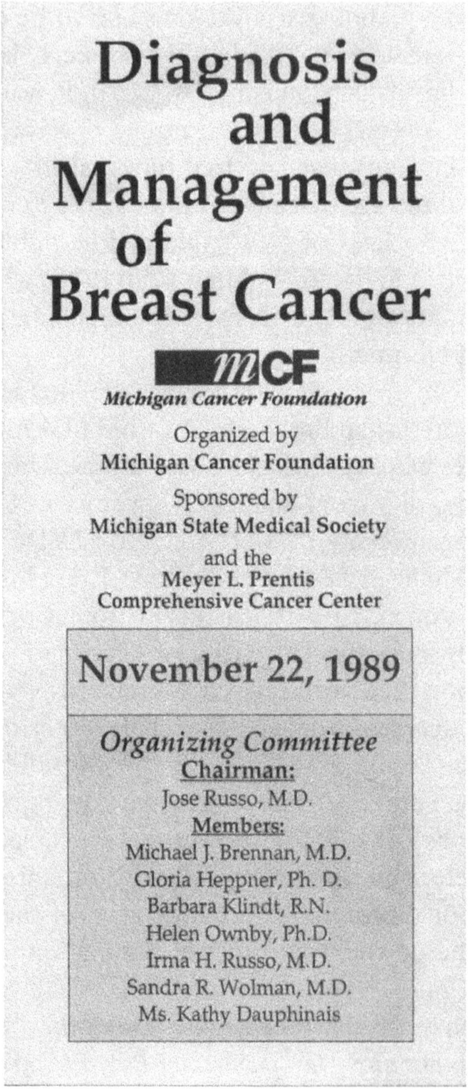

Diagnosis and Management of Breast Cancer

████*m*CF
Michigan Cancer Foundation

Organized by
Michigan Cancer Foundation

Sponsored by
Michigan State Medical Society

and the
**Meyer L. Prentis
Comprehensive Cancer Center**

November 22, 1989

Organizing Committee
Chairman:
Jose Russo, M.D.
Members:
Michael J. Brennan, M.D.
Gloria Heppner, Ph. D.
Barbara Klindt, R.N.
Helen Ownby, Ph.D.
Irma H. Russo, M.D.
Sandra R. Wolman, M.D.
Ms. Kathy Dauphinais

Figure 9.5: Facsimile of the program *Diagnosis and Management of Breast Cancer*, November 22, 1989.

a reference laboratory providing services like immunocytochemistry and electron microscopy in tumor diagnosis or in detection of hormone receptors in primary tumors. None of the local hospitals offered those services, and they used commercial vendors located out of the state to do this work. In the overall picture this kind of operation is quite common in 2018, but it was not in 1984 when we started. I was able to create a service based on a need and generate resources for our research endeavor.

The Pathology Reference Laboratory and the work in our research projects made Irma and I work close together, and we were able to expand our wings wider and wider and also to do bold things like become more entrepreneurial. For example, Irma, in addition to our work at the MCF, took the directorship of two laboratory services that provided a significant additional income, and it was her idea to buy a new home. On April 18, 1985, I wrote in my journal:

We are planning to buy a new house, and we have already made the offer and it has been accepted. It is a Tudor house located at 842 Three Mile Drive (Figure 4.2 in Chapter 4). It is a beautiful house, one that Irma and I have dreamed about for so long. For several weeks Irma was looking for a new house. And after church she enjoyed taking a ride by the Grosse Pointe houses that were on sale. One Sunday after church we were doing the routine and looking for houses, and then Irma saw that the house at 842 Three Mile Drive was for sale, and was not even listed because it was not among the houses that she had selected to see. She took the phone number and called the Realtor. Even the Realtor did not know that the house was for sale. She arranged to show us the house the next day, and as soon we entered the house we had made up our minds that this was the house that we were looking for. The price was more than we'd expected to spend but with certain restrictions from our expenditures and adjustment of our economy it will be possible. Still two major standing blocks should be overcome for us to get the house; first, is getting the mortgage approval and second, to sell the house where we are living.

In December of that year, we were already moved into the new house, and we had solved the sale and the mortgage on time. Our house on Audubon had sold for more than twice what we'd paid for it. This helped us make a significant down payment on the new house. In the new house, I located myself in the area that was called the maid quarters, three rooms in which I have put my desks and bookcases of the medical books in one and the other adjacent room, separated by a bathroom, held all the computers and graphic works that I do for the lectures and also for the manuscripts, and in the room in the back, we constructed the darkroom and archive for all the journal collections. It was an excellent setup for working. The master bedroom had another room, which Irma used for her study. It was very elegant and luminous due to the several tall windows and decorated in a very Spartan Castellan way, like all the things that she liked. Patricia was 5 years old, and she was already in kindergarten. A new laboratory at the MCF was in construction for us, and this was the period in which we received numerous invitations to lecture in several countries and American cities; that was a clear indication that our work was recognized. However, I felt a longing that I was not doing enough, that I was not putting all my energies in the right direction and that I could do more. I wrote in my journal on those days: "*I am thirsty for knowledge but I feel that I am not drinking from the sources, but looking at a mirror that reflects the water.*" This longing and thirst have not been quenched until these days but the anxiety has disappeared and I am looking at the present and future not in a mirror but in the real sources of the flowing waters.

9.4. My contribution as a breast cancer pathologist

I have contributed toward numerous publications and review articles in the pathology of the breast and made interesting contributions in the ultra-structure of tumors and in the use of immunocytochemical techniques [1–14, 19–37]. These contributions to the literature made me visible for numerous invitations as a plenary speaker in meetings and congresses on breast cancer, for teaching the state-of-the-art of those days around the country as well as in South and Central America, Europe, Japan, and the Middle East. Basically, I feel that in that period of my life I contributed to the advance of the breast pathology with my teaching.

In the histopathology of breast cancer in which hundreds of works are published in the literature every year, it is difficult to make a lasting impression in the field. However, the manuscript published in the *American Journal of Clinical Pathology* in 1987 that described the Predictor of Recurrence and Survival of Patients with Breast Cancer [10] provided an original insight into the way that primary tumors must be studied and categorized for predicting recurrence and survival using histologic grade (HG), nuclear grade (NG), mitotic grade (MG), final grade (FG), estrogen receptor (E2R) status, and patient's lymph node status (LN) at the time of surgery. In this publication, I was able to establish a patient's prognosis of recurrence-free interval and survival using one parameter or group of parameters as adequate predictors of tumor behavior. In that publication, we showed that LN, tumor size, and tumor grade were themselves significant predictors of early recurrence and breast cancer death. We showed that each unit increase in LN or MG increased the risk of death by a factor of 1.5 and 2.0, respectively.

However, prediction of time to recurrence or death was considerably more accurate when those parameters were used in conjunction, rather than individually. E_2R was also significant in predicting death. Importantly, we found that MG separated patients within a single LN group or E_2R group into two subsets having clinically and statistically different prognoses. It was found that patients who had negative lymph nodes and whose tumors were MGI had a better prognosis than those with MG2,3 tumors; in these latter patients, recurrence and death patterns were similar to those of patients with MGI tumors having one to three positive lymph nodes. Similarly we found that whereas patients with four or more positive lymph nodes had bad prognoses, those bearing MGI tumors tended to behave more like those with MG2,3 tumors and had only one to three positive lymph nodes (Figure 9.6).

The same relevance of MG was observed in those tumors that have positive or negative E_2R (Figure 9.7).

In my book *The Pathobiology of Breast Cancer*, I describe a detailed analysis of the molecular types currently used in the classification as

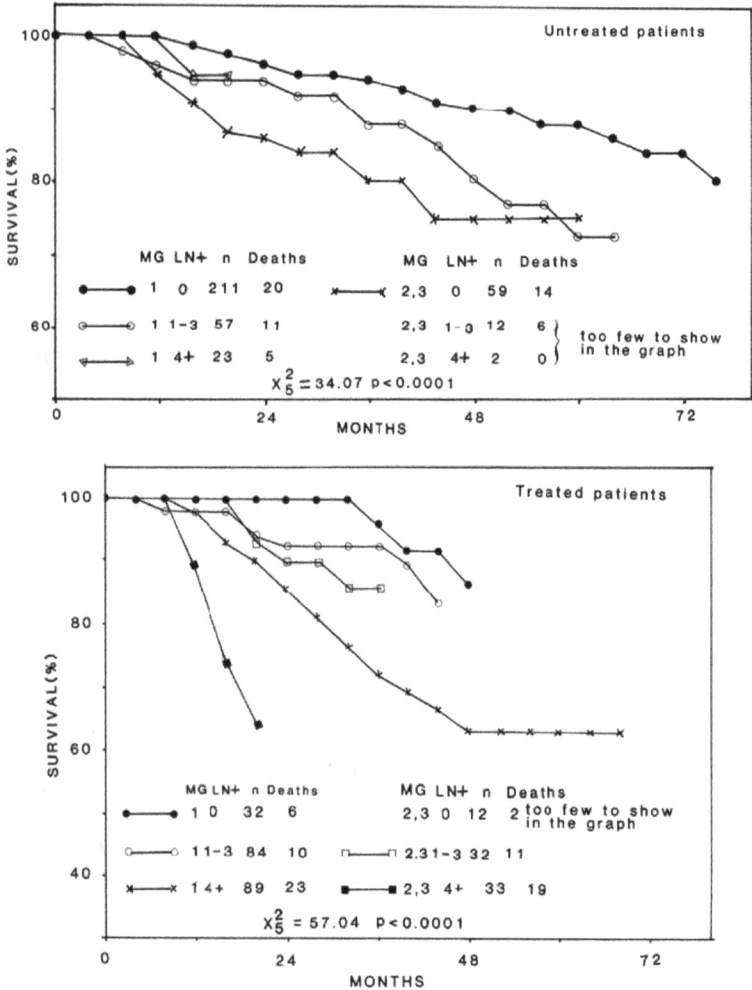

Figure 9.6: Estimated rates of death (survival %) due to breast cancer by MG and LN status. Lifetable analysis for untreated (A, upper) and treated patients (B, lower). There were no patients with four or more positive LN and MG2,3 who did not receive adjuvant treatment.

well as in the stratification of breast cancer to predict response to therapy [40]. Therefore, whereas the criteria published in 1987 are no longer used and have been replaced by molecular testing, the utilization of microscopic parameters was novel in those days and provided a better guide to stratify patients for therapy.

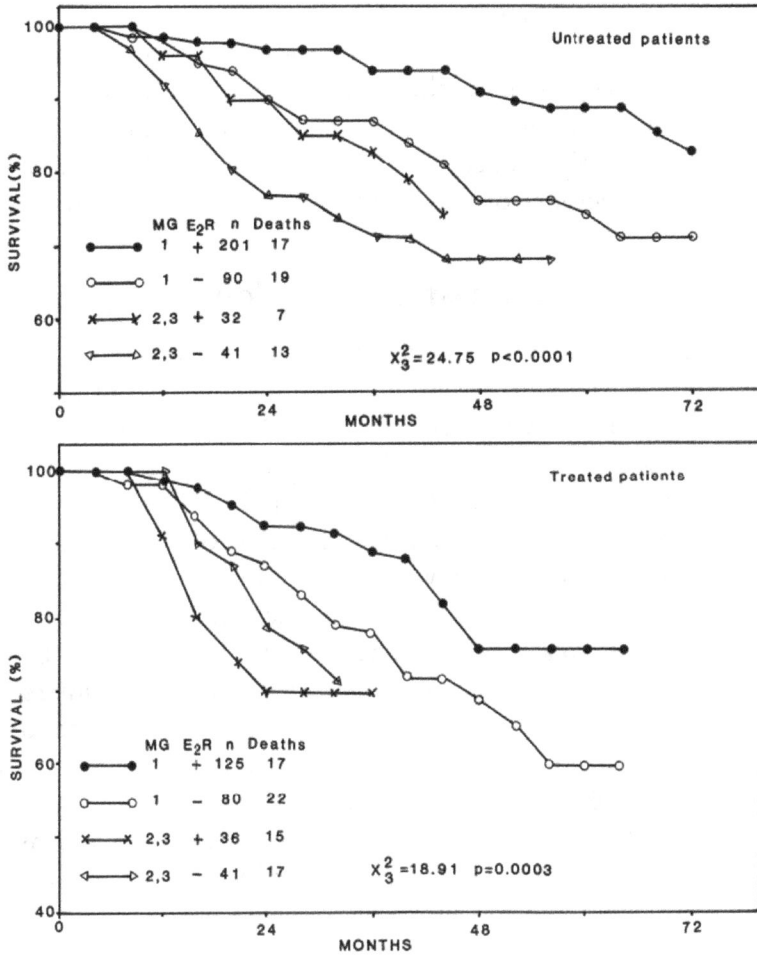

Figure 9.7: Estimated rates of breast cancer death (survival %) by MG and E_2R status. Lifetable analysis for untreated (A, upper) and treated patients (B, lower).

The experience gained in those years helped me obtain the position of Chair of the Department of Pathology at the FCCC in 1991 and to become a part of the NCI Cooperative Breast Cancer Tissue Resources (CBCTR) in 1992. The CBCTR was funded through a UO1 mechanism. The funding of the CBCTR lasted for almost 15 years, and we developed a permanent friendship and collegiality with all the members of the CBCTR. A main publication in clinical cancer research was produced in 2001 [41]. A remarkable experience for me was to work closely with John S. Meyer who, although an octogenarian at the time of the CBCTR, kept a sharp mind and a juvenile enthusiasm in his study of the breast pathology. In 2005, we published a paper in *Modern Pathology* [42] that clearly confirmed the relevance of mitotic grade in breast cancer prognosis.

9.5. The human breast as a developing organ

The question that was the main driving force in our research when we started the BCRL (Chapter 8) in 1973 was why parity produces protection against breast cancer. In those days, we were unable to initiate any study in humans, and therefore we decided to use an experimental animal system. Even though the experimental work produced a significant lead in our understanding of the mechanism of pregnancy protection that allowed us to develop a preventive strategy by using hCG (Chapter 8), still the assurance that the same biological process was taking place in the human breast must be demonstrated. As I describe in the book *Techniques and Methodological Approaches in Breast Cancer Research*, published by Springer in 2014, no other organ of the human body presents such dramatic changes in size, shape, and function as does the breast during growth, puberty, pregnancy, and lactation [43]. Although the developmental phase of the human breast starts as early as the stage of nipple epithelium during embryonic development, it is the lobule formation at puberty followed by the development and differentiation process that determines either the susceptibility to develop breast cancer or the prevention of the disease [44].

The first step in the study of the human breast was to develop a method that allowed us to see the structures of the breast in a tridimensional dimension, a concept that counterpoised the standard histological sections that give us only a two-dimensional perspective. For that purpose, we decided to use whole mount preparations like we'd used in the rat mammary gland to study the lobular composition during aging and the effect of parity. The data obtained from these studies has been widely published (see Ref. [43]).

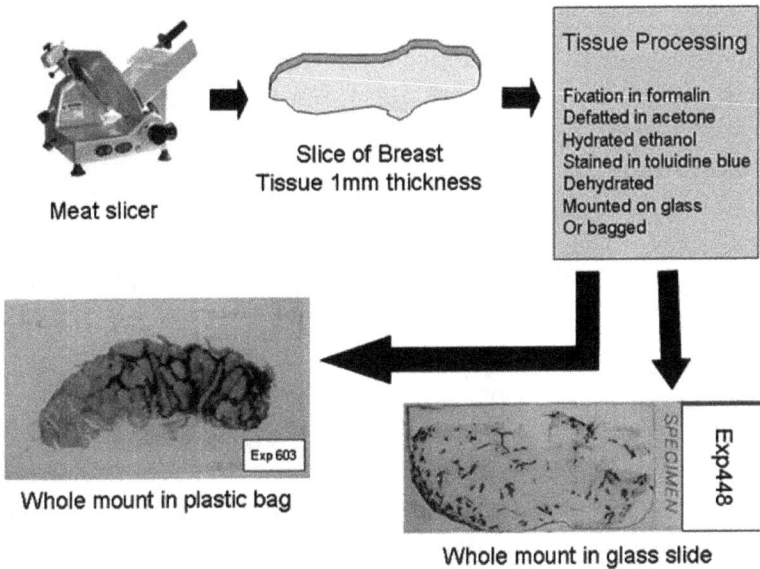

Figure 9.8: Methodological approach that we used for studying the human breast.

In Figure 9.8, I summarize the technique that we used. Basically, each breast was serially cut with a meat slicer into 1 mm thick slices. Each slice was sequentially numbered, labeled, and individually placed in a cloth bag for processing for whole mount by first defatting the tissues by immersion in acetone and then hydrating in decreasing concentrations of ethanol and staining in a toluidine blue solution [43]. The acquisition of adequate sections and staining for performing the study was laborious but nothing compared with the effort that we needed to make to acquire the tissues in the first place. This was another important task that I seldom mentioned in my early publications: how we procured the normal human breast tissue that was the source for our *in vitro* study as well as the ones that allowed to have a better understanding of the role of age and pregnancy in the lobular composition of this organ.

Our contact with plastic surgeons who were a part of the staff of the St. John Hospital was invaluable, and one of them was Dr. R. McCabe, who understood the importance of our work and for many years supplied reduction mammoplasty specimens. This surgical procedure is breast reduction by removing the excess breast fat, glandular tissue, and skin to achieve a breast size in proportion to body size, and it is a cosmetic surgery, but also therapeutic for those women who suffer the discomfort associated with overly large breasts. The adequate approval by the patient and the Internal Review Board (IRB) of the hospital as well as by the MCF was essential to use this material. The list of people that I am indebted to for their help is very large. Among them were nurses, like the ones who scheduled the surgery and let us know the day before the surgery when the tissue would be available as well as the residents and pathologists who were examining the tissue before releasing it to us and the extra burden that these tissues involved because the whole specimen was manipulated in sterile conditions, mainly the ones that were used for *in vitro* study. Added to these people were the technicians that helped transport the breast tissue to the laboratory as well as the nurses and/or technical assistants that collected the clinical information pertinent to our study, either by analyzing the clinical charts or by visiting the doctor's office to get the information on that specific donor. In many cases, the tissue was available, but we were not allowed to have the clinical data because the donor did not want to release private information in a cosmetic surgery. In many cases, Dr. McCabe provided that information by talking with the donor and making them understand the importance of the study, but in other cases the tissue could not be used because we did not have record of the pregnancy history or other clinical information. It was a highly orchestrated network that took months to put in place and worked for us for many years. When we moved to Philadelphia the network that Irma and I had painfully built up could not be reproduced, but in this case it was because the many plastic surgeons that we contacted were not interested in participating in a study that could jeopardize their interaction with the patient who wanted to keep this procedure confidential.

Another source was the use of breast tissue from autopsy material. Dr. S. Bartow was a medical examiner in Albuquerque, New Mexico, in early 1988 and years earlier had received a grant under NCI-RFP No 1-CB-84231/NO1-CN-23928 to study the presence of pre-neoplastic lesions, but after the end of her grant it was not renewed.

It was fortuitous for me to meet Dr. S. Bartow at a meeting of the American Association for Cancer Research, and the hundreds of specimens that she has collected from breast autopsy of traffic accident or other causes of death not related to any pathology were not of any use to her, and she transferred that material to me. I had in those days several grants from the NIH, such as the CA48927, CA38921 and CA06927, that allowed us to study the architectural pattern of the human breast. The hurdle was not the administrative one but the physical transport of the tissues from Albuquerque, New Mexico, to Detroit, Michigan. Irma and I are indebted to Maria Koszalka and her husband who made a special trip to bring the material in perfect condition to the BCRL in Detroit. Although the material had been packed in sealed plastic bags containing formalin, some of the bags had leaked, and the trunk of their car smelled heavily of formalin for several weeks to months after the trip. Their love for each other as well as our friendship lasted even after that ordeal.

We also used normal breast tissue samples from women who underwent surgery for benign and suspicious breast lesions; however, these excision biopsies provided only 2–6 gram of tissue and the normal breast tissue samples were dissected 2 cm distant to the lesion. They were not used for the whole mount preparation and only histological analysis was performed in these samples.

Our collaboration with Professor Henry Lynch from the University of Nebraska also provided subcutaneous mastectomies performed in carriers of BRCA1 and BRCA2 mutations finding important differences in the lobular architecture and resulting in a publication [45].

We observed hundreds and hundreds of sections of the human breast at different ages and parity conditions, counting more than 100,000 structures, and the first conclusion of our observations was that there are four different lobular structures (Figures 9.9 and 9.10). These lobular structures represent sequential developmental stages [44]. Lobules type 1 (Lob 1) are the most undifferentiated lobular structures because they are present in the immature female breast before menarche. They are composed of clusters of 6–11 ductules, or small branches, per lobule, and we compared them to the branches of a tree in winter. Lobules type 2 (Lob 2) evolve from the Lob 1 and

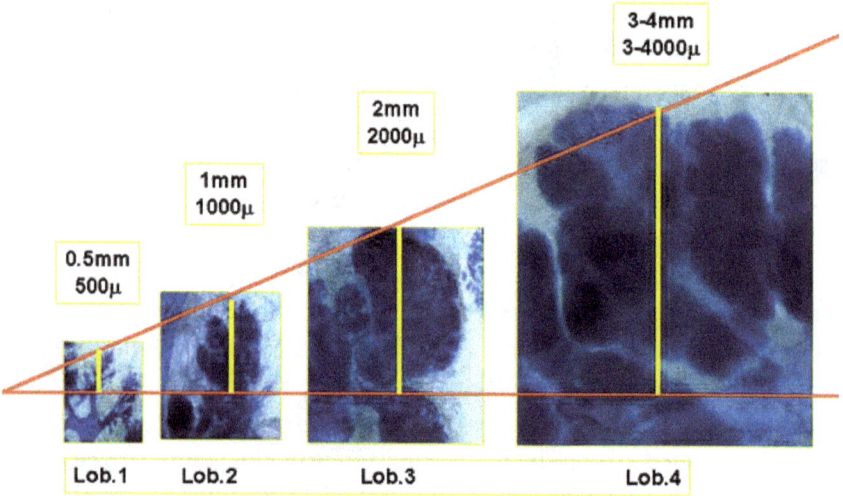

Figure 9.9: Whole mount of the lobular structures of the human breast.

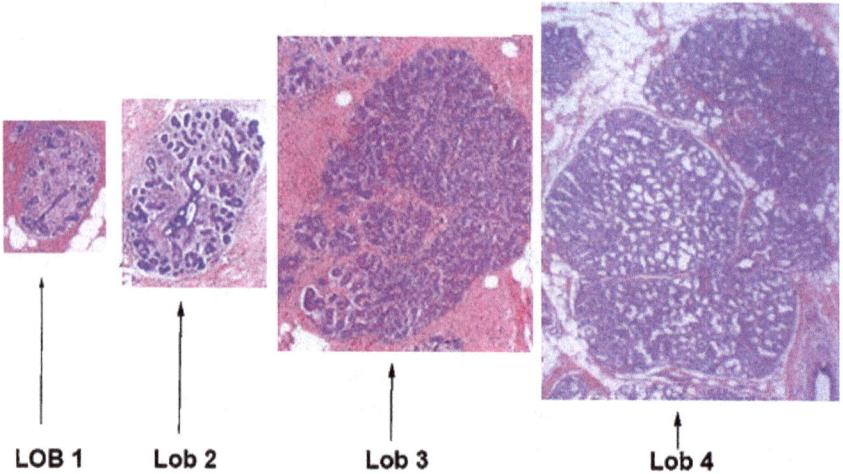

Figure 9.10: Histological sections of the lobular structures of the human breast. Stained with H&E (×2).

have a more complex morphology, being composed of a higher number of ductules or branch structures per lobule. The increase in branching is like the pattern observed in spring in which new twigs are emerging from the main branches of the winter tree.

The branching patterns continue, and the next type of lobular structure was called lobules type 3 (Lob 3). These lobules are like the summer tree characterized by having an average of 80 twigs emerging from the main branches of the winter tree. The branching patterns continue and add more ductules or alveoli per lobule; they are frequently seen in the breasts of women under hormonal stimulation or during pregnancy. A fourth type of lobule, lobule type 4 (Lob 4), has been described during the lactational period of the mammary gland but is not found in the breast of nulliparous post-pubertal women. It is considered to be the maximal expression of development and differentiation [44, 46, 47]. Each of these structures has different proliferative activity, the highest being in the structures of the terminal end bud and the lowest in the Lob 3 (Figure 9.11).

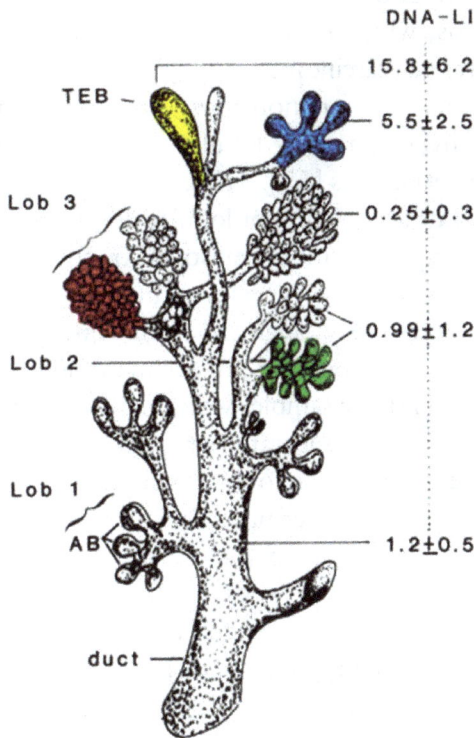

Figure 9.11: Schematic representation of the different structures of the human breast and the proliferative activity, determined as DNA labeling index. Reprinted with permission from Ref. [106].

All these structures have been observed by the old anatomists, however, nobody has defined them in a way that can be identified as *functional units,* depending on the age and reproductive history. These observations not only were novel but also acquired more meaning when all the data were separated by parity history. Based upon my previous studies in an experimental animal model, Irma and I postulated that the protective effect of pregnancy was due to differences in the degree of differentiation of the breast [46, 47], since in rodents the initiation of the neoplastic process is inversely related to the degree of differentiation of the mammary gland, which in turn is a function of age and reproductive history [48–54]. In the study of the pathogenesis of human breast cancer, it has been reported that the terminal ductal lobular unit (TDLU), which is equivalent to Lob 1 [44, 55], is the site of origin of pre-neoplastic lesions such as atypical ductal hyperplasias, which evolve into ductal carcinoma *in situ* and progress to invasive carcinoma, development of atypical lobular hyperplasia, and lobular carcinoma *in situ.* Lob 3 might originate hyperplastic or hypersecretory lobules, fibroadenomas, sclerosing adenosis, and apocrine cysts [55]. These observations suggested to us that the degree of differentiation or lobular development of the breast is influencing the type of tumors developed by this organ [55].

To study the postnatal development of the human breast, hundreds of samples were analyzed from different sources, like reduction mammoplasty, postmortem specimen and forensic pathology material [43], and all tissue samples were analyzed and plotted against age, from 14 to 58 years, separated at 4-year intervals, resulting in nine different age groups. The lobular composition of the breasts of sexually mature women is determined by numerous endogenous and exogenous factors. Principal among them are age, and hence, number and regularity of menstrual cycles, endocrine imbalances, use of exogenous hormones, environmental exposures that could act as endocrine disruptors, and pregnancy. In nulliparous women, the breast contains a moderate number of undifferentiated structures such as terminal ducts and Lob 1, although occasionally Lob 2 and Lob 3 are also present. The percentage of Lob 1 remains almost constant throughout the lifespan of nulliparous women. The fact that

Lob 2 are present in moderate numbers during the early reproductive years, and sharply decrease after age 23, while the number of Lob 1 remains significantly higher and Lob 3 are almost totally absent, suggests that a certain percentage of Lob 1 might have progressed to Lob 2, but very few or no Lob 2 have progressed to Lob 3. In parous women, on the other hand, a history of one or more full-term pregnancies between the ages of 14–20 years correlates with a significant increase in the number of Lob 3. This type of lobules remains present as the predominant structure until a woman reaches the age of 40.

The percentage of Lob 3 decreases after the fourth decade of life, the time at which they decrease in number, due to their involution to predominantly Lob 1 [44, 47]. From a biological and quantitative point of view, the regression of the breast at menopause differs in nulliparous and parous women. In nulliparous women, the predominant breast structure is the Lob 1, which comprises 65–80% of the total lobular components and their relative percentage is independent of age. Second in frequency is the Lob 2 that represents 10–35% of the total. The least frequent is the Lob 3, which represents only 0–5% of the total lobular population. In premenopausal parous women, on the other hand, the predominant lobular structure is the Lob 3, which comprises 70–90% of the total lobular component. Only after menopause, Lob 3 decline in number, and the relative proportion of the three lobular types present approach that observed in nulliparous women (Figure 9.12). These observations led us to conclude that early parous women truly underwent lobular differentiation, which was evident at a younger age, whereas nulliparous women seldom reached the Lob 3 stage, and never the Lob 4 stages. Even though during the postmenopausal years the preponderant structure in the breast of both parous and nulliparous women is the Lob 1, only the nulliparous women are at high risk of developing breast cancer, whereas parous women remain protected [47]. Since ductal breast cancer originates in Lob 1 (TDLU) [55], the epidemiological observation that nulliparous women exhibit a higher incidence of breast cancer than parous women [44, 56] indicates that Lob 1 in these two groups of women might be

CYCLE OF BREAST DEVELOPMENT AND DIFFERENTIATION

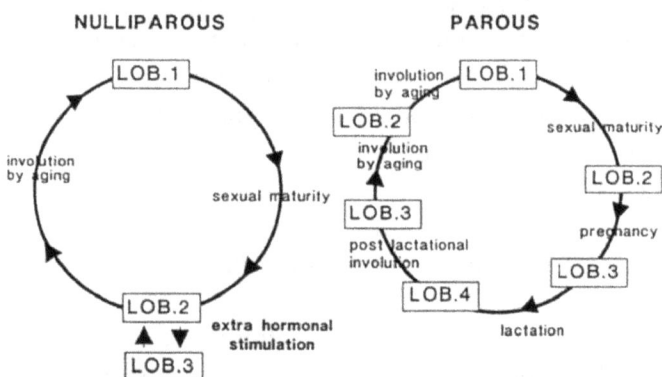

Figure 9.12: Influence of parity on lifetime breast development. Diagrammatic representation based on the relative percentage of lobules present. In nulliparous women, the breast contains primarily lobules type 1 (Lob 1) with some progression to type 2 (Lob 2), and only minimal formation of lobules type 3 (Lob 3). In parous women, pregnancy and lactation complete the cycle of lobular development through the formation of lobules type 4 (Lob 4), which regress to Lob 3 at post-weaning and to Lob 2 and Lob 1 after menopause. Reprinted with permission from Ref. [47].

biologically different, or exhibit different susceptibility to carcinogenesis [57–60]. The presence of Lob 1 in the breasts of parous women has also been interpreted as a failure of the mammary parenchyma to respond to the influences of pregnancy and lactation [47, 61]. We postulated that unresponsive lobules that fail to undergo full differentiation under the stimuli of pregnancy and lactation were responsible for cancer development despite the parity history of a woman. If this were the case, then this unresponsive Lob 1 would be as sensitive to carcinogenesis as the lobules found in the breasts of nulliparous women. We have shown that during the fourth and fifth decades of life there is a decrease in the number of Lob 2, and we postulated that this type of lobule is the site of origin of both lobular hyperplasia and carcinoma *in situ* [47, 55, 62]. Since it has been reported that the incidence of atypical lobular hyperplasia decreases significantly with advancing age, the observed diminution in Lob 2 is responsible for the decreased incidence of this type of pre-neoplastic lesions. As I will describe in the next section, these differences in proliferative activity in the three types of lobules exhibit variations in their *in vitro* growth characteristics. Lob 1 and Lob 2 grow faster; have a higher DNA labeling index, and a shorter doubling time than Lob 3 [63]. They also exhibit different susceptibility to carcinogenesis. Cells obtained from Lob 1 and Lob 2 express *in vitro* phenotypes indicative of neoplastic transformation when treated with chemical carcinogens, whereas cells obtained from Lob 3 do not manifest those changes [61, 64]. Collectively, our data have established a baseline for understanding the evolution of glandular development, and how it is influenced by age and parity. This knowledge is of utmost importance for understanding the role of differentiation in the protection of the mammary gland against carcinogenesis [62, 65–67]. In addition, these data have established well-defined endpoints for studying the response of the mammary gland to hormonal or chemopreventive agents, which could be utilized in modulating the susceptibility of the breast to carcinogenesis.

9.6. Establishing the basis of a paradigm in breast cancer prevention

The studies on the development of the human breast made up to establish thus: as long as a woman does not become pregnant, the predominant structure in her breast is Lob 1. With pregnancy and lactation, the mammary parenchyma reaches the final stage of secretory Lob 4 that forms by the end of the reproductive process and remains present during lactation (Figure 9.12). The protection conferred by pregnancy has been, to a great extent, explained by our earlier studies of DMBA-induced carcinogenesis [51, 68]. In this model, an almost complete abolition of the oncogenic response to DMBA results from the induction of differentiation of the mammary gland by either a full-term pregnancy or treatment of virgin rats with human chorionic gonadotropin (hCG), or by the administration of estrogen and progesterone, the main hormones produced during pregnancy [69–71]. Therefore, we postulated that the protection conferred by an early pregnancy is mediated by the induction of differentiation of the breast by the reproductive event, as demonstrated in the rodent experimental model [48, 54, 72, 73].

We defined differentiation as the coordinated and sequential series of events induced in the breast by the hormonal milieu of pregnancy, or pregnancy-like conditions, which culminate in the activation of genes controlling ductal and lobular development inducing a unique genomic signature. Although it took several years to demonstrate this hypothesis, which I will fully discuss in the next chapter, it was during this period of my research that I established the rational basis of this new paradigm in cancer prevention.

As it is shown in Figure 9.12, the nulliparous postmenopausal breast contains Lob 1 and these lobules are biologically different from those of early parous women. This is supported by data obtained in the rat model, in which clusters of genes remain activated in the involute gland after pregnancy, conferring a special genomic signature to the gland that is responsible for its refractoriness to chemical carcinogenesis. Thus, I postulated that the refractoriness was produced by the shifting of the compartments of stem cell 1 to another stem cell called stem cell 2 [59].

Whereas the idea of shifting of the stem cell population is a valid one, we are reinforcing the concept of stem cell 1 and 2 with our studies [74–76] that are pointing to chromatin remodeling as the main change responsible for the protective effect of pregnancy, meaning that the differentiation process induced by pregnancy is due to an imprinting of a genomic signature that remodels the chromatin responsible for the shifting of stem cell 1 to stem cell 2 creating a new paradigm in breast cancer prevention. Although these data are recently developed, they are derived from the data collected in that 1978–1991 period of my research endeavor. Only the advances of the human genome project and the availability of new tools for genomic analysis, such as cDNA array, tissue array, laser capture micro-dissection (LCM), and bioinformatics techniques, have permitted the identification of clusters of genes that are differentially expressed in populations that differ in their breast cancer risk. Furthermore, those clusters of genes whose expression may be affected by early pregnancy and that can be proven to be functionally relevant in protecting the breast from cancer could serve as markers for evaluating cancer risk in large populations.

9.7. Crossing the border of morphology

One important concept that also emerged from the study of breast development was that the Lob 1, also called terminal ductal lobular structure or TDLU, is the site of origin of the ductal carcinoma of the breast. These observations were supported by comparative studies of normal and cancer-bearing breasts that I published with Barry A. Gusterson, Adriana E. Rogers, Irma H. Russo, Sefton R. Wellings, and Mathew J. Van Zwieten, M.J, in 1991 in *Laboratory Investigation* [55]. The data published provided evidence that ductal carcinomas originate in TDLU (Lob 1) and lobular carcinomas in Lob 2, whereas Lob 3 is not associated with the development of malignancies [55]. The challenge that we faced was to experimentally demonstrate whether Lob 1 and Lob 2 were more susceptible than Lob 3 to undergoing neoplastic transformation.

From this simple question, several lines of research emerged in the BCRL that pushed us to *cross the barrier of morphology* and pursue a different type of research that I had envisioned early in 1973 but needed several years to make a reality. To make a more clear historic perspective of our findings, I divide my narrative to ten different projects: (*1*) *the study of organ culture of the human breast; (2) the isolation of mammary epithelial cells from organoids of the human breast; (3) the transformation of primary breast epithelial cells; (4) the development of an immortalized cell line or MCF10; (5) the oncogenic transformation of the human breast epithelia cell (HBEC) MCF10 by c-ha Ras oncogene; (6) the transformation of HBEC by chemical carcinogens; (7) the demonstration that estrogen was a carcinogenic substance in HBEC; (8) the molecular path of cell transformation; (9) the development of a new model of triple negative breast cancer; and (10) the control of the epithelial mesenchymal transition (EMS) and the metastatic process by regulating chromatin remodeling.*

The first six projects were developed in the period of 1978–1991 (Chapters 9 and 10) and the other ones from 1991 to the present day

(Chapter 11). Each of these projects was taken by different researchers who joined the BCRL and with whom I have developed lasting collaborations and friendship. Each of them brought different stories, some memorable and others more dramatic, but all of them were worthy of being shared. Each project pushed us to more sophisticated methodologies that made the BCRL of today.

9.7.1. *Organ culture of the human breast*

At the end of 1980, Dr. Gloria Calaf joined the BCRL. She was a professor of biology at the University of Chile, and she'd obtained her PhD at Michigan State University under Dr. Clifford Welsch. She had also visited several laboratories in Europe, and one of them was the laboratory of Richard C. Hallowes in the Imperial Cancer Research Laboratory in the United Kingdom.

Gloria Calaf was a tenacious researcher devoted to breast cancer who put so many hours and energy in the work that she was an example for other researchers in the laboratory. Together we published more than 20 papers [77–95], and in 1995 she moved to Columbia University in New York to work with Dr. Tom K. Hei. With Dr. Gloria Calaf, we worked on organ cultures of human breast tissue obtained either from reduction mammoplasty or from the normal tissue adjacent to benign lesions of excisional biopsies. In some of these experiments, Dr. Francisco Martinez, who made sabbatical rotations in the BCRL, was also part of these research projects. With Gloria, we demonstrated that estrogen affected the length of the cell cycle in the breast tissue [77] and that there was a relationship with the age of the donor, the younger ones had a higher proliferative activity [78, 79]. Importantly, we found that was a compartmentalization of the proliferative activity in the Lob 1, mainly in the terminal ductal structures entering the lobules [80–82]. In a publication in the *Journal of National Cancer Institute* in 1987, we clearly demonstrated that role of age on the cell kinetics of normal human breast tissue *in vitro* [83]. Our work originated based on the data in the experimental model that the susceptibility of the mammary gland to chemically induced carcinogenesis was directly related to the rate of cell proliferation of the gland at the time of carcinogen exposure and inversely related to its degree of differentiation. Cell proliferation, in turn, depends on the topographic location of cells within the mammary gland tree and is modulated by age, among other factors. To determine whether age and gland topography similarly influence cell kinetic parameters in the breasts of human females, we studied 15 normal human breast tissues obtained from areas adjacent to histopathologically proved benign lesions. The tissue fragments were incubated in organ culture dishes containing [3H]thymidine ([3H]-dThd) and processed for DNA labeling index (DNA-LI), length of cell cycle (Tc), and growth fraction (GF) determination; double labeling with [3H]dThd and [14C]thymidine was used for length of the S-phase determination. The mean values obtained revealed that both DNA-LI and GF were lower, with a concomitant lengthening of G1 and Tc in older women than in young women. The correlation of these values with the gland's topography revealed that in both young and older women, the highest GF and DNA-LI were observed in intralobular terminal ducts, decreasing in alveoli and ducts [83].

We were the first to point out the importance that the proliferative activity of the breast epithelial cells be normalized to the morphological functional unit of the lobular structure. Also our studies were the first ones to clearly show that age and reproductive history, like parity, affect the proliferation of the breast epithelial cells, factors that had never been considered before.

9.7.2. *Isolation of mammary epithelial cells from organoids of the human breast*

Organ culture provided good information that correlated with the morphological analysis, but it was only a small increment in our technical approach. We obtained an USPHS Grant CA38921, awarded by the NCI, for using an *in vitro* system that better reproduced the *in vivo* conditions of the breast epithelium to determine if the breast epithelium was susceptible to neoplastic transformation. For these purposes, we utilized normal breast tissues, obtained fresh and sterile from reduction mammoplasties. Upon

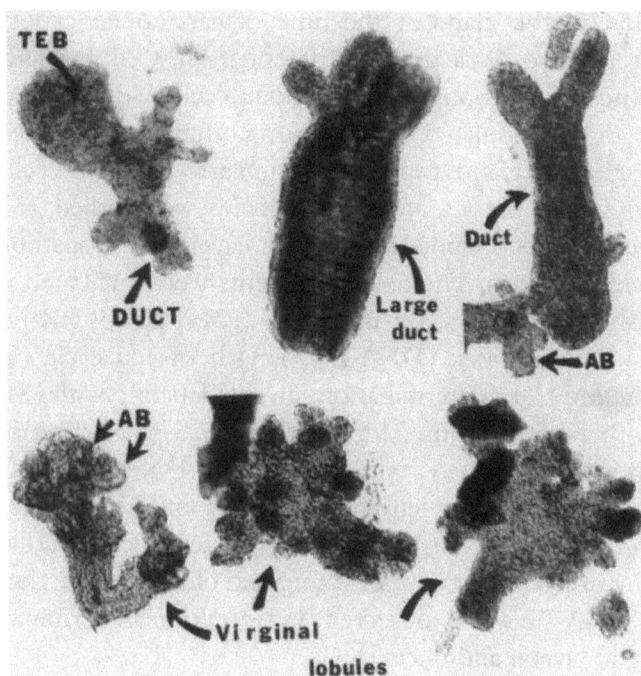

Figure 9.13:   Different organoids obtained after enzymatic digestion of the human breast and separated by micromanipulation (bright field, ×lO). *AB*, alveolar buds.

digestion of the tissues with collagenase and hyaluronidase, epithelial cells in aggregates, or organoids, are separated by micromanipulation (Figure 9.13).

Organoids were classified as Lob 1, Lob 2, or Lob 3 by applying the same criteria developed for classifying these structures in whole mount and histopathological preparations [47]. Plating each lobular type separately allows one to evaluate whether the behavior of cells in culture correlates with the specific type of lobule that originated them. Cells from Lob 1 and Lob 2, which in organ culture have shown to exhibit a higher DNA-LI, attach to the dishes promptly and start growing logarithmically, whereas cells from Lob 3, which have a lower DNA-LI, have a long lag phase before they attach to the dish and start growing. The number of doublings per lobular unit of time was also higher in Lob 1 and Lob 2 than in Lob 3 [86] (Figure 9.14).

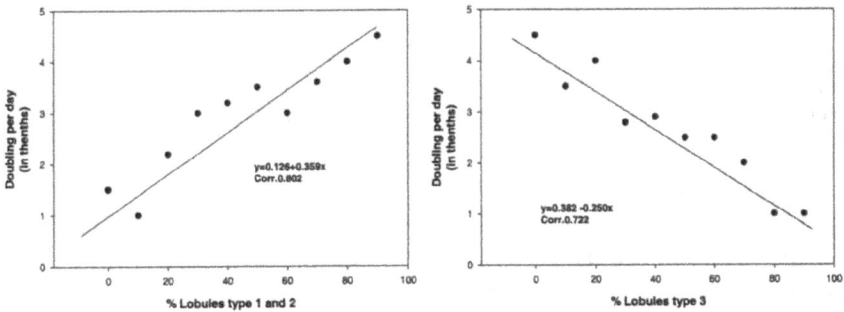

Figure 9.14: (Left) Correlation of doublings per day in Lob 1 and Lob 2 structures. (Right) Correlation of doublings per day and Lob 3 structures.

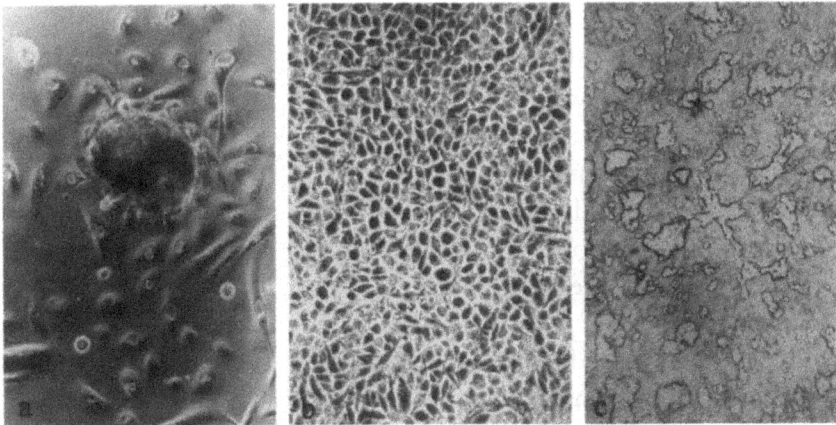

Figure 9.15: (a) Organoids of Lob 1 growing in plastic (phase contrast, ×40). (b) Confluent monolayer of Lob 1 before the formation of domes (phase contrast, ×10). (c) Dome formation (phase contrast, ×10).

Figure 9.15 depicts how the organoids are attached to the surface of the culture flask and expanded, forming monolayer and the typical formation of domes that is one of the main characteristics of human breast epithelial cells growing in the culture. This was a reproducible technique in our hands, and we decided to pursue the second step of our research that was to determine if the different physiological units, or Lob 1, Lob 2, and Lob 3, had different responses to chemical carcinogens.

9.7.3. *Transformation of primary breast epithelial cells*

We tested the susceptibility of the different lobule types to be transformed by chemical carcinogens in 52 human breast samples. For this purpose, organoids representing Lob 1, Lob 2, and Lob 3 were plated, and when the cells reached their logarithmic phase of growth they were treated with chemical carcinogens such as N-methyl-N-nitrosourea (NMU), and 7, 12-dimethylbenz(a)anthracene (DMBA), for 24 hours. We followed up the cells for several passages until they exhibited changes indicative of neoplastic transformation, such as variations in cell morphology, loss of contact inhibition, and anchorage-independent growth. The changes in cell shape induced by the carcinogens were the result of increased number of surface microvilli and decreased cell-to-cell interaction. The property to form domes when plated in plastic flasks, which is characteristic of normal breast epithelial cells, was lost in carcinogen-treated cells; I interpreted these changes to be the result of an abnormal pattern of growth caused by altered contact inhibition. Treated cells showed increased ability to survive and to form colonies in agar methocel, and to exhibit multinucleation. These types of responses, however, were observed only in the epithelial cells derived from breast tissues containing Lob 1 and Lob 2. The phenomena were not observed in the breast cells derived from Lob 3 [57, 86] (Figure 9.16).

These observations led us to conclude that primary cultures of human breast epithelial cells are susceptible to being transformed *in vitro* by chemical carcinogens and that the expression of phenotypes indicative of neoplastic transformation depends upon the stage of development of the breast and of the *in vivo* cell proliferation rate [57, 86]. The finding that Lob 1 and Lob 2 more readily express changes indicative of neoplastic transformation *in vitro* indicates that these structures are more susceptible to the transformative effect of genotoxic agents, thus supporting the observations that they are the site of origin of mammary carcinomas; it also correlates with the lack of association of the Lob 3 with the development of malignant neoplasms [55, 96]. Of greater relevance was the observation that the breasts of nulliparous women contain more Lob 1 and Lob 2 than the

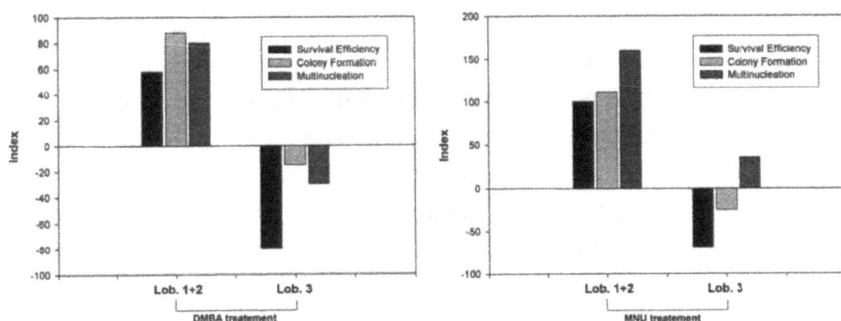

Figure 9.16: (Left) Histogram showing the expression of transformation phenotypes in primary culture of Lob 1, Lob 2, and Lob 3 treated with DMBA by 24 hour and followed up over several weeks (3–9 weeks). (Right) Histogram showing the expression of transformation phenotypes in primary culture of Lob 1, Lob 2, and Lob 3 treated with MNU (N-methyl-nitrosourea) for 24 hour and followed up over several weeks (3–9 weeks).

breasts of parous women, in which Lob 3 predominates, further emphasizing the protective effect of gland differentiation, which modulates the response of breast epithelial cells to carcinogens under *in vitro* conditions. The results of these experiments were published in *Cancer Research* in 1988 [57]. This was a difficult set of data to publish, and it took three revisions of the original manuscript, due to the demand of the reviewers for additional information, but in the end it resulted in a longer manuscript with significant new data that helped support our *original contention that human breast epithelial cells treated in vitro with chemical carcinogens manifest phenotypical changes indicative of cell transformation, and that these changes are modulated by the biological characteristics of the host, a new concept not considered before.*

The value of the publication in *Cancer Research* [57] is that it represented a methodical approach to a problem that had not been systematically studied in the past. For example: (1) We used two different carcinogens, DMBA, which requires metabolic activation, and MNU, a direct-acting carcinogen. (2) We used as a target HBEC obtained from reduction mammoplasty specimens in which normality was assessed by applying rigid histopathological criteria. (3) HBEC were derived from organoids, which are the structural units of the mammary gland that retain their architecture after enzymatic digestion, allowing us to identify whether organoids represented the types of lobules described in the whole mount preparation of the intact gland, thus permitting us to grade glandular development in both intact glands and by the proportion of the lobule type recovered after digestion. (4) Mammary development was further correlated with the patients' age and clinical history, and from these correlations emerged three categories of breast development: Low, containing Lob 1 and ducts; Medium, containing Lob 2; and High, containing Lob 3 [57]. (5) Due to the critical importance of correlating an organoid's morphology with the structure of the intact gland, the classical methodology for separation of organoids developed by Richard C. Hallowes, passing them through different size sieves [97], was modified, and organoids were separated using micromanipulation under a stereo microscope by shape as well as by size into Lob 1, Lob 2, and Lob 3, indicating increasing levels of differentiation. (6) We also found that human breast organoids plated in a serum-containing medium and changed in their first passage to serum-free medium, as has been described in the literature [98], exhibited great variability in lifespan, ranging from four to nine passages *in vitro*. However, the differences were significantly narrowed down when samples were grouped according to the degree of morphological development of the gland. Cells obtained from less developed glands were maintained *in vitro* for more passages (7.5 ± 1.5) than cells obtained from differentiated glands (4.4 ± 0.7). Demonstrating for the first time that the ability of cells to sustain a longer period of growth *in vitro* seemed to be directly related to the proliferative activity exhibited by each given structure in the intact gland [44], i.e., Lob 1 and Lob 2 had a higher mean DNA labeling index, 5.5 and 0.99, respectively, and sustained more passages than Lob 3, which had a DNA labeling index of 0.25 [44].

　　Therefore, the data published in Cancer Research *in 1988 was coherently supporting our previous observations [44, 64, 83, 99] and providing a new set of methodological criteria on how to study and interpret the study of human breast epicedial cells in vitro.*

9.7.4. *Development of an immortalized cell line,* *or MCF-10*

We have clearly demonstrated that normal HBEC have a limited capacity to divide *in vitro*, and although we have shown that the number of doublings was higher in HBEC derived from breast tissues with a lower differentiation grade, like Lob 1 and Lob 2 [57, 86], and that those cells were developing neoplastic transformation phenotypes but we were unable to make them tumorigenic, meaning that we have initiated the cells but we could not make them fully neoplastic. This led us to face the experimental problem of cell immortalization as a first step in neoplastic transformation and to accept the general prevalent concept of those days that induction of immortality, or immortalization, involved the abrogation of cellular programs for limiting the rate and the number of cell replications and as the key event of an oncogenic process. To immortalize human breast epithelial cells, many researchers were using various physical, chemical, and biological approaches, such as radiation, benzo(a)pyrene, viruses, and gene transfer. However, the most consistent approach has been the biological one, such as the use of human papilloma virus 16 (HPV-16), the oncogenes E6 and/or E7 [100, 101], and the simian virus 40 (SV 40) [102]. These two methods have successfully induced immortalization of HBEC. However, HBEC immortalized with viral oncogenes often expresses phenotypes indicative of neoplastic transformation, such as increase in anchorage-independent growth and tumorigenesis in nude mice, and the most disturbing fact was that these viruses had not been linked with the origin of human breast cancer. Therefore, I rejected these methods because it would take the BCRL out of the physiological concept of breast development, and more important, it would not provide an understanding of the early events of cancer initiation and progression. It was a difficult period for me because important laboratories around the world were discarding any way that did not use viral oncogenes for immortalization and cell transformation, and that made me feel out of context. However, I could not accept this methodology because it was basically accepting that you need a virus to immortalize HBEC. Although I accepted that was feasible and it was a likely possibility that this could be a mechanism, I was looking for a non-viral process. The solution to my dilemma started to emerge when Dr. Herbert Soule found that a mortal human breast cell, Sample #130, derived from a subcutaneous mastectomy specimen of a 36-year-old woman with no family history of breast cancer, acquired the immortal phenotype *in vitro* [103, 104]. The breast was composed of Lob 2 [44, 104] and was free of neoplasia, exhibiting only stromal fibrosis, cystic changes, and ductal hyperplasia without atypia. Original explants of the tissue, maintained for over a year, exhibited a normal diploid chromosomal pattern [103]. This cell was called MCF-10F and exhibited immortality after extended cultivation in low calcium medium [103, 104], retained the characteristics of the normal breast epithelium, such as lack of tumorigenicity in nude mice, three-dimensional growth in collagen, hormone and growth factor dependency for *in vitro* growth, lack of anchorage-independent growth, and dome formation in confluent cultures [104]. Immortalization of these cells was characterized by their continuous growth in a culture medium containing either low Ca^{++} like the MCF-10F or the conventional level of Ca^{++} (1.05 mM) like the MCF-10A without entering senescence, and without expressing phenotypes indicative of neoplastic transformation, such as colony formation in agar or in agar-methocel. *MCF-10F and MCF-10A cells (Figure 9.17) are bona fide normal HBEC in nature, expressing genetic, cytogenetic, ultra-structural, and phenotypic characteristics of normal human breast epithelium, representing the cell line closest to a normal HBEC available* [103, 104]. The phenotype of MCF-10F cells has been maintained stable for more than 118 passages *in vitro* (Figure 9.17).

Several mechanisms are considered to play a role in cell immortalization. Among them are the activation of telomerase, abrogation of cell cycle control, and activation of specific genes, and we have discussed them in length in [105, Chapter 7]. In this memoir, however, I would like to describe four studies done in the BCRL that stressed other mechanisms that we thought could also be involved in the process of immortalization of HBEC. These studies also reflect

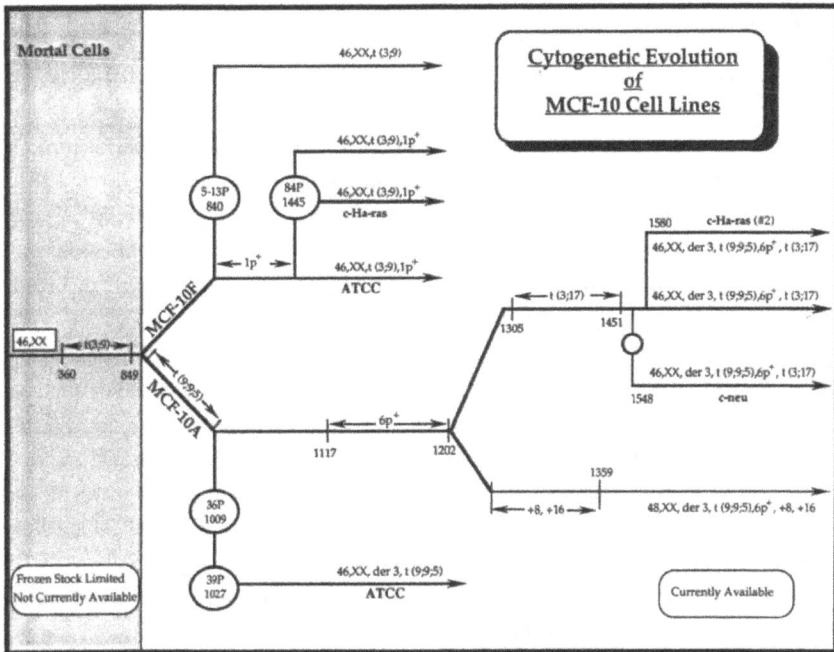

Figure 9.17: Cytogenetic evolution of MCF-10 cells. Diagram drawn by James Elliott and Jose Russo. Reprinted with permission from Ref. [105].

the work of five distinguished collaborators who were trained in my laboratory. One was the discovery of the calcium regulation of the mortal and immortal breast epithelial cells that was done with Dr. Quivo Tahin and Dr. Josiah Ochieng, the second was the discovery of a mutation in the p53 gene with Dr. Nandita Barnabas, the third one was the finding of the protein S100P with Dr. Ismael Dale Cotrin, and the last one was performed by Dr. Nadia A Higgy. All of these mechanisms were novel and significant in the understanding of cell immortalization and transformation of the MCF-10 cells. Although some of these studies were done later than 1991, when I had already moved to Philadelphia and the Fox Chase Cancer Center, I mention them here because they belong to the same theme that I started at the MCF in Detroit.

References

[1] Busch, H., Busch, R. K., Chan, P. K., Isenberg, W., Weigand, R., Russo, J. and Furmanski, P. Results of preliminary "Blind" study of the presence of the human tumor nucleolar antigen in breast carcinomas, benign breast tumors and normal breast tissues. *Clin. Immunol. Immunopath.* 18: 155–167, 1981.

[2] Weigand, R. A., Isenberg, W. M., Russo, J., Brennan, M. J., Rich, M. A. and the Breast Cancer Prognostic Study Associates. Blood vessel invasion and axillary lymph node involvement as prognostic indicators for human breast cancer. *Cancer* 50: 962–969, 1982.

[3] Fulton, A., Roi, L., Russo, J. and Brennan, M. J. Prostaglandin Activity in Patients with Primary Breast Cancer: Relationship to Clinical Parameters. *Breast Cancer Res. Treat.* 2: 331–337, 1982.

[4] Ownby, H., Martino, S., Roi, L. D., Howard, L., Russo, J., Brooks, S. and Brennan, M. J. Interrupted Pregnancy as an Indicator of Poor Prognosis in T1, 2; No, Mo Primary Breast Cancer. *Breast Cancer Res. Treat.* 3: 339–344, 1983.

[5] Fulton, A., Heppner, G., Roi, L., Howard, L., Russo, J. and Brennan, M. J. Relationship of natural killer cytotoxicity to clinical and biochemical parameters of primary human breast cancer. *Breast Cancer Res. Treat.* 4: 109–116, 1984.

[6] Ownby, H. E., Frederick, J., Russo, J., Brooks, S. L., Swanson, G. M., Heppner, G. H., Brennan, M. J. and the Breast Cancer Prognostic Study Associates. Racial Differences in Breast Cancer Patients. *J. Natl. Cancer Inst.* 75: 55–60, 1985.

[7] Ownby, D. R., Ownby, H. E., Bailey, J., Frederick, J., Tilley, B., Brooks, S., Russo, J., Heppner, G., Brennan, M. and the Breast Cancer Prognostic Study Associates. Presurgical serum immunoglobulin concentrations and the prognosis of operable cancer in women. *J. Natl. Cancer Inst.* 75: 655–663, 1985.

[8] Russo, I. H. and Russo, J. Hormone production by tumours: ectopia or gene derepression. In: Kaiser, H., (ed), *Cancer Growth and Progression. Influence of the host on tumor development*, Vol. 4, Kluwer Academic Publishers, Dordrecht. 1989, 123–132.

[9] Ownby, H. E., Frederick, J., Mortensen, R. F., Ownby, D. R. and Russo, J. Seasonal variation in tumor size at diagnosis and immunologic responses in human breast cancer. *Invasion Metastasis* 6: 246–256, 1986.

[10] Russo, J., Frederick, J., Ownby, H. E., Fine, G., Husain, M., Krickstein, H. I., Robbins, T. O. and Rosenberg, B. F. Predictors of Recurrence and Survival of Breast Cancer Patients. *Am. J. Clin. Pathol.* 88: 132–138, 1987.

[11] Huseby, R. A., Ownby, H. E., Frederick, J., Brooks, S., Russo, J. and Brennan, M. J. Node Negative Breast Cancer Treated by Modified Radical Mastectomy Without Adjuvant Therapies: Variable Associated with Disease and Recurrence and Survivorship. *J. Clin. Oncol.* 6: 83–88, 1988.

[12] Russo, J., Frederick, J. and Ownby, H. E. Predictors of Recurrence and Survival of Patients with Breast Cancer. *Oncology Journal Club* 1: 2–12, 1988.

[13] Maloney, T. M., Paine, P. L. and Russo, J. Polypeptide Computation of Normal and Neoplastic Human Breast Tissues and Cells Analyzed by Two-Dimensional Gel Electrophoresis. *Breast Cancer Res. Treat.* 14: 337–348, 1989.

[14] Ownby, H. E., Satariano, W. A., McKnight, E., McCune, R., Russo, J. and Brooks, S. Comorbidity and Breast Cancer Prognosis: A Test of Modified Cumulative Illness Rating Scale. *J. Clin. Oncol.* 1990.

[15] Foote, F. W. Jr. *Surgical pathology of cancer of the breast, Cancer of the breast.* Parsons, W. H., (ed), Springfield, Charles C Thomas. 1959, 37–38.

[16] Bloom, H. J. G. and Richardson, W. W. Histologic grading and prognosis in breast cancer: A study of 1409 cases of which 359 have been followed for 15 years. *Br. J. Cancer* 11: 359–377, 1957.

[17] Black, M. M., Opler, S. R. and Speer, F. D. Survival in breast cancer cases in relation to the structure of the primary tumor and regionallymph nodes. *Surg. Gynecol. Obstet.* 100: 543–551, 1955.

[18]   Black, M. M. and Speer, F. D. Nuclear structure in cancer tissues. *Surg. Gynecol. Obstet.* 105: 97–102, 1957.

[19] Russo, J., Tait, L. and Russo, I. H. Basic Techniques for the Ultrastructural Diagnosis of Tumors. *J. Electron Microsc. Tech.* 2: 305–351, 1985.

[20] Russo, J. Breast cancer: Adjuvant chemotherapy (Letter). *Science* 230: 886, 1985.

[21] Russo, J. Immunocytochemical Markers in Breast Cancer. In: Russo, J., (ed), *Immunocytochemistry in Tumor Diagnosis*, M. Nijhoff Publishing, Boston. 1985, 207–232.

[22] Russo, J., Tait, L. and Russo, I. H. *Guidelines in Ultrastructural Diagnosis of Tumors.* Russo, J., Sommers, S.C., (eds), Field, Wood and Associates, Inc. 1986, 15–126.

[23] Thornthwaite, J. T., Thomas, R. A., Russo, J., Ownby, H. E., Malinin, G. I., Hornieck, R. J., Wooley, T., Frederick, J., Malinin, T. T., Vazques, A. D. and Seckinger, D. A review of DNA Flow Cytometric Preparatory and Analytical Methods. In: Russo, J., (ed), *Immunocytochemistry in Tumor Diagnosis*, M. Nijhoff Publishing, Boston. 1985, 380–398.

[24] Russo, J. and Russo, I. H. Immunocytochemistry as a Tool in Cellular, Molecular Biology and Pathology. *J. Mic. Elect. Cell Biol.* 10: 1–63, 1986.

[25] Russo, J. and Jones, B. Influence of Steroid Hormones on the Growth Fraction of Human Breast Carcinomas. *Am. J. Clin. Pathol.* 88: 123–131, 1987.

[26] Russo, J. and Russo, I. H. Immunocytochemical Markers in Breast Cancer. In: DeLellis, R. A., (ed), *Advances in Immunocytochemistry*, Raven Press, New York, NY. 1988, 431–475.

[27] Russo, J., Frederick, J., Ownby, H., Fine, G., Hussain, M., Krickstein, H. T., Robbins, T. O. and Rosenberg, B. Predictors of Recurrence and Survival of Patients with Breast Cancer. In: Hickey, R. C., Saunders, G. F., Rivera, D. S., (eds), *The Yearbook of Cancer*, Yearbook Medical Publishers, Inc., Chicago, IL. 1988, 296–300.

[28] Russo, J. and Russo, I. H. Breast. In: Kovacs, K., Asa, S. L., (eds), *Functional Endocrine Pathology*, Blackwell Scientific Publications, Inc., Boston, MA. 1990, 652–669.

[29] Russo, J. and Russo, I. H. Comparative study of human and rat mammary Tumorigenesis. In: Rubin, E., Damjanov, I., (eds), *Pathology Reviews*, Humana Press. 1990, 217–251.

[30] Russo, J. and Russo, I. H. The pathology of breast cancer: staging and prognostic indicators. *J. Am. Med. Womens Assoc.* 47: 181–187, 1992.

[31] Russo, J., Rivera, M., Liang, J-D. and Russo, I. H. Undifferentiated malignant tumors. *Electron Microscopy* 3: 481–487, 1992.

[32] Russo, I. H., Rivera, M., Liang, J-D. and Russo, J. Ultrastructure of soft tissue tumors. *Electron Microscopy* 3: 485–492, 1992.

[33] El-Gendy, S., Tahin, Q., El-Merzabani, M., El-Aaser, A. A., Barnabas, N. and Russo, J. Co expression of c-erbB2 and int-2 oncogenes in invasive breast cancer. *Int. J. Oncol.* 6: 977–984, 1995.

[34] Russo, J. *Immunocytochemistry in Tumor Diagnosis*, M. Nijhoff Publishing, Boston, MA. 1985.

[35] Russo, J. and Sommers, S. C. *Tumor Diagnosis by Electron Microscopy*, Field, Wood and Associates, Inc., New York, NY. 1986.

[36] Russo, J. and Sommers, S. C. *Tumor Diagnosis by Electron Microscopy*, Vol. 2, Field and Wood, Inc., New York, NY. 1988.

[37] Russo, J. and Sommers, S. C. *Tumor Diagnosis by Electron Microscopy*, Vol. 3, Field and Wood, Inc., New York, NY. 1989.

[38] Ghadially, F. N. *Ultrastructural Pathology of the Cell and Matrix: A Text and Atlas of Physiological and Pathological Alterations in the Fine Structure of Cellular and Extracellular Components*, Butterworths, Toronto, ON. 1988.

[39] Ghadially, F. N. *Diagnostic Electron Microscopy of Tumours*, Butterworths, Toronto, ON. 1988.

[40] Russo, J. *The Pathobiology of Breast Cancer*, Springer, New York, NY. 2014.

[41] Glass, A. G., Donis-Keller, H., Mies, C., Russo, J., Zehnbauer, B., Taube, S. and Aamodt, R. The cooperative breast cancer tissue resource: Archival Tissue for the investigation of tumor markers. *Clin. Cancer Res.* 7: 1843–1849, 2001.

[42] Meyer, J. S., Alvarez, C., Lister, K., Milikowski, C., Olson, N., Russo, I. H., Russo, J., Zehnbauer, B., Glass, A. and Parwaresch, R. Breast carcinoma malignancy grading by Bloom-Richardson system vs proliferation index: reproducibility of grade and advantages of proliferation index. *Mod. Pathol.* 18: 1067–1078, 2005.

[43] Russo, J. and Russo, I. H. *Techniques and Methodological Approaches in Breast Cancer Research*, Springer, New York, NY. 2016.

[44] Russo, J. and Russo, I. H. Development of the human mammary gland. In: Neville, M. C., Daniel, C. (eds), *The mammary gland*, Plenum, New York, NY. 1987, 67–93.

[45] Russo, J., Lynch, H. and Russo, I. H. Mammary gland architecture as a determining factor in the susceptibility of the human breast to cancer. *Breast J.* 7(5): 278–291, 2001.

[46] Russo, J., Tay, L. K. and Russo, I. H. Differentiation of the mammary gland and susceptibility to carcinogenesis. *Breast Cancer Res. Treat.* 2: 5–73, 1982.

[47] Russo, J., Rivera, R. and Russo, I. H. Influence of age and parity on the development of the human breast. *Breast Cancer Res. Treat.* 23: 211–218, 1992.

[48] Russo, I. H. and Russo, J. Developmental stage of the rat mammary gland as determinant of its susceptibility to 7,12-dimethylbenz[a]anthracene. *J. Natl. Cancer Inst.* 61: 1439–1449, 1978.

[49] Russo, J. and Russo, I. H. DNA labeling index and structure of the rat mammary gland as determinants of its susceptibility to carcinogenesis. *J. Natl. Cancer Inst.* 61: 1451–1459, 1978.

[50] Russo, J., Wilgus, G. and Russo, I. H. Susceptibility of the mammary gland to carcinogenesis. I. Differentiation of the mammary gland as determinant of tumor incidence and type of lesion. *Am. J. Pathol.* 96: 721–736, 1979.

[51] Russo, J. and Russo, I. H. Influence of differentiation and cell kinetics on the susceptibility of the rat mammary gland to carcinogenesis. *Cancer Res.* 40: 2677–2687, 1980.

[52] Russo, J. and Russo, I. H. Susceptibility of the mammary gland to carcinogenesis. II. Pregnancy interruption as a risk factor in tumor incidence. *Am. J. Pathol.* 100: 497–512, 1980.

[53] Russo, J., Wilgus, G., Tait, L. and Russo, I. H. Influence of age and parity on the susceptibility of rat mammary gland epithelial cells in primary cultures to 7,12-dimethylbenz(a)anthracene. *In Vitro* 17: 877–884, 1981.

[54] Russo, J. and Russo, I. H. Is differentiation the answer to breast cancer prevention? *IRCS Med. Sci.* 10: 935–941, 1982.

[55] Russo, J., Gusterson, B. A., Rogers, A. E., Russo, I. H., Wellings, S. R. and Van Zwieten, M. J. Comparative study of human and rat mammary tumorigenesis. *Lab. Invest.* 62: 1–32, 1991.

[56] Russo, I. H. and Russo, J. Mammary gland neoplasia in long-term rodent studies. *Environ. Health Perspect.* 104: 938–967, 1996.

[57] Russo, J., Reina, D., Frederick, J. and Russo, I. H. Expression of phenotypical changes by human breast epithelial cells treated with carcinogens in vitro. *Cancer Res.* 48: 2837–2857, 1988.

[58] Hu, Y. F., Russo, I. H., Zalipsky, U. and Russo, J. Lack of involvement of bcl2 and cyclin D 1 in the early phases of human breast epithelial cell transformation by environmental chemical carcinogens. *Proc. Am. Assoc. Cancer Res.* 37: 1005a, 1996.

[59] Russo, J. and Russo, I. H. Role of differentiation in the pathogenesis and prevention of breast cancer. *Endocr. Relat. Cancer* 4: 1–15, 1997.

[60] Russo, J., Hu, Y-F., Yang, X. and Russo, I. H. Developmental, cellular, and molecular basis of human breast cancer. *J. Natl. Cancer Inst. Monograph* 27: 17–38, 2000.

[61] Russo, J. Hu, Y-F., Silva, I. D. C. G. and Russo, I. H. Cancer risk related to mammary gland structure and development. *Microsc. Res Tech.* 52: 204–223, 2001.

[62] Russo, J. and Russo, I. H. Development of the Human Breast. In: Knobil, E., Neill, J. D., (eds), *Encyclopedia of Reproduction*, Vol. 3, Academic Press, New York, NY. 1998, 71–80.

[63] Russo, J., Mills, M. J., Moussalli, M. J. and Russo, I. H. Influence of breast development and growth properties in vitro. *In vitro Cell Develop. Biol.* 25: 643–649, 1989.

[64] Mailo, D., Russo, J., Sheriff, F., Hu, Y. F., Tahin, Q., Mihaila, D., Balogh, G. and Russo, I. H. Genomic signature induced my differentiation in the rat mammary gland. *Proc. Am. Assoc. Cancer Res.* 43, 2002.

[65] Russo, J. and Russo, I. H. The cellular basis of breast cancer susceptibility. *On col. Res.* 11: 169–178, 1999.

[66] Russo, J. and Russo, I. H. Development pattern of human breast and susceptibility to carcinogenesis. *Eur. J. Cancer Prevent.* 2: 85–100, 1993.

[67] Russo, J. and Russo, I. H. Toward a physiological approach to breast cancer prevention. *Cancer Epidemiol. Biomarkers Prev.* 3: 353–364, 1994.

[68] Russo, J., Saby, J., Isenberg, W. and Russo, I. H. Pathogenesis of mammary carcinomas induced in rats by 7,12-dimethylbenz(a)anthracene. *J. Natl. Cancer Inst.* 59: 435–445, 1977.

[69] Russo, I. H., Koszalka, M. and Russo, J. Human chorionic gonadotropin and rat mammary cancer prevention. *J. Natl. Cancer Inst.* 82: 1286–1289, 1990.

[70] Russo, I. H., Koszalka, M. and Russo, J. Comparative study of the influence of pregnancy and hormonal treatment on mammary carcinogenesis. *Br. J. Cancer* 64: 481–484, 1991.

[71] Russo, I. H. and Russo, J. Role of hormones in cancer initiation and progression. *J. Mammary Gland Biol. Neoplasia* 3: 49–61, 1997.

[72] MacMahon, B., *et al.* Age at first birth and breast cancer risk. *Bull. World Health Organ.* 43: 209–221, 1970.

[73] Russo, J., Mills, M. J., Moussalli, M. J. and Russo, I. H. Influence of human breast development on the growth properties of primary cultures. *In Vitro Cell Dev. Biol.* 25: 643–649, 1989.

[74] Belitskaya-Lévy, I., Zeleniuch-Jacquotte, A., Russo, J., Russo, I. H., Bordas, P., Ahman, J., Afanasyeva, Y., Johansson, R., Lenner, P., Li, X., Lopez de Cicco, R., Peri, S., Ross, E., Russo, P. A., Santucci-Pereira, J., Sheriff, F. S., Slifker, M., Hallmans, G., Toniolo, P. and Arslan, A. A. Characterization of a Genomic Signature of Pregnancy in the Breast. *Cancer Prev. Res.* 4: 1457–1464, 2011.

[75] Peri, S., López de Cicco, R., Santucci-Pereira, J., Slifker, M., Ross, E. A., Russo, I. H., Russo, P. A., Arslan, A. A., Belitskaya-Lévy, I., Zeleniuch-Jacquotte, A., Bordas, P. Lenner, P., Åhman, J., Afanasyeva, Y., Johansson, R., Sheriff, F., Hallmans, G., Toniolo, P. and Russo, J. Defining the genomic signature of the parous breast. *BMC Med. Genomics* 5: 46–57, 2012.

[76] Russo, J., Santucci-Pereira, J., López de Cicco, R., Sheriff, S., Russo, P. A., Peri, S., Slifker, M., Ross, E., Luiza, S., Mello, M., Vidal, B. C., Belitskaya-Lévy, I., Arslan, A. Zeleniuch-Jacquotte, A., Bordas, P., Lenner, P., Ahman, J., Afanasyeva, Y., Hallmans, G., Toniolo, P. and Russo, I. H. Pregnancy-induced chromatin remodeling in the breast of postmenopausal women. *Int. J. Cancer* 131: 1059–1070, 2012.

[77] Calaf, G., Russo, I. H., Roi, L. and Russo, J. Effect of Estrogen on the length of S-phase of human breast tissue in organ culture. *Int. Res. Commun. Syst. (IRCS)* 10: 307–308, 1982.

[78] Calaf, G., Martinez, F., Russo, I. H. and Russo, J. Age-related variations in Growth Kinetics of Primary Human Breast Cell Cultures. *Int. Res. Commun. Syst. (IRCS)* 10: 551–553, 1982.

[79] Calaf, G., Russo, I. H., Roi, L. and Russo, J. Hormonal Response of Human Breast Tissue in Organ Culture. *Int. Res. Commun. Syst. (IRCS)* 10: 566–567, 1982.

[80] Calaf, G., Martinez, F., Russo, I. H., Roi, L. D. and Russo, J. The Influence of Age on DNA Labeling Index of Human Breast Epithelium. *Int. Res. Commun. Syst. (IRCS)* 10: 657–658, 1982.

[81] Calaf, G., Russo, I. H., Roi, L. D. and Russo, J. Effect of Hormones on Growth Fraction of Human Breast Tissue in Organ Culture. *Int. Res. Commun. Syst. (IRCS)* 10: 655–656, 1982.

[82] Calaf, G., Russo, I. H., Roi, L. D. and Russo, J. Effect of Peptide and Steroid Hormones in Cell Kinetic Parameters of Normal Human Breast Tissue in Organ Culture. *In vitro* 22: 135–140, 1986.

[83] Russo, J., Calaf, G., Roi, L. and Russo, I. H. Influence of Age and Gland Topography on Cell Kinetics of Normal Human Breast Tissue. *J. Natl. Cancer Inst.* 78: 413–418, 1987.

[84] Russo, I. H., Calaf, G. and Russo, J. Hormones and proliferative activity in breast tissue. In: Stoll, B. A., (ed), *Approaches to breast cancer prevention*, Kluwer, Dordrecht. 1990, 35–51.

[85] Russo, J., Calaf, G., Sohi, N., Tahin, Q., Zhang, P. L., Alvarado, M. E., Estrada, S. and Russo, I. H. Critical steps in breast carcinogenesis. *Ann. NY Acad. Sci.* 698: 1–20, 1993.

[86] Russo, J., Calaf, G. and Russo, I. H. A critical approach to the malignant transformation of human breast epithelial cells. *CRC Crit. Rev. Oncogenesis* 4: 403–417, 1993.

[87] Calaf, G., Tahin, Q., Alvarado, M. E., Estrada, S., Cox, T. and Russo, J. Hormone receptors and cathepsin D levels in human breast epithelial cells transformed by chemical carcinogens. *Breast Cancer Res. Treat.* 29: 169–177, 1993.

[88] Calaf, G. and Russo, J. Transformation of human breast epithelial cells by chemical carcinogens. *Carcinogenesis* 14: 483–492, 1993.

[89] Zhang, P. L., Calaf, G. and Russo, J. Allele loss and point mutation in codons 12 and 61 of the c-Ha-ras oncogene in carcinogen-transformed human breast epithelial cells. *Mol. Carcinog.* 9: 46–56, 1994.

[90] Calaf, G., Zhang, P. L., Alvarado, M. V., Estrada, S. and Russo, J. C-Ha-ras enhances the neoplastic transformation of human breast epithelial cells treated with chemical carcinogens. *Int. J. Oncol.* 6: 5–11, 1995.

[91] Lah, T. T., Calaf, G., Kalman, E., Shimde, B. G., Somers, R., Estrada, S., Salero, E., Russo, J. and Daskal, I. Cathepsin D, B, and L in transformed

human breast epithelial cells (HBEC). *Biol. Chem. Hoppe Seyler* 376: 357–363, 1995.

[92] Russo, J., Russo, I. H., Calaf, G., Zhang, P. L. and Barnabas, N. Breast susceptibility to carcinogenesis. In: Li, J., Nandi, S., Li, S. A., (eds), *Hormonal Carcinogenesis*, Springer-Verlag, Berlin. 1994.

[93] Wahab, I., Barnabas, N., Calaf, G. and Russo, J. Genome scanning using endogenous LTR-like elements for rapid DNA fingerprint of breast cancer and transformed human breast epithelial cells. *Int. J. Oncol.* 7: 25–31, 1995.

[94] Barnabas, N., Moraes, R., Calaf, G., Estrada, S. and Russo, J. Role of p53 in MCF-10F cell immortalization and chemically induced neoplastic transformation. *Int. J. Oncol.* 7: 1289–1296, 1995.

[95] Calaf, G., Alvarado, M. E., Bonney, G. E., Amfoh, K. K. and Russo, J. Influence of lobular development on breast epithelial cell proliferation and steroid hormone receptor content. *Int. J. Oncol.* 7: 1285–1288, 1995.

[96] Russo, J., Romero, A. L. and Russo, I. H. Architectural pattern of the normal and cancerous breast under the influence of parity. *J. Cancer Epidemiol. Biomarkers Prev.* 3: 219–224, 1994.

[97] Hallowes, R. C., Bone, E. J. and Jones, W. A new dimension in the culture of human breast. In: Richards, R. J., Rajan, K. T., (eds.), *Tissue Culture in Medical Research*, Pergamon Press, London. 1980, 56, 213–220.

[98] Hammond, S., Harn, R. G. and Stampfer, M. R. Serum-free growth of human mammary epithelial cells: rapid clonal growth in defined medium extended serial passage with pituitary extract. *Proc. Natl. Acad. Sci. USA* 81: 5435–5439, 1984.

[99] Russo, J. and Russo, I. H. Biological and molecular basis of mammary carcinogenesis. *Lab. Invest.* 57: 112–137, 1987.

[100] Band, V., Zagetowski, D., Kulesa V. and Sager, R. Human papilloma virus DNAs immortalize normal human mammary epithelial cells and reduce their growth factor requirements. *Proc. Natl. Acad. Sci. USA* 87: 463–467, 1990.

[101] Band, V., Dalal, S., Delmolino, L. and Androphy, E. L. Enhanced degradation of p53 protein in IIPV-6 and BPV-1 E6- immortalized human mammary epithelial cells. *EMBO J.* 12: 1847–1852, 1993.

[102] Yilmaz, A., Gaide, A. C., Sordat, B., Borbeny, Z., Lahm, H., Imam, A., Shreyer, M. and Odartehenko, L. Malignant progression of SV 40-immortalized human milk epithelial cells. *Br. J. Cancer* 68: 868–873, 1993.

[103] Soule, H. D., Maloney, T. M., Wolman, S. R., Peterson, W. D., Brenz, R., McGrath, C. M., Russo, J., Pauley, R. J., Jones, R. F. and Brooks, S. C.

Isolation and characterizaion of a spontaneously immortalized human breast epithelial cell line, MCF 10. *Cancer Res.* 50: 6075–6086, 1991.

[104] Tait, L., Soule, H. D. and Russo, J. Ultrastructural and immuno-cytochemical characterization of an immortalized human breast epithelial cell line, MCF-10. *Cancer Res.* 50: 6087–6094, 1990.

[105] Russo, J. and Russo, I. H. *Molecular Basis of Breast cancer*, Springer-Verlag, Berlin. 2004.

[106] Russo, J. and Russo, I. H. Development of Human Mammary Gland. In: Neville, M. C., Daniel, C. W., (eds), *The Mammary Gland Development, Regulation, and Function*, Plenum Pub. Corp. 1987, 67–93.

Chapter 10

The Breast Cancer Research Laboratory — Part 2 (Expanding the Wings 1979–1991)

10.1. Role of calcium in cell immortalization

An important property of mortal cells is their ability to control the intracellular Ca^{2+} concentration, which may explain their limited lifespan *in vitro*. The mortality of normal human breast epithelial cell (HBEC) is characterized by a progressive cessation of cell growth in culture and senescence. HBEC cultured in a standard culture medium have a lifespan comparable to that of adult human fibroblasts (30–40 doublings), before undergoing terminal differentiation and senescence. The survival of HBEC is profoundly affected by the concentration of calcium (Ca^{2+}) in the culture medium. Comparing two different culture conditions, one with a serum-free medium, in which the Ca concentration is 1.05 mM, and another containing serum, but lowering Ca concentration to 0.046 mM, significantly changes the growth properties of HBEC. Extended growth without expressing terminal differentiation is observed when the Ca^{2+} level in the culture medium is reduced from 1.05 mM to 0.046 mM (low Ca^{2+}) [1]. Under these conditions HBEC maintain their normal diploid karyotype, form domes (Figure 9.15 in Chapter 9) and duct-like structures in collagen even reproducing the morphology of the structures which they are derived from, express specific keratin filaments and milk fat globule membrane antigen, and contain all the other structural features of breast epithelial cells [2]. When the Ca^{2+} concentration is restored to 1.05 mM (also called high Ca^{2+}), the cells maintain the same phenotypic characteristics, but they stop their growth. This phenomenon is reversible by reducing the Ca^{2+} concentration in the culture medium. The response of the normal HBEC to Ca^{2+} is lost during the process of cell immortalization and transformation, and accompanied by the over expression of S100P [3]. Normal cells obtained from primary cultures do not form colonies in agar methocel; they instead form ductules in collagen matrix, and are unable to grow in athymic mice [1]. HBECs grow and can be subcultured for up to a year if the Ca^{2+} concentrations in the culture medium range from 0.03 to 0.06 mM [1]. In this culture condition, the majority of the cells assume a spherical morphology (Figure 10.1), produce duct-like structures in collagen, display all the ultra-structural features of breast epithelial cells, and maintain their normal diploid karyotype [1]. If the calcium concentration in the medium is elevated to 1.05 mM or above, the cells change their

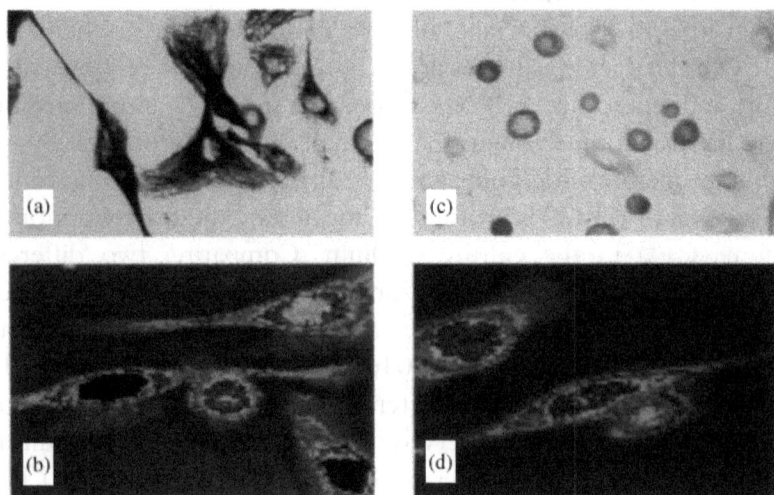

Figure 10.1: (a) Monolayer cultures of HBEC in chamber slides stained for immunocytochemistry with antibodies against tubulin and growing in high Cah medium (×40). (b) Cells stained with fura-2A. (c) Cells growing in low Ca^{2+} medium (×40). (d) Cell stained with fura-2A. The cells growing in high calcium concentrate have more intracellular Ca^{2+} (b) than those growing in low Ca^{2+} (d).

morphology to mainly elongated and flattened cells which form tight junctions and domes at confluence (Figure 10.1) [1]. This change takes place as early as 5 hours after the switch from low to high calcium medium, and the cells finally undergo terminal differentiation and stop dividing [1]. The relative calcium concentration maps using indo-1 fluorescence dye revealed that the mortal HBECs do not effectively buffer their intracellular calcium (Ca_i) against elevated levels of extracellular calcium (Ca_0). Elevation of Ca_0 from 0.04 to 1.05 mM resulted in elevated and sustained increases in Ca_i for at least 30 minutes. The immortal and transformed HBECs, on the other hand, did not show observable increase in their Ca_i subsequent to the elevation of Ca_0 to 1.05 mM. Ca_i of both mortal and immortal HBECs growing in a medium containing 0.04 mM was maintained at a very low concentration (approximately 20 nM). However, if the extracellular calcium was increased to 1.05 mM, the Ca_i+ increased two- to three-fold in the mortal cells, as depicted in Figure 10.2.

The immortal and oncogene transformed cell lines, on the other hand, did not show significant changes in their Ca_i following the elevation of Ca_0 from 0.04 to 1.05 mM. The Ca_i of both MCF-10A and MCF-10AneoT was maintained at around 20 nM regardless of the

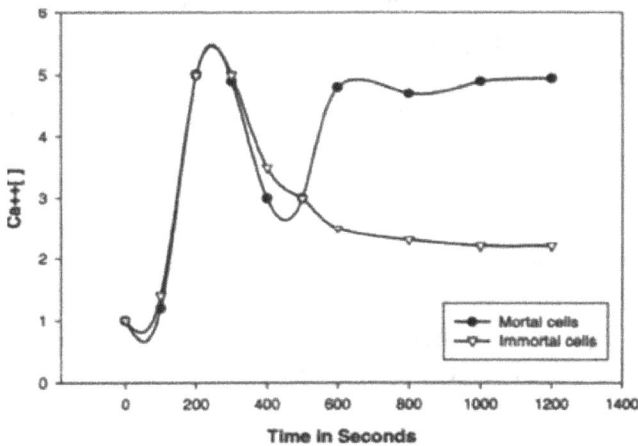

Figure 10.2: Curves showing the mobilization of Ca^{2+} in mortal and immortal cells after the switch of medium from low to high Ca^{2+}.

Ca_0 levels. To test whether or not the increased Ca_i in the mortal cells was reversible, cells that had been grown in high-calcium medium for three days were switched back to low calcium for 24 hours. Ca_i in MCF-10M cells dropped precipitously subsequent to a switch back to a low-calcium medium. The immortal and transformed cells, on the other hand, did not show a significant difference in their Ca_i levels after the switch back to a low-calcium medium as expected. Switching the mortal cells from low to high-calcium medium resulted in not only a substantial and significant increase in Ca, but also a significant increase in inositol triphosphate. The sustained increases in intracellular IP3 closely matched Ca increases over the three-day period subsequent to the switch to a high-calcium medium. The intracellular levels of IP3 in the immortal and transformed HBECs, on the other hand, did not change significantly, but remained more or less at the basal level. There is a marked difference in the manner in which mortal HBECs maintain Ca_i compared with their immortal counterpart when Ca_0 is increased. It is well established that nearly all cell types maintain their Ca at a very low concentration compared with Ca_0 [4]. To do this, cells have evolved elaborate calcium buffering systems. These include high-affinity calcium-binding proteins such as calmodulin and Ca-ATPase pump, which actively pumps calcium out from the cells against a calcium concentration gradient [1]. Opposed to these calcium buffering and export systems are the calcium influx pathways which increase intracellular calcium, such as the putative calcium channels [1, 4], the Na^+/Ca^{2+} exchanger, which drives Ca^{2+} into the cells as Na^+ is driven out, and second messenger molecules such as IP3, which mobilize calcium from its intracellular stores [1]. Therefore, we considered that any of these calcium buffering or influx pathways may be modified in either the mortal or immortal HBECs to account for the differential calcium-buffering capacity in these cells. We also have shown in calcium efflux studies differences in the rate at which Ca^{2+} is extruded from MCF-10M and MCF-10A cells subsequent to increasing extracellular calcium (Figure 10.2). However, our data tended to favor the calcium influx pathways as the ones crucial for the significant increase in Ca_i in the mortal cells. The fact is that Ca_i increases in mortal cells is closely correlated to increases in IP3, raising the possibility that increases in extracellular calcium activate phospholipase C, resulting in the hydrolysis of phosphoinositol 4,5 bisphosphate phosphate(PIP2) to diacylglycerol and IP3 [1]. Although we could not continue these studies further, it is not doubted that a detailed knowledge of these mechanisms will lead to a better understanding of growth regulation of HBECs both *in vitro* and *in vivo*.

10.2. P53 mutation in the immortalization of HBECs

Since 1980, p53, a tumor suppressor gene, has been considered extremely important in the neoplastic process [5–13], therefore, it was of relevance to us to determine whether p53 mutation played a role in not only the transformation of HBECs but also in the early phase of cell immortalization. When we received the NCI grant CA 67238, Dr. Nandita Barnabas was hired. She joined the Breast Cancer Research Laboratory (BCRL) at the end of 1990, and I assigned her the task of determining the possible role of p53 in the immortalization and transformation of HBEC. We capitalized on two previous works; one was the spontaneous immortalization of the HBEC line MCF-10F that was derived from a mortal cell designated MCF-10M [14], and second in an *in vitro* system in which HBEC treated with chemical carcinogens recapitulated sequential stages of tumor initiation and progression, culminating in the expression of tumorigenesis in a heterologous host [15–17].

In this memoir, I want to emphasize the relevance of having these two experimental systems because they were unique in the sense that a cell line that originated from a mortal cell was spontaneously immortalized and transformed using specific carcinogenic agents maintaining the original genotype, meaning that this was not a comparative work of cell lines with different genetic background but the same cell line evolving from normal to tumor allowing it to identify under the same genomic background as the genes involved in the different steps of cancer initiation and progression. Unfortunately, the relevance of this unique resource and the importance of this thinking have been overlooked in the literature.

With Dr. Barnabas, we used Southern blot, Northern blot, single-strand conformation polymorphism (SSCP), and DNA sequencing to detect mutations in the highly conserved exons 5–9 of the p53 gene [18]. Whereas no changes were detected in any of the cells tested by Southern and Northern blot, SSCP analysis showed a conformational shift in exon 7 in the MCF-10F cell line, and in clones BP1, BP1-E, D3, and D3-1, derived from DMBA and BP treated cells, respectively. This shift was absent in MCF-10M cells, the mortal cells from which the MCF-10F immortal cells were derived, and in the placental DNA used as control. Asymmetric PCR-amplified products of exon 7 revealed an insertion of thymine at codon 254, thereby causing a frame shift mutation producing a mutant p53 in MCF-10F cells and in all the clones derived from chemically transformed cells, when compared with the wild type control sequence in the mortal cells (MCF-10M), human placenta, and MCF-7 cells (Figure 10.3).

These data also indicated to us that carcinogen treatment did not induce any additional changes in the p53 gene, suggesting that the frame shift mutation took place during the process of cell immortalization. It was comforting to us to know that frame shift mutations in the p53

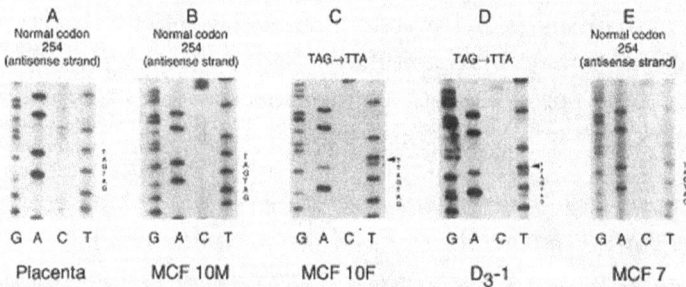

Figure 10.3: Direct DNA sequencing of the PCR-amplified products generated from exon 7 of the p53 gene of placenta, MCF-10M, MCF-10F, D3-1, and MCF-7 cells. The mortal cell line MCF-10M, placental DNA, and MCF-7 cells showed the wild-type p53 sequence. An insertional mutation of a T at codon position 254 in the antisense strand was observed in MCF-10F and D3-I cells, causing the antisense strand to read TTA instead of TAG, changing the reading frame at codon 254.

gene due to base insertions, such as the one reported in MCF-10F cells and in the transformed clones, had also been reported in breast tumors [19, 20], other tumors, and cell lines [21–27]. The sequence analysis of exon 7 of the p53 gene in MCF-10F cells revealed an additional T base at codon 254 which was not present in MCF-10M cells, which showed the wild-type sequence [28]. This mutation caused the codon 254 to change from TAG to TTA, and the amino acid sequence to read asparagine instead of isoleucine. This alteration caused the subsequent reading frame from codon 254 to codon 261 to be altered as well, thereby giving rise to a mutant p53 protein. This finding is confirmed by the positive immunohistochemistry reported previously by us in these cells [17], and the shift in this exon by SSCP analysis.

Our finding was a clear demonstration that expression of mutated p53 is associated with the immortalization phenotype. The appearance of a mutant p53 in MCF-10F cells, which was retained when the cells were transformed by chemical carcinogens, also implicates this fact. Increased proliferative activity and escape from senescence, i.e., *in vitro* immortalization, are thought to be initial events in cell transformation [29].

An important conclusion drawn from the work with Dr. Barnabas [18] *was that the phenotypical alterations indicative of neoplastic transformation induced by chemical carcinogens in MCF-10F cells are not due to changes induced in the p53 gene.*

However, carcinogen treatment of MCF-10F cells induces phenotypic alterations that are associated with loss of alleles of the *c-Ha-ras* [30] and amplification of the *c-erbB2, int-2,* and *c-myc* oncogenes [17, 31]; these are early changes observed in association with the expression of anchorage independence [17, 32]. Point mutations in codons 12 and 61 of the remaining allele of *c-Ha-ras* have been associated with clonal expansion of the transformed cells [30], whereas loss of heterozygosity of 17p in the region telomeric to p53 (17p 13.1) was a late event associated with the expression of tumorigenesis in SCID mice by BP1-E cells [1]. These observations indicate that p53 mutations might not be crucial for the emergence of the transformation phenotype, and in primary breast cancers it might be important only in a subset of human tumors. Although from our work [18] we can neither confirm nor rule out the role of p53 as the driving force in the immortalization of MCF-10F cells, it is, however, possible to speculate that the p53 mutation may lead to a genetic instability that facilitates the emergence of other genomic changes.

10.3. Discovery of S100P calcium-binding protein

With Dr. Ismael Dale Cotrin, a postdoctoral fellow from the Fundacao de Amparo a Pesquisa do Estado de Sao Paulo, Brazil, and with the award of the NCI RO1CA67238, we carried out a new set of studies using differential display techniques that allowed us to detect gene expression differences between mortal and immortal cells. As it is shown in Figure 10.4, we identified a band called 10F-D, which was differentially amplified using the primers HT 11 C and HAP-6 in the immortal cell line MCF-10F as compared to its mortal parental counterpart S130 cells or MCF-10M [33]. We isolated the band and cloned it, and 10 isolated fragments were amplified and the sequence determined. With the sequenced fragment, we were able to search for homologies in gene-bank databases (GenBank + EMBL + DDBJ + PDB) and we concluded that the cDNA band 10F-D (439 bp) showed very high homology (99%) to the *H. sapiens* mRNA encoding for the calcium-binding protein S100P. Importantly, we found that the level of S100P expression was increased nine- to ten-fold in the immortal cells including MCF-10F (spontaneously immortalized), BPlE (BP-transformed) [15], D3.1 (7, 12-dimethyl-benz(a)anthracene (DMBA)-transformed); [15] and T47D (tumor cell line) as compared to the S130 or MCF-10M mortal cells and two primary cultures, 244 and 248. The expression of S100P was also clearly up regulated (two-fold to twenty-fold) in ductal invasive carcinomas when compared to their normal adjacent tissues. Notably, a much higher increase in S100P overexpression (twenty-fold) was observed in breast cancer.

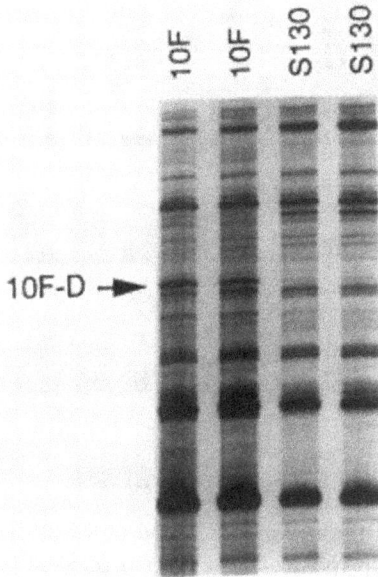

Figure 10.4: Differential display gel, in duplicate, using total RNA from the spontaneously immortalized HBEC MCF-10F (10F lanes) and its mortal parental counterpart S130 cells (S130 lanes). The arrow shows the band called 10F-D displayed only in the immortal cells.

RNA was from a poorly differentiated, lymph node-positive, ductal invasive carcinoma sample. In various normal tissues we examined, the expression of S100P was high (ten- to fifteen-fold) in full-term placenta; low in lung, breast, and colon; and essentially absent in other tissues.

Immunocytochemical localization of S100P with monoclonal antibodies was absent in all the normal breast tissues analyzed. All the ductal hyperplasias, typical and atypical, ductal carcinomas *in situ*, and invasive carcinomas were positive. Interestingly, in cases of morphologically normal breast tissues adjacent to five ductal hyperplasias, two of the carcinomas *in situ* and three of the invasive carcinomas were slightly positive for S100P [33]. The S100P protein

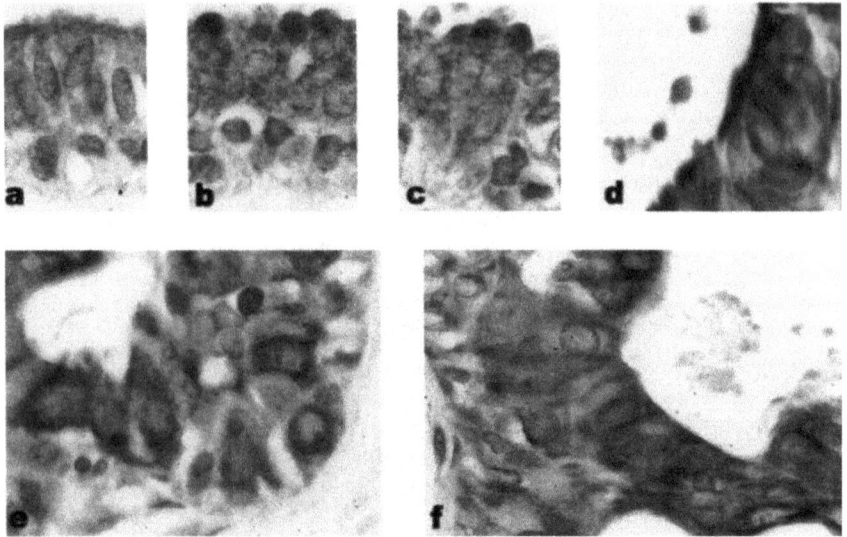

Figure 10.5: (a) immunocytochemical localization of S100P in the cytoplasm of epithelial cells from a ductal hyperplasia of the breast. (b), (c) Show the immunoreacted protein migrating toward the apical portion of the cells and extruding in the lumen (d). (e), (f) Strong reactivity in the cytoplasm of invasive ductal carcinoma (×40).

was localized in the cytoplasm of the epithelial cells and tended to accumulate at high concentrations in the apical and supranuclear regions (Figure 10.5).

The S100P calcium-binding protein was first isolated from the human placenta [34, 35] and belongs to the family of S100 calcium-binding proteins [36] characterized by a common structural motif, the EF-hand domain, which binds to calcium with high affinity and specificity [37]. Calcium is an essential component of cell membrane structures and a major second messenger in the control of a variety of biological processes, such as cell cycle progression, differentiation, and cell death [38]. It has already been demonstrated that an increase in the concentration of calcium in the culture media decreases cell proliferation and induces cell differentiation in the HBEC [39, 40], whereas lowering concentration of calcium in the culture media extends the lifespan of primary cultures and mortal HBEC [2, 14]. Therefore, the discovery of S100P allowed us to speculate that the increase in calcium-binding proteins could conceivably diminish the intracellular pool of free calcium, and the fact that S100P is overexpressed during the process of cell immortalization could explain our observation that the intracellular concentration of free calcium is higher in mortal cells as compared to immortal cells [41]. The preferential expression of S100P mRNA in immortal cells, but not in their mortal parental counterparts or primary HBEC cultures, regardless of different calcium concentrations, suggests that the S100P protein might be one of the molecules involved in specific pathways of cell cycle control whose imbalance might enable cells to escape from senescence reaching therefore the immortal cell status.

Based on these results we developed a hypothetical model (Figure 10.6) explaining how S100P could be involved in the mechanisms of immortalization and transformation of HBEC. S100P shares considerable homology with the mts-1 gene (metastasis-associated gene), which was postulated to be involved in p53 sequestration, tubulin depolymerization, and G 1-S transition. S100P is also very

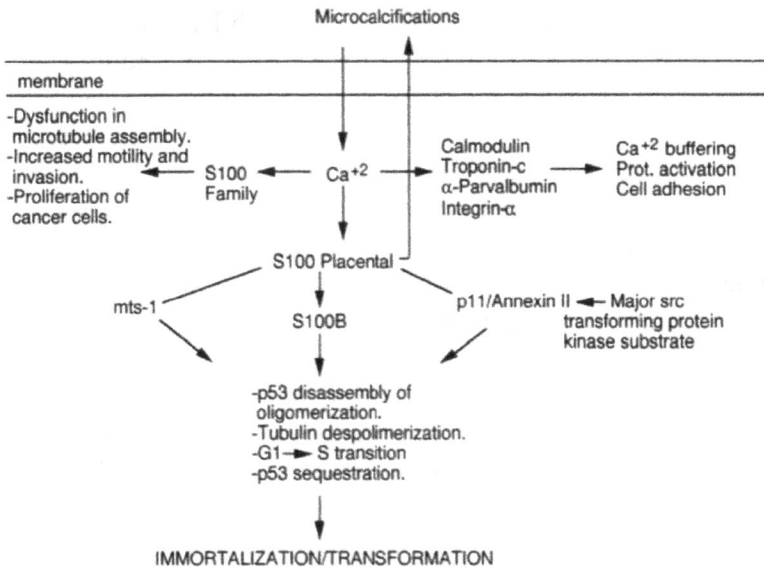

Figure 10.6: Hypothetical model explaining how S100 could be involved in the mechanism of immortalization and transformation of the HBEC.

similar to pll, the regulatory subunit of annexin 11, and the major cytoplasmic avian sarcoma viruses (src) transforming protein kinases substrate. At the amino acid level, S100P shares 50.6% homology with S100B that binds p53 and not only induces total inhibition of p53 oligomerization but also promotes disassembly of the p53 oligomerization making this protein a cellular target for the S100 family members involved in cell cycle control at the GO-GI/S boundary.

Because S100P calcium-binding protein overexpression is a very early event in the carcinogenic process, we postulated that this imbalance in the calcium metabolism might explain not only the involvement in immortalization but also the process of micro-calcification phenomena, a very important signal found in the early stages of malignancy [33].

10.4. Human ferritin H in the immortalization of the HBEC

Using the same technique of differential display that I used with Dr. Ismael Dale Cotrin [33], we discovered with Dr. Nadia Higgy the cDNA clone (233 bp) isolated by subtractive hybridization between the mortal HBEC S-130 or MCF-10M and its immortal counterpart MCF-10F. The fragment was cloned, purified, and sequenced, and the sequence comparison in the GenBank database revealed it to be 100% homologous at the nucleotide level to the coding sequence (exon 4) of human ferritin H chain gene [42]. The importance of this finding was that the expression of ferritin H chain increased with the progression of cell immortalization and it is highly expressed in the neoplastic cells. *In situ* hybridization using an antisense ribo probe for ferritin H chain showed no signal in normal breast lobules; an increased localized signal was observed in areas with ductal hyperplasia [1, 42]; we described this in detail in the original publication on the importance of ferritin H [42], but suffice it to say that the increase of ferritin H chain gene may provide iron necessary for the clonal selection and uncontrolled growth of cells as is summarized in Figure 10.7. The pathway that we published with Dr. Higgy was featured on the cover of *Molecular Carcinogenesis* [42].

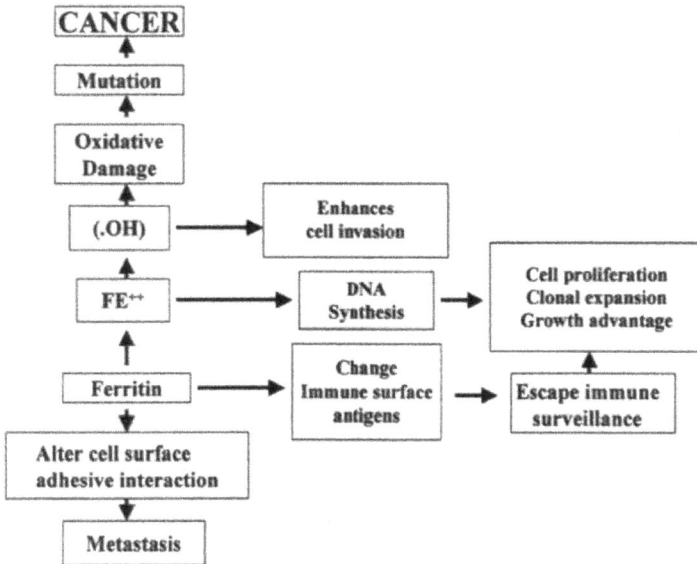

Figure 10.7: The possible role of increased ferritin H chain gene in HBEC immortalization and malignancy. Reprinted with permission from Ref. [42].

We postulated that the increased ferritin H chain gene transcription may contribute to immortalization of HBECs through several possible mechanisms; it may be a source of iron required by rapidly dividing cells for clonal expansion; it may provide iron capable of participating in free radical reactions leading to oxidative DNA damage and mutation [43]; or it may affect immune surface antigens and provide immortal cells with growth advantage by escaping immune surveillance. Ferritin H chain gene induction may either be a consequence of or an inducer of cell immortalization. In either instance, it may prove to become a valuable marker of cell immortalization and/or an early indicator of malignant transformation.

All these studies involving understanding the mechanism of cell immortalization led us to postulate that the phenotypic alterations induced by the immortalization process, which is associated with a lack of calcium buffering system, overexpression of S100P protein, and ferritin H, are all linked. The low Ca_i may result in stimulation of cell *proliferation that, associated with the high level of ferritin H, will increase the formation of more free radicals, resulting in DNA damage that explains the formation of micro satellite instability (MSI), as has been demonstrated in breast cells in culture* [43, 44] *as well as in early lesions of the breast* [45].

10.5. Transformation of the HBEC MCF-10 by *c-Ha-ras* oncogene

A significant discovery in cancer research has been the identification and subsequent characterization of oncogenes *in both human and experimental animal tumors* [46–49]. Activation of the *ras* gene family has been found in human and animal tumor model systems [47–51] and a point-mutated *c-Ha-ras* proto-oncogene may be involved in the development of mouse and rat mammary tumors induced by treatment with chemical carcinogens [52, 53]. The HBECs previously immortalized with benzo (a) pyrene have been transfected with *v-Ha-ras* oncogene using a retrovirus vector, but the expression of the fully malignant phenotype in those cells required the cooperation of two oncogenes, *v-Ha-ras* and large T antigen [54]. It was at this stage of our knowledge when Dr. Fulvio Basolo and his wife, Dr. Gabriela Fontanini, came from the University of Pisa, in Italy, to work at the BCRL. Both of them were highly driven researchers who found in our laboratory the completion of their scientific formation as medical researchers. The assignment for them was to carry on the next step in our research agenda, namely to determine if the HBEC MCF-10A [14] could be neoplasticallly transformed with an activated Ha-ras oncogene alone. For this purpose, MCF-10A cells were transfected with the *c-Ha-ras* oncogene contained in the plasmid pHo6-Tras [56] that was generously provided to us by Demetrio Spandidos. We found that *c-Ha-ras* gene transfected into MCF-10A cells was inserted in the DNA of the cells and expressed itself by the production of the mutated p21 protein. This insertion did not result in activation, rearrangement, or amplification of other oncogenes known to be associated with breast carcinoma, such as *c-erbB-2/HER-2lneu* and *int-2* [56–59]. We found that the insertion of the *c-Ha-ras* has been mainly localized in chromosome 11 using *in situ* hybridization [1] and the malignant phenotypes expressed by transfected MCF-10A cells were anchorage-independent growth, hormone and growth factor independence, alterations in the tridimensional pattern of growth in collagen matrix, increased invasiveness and collagenolytic activity, and tumorigenesis in nude mice, all properties observed in transformed cells [16, 54, 60–62]. One of our more remarkable experiences was to see the cells growing in an anchorage-independent manner (Figure 10.8), which was detected as early as the third passage *in vitro*. This phenomenon was never observed before when we used primary culture of HBECs. This pattern of growth was so evident that we really knew for the first time that we were on the right path of understanding the transformation event [63].

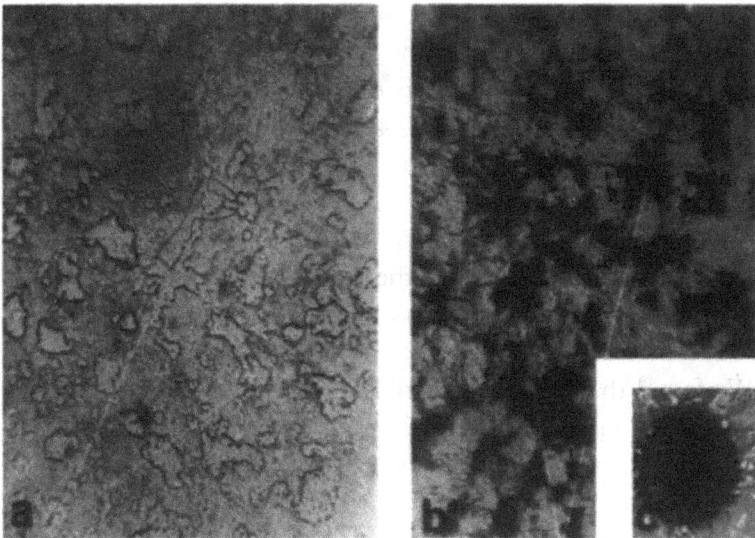

Figure 10.8: (a) Morphology of post-confluent MCF-10A cells (×40). (b) Morphology of post-confluent MCF-10AneoT cells showing loss of contact inhibition; growing cells overlap forming foci (×40). (c) Enlargement of an individual focus from panel (b) (×100). All the photographs were taken under phase contrast microscopy.

Although we have published in detail these observations [1,63], I would like to emphasize that the altered morphology *in vitro* could explain the undifferentiated pattern of tumors developed *in vivo* and the alterations in the morphogenetic properties of the mammary epithelium. We also found that the *c-Ha-ras*-transfected cells had a reduced requirement for epidermal growth factor (EGF), as has been reported in other systems. In the rodent model, transfected cells synthesize and secrete their own transforming growth factor (TGF-α), which binds the EGF receptor [64, 65]; this mechanism also appears to operate in transfected MCF-10A cells [66], in which transfection induces an increase in TGF-α-mRNA expression and TGF-α protein secretion [67]. This increase in TGF-α production may partly account for the enhanced growth rate of these cells in hydrocortisone- and cholera toxin-deprived medium or in serum-free medium and for their ability to grow in soft agar [67]. Our results on *ras* transformation and TGF-α production in MCF-10A cells contrasted with those reported in another human mammary epithelial cell line [68] in which no significant change in the levels of TGF-α production could be detected in *v-Ha-ras*-infected cells or in cells transformed by a combination of *v-Ha-ras* and SV40T oncogenes as compared with their parental cells [68]. In separate experiments that we published elsewhere [66, 67], MCF-10AneoT cells expressed a five- to ten-fold increase in the level of 1.4-kb *c-Ha-ras* RNA transcripts in comparison with the parental cell line and the other transfectants. In addition, there was a corresponding increase in p21 *ras* protein expression and in TGF-α production.

We found that these data could explain the biological differences in anchorage-independent growth in the absence of EGF and may be functionally relevant in the process of ductulogenesis. Transfection of MCF-10A cells with the activated *c-Ha-ras* oncogene induces the expression of invasive characteristics similar to those of tumorigenic or transformed cells of intermediate malignancy [69, 70] or of NIH 3T3 and 10T1/2 *ras* oncogene-transformed cells [71–78]. In an *in vitro* chemoinvasive assay, MCF-10AneoT cells were more invasive than MCF-10A cells transfected with the neomycin-resistant gene alone or with the proto-oncogene, but less invasive than metastatic melanoma cells [78] or ras transfected NIH 3T3 cells. Like NIH 3T3 cells [79] and human bronchial epithelial cells [62], MCF-10AneoT cells also produced more type IV collagenase than non-transfected cells, an important property in the process of invasion and metastasis. MCF-10AneoT cells exhibited greater chemotaxis than cells transfected with the neomycin-resistant gene alone or the *ras* proto-oncogene, although chemotactic activity was not significantly different from that of MCF-10A parent cells, a phenomenon also observed in immortalized human bronchial epithelial cells [62]. *Ras* transfection of immortalized HBEC MCF-10A cells can also be involved in early steps of tumor progression *in vitro*. This observation agrees with a study reporting that activation of the *ras* oncogene preceded the onset of mammary neoplasia [80], although in that case the presence of the activated oncogene alone did not suffice to induce the expression of malignancy, since it was first necessary that active cell proliferation be induced by estrogenic hormones for the neoplastic phenotype to be manifested [80].

Our findings clearly indicated that MCF-10A cells, which are immortal and actively proliferating, express the fully malignant phenotype upon insertion of the activated oncogene. This turns out to be an excellent model for understanding the mechanisms whereby the c*Ha-ras* oncogene induces malignant phenotypes and collectively, all of these data support the concept that *c-Ha-ras* oncogene could be involved in both early and late stages of mammary carcinogenesis [63].

10.6. Transformation of HBEC by chemical carcinogens

My quest to transform normal HBECs was not easily accomplished because under ideal conditions, the evaluation of an etiological agent or a carcinogen requires that the target cells have not been previously affected by viral or chemical agents either *in vivo* or *in vitro*. Only under these conditions we will ensure that the effect measured is truly that of the carcinogen tested. The availability of MCF-10A or MCF-10F, the cells closer to normal, provided again the opportunity to demonstrate whether chemical carcinogens were able to transform breast epithelial cells. We initiated these studies with Dr. Gloria Calaf, and we decided to treat MCF-10F cells using two carcinogenic compounds that require metabolic activation, DMBA and B(a)P, and two direct-acting carcinogens, NMU and MNNG [32, 81, 82]. I need to emphasize the importance of these experiments because MCF-10F cells, in addition to expressing the normal phenotype of HBEC, are pseudodiploid and express minimal chromosomal alterations [46xx,lp+,t(3;9)(p13:p22)] [14]. MCF-10F cells in that sense are unique because even though they are long lived, they have retained the features of normal differentiation that allow one to test small deviations after they are treated with chemical carcinogens *in vitro*. MCF-10 M, also called sample #130, the cells that gave origin to the immortal MCF-10F and MCF-10A cells, exhibited increased survival efficiency in agar methocel after treatment with chemical carcinogens *in vitro*. However, neither these cells nor other breast primary cultures exhibited a progression in the expression of phenotypes associated with neoplastic transformation. Since *in vitro* treatment of HBEC primary cultures with chemical carcinogens did not succeed in inducing the full expression of transformation phenotypes, we decided with Dr. Calaf to use the protocol developed for primary cultures of breast epithelial cells for testing the response of the spontaneously immortalized cells MCF-10F to the same carcinogens, in order to elucidate whether immortalization is required for the expression of the fully transformed phenotype [16, 32].

MCF-10F cells treated with carcinogens *in vitro* (Figures 10.9 and 10.10) express phenotypes indicative of neoplastic transformation, such as increased total number of doublings and decreased DT, expression of anchorage-independent growth, *in vitro* invasive capability, altered cell growth patterns in collagen matrix and tumor formation in SCID mice. MCF-10F cells treated with either DMBA, MNNG, NMU, or B(a)P express an early increase in growth and changes in the rate of cell proliferation, as indicated by a shorter doubling time (DT), which becomes progressively shorter with the number of passages.

This phenomenon suggests that in each passage there is a selection of highly proliferating cells that booster cell growth advantage, thus

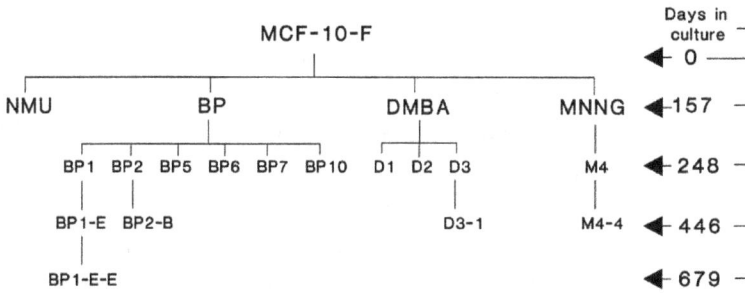

Figure 10.9: Flow chart showing the evolution of MCF-10F cells after treatment with the carcinogens NMU, B(a)P, DMBA, or MNNG. Days in culture indicate the number of days *in vitro* that it took each cell line to emerge. Reprinted with permission from Ref. [15].

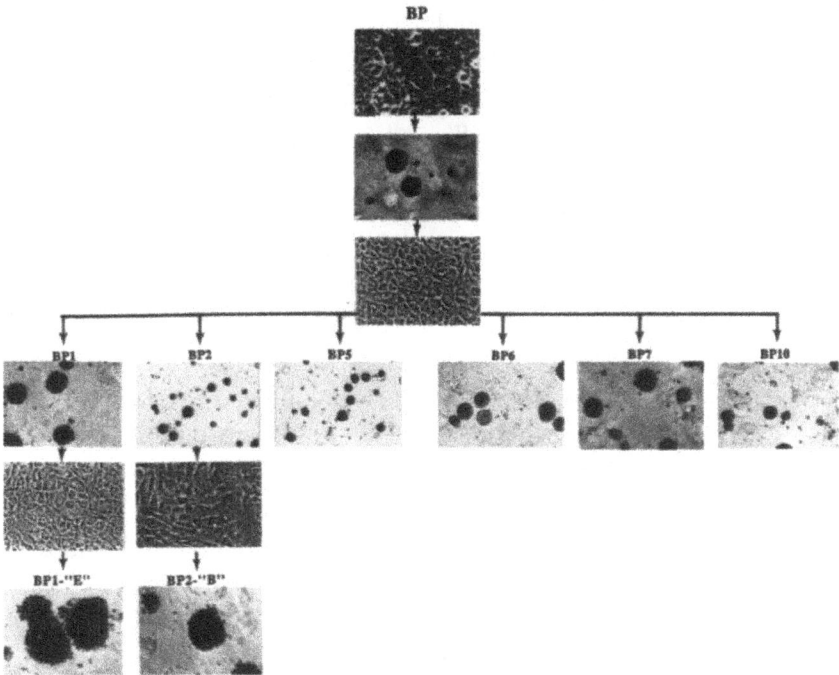

Figure 10.10: BP-treated MCF-10F cells (phase contrast) formed colonies that isolated and expanded and were reseeded in agar methocel originating the cell lines, BP1, BP2, BPS, BP6, BP7, and BP10. From BP1 and BP2 originates the clones BP1-E and BP2-B. BP1-E is the clone that will induce tumors in heterologous host. Reprinted with permission from Ref. [15].

each passage resulted in the selection of more aggressive phenotypes. There are clear morphological changes observed either by light microscopy or by ultra-structural means.

We clearly show that neoplastic transformation *in vitro*, like neoplastic development *in vivo*, is a progressive process. In the case of MCF-10F cells treated with chemical carcinogens, alterations in the ductulogenic pattern in collagen gel preceded morphological changes observed in monolayers. These morphologically transformed cells were able to grow in agar methocel, and this latter phenotype was expressed with more intensity in later passages (Figure 10.9). In the case of MCF-10F cells, the acquisition of anchorage independence was manifested at 157 days in culture, and the efficiency varied from carcinogen to carcinogen, being the highest for DMBA and B(a)P. NMU was the least efficient in inducing colony formation and did not originate clones; MNNG originated four colonies from which only one clone, M4, emerged at 248 days post treatment. M4 exhibited greater CE than the parental cells, and generated other subclones that emerged by 446 days in culture. We observed that the apparent refractory nature of HBECs to express the phenotypes of neoplastic transformation upon treatment with carcinogens *in vitro* could be overcome by isolating and reseeding the colonies formed in agar methocel, which are further selected by reseeding in semisolid medium. Whereas this selective pressure *in vitro* may not represent the same forces that are operational *in vivo*, our observations indicate that the emergence of neoplastic phenotypes is a continuum expressed only in those cells that exhibit further growth advantage. For example chemoinvasion, or the ability of cells to cross basement membranes *in vitro*, as well as chemotaxis, or the ability of the cells to respond to a chemo attractant, are cell properties that are enhanced in transformed cells and correlate with malignant characteristics *in vivo* [83–88]. The clones derived from DMBA- and B(a)P-treated cells, i.e., D3-1 and BP1-E, respectively, exhibited greater invasive and chemotactic capabilities than MCF-10F control cells, and both parameters were similar to those of the tumorigenic T24 cells. The clones BP5, BP7, and BP10 presented greater values for invasion and chemotaxis than MCF-10F control cells, but less than BP1-E, D3-1, and T24 cells.

The higher chemoinvasive and chemotactic capacity of BP1-E and D3-1 cells was observed in late passages and correlated with their higher CE in agar methocel.

For testing tumorigenicity, we used the SCID mice as heterologous hosts. SCID mice have an autosomal dominant recessive defect that impairs the rearrangement of antigen receptor genes in both T and B lymphocyte progenitors. SCID mice also lack functional T and B cells, which make these animals a suitable host for hetero-transplantation. Tumorigenesis in heterologous hosts is considered to be the final reliable criterion for assessing complete transformation of human cells [79], even though the validity of this model has been questioned, since many human malignancies or cell lines derived from them are not tumorigenic in the nude mouse [89]. The adequacy of SCID mice for testing tumorigenicity has been validated by the observation that 100% of the mice inoculated with either T24 or MCF-7 cells developed tumors with a short latency period. SCID mice proved to be more adequate as a host for MCF-7 cells than nude mice, since in our model they did not require estrogen supplementation [90]. The tumors developed in inoculated SCID mice were proven to be of human origin by determination of Alu sequences [91], which showed that they were derived from the cells inoculated and not a host reaction. T24 and BPIE, the two cell lines expressing tumorigenesis in SCID mice, exhibited the highest in agar methocel in MNNG-treated cells. BP1-E cells also exhibited a higher CE, larger CS and higher CN than the other non-tumorigenic clones, which indicated that these phenotypes need to be sequentially expressed prior to the manifestation of the tumorigenic phenotype. Although anchorage-independent growth is considered to be a predictor of tumorigenesis in other cell systems [79], in the experimental model neither anchorage independence nor any of the other parameters served, when considered individually, as an indicator of the tumorigenic potential of a cell. These observations are supported by results on HBECs obtained from milk, which have been reported to acquire anchorage-independent growth and immortalization after SV 40 infection, but do not elicit tumorigenesis in nude mice [14, 79] and by the observation that the extended lifespan induced in HBECs treated with B(a)P *in vitro* was not accompanied by the expression of anchorage independence or tumorigenicity [92]. The ultimate mechanism that determines the expression of the tumorigenic phenotype by cells derived from chemically treated HBECs is not known, but we have concluded that tumorigenesis in a heterologous host emerges in chemically treated immortal cells as a consequence of clonal expansion, in which phenotypes indicative of neoplastic transformation are cumulatively expressed through successive processes of selection over long periods of time. During the process of neoplastic transformation, no chromosomal changes were detected. The molecular events that are operational in each phase of the transformation process indicate that each carcinogen induces different degrees of point mutations in codons 12 and 61 of the c-Ha-ras oncogene [93, 94] as an event detectable by the 10th passage post carcinogen treatment. Other genes such as p53, Rb, and erbB2 were differently expressed by the various clones derived from carcinogen-treated cells [94, 95].

Although we have shown that mutated *cHa ras* oncogene was able to transform the HBEC, it still did not prove that this oncogene was the driver of the initiation of cancer. Therefore, one way to evaluate the contribution of *ras* genes in the development of the tumorigenic phenotype is to introduce this gene into suitable acceptor cells. For this purpose, we transfected the non-tumorigenic cell lines, clones D3-1 and BP1, derived from the carcinogen-treated MCF-10F cell lines, and we observed that the *cHa-ras* oncogene not only enhanced colony formation in agar-methocel and invasiveness but induced tumorigenicity with a short latency period in SCID mice. The MCF-10F cells, DMBA or BP-treated cells and the clones D3-1 and BP1 did not exhibit tumorigenicity in SCID mice. We have already shown that the subclone BP1-E derived from BP1 expressed the tumorigenic phenotype after 101 days of inoculation whereas the MCF-10F-Tras had lower tumorigenicity because it took 99 days to induce tumors in 3 of 14 animals, the clones D3-1-Tras and BPI-Tras were highly tumorigenic and the tumors appeared between 47 and 60 days post inoculation, in 4 out of 4 animals and 11 out of 14 animals, respectively.

All the tumors derived from D3-1-Tras and BP 1-Tras cells were poorly differentiated adenocarcinomas. Tumor cell lines derived from the tumors thus originated have been an important resource for understanding the molecular basis of mammary carcinogenesis.

Altogether our work has demonstrated that an in vitro model of breast cancer, in which the final malignant phenotype of tumorigenesis can be induced in HBEC by carcinogen treatment alone or in combination with ras oncogene, provided that the treated cells are previously immortalized and enough time and clone selection are allowed for its expression. This model provided clones of cells expressing different stages of progression to malignant transformation, which are useful for determining whether specific phenotypes are the result of specific genotypic alterations (Figure 10.11).

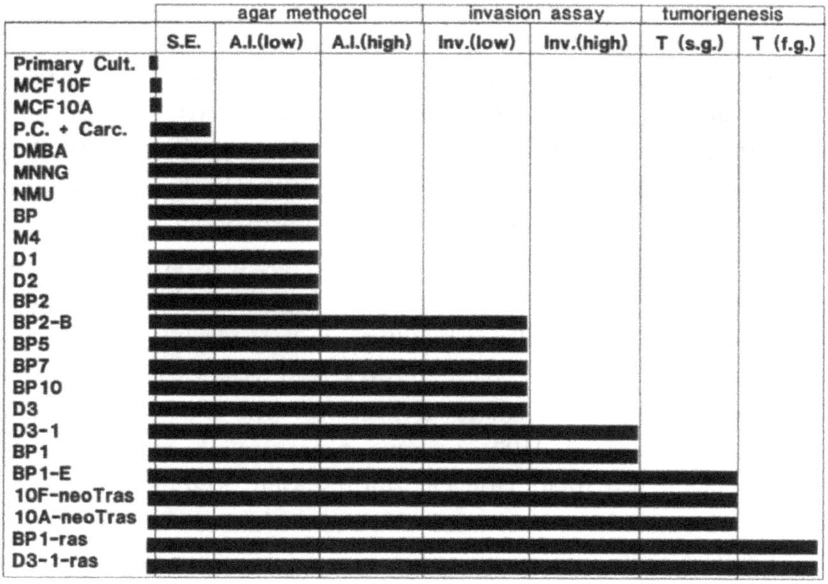

	agar methocel			invasion assay		tumorigenesis	
	S.E.	A.I.(low)	A.I.(high)	Inv.(low)	Inv.(high)	T (s.g.)	T (f.g.)
Primary Cult.							
MCF 10F							
MCF 10A							
P.C. + Carc.							
DMBA							
MNNG							
NMU							
BP							
M4							
D1							
D2							
BP2							
BP2-B							
BP5							
BP7							
BP10							
D3							
D3-1							
BP1							
BP1-E							
10F-neoTras							
10A-neoTras							
BP1-ras							
D3-1-ras							

Figure 10.11: Expression of malignant phenotypes. Comparison of HBEC primary cultures, MCF-10A and MCF-10F, carcinogen-treated cells, derived clones, and c-ras transfected cells, respectively. S.E. survival efficiency, A.I. anchorage-independent growth, Inv. invasiveness, T tumorigenesis, s.g. slow growth, f.g. fast growth. Reprinted with permission from Ref. [17].

10.7. My last years at the Michigan Cancer Foundation

On June 20, 1991, I left the Michigan Cancer Foundation (MCF) to take the position of Chairman of the Department of Pathology at the Fox Chase Cancer Center (FCCC) in Philadelphia. The decision to leave the MCF was multifactorial but probably triggered by a single event that took place after a lecture that I gave to the faculty on May 12, 1990. I will place this incident in a historical perspective describing several events before and after that lecture.

On August 31, 1988, I wrote in my journal that the grant on cell transformation was funded with a high priority score of 1.20, one of the highest registered at the MCF, and the funding was for 5 years and allowed me to hire new people among them molecular biologist Dr. N. Nass, biochemist Dr. Josiah Ochieng, and cell biologist Dr. Gloria Calaf. These plus newcomers Dr. Fulvio Basolo and Dr. Gabriela Fontanini were a great addition to the team of Drs. Quivo Tahin, Pei Li Zhang, Nandita Barnabas, Ismael Dale Cotrin, and James Elliott who were already working on cell transformation, meaning that I had at that specific moment a powerhouse of dedicated investigators at the BCRL; they shared with me the same passion and interest in the mechanism of cell transformation of HBECs. All of them were highly motivated and generating such great amounts of data that took me several years to publish all of them. The results of our work were spreading, and I received numerous invitations to seminars, plenary lectures, and as keynote speaker in different national and international meetings. One of those invitations was in December of 1989 to give a lecture at the FCCC in Philadelphia. I was invited by Dr. Andres Klein Szanto, one of the senior members of that institution and also we had served together in the chemical pathology study session of the NCI. During the visit to FCCC, Andres explained to me that there was an active search for a chair in the Department of Pathology at the FCCC, and he asked me if I was interested because if so he would submit my curriculum to the search committee. I agreed and because he already had a copy that I sent him before my lecture, I forgot about this issue until the early days of February of 1990 when he called me back. Andres told me again that the search for a Chairman of the Department of Pathology was at its peak and that the candidates that they had were not matching with the objectives of the FCCC which meant that I had a significant chance to be selected for that position.

After Andres's call, I felt ambivalent because the research work at the MCF, our private life, and the education and raising of Patricia were filling our existence. The idea of leaving Grosse Pointe and the daily work that we had been doing for almost 19 years were not part of our plans. On the other hand, I felt that Irma had suffered a lot in the MCF and was never considered for a promotion — even to Associate Professor. She had more publications and received more external support than other female scientists at the institution but there was a blind spot about recognizing her. Irma laughed about their pettiness and used her wittiness to make them seem ridiculous. But I knew that she suffered for this inequality, and it made me feel bad.

On March 21 of 1990, I was selected Chair of the Research and Development Advisory Committee (RDAC) at the MCF. That was, as the words indicated, an advisory committee to the Scientific Director, Dr. Gloria Heppner, and the President of the MCF, Dr. Michael Brennan. That position entitled me to be aware of the ins and outs of what was already going on in the institution, and it was an important distinction. I felt pleased by that honor, however deep inside of me they were hurting me by not recognizing Irma, therefore the chairing of the RDAC did not inspire much excitement in me; on the contrary, it left me feeling a great deal of uneasiness.

At the same time, I was fighting not only for the grants to support the research of the BCRL but also by publishing our data in the most competitive journals. In April of that year, I contacted three members of the National Academy to sponsor the manuscript on cell transformation to be considered for publication at the *Proceedings of the National Academy of Sciences*, and all of them said no. The idea of asking for sponsorship made me nervous and uneasy, and after those negative responses I felt extremely mortified with myself for having *broken my rule of never asking for any favor, honor, position, merit award, or invitation to be a speaker in a meeting.* I strongly believed that if I was good, the recognition would come. The support for this concept came when Dr. Lea Sekely, a Program Director of the breast cancer program at the NCI, called Irma indicating that I was being considered as a candidate for the study session on chemical pathology. One day later, Charles King mentioned to me that Dr. Edmond Copeland, the Secretary of the study session of chemical pathology at the NCI, told him the same message, and on April 9, 1990, I received a letter from Dr. J. Green of NCI inviting me to be a member of the study session of chemical pathology. I felt very good about this distinction because it was an honor to be part of the study session that distinguished scientists such as Emanuel Farber had been a part of. To be member of the study session was a continuous source of intellectual reward and challenges during the 4 years that I served.

Coming back to my function as a chair of the RDAC, it is important to mention that part of my duties was also to be a member of the search committee for selecting the replacement of Dr. Michael Brennan, giving me significant weight to express opinions about the future course of the institution. As expected, there were several external and internal candidates for the position of Michael Brennan. Among the external candidates was Dr. Craig Jordan, an outstanding one who was selected and offered the position, but after it was offered to him the MCF board of directors annulled the offer, leaving us and the candidate extremely confused about what was going on. An explanation was never received or given. After that incident, the search for external candidates ceased and the internal ones started competing for the position. I entered the following reflection in my journal:

> *I feel that those internal candidates are in a certain way the cause of all the problems of the MCF. Many of them have been far from been leaders and instead very destructive, not only being unfair with many people but also causing most of the deficit of the MCF. In addition I feel that they are not really interested in science and have a cynical attitude about the important values that a human being must have in medical research. I never felt like this before, a sudden realization that*

there are people at the MCF who are cynics, and they are the opposite of
my Christian values. I feel that is a vacuum in science, and in the need
for strong values.

I am not sure if the "feelings" that I depicted in those months
of 1990 were just, neither am I sure that my perception of the
situation at the MCF was accurate. But when I remember and see in
my journal what was happening I realized why the heroes and
leaders of a revolution emerge. It is because it is morally intolerable
to sustain the system, it's like a need to stop something that is
beyond the tolerance level, and I heartily wished to find a way to
solve it but I did not know how.

Finally on May 12, 1990, I gave my annual lecture to the faculty
of the MCF. I had spent almost six months preparing for that
conference at which I presented all our accomplishments, published
and unpublished, on cell transformation in primary culture of the
human breast as well as in the MCF-10F and A cells. I considered it
a scholarly presentation, providing almost what I have described in
this and previous chapters. I had crafted every slide to be sure that it
described each experiment clearly and perfectly. The whole conference
was rehearsed several times to be sure that every enunciation was
clearly understood and that each concept and conclusion were
supported by solid data. Irma witnessed all the energy that I put into
the preparation of that lecture; it was an act of dedication and love to
be sure that each of the people who had been helping me obtain the
data were properly acknowledged. Although I never expected a
standing ovation, I was unprepared for the reaction of my colleagues.
The lecture elicited a negative reaction, and I was accused of my work
being so extensive that I had curtailed or left out any possibility of
further work by any of the scientific staff at the MCF. Basically I was
guilty of having covered all the possibilities and made my research so
broad that I had taken away any possibility of them using the MCF-
10A or MCF-10F cells. The reaction was led by the breast cancer
group and carried on by the Scientific Director, Dr. Gloria Heppner;
it was some kind of impeachment or judgment of my work as a
scientist. It was a devastating experience to feel the mediocrity

personified in my colleagues who reacted this way, and they are unworthy to mention in this memoir. This expression of mediocrity took me some time to understand until I was finally summoned by Dr. Samuel Horowitz, who had been selected by a committee created to study my misbehavior and punish me. Dr. Samuel Horowitz articulated what I described above as the main reason for the negative reaction to my lecture. After listening to him be a messenger for their ridiculous critiques, I explained that my only defense against those accusations was that: *"I was doing what a scientist needs to do to solve a scientific problem; my problem was to understand the mechanism of cell transformation of human breast epithelial cells and all the experiments that I had done in my laboratory or in collaboration with others were fully proposed and funded by the NIH. Therefore I was driven to solve a scientific problem."* Samuel Horowitz understood my explanation, and he took care of dissipating the black clouds around me, agreeing that I had been wrongly accused and misinterpreted. However for me, it was the most painful experience in my scientific career to be accosted by mediocre scientists only for doing what a research scientist was supposed to do. The feeling of being so wrongly accused was the turning point; I decided that we must move the BCRL to another place. That was the last drop that filled the cup.

On Monday, May 14, only two days after my lecture at the MCF, I received a letter from Dr. Robert Comis, Vice President for medical sciences of the FCCC asking me to present my CV for the position of Chairman of the Department of Pathology. This concrete request came at just the right moment for us, and I accepted the challenge that followed that letter. The FCCC needed somebody to organize a department and at the same time expand and modernize the surgical pathology. I submitted my CV with a letter indicating my interest. I knew that I needed to wait and study what I wanted but the fact was that I traced an organizational chart that would allow me to expand into what I considered an ideal Department of Pathology should be.

Because we did not know at that time the final outcome of this initial letter, we decided to act extremely discreetly and continue our normal activities in our jobs as well as in our family life. We followed our schedule of experiments, participating in national and international meetings, I did my work in the study sessions, chaired the RDAC as if nothing important had happened in our life. On Thursday, June 13, I received a reply from the FCCC, wanting to arrange a personal interview on July 30–31 and August 1.

My feelings were again mixed because when I saw Patty, Irma, and my mother-in-law, Carmen, enjoying Grosse Pointe as much as they did, and looking at our house and environment, the idea of looking for another place was inconceivable. I wanted to stay but at the same time I realized that this could be the right opportunity to leave the MCF, which was being run more anarchically every day. All of that plus the setup that we had organized made me feel uneasy. However, the idea of a better Department of Pathology with new laboratories and the possibility of a more permanent position for Irma and I was the other side of the coin. Our first visit to FCCC was promising, but it was too early for a final impression. My basic question was: How sincere they were about rebuilding the Department of Pathology? The current situation was that the department was in disarray because it lacked a chair, however, most of the people honestly expressed a trust in the administration and belief in the seriousness of the institution's commitments. What I saw there indicated the possibility of 11,000 square feet of lab space to accommodate both the research and service areas. The electron microscopy facility was discussed but nothing agreed upon. The first visit was exploratory but I detected the possibility of a real and a full Department of Pathology. The pathologists sounded positive about the idea of a new chair and the position of director of surgical pathology might be ideal for Irma. Robert Comis asked for her CV.

In the middle of these negotiations, I was preparing a trip to Argentina, the reviews of the grant applications for the next study session, and coping with the taxing situation of the budget at the MCF, struggling every single day to keep my people in the laboratory and battling the continuously menacing attitude of the administration trying to shorten the budget or dismiss people. Above all these distractions, my main concern was how to more efficiently gear the research projects. I knew that the research on hormone prevention was on solid ground but I was worried about how to push the subject to the next step. I also was conscious that although we had generated important data on cell transformation and the susceptibility to transformation, it required more thinking and maturation about what was the meaning of our data as well as what to do next.

Our second visit to FCCC, and this time with Irma, was scheduled for September 25–27, 1990 that turned out to be a very promising one because we started the negotiation of salary, funds for organizing the department, space, and equipment. We thought that whatever the outcome we felt good about ourselves and we could not have done better. I personally was very impressed with Irma, she did a very good job, and she was smashing in all the interviews in how she managed herself and how she foresaw the organization of the surgical pathology. We hoped the FCCC offer would become a reality and give us the opportunity to start a more clean operation, to have better laboratories, a department of pathology with direct access to human material, and a more consolidated place of work for both of us. However, the negotiations progressed at a very slow pace for my taste, probably due to the instability at the MCF and in my role as a Chairman of RDAC. As such my interaction with the other chairmen, with Brennan and Gloria Heppner, the lab services, and the Detroit community, made the whole situation disturbing at some moments. There were also a few aspects beyond our control, like the visit of MacKay, the Vice President of the FCCC, to review the administration of the MCF, the call of Dr. Ila Merchandani, telling all the gossip about the Department of Pathology in FCCC and the Jennie's Hospital, all of these were a continuous distracting force of concern, rationalization, and hope that made it extremely difficult to focus my days. Adam Frankenfield, the publisher of the three volumes of *Electron Microscopy in Tumor Diagnosis,* sent us the offer for a contract for a book about the new perspective of breast cancer outlook for the twenty-first century, and he was also interested in Irma and I starting a new journal on tumor diagnosis, with she and I as executive editors. We were undecided but the idea was tantalizing. We were waiting to see how the situation with the FCCC's offer evolved before more seriously considering that proposal.

The response to our letter, in which we described the space needed as well as the budget required for new equipment and a new electron microscope, arrived on October 13. The space offered and the money for equipment was less than requested, and we sent a counteroffer for the equipment budget plus a new electron microscope. This time the answer took several weeks and although I received calls from Andres Klein Szanto saying that they were interested in us and counting on bringing us aboard, I started to feel that the whole negotiation was cooling off. This was the time that I received an invitation to present my application as a Chair of the Department of Pathology at the University of Pittsburgh, but studying the environment of the place I decided not to apply and on November 8, I received a call from Robert Comis that the FCCC was extremely interested in us, and we scheduled the next meeting for November 20. In the intervening two weeks several events took place. One was to prepare the new budget and organizational plans for the Department of Pathology at the FCCC, but we were not optimistic of the outcome of the next meeting because Irma had a bad feeling during her interview with Robert Young, the President of the FCCC, and J. MacKay, the Vice President; she was not sure but she felt that something was not clear, something was hidden that neither she nor I could find what it was, a perception that later on we confirmed was right (see Chapter 11). The second event was that as the chair of the RDAC at the MCF every day I realized that the situation, especially the financial deficit of the MCF, was increasing exponentially. I could not see clearly how the MCF situation could be solved. There was so much bitterness and resentment that it was difficult to find the way. A clear fact was that many of the senior staff wanted that Gloria Heppner step down; she must either leave or go back to being Chairman of immunology, the position that she had before. It was also suggested that the Research Division could be managed through RDAC and a director that reported to the board on a yearly basis. I could not sleep many nights during this entanglement that also involved rumors of merging with, or more accurately, becoming part of Wayne State University. The third incident was when Gloria

Heppner asked me if I could also be the principal investigator in the program project for MCF-10, and I told her that I needed to think about it. The last unexpected incident was when Gloria Calaf vented her impatience about her visa situation and salary, and then I needed to break the silence and indicate to her that we were negotiating with FCCC.

On November 20, we went to FCCC and they agreed to our budget and space requests. The electron microscope laboratory was better understood, and I presented to them three options: one was to buy a new microscope, second, to move the Philips 400 from the already existing location, or the last option was that I be named co-director of the EM facility directed by Dr. Bayer and have equal say in the way that the operation was run. The creation of the two laboratories of cell markers and molecular pathology were also accepted and with that the positions involved. The other points like salaries, payment of moving expenses, and space were also negotiated. Comis promised a written letter for the following week. I had a better chance to review one by one the laboratories and without being overenthusiastic, everything looked good. *Although my enthusiasm was tempered by doubts that the FCCC would honor everything that they promised.*

There was also some anxiety from Irma and I about all the new things that we needed to face up to. For example, we needed to relocate all the people of our laboratory and to hire new ones; we would lose certain things that we know were working well, like the human breast sample collection; we needed to sell the house that we loved and find another one; to change the habitat of Patricia; and all of these plus the uncertainty of new things were not easy to overcome. I had reservations about how Bayer, the Director of the EM facility, would react to the part of negotiations that concerned him. I wished for a solution that did not affect him, like acquiring a new EM. At the end, the FCCC acquired for the Department of Pathology a new Zeiss EM together with all the ancillary equipment. This was a real relief for me. In the middle of these negotiations, Gloria Heppner approached me again and asked me to be the PI for the MCF-10 grant and the request came from the whole Breast Program

Membership, and it was the most open declaration that *they wanted me to be the PI because I was the only one with the authority to take command.* I was really touched because many of them were the same ones that complained at my lecture on May 12, 1990, and they were in one way or another responsible for my decision to leave the MCF. The following morning I faced Gloria Heppner, and I explained that I would be unable to be PI because "*I have been offered a new position, and even though I have not yet accepted the new position, I do not want to put the MCF in a bad position nor any of the people who were involved in the project.*" Also, I mentioned that I wanted her to be the first one to know about this, and she replied that she already knew because Dr. Sandra Wollman told her of the position that I had been offered at the FCCC. She said that she understood, and we started to discuss her position; it was a tense situation holding the research direction of the MCF amidst the opposition that she had from the staff. When G.H. asked me to be the PI of the MCF cell project she already knew about the offer from the FCCC, therefore it was a futile exercise to entice me to stay at the MCF. The situation in the MCF was deteriorating, and the same day 12 people were fired, including senior members. The measure was taken to compensate the budget. All of these events made me feel that our decision to move to FCCC was the right one.

On December 2, I communicated to the members of the BCRL our plans of moving. Among those I spoke to were Larry Tait, Quivo Tahin, Gloria Calaf, James Elliott, and Nerio and Maria Elena Alvarado. The offer of the FCCC was *vox populis*, in Harper Hospital, the medical school, and the MCF were all aware and certain that we would be gone by July 1, 1991; also we received a call from John Crissman, the Chair of the Department of Pathology at Harper Hospital, congratulating us and telling us that he was interested in buying our home.

Robert Comis personally called and assured me that everything was fine but that the letter was delayed because the President, Robert Young, was out of the country until December 10. He promised to me that on December 11 the letter would be mailed. I had talked with different members of the lab, and there was a good feeling toward coming with us. We felt, along with Irma, that the process was becoming irreversible, and we had the vivid impression that everybody knew that we were leaving. The official letter arrived on December 13, and everything was spelled out as we had negotiated, and we signed and mailed the letter back. With the acceptance letter a new episode began in our life. The same day I decided to let Gloria Heppner and Michael Brennan know that we were leaving. It was a smooth talk. The Brennan meeting was very warm and he congratulated us on our move.

I divided our move to Philadelphia into 10 phases. Phase one implied organizing the offices and establishing an agenda of priorities that would enable us to have the labs in order when we moved. We planned to be in the FCCC one day a week starting January 16, 1991. This allowed us to get a closer look at the organization and make changes in the department, and also to buy equipment and hire the right people. Suffice it to say that I was afraid that in assuming this responsibility I would escalate to a level of incompetence.

We did not want a farewell party at the MCF and after almost 20 years we finished as good friends, and every group in their own way offered their friendship and farewell. Dr. Michael Brennan came to our office and gave us a plaque in the name of the MCF thanking us for all our services to the institution. Gloria Heppner, Fred Miller, Stut Ratner, and Wei Zeng Wei took us for dinner to the 123 restaurant of Grosse Pointe, Paula and Jhon Kin took us for lunch to the Rattle Snake on the Detroit River. Josiah Oschieng, Larry Tait, and Terry Maloney also took us for lunch. Additionally, Aby Raz, Charles Kin, and Judy Christmas took us for lunch to a Detroit restaurant.

June 14, 1991, was our last day, and at 10 a.m. we signed our finalization papers and the chapter of our life at the MCF was closed forever. On July 1, 1991, the MCF lost its freestanding status and became part of the Wayne State University, and Dr. Michael Brennan was replaced by Prof. V. Vaitkevicius, the Chairman of the Department of Oncology. In 1995, the cancer center was named after Barbara Ann Karmanos, the late wife of Peter Karmanos Jr., former Chairman and Chief Executive Officer of Compuware Corporation, and on October

30, 2013, Karmanos Cancer Institute and McLaren Health Care signed an agreement, finalized in January of 2014, creating the largest cancer research and provider network in Michigan.[a]

References

[1] Russo, J. and Russo, I. H. *Molecular Basis of Breast cancer*, Springer-Verlag, Berlin. 2004.

[2] Tait, L., Soule, H. D. and Russo, J. Ultrastructural and immunocytochemical characterization of an immortalized human breast epithelial cell line, MCF-10. *Cancer Res.* 50: 6087–6094, 1990.

[3] Slater, C. M., Lareef, M. H., Russo, I. H., Tomaz, J., Band, V. and Russo, J. S100p is a marker of cell immortalization, preceding phenotypic expression of neoplastic transformation in human breast epithelial cells. *Proc. Am. Assoc. Cancer Res.* 42: 4784a, 2001.

[4] Russo, J., Barnabas, N., Higgy, N., Salicioni, A. M., Wu, Y. L. and Russo, I. H. Molecular basis of human breast epithelial cell transformation. In: Calvo, F., Crepin, M., Magdelenat, H., (eds), *Breast Cancer. Advances in biology and Therapeutics*, John Libbey, Eurotext. 1996, 33–43.

[5] Chang, F., Syrjanen, S. and Syrjanen, K. Implications of the p53 tumor-suppressor gene in clinical oncology. *J. Clin. Oncol.* 13: 1009–1022, 1995.

[6] Mercer, W. E., Nelson, D., Deleo, A. B., Old, L. J. and Baserga, R. Microinjection of monoclonal antibody to protein p53 inhibits serum-induced DNA synthesis in 3T3 cells. *Proc. Natl. Acad. Sci. USA* 79: 6309–6312, 1982.

[7] Baker, S. J., Fearon, E. R., Nigro, J. M., Hamilton, S. R., Presinger, A. C., Jessup, J. M., van Tuinen, P., Ledbetter, D. H., Barker, D. F., Nakamura, Y., White, R. and Vogelstein, B. Chromosome 17 deletions and p53 gene mutations in colorectal carcinomas. *Science* 249: 912–915, 1990.

[8] Diller, L., Kassel, J., Nelson, C. E., Gryka, M. A., Litwak, G., Gebhardt, M., Bressac, B., Ozturk, M., Baker, S. J., Vogelstein, B. and Friend, S. p53 functions as a cell cycle control protein in osteosarcomas. *Mol. Cell. Biol.* 10: 5772–5781, 1990.

[9] Gerbes, A., Caselman, W. H. Point mutations of the p53 gene, human hepatocellular carcinoma and afflatoxins. *J. Hepatol.* 19: 312–315, 1993.

[10] Fearon, E. R. and Vogelstein, B. A genetic model for colorectal tumorigenesis. *Cell* 61: 759–767, 1990.

---

[a] http://www.karmanos.org

[11] Van Dongen, J. A., Harris, J. R., Peterse, J. L., Fentiman, I. S., Holland, R., Salvadori, B. and Steward, H. J. In situ breast cancer: the EORTC concensus meeting. *Lancet* 25: 28, 1989.

[12] Finlay, C. A., Hinds, P. W. and Levine, A. J. The p53 proto-oncogene can act as a supressor of transformation. *Cell* 57: 1083–1093, 1989.

[13] Levine, A. J., Momand, J. and Finlay, C. A. The p53 tumor suppressor gene. *Nature* 351: 453–456, 1991.

[14] Soule, H. D., Maloney, T. M., Wolman, S. R., Peterson, W. D., Brenz, R., McGrath, C. M., Russo, J., Pauley, R. J., Jones, R. F. and Brooks, S. C. Isolation and characterization of a spontaneously immortalized human breast epithelial cell line, MCF 10. *Cancer Res.* 50: 6075–6086, 1991.

[15] Calaf, G. and Russo, J. Transformation of human breast epithelial cells by chemical carcinogens. *Carcinogenesis* 14: 483–492, 1993.

[16] Russo, J. and Russo, I. H. *Techniques and Methodological Approaches in Breast Cancer Research*, Springer, New York. 2014.

[17] Russo, J., Calaf, G., Sohi, N., Tahin, Q., Zhang, P. L., Alvarado, M. E., Estrada, S. and Russo, I. H. Critical steps in breast carcinogenesis. *Ann. NY Acad. Sci.* 698: 1–20, 1993.

[18] Barnabas, N., Moraes, R., Calaf, G., Estrada, S. and Russo, J. Role of p53 in MCF-10F cell immortalization and chemically induced neoplastic transformation. *Int. J. Oncol.* 7: 1289–1296, 1995.

[19] Cornelisi, R. S., van Vliet, M., Vos, C. B. J., Clenton-Jansen, C., van de Vijver, M. J., Peterse, J. L., Khan, P. M., Borrensen, A. L., Cornelisse, C. J. and Devilee, P. Evidence for a gene on 17pl3.3, distal to TP53, as a target for allele loss in breast tumors without p53 mutations. *Cancer Res.* 54: 4200–4206, 1994.

[20] Dunn, J. M., Hastrich, D. J., Newcomb, P., Webb, J. C. J., Maitland, N. J. and Farndon, J.R. Correlation between p53 mutations and antibody staining in breast carcinoma. *Br. J. Surg.* 80: 1410–1412, 1993.

[21] Hamelin, R., Jego, N., Laurent-Puig, P., Vidaud, M. and Thomas, G. Efficient screening of p53 mutations by denaturing gradient gel electrophoresis in colorectal tumors. *Oncogene* 8: 2213–2220, 1989.

[22] Boyle, J. O., Hakim, J., Koch, W., van der Riet, P., Hruban, R. H., Roa, R. A., Correo, R., Eby, Y. J., Ruppert, J. M. and Sidransky, D. The incidence of p53 mutations increases with progression of head and neck cancer. *Cancer Res.* 53: 4477–4480, 1993.

[23] Imazeki, F., *et al.* p53 gene mutations in gastric and esophageal cancer. *Gastroenterology* 103: 892–896, 1992.

[24] Rissinger, J. I., *et al.* p53 gene mutations in human endometrial carcinoma. *Mol. Carcinog.* 5: 250–253, 1992.

[25] Scarpa, A., *et al.* Pancreatic adenocarcinomas frequently show p53 gene mutations. *Am. J. Pathol.* 142: 1534–1543, 1993.

[26] Sugimoto, K., *et al.* Mutations of the p53 gene in lymphoid leukemia. *Blood* 77: 1153–1156, 1991.

[27] Bennett, W. P., *et al.* Archival analysis of p53 behaves as a tumor suppressor gene in sporadic breast tumors. *Oncogene* 6: 1779–1784, 1991.

[28] Hollstein, M. C., *et al.* Genetic analysis of human esophageal tumors from two high incidence geographical areas: frequent p53 base substitutions and absence of ras mutations. *Cancer Res.* 51: 4102–4106, 1991.

[29] Gonos, E. S. and Spandidos, D. A. Oncogenes in cellular immortalization and differentiation. *Anticancer Res.* 13: 1117–1122, 1993.

[30] Zhang, P. L., Calaf, G. and Russo, J. Allele loss and point mutation in codon 12 and 61 of the *c-Ha-ras* oncogene in carcinogen transformed human breast epithelial cells. *Mol. Carcinog.* 9: 46–56, 1994.

[31] Zhang, P. L., Chai, Y. L., Ho, T. Y., Calaf, G. and Russo, J. Activation of c-myc, c-neu and int-2 oncogenes in the transformation of the human breast epithelial cell line MCF-10F treated with chemical carcinogens in vitro. *Int. J. Oncol.* 6: 963–968, 1995.

[32] Russo, J., Calaf, G., and Russo, I. H. A critical approach to the malignant transformation of human breast epithelial cells. *CRC Crit. Rev. Oncogenesis* 4: 403–417, 1993.

[33] Dale Cotrin, G., Silva. I., Hu, Y. F., Russo, I. H., Ao, X., Salicioni, A. M., Yang, X., and Russo, J. S100P Ca^{+2}-binding Protein Overexpression is Associated with Immortalization and Neoplastic Transformation of Human Breast Epithelial Cells *in vitro* and Tumor Progression *in vivo*. *Int. J. Oncol.* 16: 231–240, 2000.

[34] Becker, T., Gerke, V., Kube, E. and Weber, K. S1OOP: a novel calcium-binding protein from human placenta. eDNA cloning, recombinant protein expression and calcium-binding properties. *Eur. J. Biochem.* 207: 541–547, 1992.

[35] Emoto, Y., Kobayashi, R., Akatsuba, H. and Hidaka, H. Purification and characterization of a new member of the S 100 protein family from human placenta. *Biochem. Biophys. Res. Comm.* 182: 1246–1253, 1992.

[36] Moore, B. E. A soluble protein characteristic of the nervous system. *Biochem. Biophys. Res. Commun.* 19: 739–744, 1965.

[37] Sherbet, G. V. and Lakshmi, M. S. AlOOA4 (MTS1) calcium binding protein in cancer growth, invasion and metastasis. *Anticancer Res.* 18: 2415–2422, 1998.

[38] Schafer, B. W. and Heizmann, C. W. The S1OO family of EF hand calcium-binding proteins: functions and pathology. *Trends Biochem. Sci.* 21:134–140, 1996.

[39] McGrath, C. M. and Soule, H. D. Calcium regulation of normal human mammary epithelial cell growth in culture. *In vitro Cell Dev. Biol.* 20: 652–662, 1984.

[40] Soule, H. D. and McGrath, C. M. A simplified method for passage and long-term growth of human mammary epithelial cells. *In vitro* 22: 6–12, 1985.

[41] Ochieng, J., Tahin, Q. S., Booth, C. C. and Russo, J. Buffering of intracellular calcium in response to increase levels in mortal, immortal and transformed human breast epithelial cells. *J. Cell. Biochem.* 46: 250–254, 1993.

[42] Higgy, N. A., Salicioni, A. M., Russo, I. H., Zhang, P. I. and Russo, J. Differential expression of human ferritin H chain gene in immortal human breast epithelial MCF-10F cells. *Mol. Carcinog.* 20: 332–339, 1997.

[43] Huang, Y., Bove, B., Wu, Y. L., Russo, I. H., Yang, X., Zekri, A. and Russo, J. Microsatellite instability during immortalization and transformation of human breast epithelial cells in vitro. *Mol. Carcinog.* 24: 118–127, 1999.

[44] Wu, Y., Barnabas, N., Russo, I. H., Yang, X. and Russo, J. Microsatellite Instability and Loss of heterozygosity in chromosomes 9 and 16 in human breast epithelial cells transformed by chemical carcinogens. *Carcinogenesis* 18: 1069–1074, 1997.

[45] Russo, I. H., Tahin, Q., Huang, Y. and Russo, J. Cellular and molecular changes induced by the chemical carcinogen benzo(a)pyrene in human breast epithelial cells in association with smoking and breast cancer. *J. Womens Cancer* 3: 29–36, 2001.

[46] Bishop, J. M. The molecular genetics of cancer. *Science* 235: 305, 1987.

[47] Zarbl, H., Sukumar, S., Arthur, A. V., Martin-Zanca, D., Barbacid, M. Direct mutagenesis of Ha-ras-1 oncogenes by Nnitroso-N-methylurea during initiation of mammary carcinogenesisin rats. *Nature* 315: 382–385, 1985.

[48] Balmain, A. and Pragnell, L. B. Mouse skin carcinoma induced in vivo by chemical carcinogens have a transforming Harvey-ras oncogene. *Nature* 303: 72–74, 1983.

[49] Barbacid, M. Ras genes. *Annu. Rev. Biochem.* 56: 779–827, 1987.

[50] Bos, J. L. The ras gene family and human carcinogenesis. *Mutat. Res.* 195: 255–271, 1988.

[51] Sukumar, S. Ras oncogenes in chemical carcinogenesis. In: *Current Topics in Microbiology and Immunology*, Vol.148, Springer-Verlag, Berlin. 1989, 93–114.

[52] Sukumar, S., Notario, V., Martin-Zanca, D. and Barbacid, M. Induction of mammary carcinomas in rats by nitrosomethylurea involves malignant activation of H-ras-locus by single point mutations. *Nature* 306: 658–661, 1983.

[53] Dandekar, S., Sukumar, S., Zarbl, H., Young, U. T. and Cardiff, R. D. Specific activation of the cellular Harvey-ras oncogene in dimethylbenzanthracene-induced mouse mammary tumors. *Mol. Cell Biol.* 6: 4104–4108, 1986.

[54] Clark, R., *et al.* Transformation of human mammary epithelial cells by oncogenic retroviruses. *Cancer Res.* 48: 4689–4694, 1988.

[55] Spandidos, D. A. and Wilkie, N. M. Malignant transformation of early passage rodent cells by a single mutated human oncogene. *Nature* 310: 469–475, 1984.

[56] Liderau, R., Callahan, R., Dickson, C., Peters, G., Escot, C. and Ali, I. U. Amplification of the int-2 gene in primary human breast tumors. *Oncogene Res.* 2: 285–291, 1988.

[57] Slamon, D., *et al.* Studies of HER-2/neu proto-oncogene in human breast and ovarian cancer. *Science* 24: 707–712, 1989.

[58] Yamamoto, T., *et al.* Similarity of protein encoded by the human c-erbB-2 gene to epidermal growth factor receptor. *Nature* 319: 230–234, 1986.

[59] Casey, G., Smith, R., McGillivray, D., Peters, G. and Dickson, C. Characterization and chromosome assignment of the human homolog of int-2, a potential proto-oncogene. *Mol. Cell Biol.* 6: 502–510, 1986.

[60] Chang, S. E., Ken, J., Lane, E. B. and Taylor-Papadimitriou, J. Establishment and characterization of SV 40-transformed human breast epithelial cell lines. *J. Cancer Res.* 42: 2040–2053, 1982.

[61] Yoakum, G. H., *et al.* Transformation of human bronchial epithelial cells transfected by Harvey-ras oncogene. *Science* 227: 1174–1179, 1985.

[62] Ura, H., *et al.* Expression of type IV collagenase and procollagen genes and its correlation with the tumorigenic, invasive and metastatic abilities of oncogene-transformed human bronchial epithelial cells. *Cancer Res.* 49: 4615–4621, 1989.

[63] Basolo, F., Elliott, J., Tait, L., Chen, X. Q., Maloney, T., Russo, I. H., Pauley, R., Momiki, S., Caamano, J., Klein-Szanto, A. J. P., Koszalka, M. and Russo, J. Transformation of Human Breast Epithelial Cells by *c-Ha-ras* oncogene. *Mol. Carcinog.* 4: 25–35, 1991.

[64] Salomon, D. S., Perroteau, I., Kidwell, W. R., Tam, J. and Derynck, R. Loss of growth responsiveness to epidermal growth factor and enhanced production of alpha-transforming growth factors in ras-transformed mouse mammary epithelial cells. *J. Cell Physiol.* 130: 397–409, 1987.

[65] Derynck, R. Transforming growth factor-alpha. *Cell* 54: 593–595, 1988.

[66] Saeki, T., Ciardello, F. and McGeady, M. Transformation of a human mammary epithelial cell line following overexpression of a human transforming

growth factor-alpha (TGFalpha) gene. *Proc. Am. Assoc. Cancer Res.* 31: 228a, 1990.

[67] Ciardello, F., McGeady, M. L., Kim, N., Basolo, F., Hynes, N., Langton, B. C., Yokozaki, H., Saeki, T., Elliott, J., Mauri, H., Mendelsohn, J., Soule, H., Russo, J. and Salomon, D. Transforming growth factor alpha expression is enhanced in human mammary epithelial cells transformed by an activated *c-Ha-ras* protooncogene but not by the c-neu protooncogene, and overexpression of the transforming growth factor alpha complementary DNA leads to transformation. *Cell Growth Differ.* 1: 407–420, 1990.

[68] Valverius, E. M., Bates, S. E. and Stampfer, M. R. Transforming growth factor-alpha production and epidermal growth factor receptor expression in normal and oncogene transformed human mammary epithelial cells. *Mol. Endocrinol.* 3: 203–214, 1989.

[69] Koszlowsky, J. M., McEvan, R. and Keer, H. Prostate cancer and the invasive phenotype: Application of new in vivo and in vitro approaches. In: Fidler, I. J., Nicholson, G., (eds), *Tumor Progression and Metastasis.* Alan R. Liss, Inc., New York, NY. 1988, 189–231.

[70] Albini, A., Iwamoto, Y. and Kleinman, H. K. A rapid in vitro assay for quantitating the invasive potential of tumor cells. *Cancer Res.* 47: 3239–3245, 1987.

[71] Egan, S. E., *et al.* Expression of H-ras correlates with metastatic potential: Evidence for direct regulation of the metastatic phenotype in 1 OTl/2 and NIH/3T3 cells. *Mol. Cell Biol.* 7: 830–837, 1987.

[72] Varani, J., Fliegel, S. E. G. and Wilson, B. Motility of ras-H oncogene transformed NIH/3 T3 cells. *Invasion Metastasis* 6: 335–346, 1986.

[73] Bolscher, J. G. M., van der Bijl, M. M. W., Neefjes, J. J., Hall, A., Smets, L. A. and Ploegh, H. L. Ras (proto) oncogene induces Nlinked carbohydrate modification: Temporal relationship with induction of invasive potential. *EMBO J.* 7: 3361–3368, 1988.

[74] Bondy, G. P., Wilson, S. and Chambers, A. F. Experimental metastatic ability of H-ras transformed NIH/3T3 cells. *Cancer Res.* 45: 6005–6009, 1985.

[75] Greig, R. G., *et al.* Tumorigenic and metastatic properties of "normal" and ras-transfected NIH/3T3 cells. *Proc. Natl. Acad. Sci. USA* 82: 3698–3701, 1985.

[76] Collard, J. G., Schijven, J. F. and Roos, E. Invasive and metastatic potential induced by ras-transfection into mouse BW5147 T-lymphoma cells. *Cancer Res.* 47: 754–759, 1987.

[77] Egan, S. E., Broere, J. J., Jarolim, L, Wright, J. A. and Greenberg, A. H. Coregulation of metastatic and transforming activity of normal mutant ras genes. *Int. J. Cancer* 43: 443–448, 1989.

[78] Albini, A., Aukerman, S. L. and Noonan, D. M. The in vivo invasiveness and interactions with laminin of K-1735 melanoma cells. *Clin. Exper. Metastasis* 7: 436–451, 1989.

[79] Greene, H. S. N. The Significance of the Heterologous Transplantability of Human cancer. *Cancer* 5: 24–44, 1952.

[80] Kumar, R., Sukumar, S. and Barbacid, M. Activation of ras oncogene preceding the onset of neoplasia. *Science* 248: 1101–1104, 1990.

[81] Russo, J., Tay, L. K. and Russo, I. H. Differentiation of the mammary gland and susceptibility to carcinogenesis. *Breast Cancer Res. Treat.* 2: 5–73, 1982.

[82] Gullino, P. M., Pettigrew, H. M. and Grantham, F. H. N-Nitrosomethylurea as mammary gland carcinogen in rats. *J. Natl. Cancer Inst.* 45: 401–404, 1975.

[83] Ochieng, J., Basolo, F., Albini, A., Melchiore, A., Watanabe, H., Elliott, J., Raz, A., Paredi, S. and Russo, J. Increased invasive chemotactic and locomotive abilities of *c-Ha-ras* transformed human breast epithelial cells. *Invasion Metastases* 11: 38–47, 1991.

[84] Liotta, L. A. Tumor invasion and metastases: the role of basement membrane. *Am. J. Pathol.* 117: 339–348, 1984.

[85] Bonfil, R. D., Reddel, R., Ura, H., Reich, R., Fridman, R., Harris, C. C. and Klein-Szanto, A. J. P. Invasive and metastatic potential of a v-Ha-ras transformed human bronchial epithelial cell line. *J. Natl. Cancer Inst.* 81: 587–594, 1989.

[86] Zimmermann, A. and Keller, H. V. Locomotion of tumor cells as an element of invasion and metastasis. *Biomed. Pharmacother.* 41: 337–344, 1987.

[87] Mensing, H., Albini, A. and Kreig, T. Enhanced chemotaxis of tumor derived and virus transformed cells to fibronectin and fibroblasts conditional medium. *Int. J. Cancer* 33:43–48, 1984.

[88] MacCarthy, J. B., Basara, M. l., Palon, D. F. and Funcht, L. T. The role of cell adhesion proteins, laminum and fibronectin in the movement of malignant and metastatic cells. *Cancer Metastases Rev.* 4: 12–152, 1988.

[89] Smith, H. S., Wolman, S. R. and Hackett, A. J. The biology of breast cancer at the cellular level. *Biochem. Biophys. Acta.* 738: 103–123,1984.

[90] Russo, J., McGrath, C. M., Russo, I. H. and Rich, M. A. Tumoral growth of a human breast cancer cell line (MCF-7) in athymic mice. In: Nieburgs, H.E., (ed.), *3rd Int. Symp. on Detection and Prevention of Cancer*, 1976, 617–626, New York, NY.

[91] Cooper, C. S., Blair, D. G., Oskarsson, M. K., Tainsky, M. A., Eader, L. A. and Vande Woude, G. F. Characterization of human transforming genes from chemically transformed teratocarcinoma, and pancreatic carcinoma cell lines. *Cancer Res.* 44: 1–10, 1984.

[92]   Stampfer, M. R. and Bartley, J. C. Induction of transformation and continuous cell lines from normal human mammary epithelial cells after exposure to benzo[a]pyrene. *Proc. Natl. Acad. Sci. USA* 82: 2394–2398, 1984.

[93]   Zhang, P. L., Calaf, G. and Russo, J. Point mutation in codons 12 and 61 of the *c-Ha-ras* gene in carcinogen-treated human breast epithelial cells (HBECs). *Proc. Am. Assoc. Cancer Res.* 33: 669a, 1992.

[94]   Abarca-Quinones, J., Calaf, G., Estrada, S., Barnabas-Sohi, N., Zhang, P. L., Garcia, M. and Russo, J. Phenotypic progression of human breast epithelial cells (HBECs) transformed with chemical carcinogen. *Proc. Am. Assoc. Cancer Res.* 33: 670a, 1992.

[95]   Calaf, G. and Russo, J. Emergence of progressive neoplastic phenotypes of human breast epithelial (HBEC) treated with chemical carcinogens in vitro. *Proc. Am. Assoc. Cancer Res.* 33: 1141a, 1992.

Chapter 11
The Peak of the Mountain
(1991–2002)

11.1. Our arrival in Pennsylvania

We humans cannot see or predict the future; we can only understand the present by viewing the events of our past. In this chapter, I will describe the events that took place from 1991 to 2002, a period of my life rich in vital experiences, some of them painful and many others rewarding. I called this chapter *The Peak of the Mountain* because it is reminiscent of my experience climbing the pre-Andean Mountains of my native Mendoza. For those who have had that experience or a similar one, the feeling is the same. First, the great space around you and the path walked by many others like you, then the walking until you reach the foot of the climbing site, and then the climbing starts. First you take solid and firm steps, but the more you climb, the shorter the steps, and with that the air thins and your breathing becomes labored. You slow down and make a short stop contemplating the peak and also to look down and see how far you have walked. The more you climb, the more you need to stop and rest, and when the peak nears you, rest a little longer for the last stretch. Finally, you reach the peak, heart pumping not only from the effort but also from the excitement that you made it. You have reached the top of the mountain. You would like to stay there as long as you can. Your senses feel more alive with all the views, the silence, the air, watching every single speckle in the southern blue skies, and if you are lucky the pass of a condor will make your day. You feel good, and when nothing else can be said you start in descending silence. The climbing is arduous, and only if you reach the top of the mountain will you have a true appreciation of the path taken and see the world in a different dimension.

11.2. Rydal

We arrived at Rydal, the site of our new home, on June 26, 1991, and we started work at the Fox Chase Cancer Center (FCCC) on July 1, that was the day that I was officially a Chairman in charge of the Department of Pathology at the FCCC in Philadelphia. We had several fronts to cover, one was the organization of our home, the stabilization of Patricia in the school and the new environment; the other two fronts were the organization of the service area or the surgical pathology, and the most important from the perspective of my memoirs, my research endeavor.

After almost three weeks in our new home in Rydal, I was able to retreat a bit and see how all the quarters of the house were starting to look. The house is a three story stone colonial building, with 7,500 square feet of living area, including a basement and attic. The main house is placed in the center of a five-acre piece of land. There are gardens all around the house with many paths conducting to the upper and lower garden, making the whole property a beautiful one but a difficult task to maintain. The upper garden is in the front of the main entrance of the house which is more than a hundred yards from the main gate at the street level. At the same level are the garages, the tennis court, and the swimming pool, which was the main attraction to Irma. The lower garden is covered with pachysandras and has a creek that runs north to south and is interrupted by a reflection pool 30 feet in diameter, bordered by a stone path that runs in the same direction as the driveway. In the southern side of the lower garden is a pond where the water is renewed by a natural spring that in older days was the source of water for the whole state. The water was collected in gigantic tanks that are still grounded and connected to the basement. The water from the spring was pumped to the reservoirs that were large enough to cover the water needs of the house. Now the tanks are emptied and storage shelves cover their walls, a reminder of times past.

The house was built around 1900, and we found it after visiting 60 other houses during the six-month period from January to June 1991. Irma loved this property on sight, and although I complained at the beginning that was too large for us and it would be difficult to maintain, the property started to grow on me, and this is the house where I am writing these memoirs. It is filled with the echoes of Irma, Patricia, Carmen, and all the members of the family that at one time or another were here before I was the only occupant.

When we moved into the house, I transformed the maid quarters into my own working space, leaving only a set of bells with different chimes indicating where the lady of the house was calling from. Now it is a nice conversation piece. The quarters are separated from the house by two doors, one that connects with the stairs down to the kitchen, and the other one with the bedrooms on the second floor. If these two doors are closed, the quarters are isolated from the rest of the house. It can be connected to the attic by a folding pull-down stair. The door to the attic stairs is located in a narrow hall that connects the two rooms and the bathroom. The larger room, which was used as a sitting room, became my work space, where the computers, fax, copy machine, phones, microscope, and the rest of the drawing material were located. The second room I transformed from a bedroom into a dark room. The main area for reading was the library on the first floor. This is one of the largest rooms in the house, and all the books and collections are there. In 1996, we transformed the solarium in my office, together with the library, to make the work space that I am using presently. The dark room was moved to the basement, and the place that had been used as my work space in the maid quarters is now the atelier where I paint. Other changes in the house were the building of a fence around the property with a main gate that controlled the access to the estate. Irma was very good at maintaining the home, and she ran it like a ship. I continue to enjoy walking in the garden during the morning, at practically every hour of the day, and feeling the space in my whole body, the surrounding tall trees and the rhododendron that grow in every inch of the garden. The Rydal Estate, like Irma wanted to call it, is the testimony of our life and all the perils that we as a family had been going through. On two occasions we were afraid of losing the house but Irma's skills at remortgaging and working with the bank allowed us to keep the house as part of the inheritance for my daughter.

The first six months in Rydal were complicated not only by our need to adapt to the East Coast, which was so different to the Midwest in which a *Yes is a Yes* and a *No is a No*, but also the organization of the surgical pathology services and our trip commitments to Detroit, San Antonio, Washington, D.C., the Netherlands, and three trips to Argentina, two related to an invitation of the Academy of Pathology and one, most sadly, to the sickness and death of my mother. My mother started to suffer a pneumonitis in September of 1991, and she was getting worse every week. On October 19, I arrived in Mendoza, and found that my mother was in the hospital and in a very poor condition. She developed a left ventricular insufficiency and subendocardic infarction, and I was with her when she started to agonize. I gave her water and started talking to her, expressing how much I love her; she heard me, pressed my hand, and then I felt that she was going. I called my sister, and after that our mother's heart started showing arrhythmia, she stopped breathing, her eyes became fixed, and she died on November 1, All Saints Day. She was buried in the CAMPO DEL DESCANZO on November 2, the Day of All Deaths at 6 p.m. My mother, the most loving being that I have ever met, was the first person who died in my arms. Her death was the culmination of 50 years of sickness and a continuous physical deterioration. Her organs were exhausted and that was more powerful than her strong will to live. It was a Christian funeral. My father was devastated, and he could not make it to the rest of the burial. To put her in the ground and leave her there was not easy. That night we had dinner at my sister's house. The following day we went to Mass and had lunch in my parents' house. My father never again returned to his home and stayed with my sister until his death. When nothing else could be done, I returned to Philadelphia. In my journal, I wrote: "*I am so afraid of the coldness of death that it is difficult to think of an afterlife when the death itself is so real to me. I see death not as an ending of life but as the major failure of our existence."* The Rydal home witnessed my sorrow and crying until my tears were no more. This home keeps all the memories of our life. There are so many events that I would like to narrate in which the Rydal home played a central part and one of them was LOWAC or the League of Women Against Cancer.

11.3. The League of Women Against Cancer

Irma, my wife and companion and a real partner in research, was a great woman. She was the salt of the earth, precious to her mother, Carmen, and of course to Patricia and me.

Irma was an extraordinary woman, and in the middle of all our professional activities she foresaw that we would need to have something else, something bigger than us that could persist after our jobs were gone and even after our deaths. On May 27, 1994, I wrote in my journal that Irma had created the League of Women Against Cancer, or LOWAC (Figure 11.1). The logo was created by Patricia, who in those days showed signs of being a budding artist. The image is of a woman who has lost her hair due to chemotherapy, and she was emerging with a world of new hopes for the future.

Irma was extremely happy with LOWAC, and she worked very hard to create the bylaws, a board that supervised and advised the management of the new foundation, and even obtained non-profit status from the state of Pennsylvania, which allowed her to receive donations. The mission of LOWAC was clear: *It was a nonprofit organization comprised of professionals and community individuals dedicated to the promotion of cancer awareness, prevention, and early detection.*

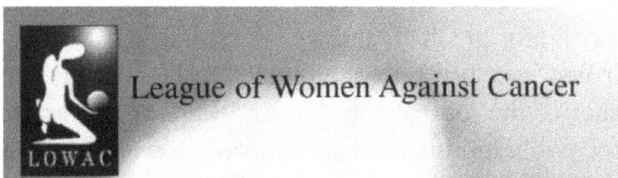

Figure 11.1: Logo of the League of Women Against Cancer.

The Function of LOWAC was: (1) to educate women and their families about women's cancer, (2) to create culturally and linguistically appropriate literature on the subject of women's cancer education and awareness, (3) to motivate women to adopt preventative behaviors with regard to cancer, (4) to inform women of the most modern methods for early detection, prognostic indicators, and modern therapeutic modalities, (5) to support cancer research at the basic clinical and social levels, and (6) to alleviate the suffering of women affected by the disease through support groups and assistance.

Irma's vision was to create our own institution that would allow us to pursue our dreams independently of the FCCC, universities and the restrictions of government grants. It was the most American thought of self-determination and reliance that you could expect.

One of the first accomplishments was a contract with the International Life Sciences Institute through a cooperative agreement between Risk Science Institute and the U.S. Environmental Protection Agency (EPA), Office of Pesticide Programs (Figure 11.2).

The contract was for writing a manuscript that was fully published in *Environmental Health Perspectives* on September of 1996. The publication resulted in a monumental review of our work and was featured on the cover of the journal (Figure 11.2). This success generated the idea of a newsletter that saw the light on May 16, 1996. Following this path, Irma organized a meeting of LOWAC in Mendoza, Argentina, in June of the same year with Dr. Ricardo Deis, the Director of the Institute for Reproduction and Lactation. The meeting in Mendoza was a success, and all the speakers were outstanding, and the general perception of the meeting was excellent. Many other meetings were organized by LOWAC and the list is too long to be discussed here.

The next endeavor of LOWAC emerged on October 15, 1997, with the creation of *The LOWAC Journal Women and Cancer* (Figure 11.3). I was the Co-Editor in Chief, and we selected an outstanding editorial board. Our first issue was published in 1998 (Figures 11.3 and 11.4). The publisher of the journal was Atlantic Ring. However, due to the high cost of publication with that company, we decided to stop the contract with them by a decision of the LOWAC board of directors on November 15, 1999, and continue with the journal with another name,

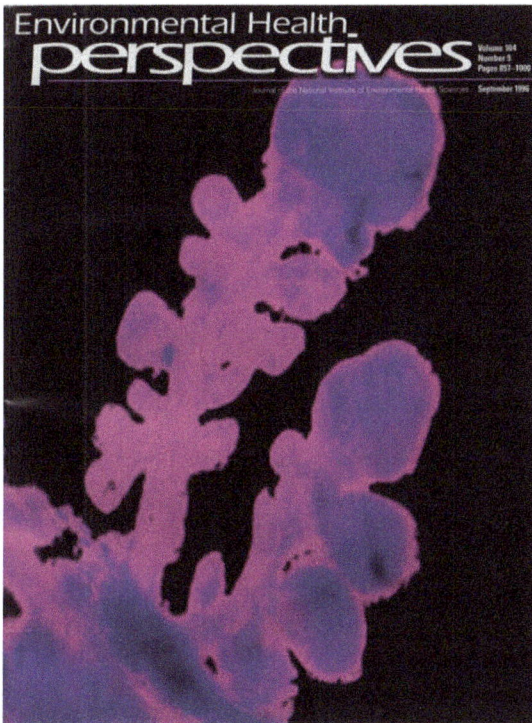

Figure 11.2: On the cover: Intraductal proliferation that forms from the terminal end buds of the rat mammary gland becoming enlarged after DMBA administration (Russo and Russo p. 938).

Journal of Women's Cancer, suggested by one of the members of the board, Mr. Frank Monaghan. Also the board decided to utilize other local printers, significantly reducing the cost. The Volume 2 Issue 1 was published in 2000, and the Editorial Assistant was Darcy Quillen, who was featured with her mother, a breast cancer survivor, on the cover of that issue (Figure 11. 5). This decision by LOWAC's board of directors allowed us to maintain the journal with the subscriptions, advertisements, the reprint and page charges, and most importantly the donations that Irma solicited plus the one that I obtained from Bristol-Meyer-Squibb.

The history of LOWAC and the journal could be the subject of a separate memoir because it is ingrained with so many members of our family, friends, and colleagues that there is too much to describe in

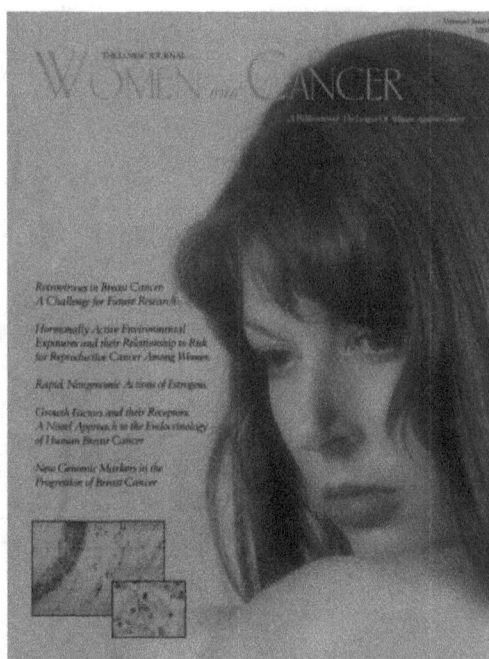

Figure 11.3:   Cover of the first issue of the LOWAC Journal Women and Cancer.

this book. When Irma's health started to deteriorate at the end of 2012, and I was slowly recovering after my subdural hematoma, which also put my own mortality in check (see Chapter 13), Irma decided to close LOWAC and the journal. Nobody could replace her, even me; she saw all the steps from its creation to the end. After her death in June 2013, I collected what was left from LOWAC, and it is all kept in sealed boxes and storage in our Rydal home, expecting a writer to tell the story of that unique grassroots movement.

11.4. The organization of my research work at the FCCC

The research environment at the FCCC turned out to be unique not only because one institution had such a variety of technological resources, but more important because of the research and the

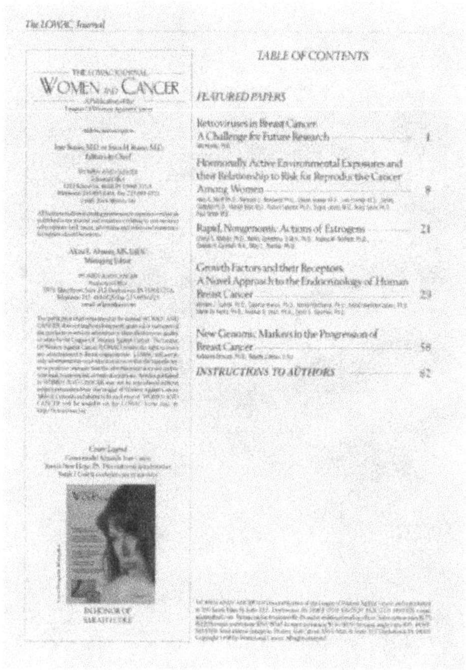
The LOWAC Journal

THE LOWAC JOURNAL

WOMEN AND CANCER

TABLE OF CONTENTS

FEATURED PAPERS

IN HONOR OF SARAH STOKE

Figure 11.4: Table of contents of the first issue of the LOWAC Journal Women and Cancer.

researchers that had significantly contributed to the advancement of our understanding of the nature of cancer. The place inspired a sense of transcendence and history. The *FCCC* is a National Cancer Institute-designated Comprehensive Cancer Center research facility and hospital. The center was formed in 1974 by the merger of the *American Oncologic Hospital*, which was founded in 1904 as the first cancer hospital in the United States [1], and the *Institute for Cancer Research*, founded in 1927. The center was an independent, non-profit institution until it became part of the Temple University Health System (TUHS) specializing in the treatment and prevention of cancer in July 1, 2012.

There are several landmark discoveries at FCCC that have made this place a remarkable one and which are living examples of the institution that hired me. Although the objective of this chapter is not

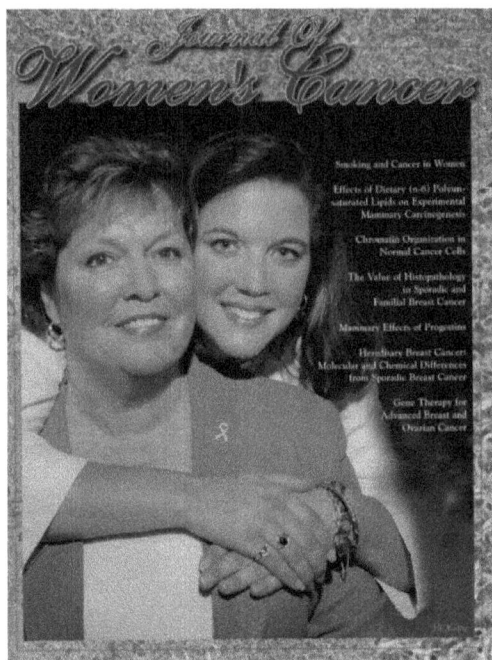

Figure 11.5: Cover of Volume 2 of the issue, number 1 of LOWAC's journal with the name *Journal of Women's Cancer.*

a full description of what FCCC has accomplished, it is still important to mention some landmark discoveries, like the Philadelphia chromosome, the hepatitis virus, and the two hit hypothesis that are important scientific discoveries in our understanding of cancer.

The so-called Philadelphia chromosome is a defect that results from a translocation, in which parts of two chromosomes, 9 and 22, swap places. This creates a fusion gene by juxtaposing the *ABL1* gene on chromosome 9 (region q34) to a part of the *BCR* (breakpoint cluster region) gene on chromosome 22 (region q11). This process is called reciprocal translocation, creating an elongated chromosome 9 and a truncated chromosome 22 that is the *Philadelphia chromosome* [2, 3]. The Philadelphia chromosome was first discovered and described in 1959 by David A. Hungerford from the FCCC and Peter Nowell from the University of Pennsylvania School of Medicine and was therefore named after the city in which both facilities are located [2, 4, 5]. Hungerford was a graduate student writing his doctoral thesis on chromosomes at the FCCC when he detected that certain leukemia cells had an abnormally short chromosome 22. Nowell, a pathologist at the University of Pennsylvania, had noticed that leukemic cells have altered chromosomes that made him look for Hungerford. The relevance of this discovery is that it was the first genetic defect linked to a specific human cancer. The results of these finding were published in *Science* in 1960 [5] with a descriptive title: *"A minute chromosome in chronic granulocytic leukemia."* The mutation became known as the Philadelphia chromosome. Although I never met Hungerford, because he died before I joined the FCCC, his wife was still working in the Department of Pathology that I chaired, and I learned this remarkable story from her as well as sharing our mutual interest in gardening and her advice on how to best kill poison ivy.

Another iconic work done at the FCCC was the one developed by Dr. Baruch S. Blumberg, who in 1976 received the Nobel Prize in Physiology and Medicine for *"discoveries concerning new mechanisms for the origin and dissemination of infectious diseases."* Blumberg identified the hepatitis B virus, and later developed its diagnostic test and vaccine [6]. He studied the genetic variations in human beings by focusing on the question of why some people contract a disease in a given environment while others do not. Blumberg discovered a surface antigen for hepatitis B in the blood of an Australian aborigine and demonstrated that the virus could cause liver cancer [7]. He and his team were able to develop a screening test for the hepatitis B virus, to prevent its spread in blood donations, and also developed a vaccine. Blumberg later freely distributed his vaccine patent in order to promote its distribution by drug companies. Development of the vaccine reduced the infection rate of hepatitis B in children in China from 15% to 1% in 10 years [8]. Although Irma had frequent talks with Blumberg and shared common areas of interest on demographic differences and disease, I only spoke with him on a few occasions, most of the time at social gatherings.

Alfred Knudson was at the FCCC from 1976 until 2016 [9, 10]. He was an affable man that I had the privilege to know and to talk with many times over the course of his years at the institution. I revised many manuscripts for him that reached his hands as a member of the editorial board of the Proceeding National Academy of Sciences. We met several times with him and Irma to discuss our concepts on breast development and cancer. Knudson is best known for his "two-hit hypothesis," explaining the incidence of hereditary cancers, such as retinoblastoma. The inherited mutation is the "first hit." Over time, a mutation may arise in the normal version in one cell, thus producing the "second hit," which leaves the cell unable to control the process of cell division in an orderly manner, leading to cancer [11]. Knudson's insight was to compare the incidence of retinoblastomas, including the number of tumors, the ages of occurrence, and whether tumors occurred in both eyes, among children in families with and without hereditary predisposition to retinoblastomas. Children in families with a hereditary predisposition have more tumors at a younger age and usually have tumors in both eyes. Children in families without the hereditary predisposition usually have only one tumor at a later age. Knudson subsequently showed that the model was not only applicable to retinoblastoma but also to Wilms's tumors of the kidney [12]. These studies led to the concept of tumor suppressor genes, which Knudson called "anti-oncogenes" [11].

There were many other outstanding researchers at the time of my arrival at FCCC, such as Beatrice Mintz, who produced the first mouse model of human malignant melanoma, in which the disease resembles the human malignancy; Irwin Rose, who was awarded the Nobel Prize in Chemistry in 2004 for the discovery of ubiquitin-mediated protein degradation; Melvin Bosma, who discovered the SCID mouse, a strain of mouse with no natural immunity; Robert Perry, who discovered that the messenger RNAs of mammalian cells and their precursors contain a novel structure at their leading ends and that ribosomal RNA is synthesized in the nucleolus as a large precursor molecule that is subsequently processed into mature components. There was also Jenny Glusker, who worked in the crystal structure of a nucleic acid–drug complex as a model for anti-tumor agent and mutagen action. She was the successor of Lindon

Patterson's Department of Crystallography who helped Rosalyn Franklin in her formation as crystallographer and to elucidate the DNA structure. These are only few of the many extraordinary researchers, like Thomas London and Sam Sorof, who have contributed so much to the institution that is a part of the history of scientific discovery. Both Thomas and Sam were very kind to Irma and I, making sure that we were integrated into the research community of the FCCC. Of significance was also the positive impact of one message written on the altar of our church: *Bloom where you are planted.*

The most important part of this narrative in my memoirs is to record that I felt welcomed in that research environment, and every time I needed a scientific opinion they were extremely helpful and generous with their time. Upon my arrival in 1991, the research organization of FCCC was well integrated, and all the facilities and the administration were centered to make research the centerpiece of the institution's objectives. I finally found in the FCCC the cancer research environment that I was looking for; the researchers were seasoned and understood the priorities of generating new ideas, first-class publications and how to procure funding for performing the research. I was offered many other positions and invitations at other places around the country during my tenure at FCCC, but the balance all the time tilted in favor of FCCC, and we always preferred to stay.

The FCCC was an ideal intellectual environment, and I found myself without restriction, able to think as big as I could, meaning that it was not enough for me to generate good results for the competing grant renewal and to generate new ideas for research grant applications and publish my work, but I wanted to make a Breast Cancer Program in the BCRL a self-contained Institute of Breast Cancer. At this institute, many different projects would cover all the main fields of breast cancer that were of my interest and establish the largest network of collaboration possible to help me fly even further. These objectives required a more concentrated effort from me, and I developed 10 integrated research projects that are the signature of the BCRL. The research projects proved to be a fertile ground for obtaining competitive external support mainly by the National Cancer Institute, the Department of Defense, the Barbara Komen Foundation, and the Avon Foundation. In addition, I obtained support from private donations and contracts with pharmaceutical company. From 1997 to 2004, I was the best funded researcher after the president of the FCCC (Figure 11.6). Although this fact was never acknowledged publicly or in any report of the FCCC, it was reported by a non-governmental institution (Research Crossroads) that kept record of funding as it is shown in Figure 11.6.

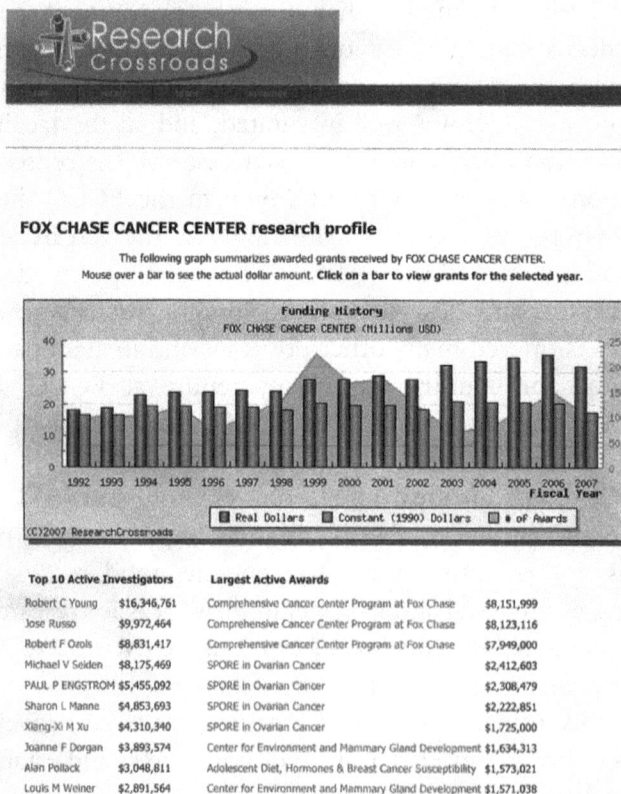

Figure 11.6:   The research funding at the FCCC.

11.5. My research programs at the FCCC

I developed 10 research projects at the FCCC, and although some of them are closed at the time that I am writing this, many of them are active and driven. For the purpose of this memoir, I will describe them as: (1) FCCC Breast Cancer Tissue Resources; (2) Breast Cancer and Environmental Factors; (3) Genomic Basis of Reproductive History in Breast Cancer; (4) Breast Cancer Therapy by Differentiation Gene Activation; (5) Estrogens and Breast Cancer; (6) Epigenetic Control of Estrogen Induced Cell Transformation; (7) Prevention Trial in the Use of r-hCG in Women of High Risk of Developing Breast Cancer; (8) Circadian Rhythm and Mammary Gland Development; (9) Chromatin Remodeling in Breast Cancer and Prevention; and (10) the developing of new peptides that could be used in replacing the whole molecule of hCG. In this chapter, I will describe the first eight programs and the last two will be part of Chapter 14.

11.5.1. *FCCC breast cancer tissue resources*

The major goal of this project was to have a tissue bank of primary breast cancers with a detailed follow-up and histopathological characterization. The opportunity opened to me on March 24, 1993, when I met the pathologists of the FCCC network. This network had been previously organized by Dr. Paul F. Engstrom. His suggestion was that I could use this network and the pathologists as potential participants for answering the RFA of the NCI for constructing a tumor registry. Almost a month later, I submitted the application and was funded on August 20 of that year. As a Principal Investigator (PI) I have been able to maintain this resource for 13 years with a continuous support from the NCI since 1993 (UO1-CA62772) and after that with our general funds of the BCRL. When we were under the NCI funding, one of the aims of this project was to provide tissue sections and pertinent clinical data to investigators and construct tissue microarrays for our use and also for further distribution to investigators. The Fox Chase Breast Cancer Tissue Resource has

422   *Memoirs of a Cancer Researcher*

stored the largest amount of primary breast cancer totaling 1,850 cases, and we were initially one of four geographically diverse facilities across the nation participating in the National Cancer Institute's Cooperative Breast Cancer Tissue Resource. The other three institutions working in consortium with FCCC were Kaiser Permanente in Portland, Oregon; University of Miami; and the University of Missouri. A computerized central database was maintained in Silver Spring, Maryland. Our Fox Chase Breast Cancer Tissue Resource maintained this collaborative effort with the hospital of the FCCC and 11 other Fox Chase Network Hospitals. We were able to publish seven manuscripts from this project [13–19], and we still use this tissue bank for any of the other projects that need evaluation in primary breast cancer [20]. This project allows me to keep up to date on the major discoveries and trends in the prognostic markers of breast cancer. Through these resources, we were able to provide the material needed to validate the use of Her 2 evaluation in paraffin sections of breast cancer and its further clinical application as a tumor marker and a prognostic indicator of tumor response to treatment.

11.5.2. *Breast Cancer and the Environment Research Center*

Although the Breast Cancer and the Environment Research Center (BCERC) was created in 2004, it began almost 10 years earlier.

On July 26, 1994, I wrote in my journal:

> *Dr. Lea Sekely from the NCI called this morning. The RFA on timing of carcinogenesis has received a very good score. Therefore the chances of funding are good. Lia said that is was the best.*

On August 29, I wrote:

> *I received the pink sheet from the RFA on timing of carcinogenesis, and I called the secretary Dr. Gwen Collman, and she indicated to me that it will be funded, and on October 15 I wrote: The grant under the RFA on timing in carcinogenesis has been granted and is already activated.*

This document affirmed my long-lasting interest in carcinogenesis and susceptibility to mammary cancer, making us a strong contender when the RFA from the NIEHS and NCI for forming the BCERC was called in 2004. Our application was funded and constituted a consortium composed of FCCC, University of Alabama at Birmingham, and Mt. Sinai School of Medicine. I was the PI of that consortium which was maintained for 8 years, and when the funding was discontinued I was able to maintain the center at FCCC by extending my collaboration first with Dr. Coral Lamartiniere at the University of Alabama and presently with Dr. Karin Michels from the University of California.

From 2004 to 2011, the NCI-NIEHS supported our Environment Research Center and was one of the four consortiums working together to investigate the relationship between the environment and breast cancer. The University of Cincinnati, University of California at San Francisco, and Michigan State University are the other three leaders of this effort. Our BCERC consisted of two research projects and two cores. The goal of our research project (Project 1) was to investigate the potential of known endocrine disruptors, and one nutritional agent that has been demonstrated to protect against breast cancer and alter mammary cancer susceptibility when exposure occurs alone and in combination with each other. The goal of Project 2 was to examine the relationship between environmental exposures and pubertal milestones, taking into consideration hormonal determinants, oxidative stress, and obesity. The purpose of the Administrative Core was to provide leadership, direction, evaluation, organization, and integration of the center. The goals of the Community Outreach and Translation Core were to develop and coordinate onsite workshops for study participants, and to publish and distribute a biannual newsletter on relevant topics. Through this center, we have taken the leadership of offering training in laboratory research to breast cancer advocates. I instituted an External Advisory Board that helped to gauge the yearly progress of our research endeavor.

The central hypothesis of our work was that exposure to estrogenically active chemicals alone, or in combination with each other, during early critical periods of development could alter predisposition for breast cancer. Our goal was to investigate the potential ability of environmental chemicals that are known endocrine disruptors, to alter morphology and genomic/proteomic expressions that can alter mammary gland differentiation and therefore create a predisposition to breast cancer. To reach this goal, we studied three compounds: Bisphenol A (BPA) — A monomer used to manufacture polycarbonate plastic, the resin used for most food and beverage cans, dental sealants and more. Butyl Benzyl Phthalate (BBP) — A plasticizer used in PVC, vinyl foams, traffic cones, food conveyor belts, artificial leather, plastic foams. It can also be found in some cosmetics, and 2,3,7,8 Tetrachlorodibenzo-p-dioxin (TCDD) — A highly toxic dioxin produced mainly by combustion, including incineration of waste and burning fuels. It is also found in some herbicides. These compounds were used separately to treat the rats at two early periods of development: *prenatal* (while the rats were developing intrauterus, the compound was received through the placenta) and *prepubertal* (during lactation, the compound was received through the milk of the mother). The study of the female offspring was performed when they reached 21, 35, 50, or 100 days (Figure 11.7).

After the mammary glands of the animals were collected, they were used for morphological analysis utilizing whole mount preparations and cell proliferation studies. In addition, RNA was extracted from the mammary glands, which was used for gene expression analysis through microarray analysis and real time RT-PCR (Figure 11.8). Biostatistics and bioinformatics analysis have been

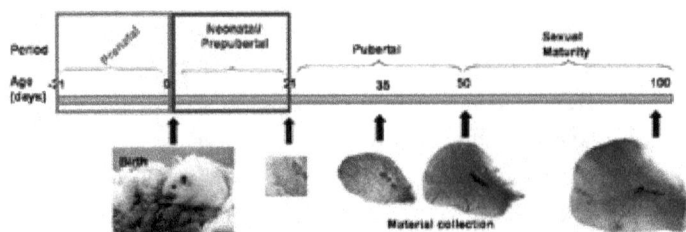

Figure 11.7:   Experimental protocol.

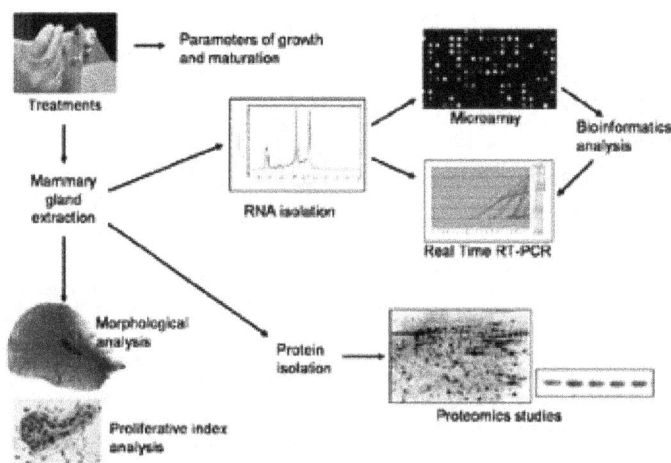

Figure 11.8: Design of the experiments realized for each treatment.

done with the microarray results to determine gene expression profiles of exposure, as well to predict or explain changes in the development or cancer susceptibility.

This project required a close interaction between the animal studies performed at the University of Alabama at Birmingham (UA) and the genomic studies performed in the BCRL at the FCCC. At UA, the animals were treated according to the protocol described in Figure 11.7 and the mammary glands were collected and shipped to the FCCC, where the morphological, cell kinetics, and genomic studies were performed. The informatics cores of the FCCC and the UA were extremely important for the data analysis and interpretation for the genomic and proteomic data, respectively, and more than 70 publications were originated from this project [21–87]. The main concept that emerged from these studies was that Bisphenol A (BPA), *n*-butyl benzyl phthalate (BBP) and 2,3,7,8-tetrachl orodibenzo-*p*-dioxin (TCDD), endocrine disruptors widely present in the environment, affect the global gene expression profile of the rat mammary gland at different ages. Each compound has a specific action on the gene expression of the mammary gland. Moreover, the changes observed also vary with dose administered, stage of life at the time of exposure, and the age studied. It was observed that transcription and DNA-related genes, including estrogen and DNA damage response signaling pathways and developmental genes, were mainly affected upon BPA action. TCDD had the greatest effect on the tumor suppressor genes. Several genes related to the lipid metabolism were regulated by BBP and TCDD treatments, but not by BPA. Immune-related genes were modulated by TCDD at several conditions and were suppressed by BBP in early puberty (Figure 11.9).

The relevance of these data is that each endocrine disruptor induces a set of specific changes in the mammary gland, leading to different biological responses [88]. The data that we were able to collect from these studies allowed us to conclude that epigenetic changes were also responsible for the gene transcription modifications induced by the environmental agents. Using the list of genes that might be

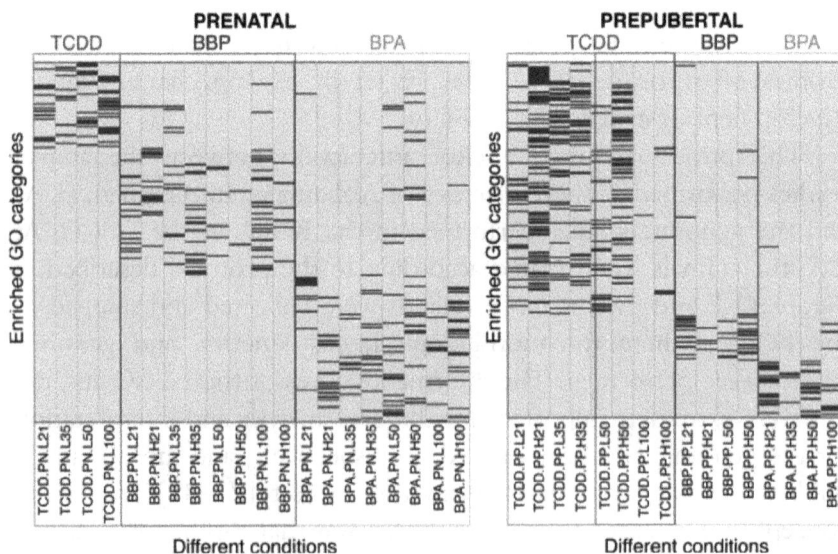

Figure 11.9: Distribution of enriched GO terms in prenatally or prepubertally exposed animals with every available combination of compound (BPA, BBP, TCDD), dose level (low, high), and age (21, 35, 50, 100 days). Blue indicates that specific GO terms (rows) were overrepresented among genes differentially expressed at specific conditions (columns). Little overlap of GOs was observed for the three compounds, emphasizing that each compound induces a specific genomic signature.

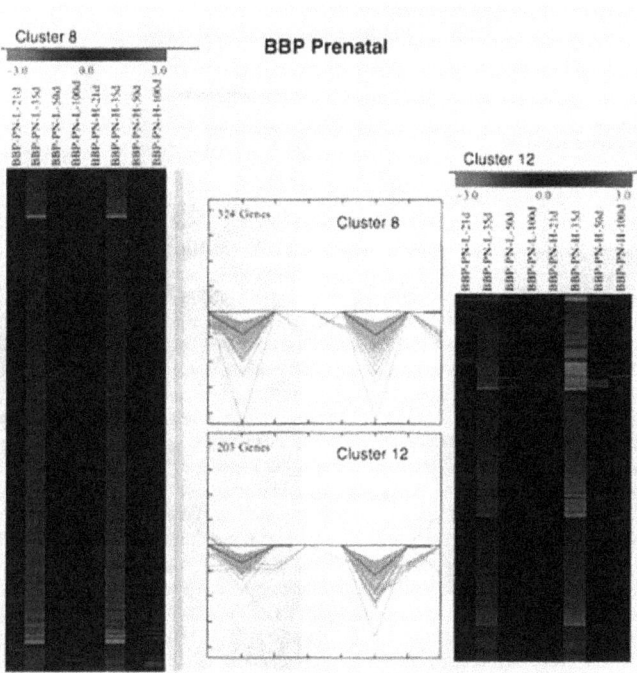

Figure 11.10: Clusters of genes down-regulated at 35 days of age after prenatal exposure to BBP. The pink line represents the average expression and gray lines represent the expression of each selected gene.

methylated, through k-means clustering, we divided the expression profiles of all doses and ages studied into 12 patterns of expression, and in this way, observed clusters of genes that had peaks of down regulation by one of the compounds at certain time points after which their expression returned to normal or it became up-regulated. For example, prenatally BBP-exposed animals had two clusters of genes (Figure 11.10), which were down-regulated at 35 days, independently of the doses. A list of 38 genes that were at least two-fold down-regulated compared to the control group was identified with methylation sites in their promoter or exon 1. Among the patterns of expression found after the prenatal treatment with BPA, three clusters were considered to have potential methylated genes (Figure 11.11). TCDD-prenatally exposed animals induced the down regulation of

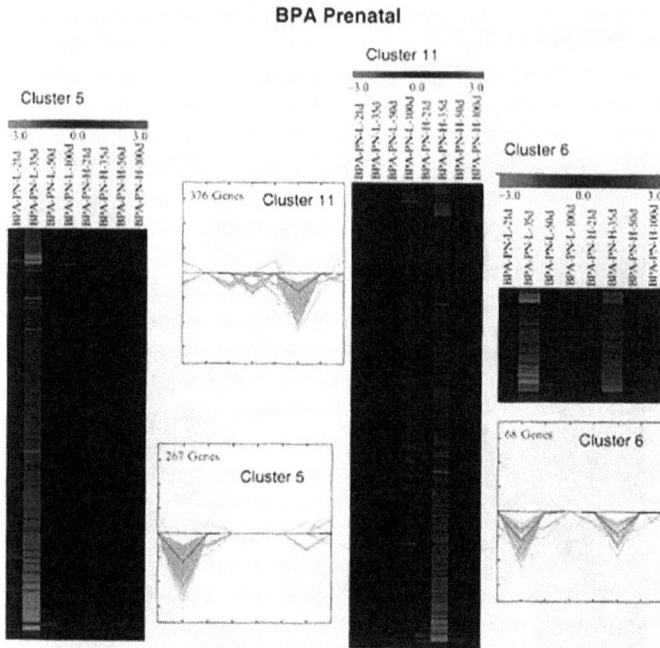

Figure 11.11: Clusters of genes down-regulated at 35 days of age after prenatal exposure to BPA. The pink line represents the average expression and gray lines represent the expression of each selected gene.

83 genes clustered at 35 days of age and other cluster of 85 genes at 100 days of age (Figure 11.12).

In summary, these findings suggested that the compounds, when administered prenatally, induced at the time of puberty (35 days of age) down regulation of genes that are specific to BBP and BPA. The fact that this effect disappears at 50 and 100 days of age and returns to the same values observed at 21 days indicates that at puberty a series of events not yet identified regulate the transcriptional pattern of the mammary gland. The same effect is observed with TCDD-prenatally treated animals, in which a different cluster of down-regulated genes appears at 100 days. These observations allowed us to postulate that this transcription pattern could be epigenetically controlled.

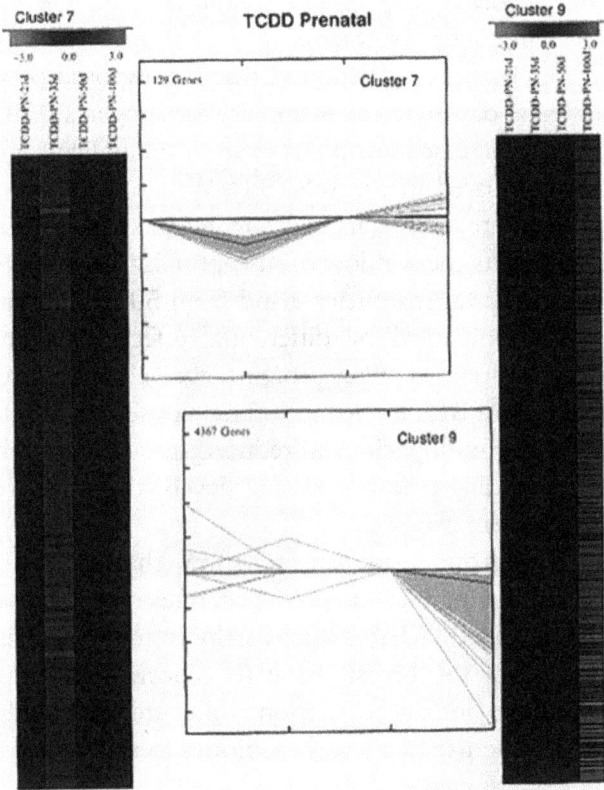

Figure 11.12: Pattern of expression of two clusters of genes after prenatal exposure to TCDD. The pink line represents the average expression and gray lines represent the expression of each selected gene.

We further made a correlation between these genetic and epigenetic changes with the susceptibility to develop mammary cancer. In animals exposed to BPA in the lactation period, a significantly increased cell proliferation in TEBs of 50-day-old but not 21-day-old rats was observed. Interestingly, apoptosis was significantly decreased in the mammary gland of 50-day-old but not 21-day-old BPA exposed rats [38]. *The data clearly indicated that genomic and proteomic changes detected in the mammary glands of prepubertally exposed animals show signatures that predict the response to a carcinogen challenge. Indeed, this assumption was supported by experimental data published by our group* [38]. In that publication, we reported that rats exposed prepubertally to BPA and then at day 50 to the mammary carcinogen DMBA showed a dose-dependent increase in mammary tumor multiplicity and reduced tumor latency compared to controls [38]. We also reported [42] that oral prenatal exposure to BPA increases mammary cancer susceptibility in offspring and shifts the window of susceptibility for DMBA-induced tumorigenesis in the rat mammary gland from 50 to 100 days. These changes were accompanied by differential effects of prenatal BPA exposure on the expression of key proteins involved in cell proliferation [42]. Thus, effects of BPA in rats, including a dose-dependent increase in mammary tumor multiplicity and reduced tumor latency, have been observed at exceedingly low exposure levels that are well below environmental human exposure.

The impact of our work was to show that these ubiquitous compounds produce significant specific changes on the transcriptome of the mammary gland. What is noteworthy is genomic changes alter the susceptibility of the breast tissue to cancer. The translation of these studies to the human population is that this knowledge can be used to regulate the use of these xenobiotics in our society to lessen the burden of breast cancer.

In May 2009, Julia Pereira, who was working on this project, received her PhD degree by studying the role of TCDD in the mammary gland and in 2011, Springer, New York published my book titled *Environment and Breast Cancer* that summarized not only the work of our group but also the other members of the NICI-NIEHS consortium (Mary Helen Barcellos-Hoff, Angela M. Betancourt, Frank M. Biro, Irineu Illa Bochaca, Deborah J. Clegg, Ricardo López de Cicco, Suzanne E. Fenton, Sandra Z. Haslam, Robert A. Hiatt, Sarah Jenkins, Coral A. Lamartiniere, Maricel V. Maffini, James A. Mobley, Raquel Moral, David H. Nguyen, Suraj Peri, Jennifer L. Rayner, Irma H. Russo, Patrícia A. Russo, Stephen Safe, Julia Santucci-Pereira, Michael Slifker, Carlos Sonnenschein, Ana M. Soto, Kelcey Walker, Jun Wang, Richard Wang, Sally S. White, Mary S. Wolff, Yong Xu, Chengfeng Yang, and Shu Zhang [88]. I dedicated this book to Dr. Kenneth Olden, the Director of the NIEHS, whose efforts made possible the study of the role of the environment and breast cancer.

11.5.3. *Genomic basis of reproductive history in the prevention of breast cancer*

We already knew that breast cancer risk has traditionally been linked to nulliparity, or late first full-term pregnancy, whereas young age at first childbirth, multiparty, and breastfeeding are associated with a reduced risk. We demonstrated that early pregnancy confers protection by inducing breast differentiation, which imprints a specific and permanent genomic signature in experimental rodent models, as I have described in previous chapters. However, the main question in my mind was: *Is the same phenomenon detectable in the involuted breast of postmenopausal parous women?* As I described in Figure 9.12 in Chapter 9, if our hypothesis was correct, the parous postmenopausal breast must have not only a signature different from the postmenopausal nulliparous women but also reflect the expression of genes indicative of cell differentiation. The challenges were enormous because it would require a large budget, a protocol design with a statistical power that be conclusive, a personal questionnaire that could be administered to the participants and that contained the information needed, mainly parity, age at the first pregnancy, and any treatment that could affect the outcome of the breast development and differentiation. We needed a good population of normal human breast tissue with solid information regarding their pregnancy history. We also required a network of surgeons and hospitals that were interested in accepting our protocol and collaborating on this project that was supposed to last for a minimum of 5 years. Besides this logistic problem, we were proposing to study gene expression profile using cDNA array, an emerging technique in those days, and we must target our sample to the breast epithelia, implying that we must also use another merging technique that was the laser capture micro dissection. For this purpose, we designed a case control study for the analysis of the gene expression profile of RNA extracted from epithelial cells micro dissected from normal breast tissues. Finally, we obtained an RO1 grant that I received from the NCI (CA093599) that made this study feasible. The study that we proposed to the NCI was to determine the specific gene expression profile of women at "low" and "high" risk of developing breast cancer due to reproductive history and to determine if gene clusters differentially expressed in women at risk of developing breast cancer due to reproductive history are also differentially expressed in the breast tissue of postmenopausal women with breast cancer, and to examine these clusters in comparison to postmenopausal women who do not have breast cancer. The collection of the normal breast tissue was made possible by a collaboration with Dr. Emily Penman and Dr. Nicholas J. Petrelli, from the Helen F. Graham Cancer Center, Christiana Care Health System, Newark, Delaware; Dr. Angela Lanfranchi from Somerset Medical Center, Somerville, New Jersey; Dr. Kathryn Evers from the Diagnostic Imaging, American Oncology Hospital, Philadelphia, Pennsylvania. Using these resources, I was able to obtain breast tissue from 18 parous and 7 nulliparous women free of breast pathology (controls), and 41 parous and 8 nulliparous women with history of breast cancer (cases), suffice to say that the whole conception of the idea was developed with Irma and that allowed us to gather many collaborators, among them Dr. Joana Dorgan, who was pivotal for developing the questionnaire and designing the case control study. We also recruited Dr. Gabriela Balogh, who was a young investigator that was working in Buenos Aires at the Campomar Institute performing all the cDNA array and RNA extraction of the samples, and Daniel Mailo, a graduate student recruited to perform bioinformatics analysis. He used his training in our laboratory and mentored his doctoral thesis at the University of Bahia Blanca in Buenos Aires. My daughter, Patricia, was hired after receiving her BA from Bennington College, and she was instrumental in the setting of the laser micro dissection in frozen and paraffin embedded sections. We had been working with all these techniques for almost a year but adjustments and adaptations of them were needed before we could present this project to the NCI. Gabriela Balogh was an important addition to the BCRL because she was an energetic and ambitious young woman who had a good training at the University of Buenos Aires and updated our laboratory and trained many technical and young investigators working in the BCRL. Both Gabriela and Daniel trained other researchers, like Dr. Raquel Moral and Julia Pereira, in the techniques of cDNA array and bioinformatics; later on, these two investigators developed them even further. We used the laser micro dissected normal breast epithelia for isolating the RNA that was hybridized to eDNA glass microarrays containing 40,000 genes. Each slide array was scanned and the images were analyzed using ImaGene software and the normalization and statistical analysis were carried out using Linear Models for Microarrays and GeneSight software for hierarchical clustering. The specific methodology can be obtained from our main publications [89–94].

The parous control group had 126 genes up-regulated and 103 down-regulated genes with respect to the nulliparous control and case groups and to the parous group with breast cancer (cases). We found that the unsupervised hierarchical clustering done using the expression profiles of 2,541 globally varying genes across the nulliparous and parous data sets representing the four groups revealed that samples clustered primarily based on parity status (Figure 11.13). This suggested that the principal source of global variation in gene expression across these data sets was due to genetic differences between women due to reproductive history. *This observation suggested that determining which parity-induced gene expression changes were conserved among these highly divergent groups could represent a powerful approach to defining a parity-related gene expression signature.*

Results of clustering sets depicted in Figure 11.14 indicated that the combined parity and absence of breast cancer data generate a distinct genomic profile that differs from the breast cancer groups, irrespective of parity history, and from the nulliparous cancer-free group, which has been traditionally identified as a high-risk group. We measured the relevance of gene ontology (GO) terms [95] belonging to the category of biological processes in the breast epithelium of parous women and analyzed the biological significance of those terms that were found to be deregulated in response to an early reproductive event with high statistical significance. Among the

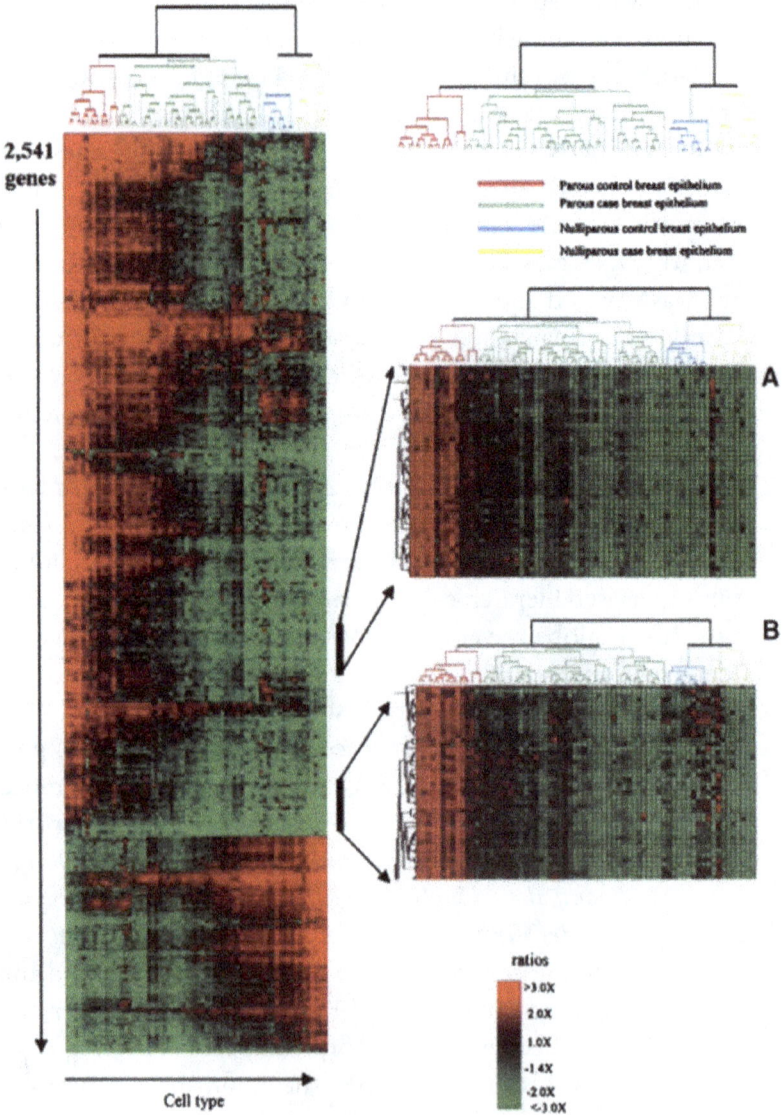

Figure 11.13: Unsupervised hierarchical clustering analysis using the expression profiles of 2,541 globally varying genes across the nulliparous and parous data sets representing parous controls (red lines), parous cases (green lines), nulliparous controls (blue lines), and nulliparous cases (yellow lines).

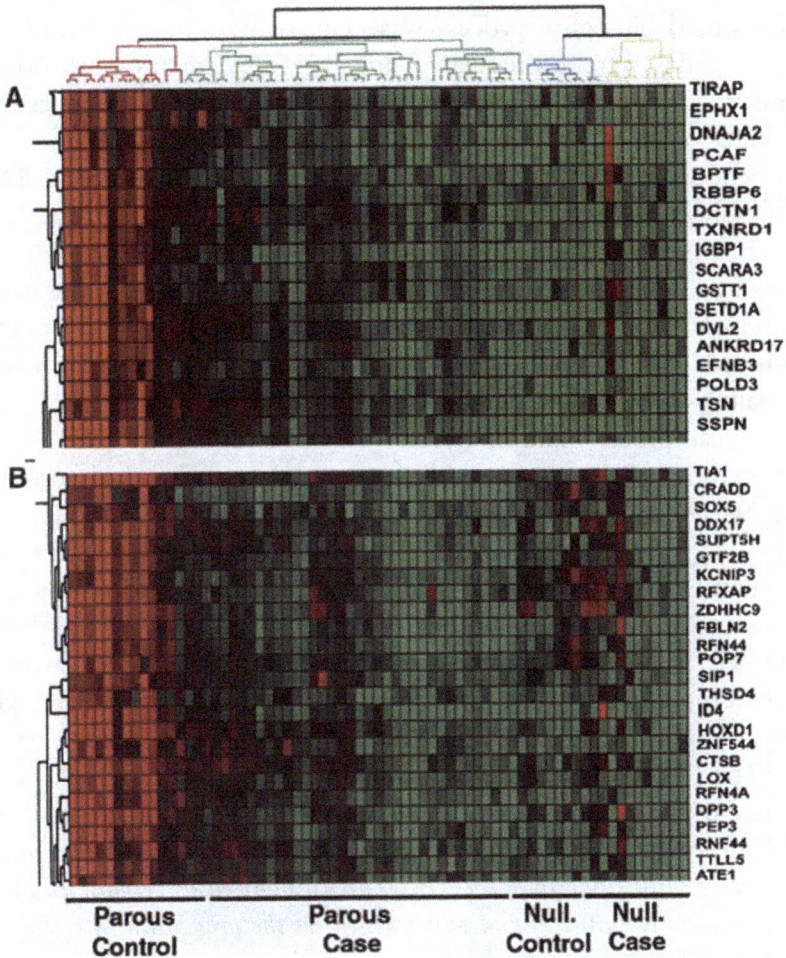

Figure 11.14: A and B, unsupervised hierarchical analysis of subsets of 18 matched breast epithelia from the parous control specimens shown in Figure 11.13 that were micro dissected and hybridized independently as biological replicates. The combined parity/absence of breast cancer data generated a distinct genomic profile that differed from those of the breast cancer groups, irrespective of parity history, and of the nulliparous cancer-free control group. Groups identified as for Figure 11.13.

18 categories identified to contain deregulated genes, the most highly represented biological process was gene transcription, in which 21 (64%) genes were up-regulated and 12 (36%) genes were down-regulated. Higher gene expression was observed in 11 processes that included proteolysis and ubiquitination cell adhesion, response to exogenous agents, metabolism, DNA repair and replication, RNA processing, apoptosis, miscellaneous processes, antiapoptosis, and chromatin modification, in which the ratios of up-regulated to down-regulated genes ranged from 1.75 to 11. A greater number of genes with lower level of expression were observed in various processes that included: cell transport, protein biosynthesis and metabolism, cell signaling-signal transduction, biological process unknown and biological process and molecular function unknown [89]. With Dr. Gabriela Balogh, we published several papers and almost half [89–94, 96–98] were related to the genomic signature of pregnancy. One of them [97] was particularly novel and was related to the role of immune surveillance. The study was done using a micro fluid card for genes related to the immune system and programmed cell death, and we found that breast epithelial cells from parous women significantly overexpressed 17 out of 20 genes (p < 0.001) with respect to the nulliparous breast.

The 17 genes that were over expressed in the parous samples were related to the immune surveillance system and programmed cell death [97]. *These data allowed us to postulate that an early pregnancy makes the breast epithelial cells of the parous breast more easily recognized by the immune surveillance system which initiates the programmed cell death pathway if exposure to toxic or carcinogenic agents occurs.* This paper was published in 2007 and has significance with the new data that we published with Dr. Julia Pereira, stating that an increment in the expression of immune surveillance genes takes place in the first 5 years post pregnancy [99].

Although a larger study (Chapter 14) was necessary to demonstrate categorically our hypothesis, the data obtained through this project indicated in 2008 that the first full-term pregnancy induces in the breast epithelium a specific genomic profile that is still identifiable in parous women at postmenopause. Furthermore, this genomic signature is manifested by genes that cluster differently than those genes expressed in the epithelial cells of parous and nulliparous women with breast cancer as well as from nulliparous women without cancer. This genomic signature confirmed our hypothesis and allowed us to evaluate the degree of mammary gland differentiation induced by pregnancy. Of importance was the fact that this signature serves for characterizing at molecular level the fully differentiated condition of the breast epithelium that is associated with a reduction in breast cancer risk, thus providing a useful molecular tool for predicting when pregnancy has been protective, for identifying women at risk irrespective of their pregnancy history, and for its use as an intermediate biomarker for evaluating cancer preventive agents [89].

11.5.4. *Developing a new paradigm in breast cancer prevention*

Irma and I had written numerous articles indicating that sporadic breast cancer is the fatal disease most frequently diagnosed in American women from all ethnic groups. The incurability of the disease, in association with the worldwide increase in incidence, indicated that primary prevention was and is the ultimate goal for breast cancer control. However, the possibility of developing strategies for preventing the initiation of cancer are hindered by the multistep nature of the process, and the fact that only inheritance of cancer-predisposing genes and radiation exposure at a young age have been identified as a mechanism or causal agent associated with cancer initiation. Current strategies to prevent breast cancer have focused on a unique feature of this disease, its endocrine, namely estrogen, dependence, which can be manipulated to control growth or prevent tumor development utilizing either selective estrogen receptor modulators (SERMs), such as tamoxifen, or aromatase inhibitors (AI's), such as Arimidex, letrozole, and exemestane. However, these strategies are not widely acceptable to a majority of treated women who would not have developed breast cancer even if untreated. Therefore, what we saw clearly was that we needed to develop a new paradigm in breast cancer prevention and treatment. As I narrated earlier, this new paradigm has emerged from epidemiological observations of a direct association of breast cancer risk to nulliparity and of protection conferred by an early first full-term pregnancy. However, the novelty of this paradigm did not germane from the knowledge that an early first full-term pregnancy protects the breast against neoplastic transformation, but from our studies that unveil the biological principle underlying the protection conferred by an early first full-term pregnancy and by demonstrating that it induces in the breast the expression of a specific signature that results from the completion of a cycle of this organ's differentiation driven by the reproductive process. More importantly, we have demonstrated that a short treatment with human chorionic gonadotropin (hCG), a placental hormone secreted during pregnancy, induces the same genomic signature as pregnancy, inhibiting not only the initiation but also the progression of mammary carcinomas, stopping the development of early lesions, such as intraductal proliferations and carcinomas *in situ. These observations indicated that hCG administered for a very short period of time has significant potential as a chemo preventive agent, protecting the normal cell from becoming malignant. This new biological concept also implies that when the genomic signature of protection or refractoriness to carcinogenesis is acquired, the hormonal treatment with hCG is no longer required.* This was and is still a novel concept that is a clear contraposition to the current knowledge that a chemo preventive agent needs to be given for a long period to suppress a metabolic pathway like the case of SERMs and AI's, or abrogate the function of an organ like ovariectomy (castration) in the case of BRCA1/2 carriers.

Our concept that hCG can be used for breast cancer prevention was, however, not accepted by everybody. One example of this is reflected in my May 23, 1993, journal entry:

> *Pelayo Correa, the editor of one of the American Association for Cancer Research's journals, approached me in the AACR meeting and he gave me some feedback about the President Panel meeting that he had been part of it. He told me that the idea of hCG was in a way considered ridiculous, and he advised me to be more simple and focused*

in the idea. He asked me to write an editorial for the Journal of Epidemiology and Prevention, in order to help to clarify the issue. It was a good feeling to have positive people that wanted to help us.

Following his advice and request, we published a 1994 article titled: *"Toward a physiological approach to breast cancer prevention"* [100].

11.5.4.1. *Epidemiological basis for the new paradigm in prevention*

It has long been known that the incidence of breast cancer is greater in nulliparous than in parous women and also that changes in lifestyle can in turn influence the endocrinology of women; this has been observed in American women during the last decades, namely a progressive decrease in the age of menarche and a progressive increase in the age at which a woman bears her first child. The significance of these changes is highlighted by the reduction in breast cancer risk associated with late menarche and the completion of a full-term pregnancy before age 24, with further reduction in the lifetime breast cancer risk as the number of pregnancies increases. Women who undergo their first full-term pregnancy after age 30, on the other hand, appear to be at higher risk of breast cancer development than nulliparous women, suggesting that parity-induced protection against breast cancer is related to the *timing* of a first full-term pregnancy. Although pregnancy appears to have a dual effect on breast cancer risk, a transient increase (relative to nulliparous women) lasting 10–15 years, followed thereafter by a decreased risk, the protection conferred lasts a lifetime. Of interest is the fact that women from different countries and ethnic groups exhibit a similar degree of parity-induced protection from breast cancer, regardless of the endogenous incidence of this malignancy. This observation suggests that the reduction in breast cancer risk associated with early first full-term pregnancy does not result from factors specific to a particular environmental, genetic, or socioeconomic setting, but rather from an intrinsic effect of parity on the biology of the breast (which nevertheless may be modified by environmental, genetic, or other factors). These observations indicate that an early first full-term pregnancy modifies specific biological characteristics of the breast that result in a decreased lifetime risk of cancer development. We attribute this protection to the induction of terminal differentiation of the mammary gland, a mechanism that has been found to reduce the susceptibility of the mammary epithelium to carcinogenesis. These observations indicate that the terminally differentiated state of full-term pregnancy should be reached for attaining protection, although other mechanisms have been proposed for the protective effect of early first full-term pregnancy, including the occurrence of sustained changes in the level or regulation of hormones that affect the breast. Regardless of the intervening mechanism, the end result of the first pregnancy is a dramatic modification of the architecture of the breast. The direct association of breast cancer risk with nulliparity, as well as the protection afforded by early first full-term pregnancy has been in great part explained by experimental studies as has been described in previous chapters.

11.5.4.2. *Experimental animal studies*

The direct association of breast cancer risk with the prolongation in the period encompassed between menarche and the first full-term pregnancy, as well as the protection afforded by pregnancy has been explained by experimental studies performed in our laboratory. It has been demonstrated that mammary cancer in rodents can be induced with the polycyclic hydrocarbon 7, 12-dimethylbenz (a) anthracene (DMBA) preferentially when the carcinogen is administered to young nulliparous females. Those females who have completed a full-term pregnancy prior to carcinogen exposure fail to develop carcinomas. Pregnancy, alone or followed by lactation, induces in the mammary gland a permanent protective effect from chemically-induced carcinogenesis, since administration of a carcinogen to parous rats when the glands have regressed to a resting stage either fails to induce carcinomas or considerably lowers their incidence, whereas mammary glands showing gestational or lactational hyperplasia are moderately refractory to DMBA-induced carcinogenesis. This indicates that it is not the transient hormonal status occurring during pregnancy and lactation that protects the mammary gland, but the permanent changes induced in the gland structure and in the biological properties of the glandular epithelium by the reproductive phenomenon. The observation that pregnancy before carcinogen administration seems to be the only truly protective factor in chemically-induced mammary gland carcinogenesis suggests that placental hormones play an important role in mammary growth and development during pregnancy. The main placental hormone, hCG, has a stimulatory effect on the mammary gland when administered exogenously, producing either a gestational or a lactational type of mammary development that considerably reduces the incidence of tumors. The fact that the hormonal changes of pregnancy accelerate DMBA-induced mammary tumor growth when mating occurs after carcinogen administration indicates that the most important event in determining the role that this hormone plays in either preventing initiation or in promoting tumor growth is the sequence in which it reaches the mammary gland.

Up to now, the main known physiological function of hCG in the female is the maintenance of the corpus luteum of pregnancy through its interaction with the ovarian lutropin-choriogonadotropin-receptor (LH-CG-R), which has been described in the human breast [101]. This interaction activates a cascade of effects that results in increases in serum levels of estrogen and progesterone. Administration of hCG to virgin rats elicits a similar response [102–107]. In addition, our studies have shown that hCG has a direct effect on the rat mammary epithelium and on HBEC *in vitro* [108]; hCG is currently used in the treatment of infertility and hypogonadotropic hypogonadism in males [109–112]. It has also successfully been used for the treatment of obesity [113] and in Phase I/II trials in the United States for the treatment of Kaposi's sarcoma lesions in acquired immune deficiency syndrome (AIDS) patients [114–116]. A drawback in these studies is the fact that the most common source of all commercially available hCG preparations is the urine of pregnant women, which carries numerous bioactive ovarian and placental hormone and peptide metabolites. The assessment of the specific effects of hCG, therefore, requires the use of a pure form of the hormone, such as a recombinant preparation. Pregnancy can be considered the most physiological mechanism for protecting the mammary gland from malignant transformation, a conclusion supported by epidemiological data [117, 118]. The fact that hCG appears to mimic the effect of pregnancy makes the use of this protocol for cancer prevention an appealing idea. Our experimental results constitute the rationale for proposing to evaluate both the therapeutic efficacy of hCG in newly diagnosed breast cancer and its potential to prevent the development of new malignancies in the patients treated with hCG for primary breast cancer. In order to identify the ultimate mechanisms responsible for pregnancy/hCG-mediated protection, we compared the mammary cancer preventive and therapeutic effects of hCG obtained from the urine of pregnant women (urinary hCG or u-hCG) with those of the pure hormone, recombinant hCG (r-hCG). These studies were possible by a support that we received from the Serono Pharmaceutical Company in Geneva, Switzerland.

Figure 11.15 shows the experimental protocol in which 450 animals were separated into nine different groups. Through these studies we aimed to, first, evaluate the efficacy of r-hCG in comparison with that of u-hCG and placebo in the prevention of mammary cancer by determining the potential of these hormones to inhibit the initiation of DMBA-induced rat mammary carcinomas. The second purpose was to evaluate the therapeutic efficiency of r-hCG on mammary cancer. For this objective, the tumoristatic and tumoricidal efficacy of r-hCG and u-hCG on early and advanced mammary cancer was tested in intact virgin rats that had received DMBA 20 days prior to the initiation of the hormonal treatments. The effect on advanced tumor development was evaluated by starting the hormonal treatment 60 days after DMBA administration, or when tumors were already palpable. The complete report of these studies were published in detail elsewhere [101]. Our findings demonstrated clearly that a 21-day treatment of young virgin rats with r-hCG (Ovidrel) prevents the initiation and inhibits the progression of DMBA-induced tumors. A 21-day treatment with Ovidrel produces a preventive effect similar to that previously demonstrated by u-hCG, even when the treatment had been terminated 21 days prior to carcinogen administration. Only 8% of Ovidrel-treated animals developed tumors (the total

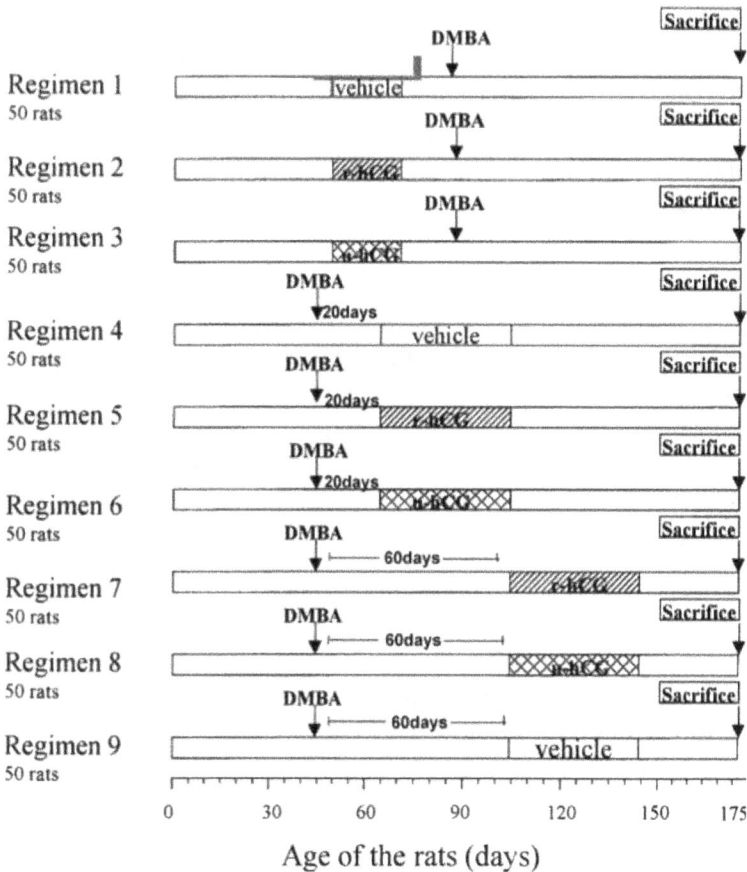

Figure 11.15: Experimental protocol designed for testing the preventive and therapeutic efficacy of hCG on rat mammary cancer. Final tumorigenic response was evaluated 18 weeks after administration of DMBA.

number of tumors developed was five), whereas 44.9% of placebo-treated animals developed tumors, 44 tumors in all, at an average of 0.89 tumors per animal. The group receiving u-hCG also exhibited an inhibitory effect on tumorigenesis, although the reduction was less significant than that induced by the r-hCG.

R-hCG treatment of rats previously inoculated with DMBA inhibited the development of early mammary lesions, since initiation of the hormonal treatment 20 days after carcinogen administration significantly reduced both tumor incidence and tumor burden. Both r-hCG and u-hCG exhibited similar tumor inhibitory effects. These data have a significant clinical implication, because they indicate the usefulness of the utilization of this hormonal treatment on early as well as on premalignant lesions. *The lesson here is that the sooner a treatment is started the more efficient is the therapeutic effect of these hormones.* When the hormonal treatments were initiated 60 days after administration of DMBA, the reduction in tumor incidence was less pronounced, but the tumor burden, expressed as the number of tumors per animal, were significantly depressed. Both r-hCG and u-hCG reduce the tumor burden significantly and reduce the growth of tumors, as evidenced by the lower number of tumors per animal after cessation of the hormonal treatments. The analysis of the final tumorigenic response demonstrated that the placebo-treated animals had 40% more tumors than those treated with either hormone. It is important to analyze the slope of the curve between the initiation (start) and finalization (stop) of the treatment shown in Figure 11.16. Both hormones induce a decline in the slope of the curve due to the direct effect of the hormones on tumorigenesis. At the end of treatment, the slope of the curve becomes steeper, but it never reaches that of the animals that received the placebo, an indication that both hormones have an efficient therapeutic effect by reducing tumor burden by 40%. These observations suggest that r-hCG would be more efficient as a therapeutic tool when used in not only one but probably multiple cycles of treatment in order to be fully curative.

The important message is that hCG treatment of virgin rats for 21 days with a daily intraperitoneal injection of this hormone prior to carcinogen administration exhibits a dose-related reduction in tumor incidence and number of tumors per animal. This phenomenon is mediated by the induction of mammary gland differentiation, inhibition of cell proliferation, increase in the DNA repair capabilities of the mammary epithelium, decrease binding of the carcinogen to the DNA, and activation of genes controlling programmed cell death (PCD) [101]. The activation of these genes by hCG is of great relevance because PCD is a physiological and phylogenetically

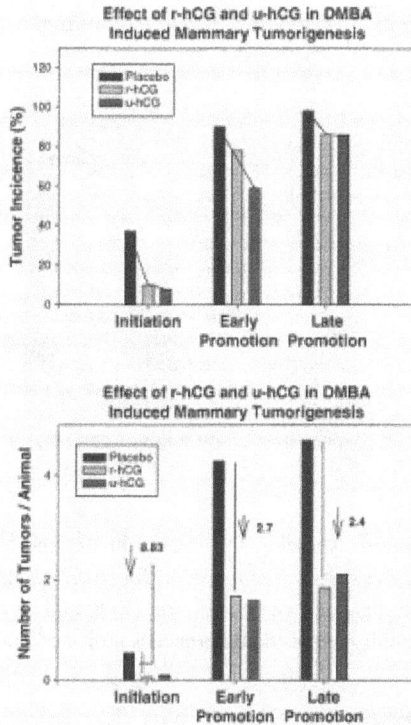

Figure 11.16: (Upper) Histogram showing in the ordinate tumor incidence in the mammary gland of virgin rats treated with placebo (Regimen 1), r-hCG (Regimen 2), or u-hCG (Regimen 3) 21 days prior to DMBA, initiation; 20 days after DMBA early promotion (Regimens 4, 5, and 6), or 60 days after DMBA administration, late promotion (Regimens 7, 8, and 9), according to the protocol shown in Figure 11.14. (Lower) Histogram showing in the ordinate the number of tumors per animal and in the abscissa the regimens for studying initiation (Regimens 1, 2, and 3), early promotion (Regimens 3, 4, and 5), and late promotion (Regimens 7, 8, and 9), as described in Figure 11.14. The arrows and the numbers indicate the rate of tumor reduction as the result of treatment of the animals with r-hCG.

conserved form of active cell death (or apoptosis) that has been associated with specific phases of development that control cell proliferation and differentiation. Interestingly enough as it is shown in Figure 11.17, the PCD or apoptosis induced by hCG is observed not only in the early phase of initiation and promotion as well as in

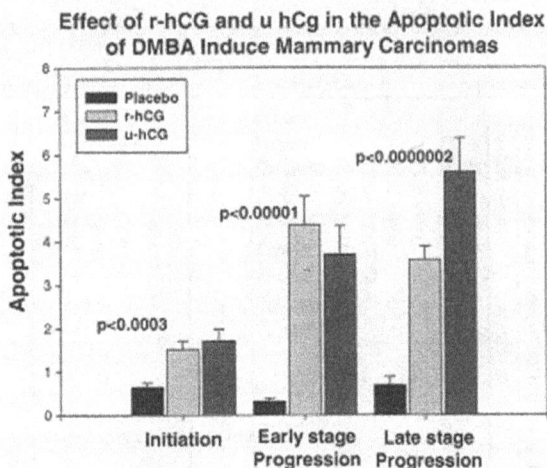

Figure 11.17: Histogram showing in the ordinate the Apoptotic Index of adenocarcinomas and in the abscissa the regimens for studying initiation (1, 2, and 3), early promotion (3, 4, and 5), and late promotion (7, 8, and 9) of protocol described in Figure 11.14. The significance of the difference is indicated above the bars.

the tumors observed in the few animals that received the hormone previous to the carcinogen treatment.

11.5.4.3. *Clinical studies*

On June 19, 1996, I wrote in my journal:

> *Irma and I are going to Elbingealp in the Austrian Tyrol to a meeting organized by the European Cancer Prevention Organization and chaired by Jaak Janssens. We are invited to talk about our work of gland development and cancer susceptibility and the role of hCG. I had met Jaak at a previous meeting that he organized in Limburg on June of 1993 for talking about "Premalignant Lesions of the Breast."*

It was at that opportunity that we presented our concepts of hCG, and Professor De Ward made important remarks on the significance of our work. Therefore, the relation with the European

Cancer Prevention Organization was not new for us. At the end of the meeting in the Elbingealp, Jaak drove us to Brussels very early in the morning, and Irma and Magda were sleeping in the back of the car and I was talking with Jaak about the meeting and, most important for me, how he could help us in the clinical part of our work. Based on that talk with Jaak and our preclinical data that had demonstrated that hCG treatment of virgin rats prevented the initiation and inhibited the progression of DMBA-induced mammary carcinomas, we decided to test this in humans with his collaboration. At this time, Jaak Janssens was a professor at the University of Hasselt in Belgium [119]. Our initial protocol was to use r-hCG or Ovidrel (Serono Pharmaceutical Company) on primary breast cancer in postmenopausal patients. For this purpose, we recruited 25 postmenopausal women with newly diagnosed breast cancers larger than 1.5 cm in diameter. They received multiple tru-cut needle biopsy of the primary tumor for morphological, immunohistochemical, and biochemical analyses. Large core biopsy methods were not available at this time. A blood sample was taken as well. Twenty patients were given r-hCG and five patients received placebo. Randomization was done immediately after histological confirmation of malignancy in a 4:1 ratio. Then 500 μg of r-hCG or saline was injected IM every other day. Each patient received seven injections. We evaluated the tumor response and side effects according to contemporary standards [120, 121]. Two weeks after the start of the treatment, surgery was performed with either lumpectomy or mastectomy according to the clinical presentation and choice of the patient. Each patient had axillary dissection. The study was terminated after surgery. None of the patients had metastatic disease. Post-surgical treatment was given according to the institutional guidelines with adjuvant radiotherapy, chemotherapy or/and hormone therapy. We studied seven intermediate end points of hCG effects on breast cancer. A decrease in cell proliferation (inhibition) was expected with down-regulation of the alpha estrogen receptor and progesterone receptor. Activation of programmed cell death genes, p53 and p21 tumor suppressor genes, c-myc oncogene and inhibin growth factor was hypothesized as well. All patients treated with r-hCG showed a decrease in proliferative index (Ki67) between the start and the end

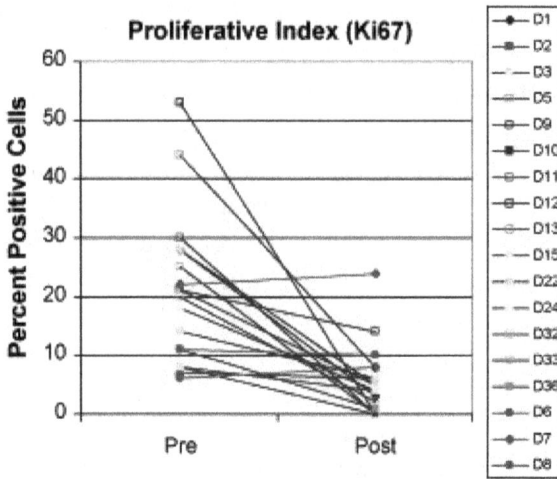

Figure 11.18: Treatment of primary breast cancer with 500 μg r-hCG decreases the proliferation index, as measured with Ki67 antibodies.

of treatment. No effect was seen in the placebo (red lines in the figure) treated patients (Figure 11.18).

The proliferation index dropped from an average of 20% of labeled cells up to 5, meaning a 75% overall reduction. The placebos had an average of 10% and remained at this level after treatment. Both progesterone (PgR) and estrogen (ER) receptors decreased from an average of 34–10% labeled cells to give an overall reduction of 74%. During the r-hCG treatment, the estradiol level in the plasma remained about 8 ng/dl and was identical for the placebo and r-hCG group. This observation excludes the possible interference of endogenous estrogen change as an explanation of r-hCG activity. No change was also observed for inhibin, progesterone and follicle-stimulating hormone (FSH) concentration during the treatment period. In contrast, luteotrope hormone (LH) concentrations were increased. From this study, we concluded that r-hCG reduces significantly the proliferative index in primary breast cancers; r-hCG reduces also the expression of both ER and PgR but does not modify the hormonal level of estradiol, progesterone, inhibin, or FSH. The levels of LH seemed significantly increased but here an interference with r-hCG can be expected. We published these studies in 2007 [119].

Encouraged by the subclinical effects of r-hCG, we continued teaming up with Jaak Janssens and decided to make an open-label, single center study testing the inhibitory effect of r-hCG on metastatic breast cancers in postmenopausal women. The primary objective was to assess the effect of r-hCG on the tumor response rate. Secondary objectives were to assess the effect on symptoms of the tumors, to assess the adverse systemic effects, to measure time to tumor progression and to assess the effects of endocrinology and tumor markers. All 13 postmenopausal breast cancer patients with metastatic breast cancer were treated every other day with 500 µg r-hCG IM. Every 60 days, a clinical evaluation was performed with study of the tumor parameters. Tumor response was on radiological or clinical measurable tumor lesions according to the WHO-criteria [121].

In this pilot clinical trial that we published with Jaak in *Molecular and Cellular Endocrinology* in 2007, we clearly showed that in four patients who had progressive disease, after 60 days, seven patients had stable disease and two patients had a decrease of the soft tissue localizations for more than 50% of the initial diameters. No complete remission was seen partly as a result of the high percentage of patients with bone lesions.

The longest remission in a patient with partial remission was 240 days. The response in the liver was evaluable in nine patients: two with progressive disease, two partial remissions, and five stable diseases. Our final conclusion was that the r-hCG was active in the treatment of postmenopausal metastatic breast cancer. The response duration was relatively short but most of the patients had extensive prior treatments. A response to previous hormonal treatment is indicative for response to r-hCG [119].

From the evidence that r-hCG produced clinical responses in both early and metastasized breast cancer, there was reason to believe that r-hCG might be active in cancer prevention trials. It was at this point that Jaak, Irma, and I started to receive support from the Serono Company in Geneva, Switzerland, for our study. Although Serono supported our initiative, they were not interested in the prevention part of r-hCG, and they saw an economical potential in the treatment of breast cancer using the r-hCG. The Serono Company supported our research and was basically interested in comparing the u-hCG and r-hCG and demonstrating that the effect we had observed initially using the u-hCG was due to the hormone and not to a contaminant/s that could be present in the u-hCG.

Our studies not only demonstrated that r-hCG was the real hormone involved in the prevention of breast cancer but also had the potential for treating the disease. The data were published few months before Irma's death in 2013 [101]. Serono also decided to make a larger clinical trial to test the treatment property of r-hCG, however, none of us participated in the final conclusion of their data. Ironically, a patent was granted by the United States Patent office on February 27, 2007 for the use of r-hCG in the treatment of breast cancer (Figure 11.19).

Our goal of using r-hCG in prevention and having a large pharmaceutical company support us vanished when Serono Pharmaceutical decided not to continue supporting this line of research. It took almost 10 more years to develop a clinical trial (see Chapter 14).

11.5.4.4. *Comparative effects of the preventive effect of pregnancy, steroidal hormones, and hCG*

It was of utmost importance for us to pursue our ideas further and identify the molecular pathways that were responsible for the hormonally-induced prevention. We presented a grant application to the Barbara Komen Foundation for the Cure postulating that chromatin remodeling was the mechanism by which pregnancy and hCG induce breast cancer prevention. This was a well-crafted proposal involving animal studies followed by a detailed clinical protocol. Unfortunately, they did not fund the clinical part but they awarded me the grant KG101080 for conducting a detailed transcriptomic analysis of the resting mammary glands of Sprague Dawley rats that had been treated for 21 days with hCG, full-term pregnancy or treatment with a pellet of estrogen and progesterone (pellet). The data demonstrated that the three protocols induced differentiation of

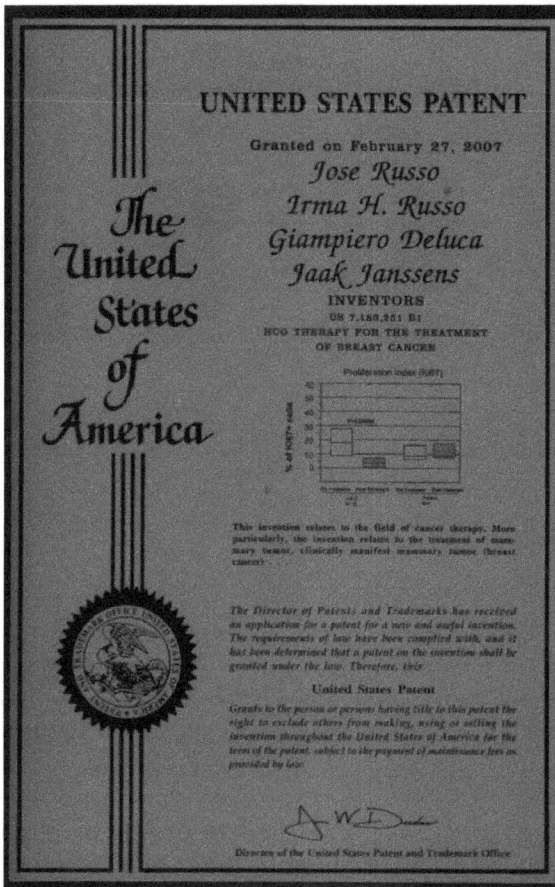

Figure 11.19: Patent for the use of r-hCG in the treatment of breast cancer.

the mammary gland, and there were common genes that constituted the genomic signature explaining the preventive effects of these approaches (Figure 11.20). Importantly enough, the transcriptomic profile induced by hCG provided a new insight in the use of this hormone as a preventive agent in human breast cancer. The genomic signature of the mammary gland induced in virgin animals by exogenous administration of hCG was similar to that induced by pregnancy, and those specific genomic profiles are still manifested 42 days post termination of treatment (Figures 11.21 and 11.22) [108].

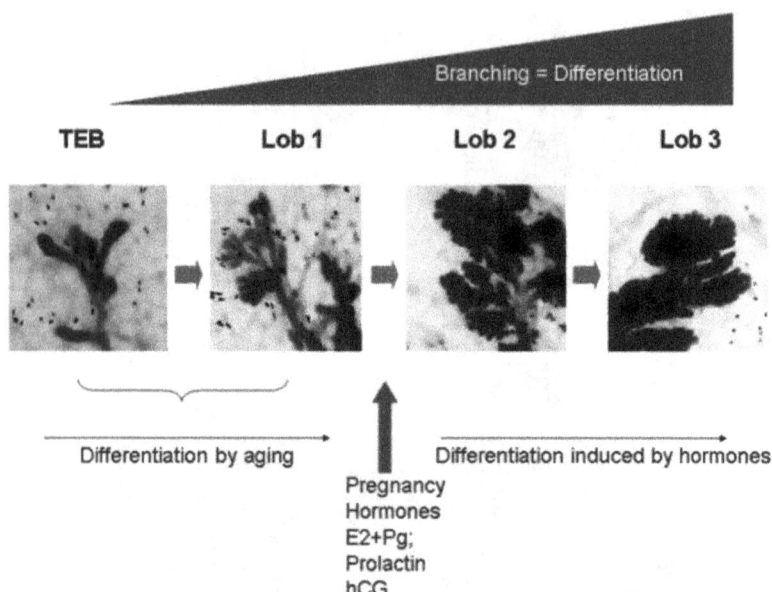

Figure 11.20: Pathway of mammary gland differentiation from the terminal end buds (TEB) to the formation of lobules type 1, 2, and 3. Differentiation and branching occurring from lobules type 1 to 2 and 3 are mainly driven by an endogenous hormonal stimulation like pregnancy of exogenous hormonal treatment.

The importance of these specific signatures was highlighted by the fact that administration of carcinogen to hCG-treated or control virgin rats whose mammary glands appear morphologically similar will induce a markedly different tumorigenic response, supporting the concept that the differentiation induced by hCG was expressed at the genomic level and resulted in a shifting of the susceptible cells to refractory stem cells. The permanence of these changes, in turn, makes them ideal surrogate markers for the evaluation of hCG effect as a breast cancer preventive agent [85, 91, 96, 122–151]. There is a group of genes that is up-regulated in the three preventive modalities tested that are related to the inflammatory response. As depicted in Figure 11.22, the preventive signature of the mammary gland is related to the up-regulation of genes controlling cell differentiation, innate immune defense, inhibition of cell proliferation, angiogenesis,

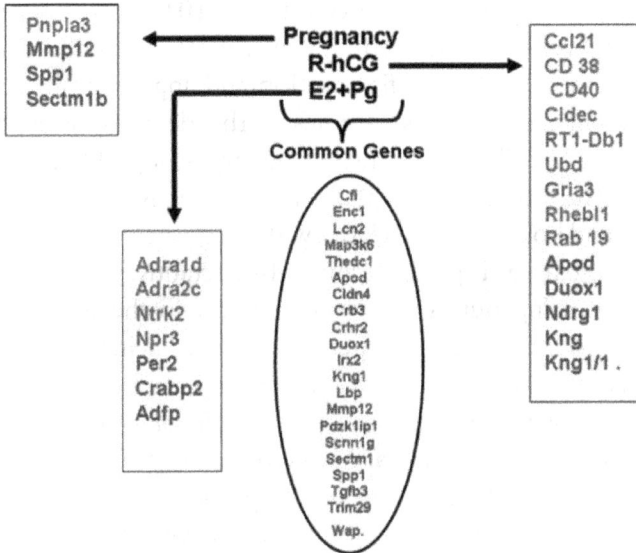

Figure 11.21: Common genes and specific transcripts expressed in the rat mammary gland following pregnancy, hCG and pellets using a p < 0.01 and FC of 2.0.

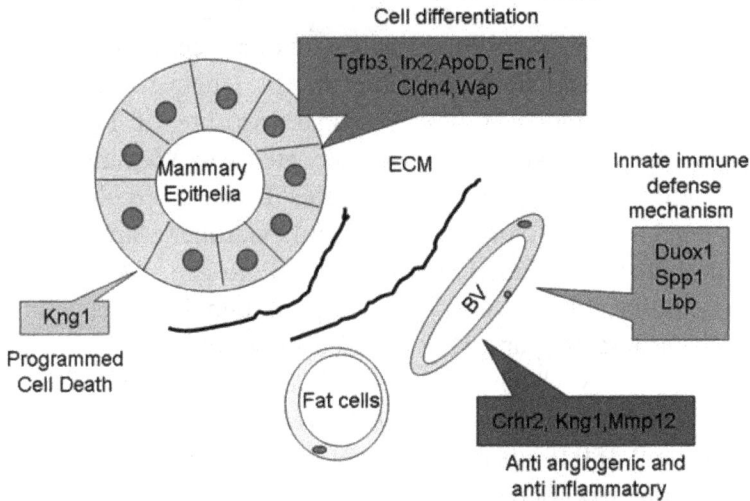

Figure 11.22: Schematic representation of the different biological processes involved in the prevention signature.

inflammation, and programmed cell death [101]. This indicates that the epithelial cells are interacting very actively with the stroma by halting many stressors like inflammation and angiogenesis.

The significance of these studies is the demonstration that the transcriptomic profile of the rat mammary gland displays a set of common genes that can explain the protective effect of hCG, pregnancy, and hormones associated with pregnancy, like the combined use of estrogen and progesterone. Importantly, these preventive strategies occurring during a narrow window in the development of the breast would succeed in permanently inducing the molecular changes that will make the mammary gland resistant to develop cancer.

Of relevance is that hCG induces specific set of genes and wider transcriptomic changes that could be extremely important to control the progression of the differentiation pathway, and that these changes are permanently imprinted in the mammary gland, regulating its long-lasting refractoriness to develop cancer.

11.6. Demonstrating that estrogens are carcinogenic

On Monday, April 22, 1996, I was a part of a meeting organized by Dr. David G. Longfellow, the Chief of the Chemical and Physical Carcinogenesis Branch of the National Institute of Health. The meeting took place at the Renaissance Hotel in Washington, DC. Also invited to the meeting were Maarten Bosland, Ercole Cavalieri, Bob Creveling, Krystyna Frenkel, Hank Gardner, Shuk-Mei Ho, Joachim Liehr. Leo Liu, Don Malins, Elli Rogan, Deodutta Roy, Thomas Sutter, Judith Weisz, Jim Yager, Colin Jefcoate, Shutsung Liao, Richard Santen, and Richard Weinshiboum. All of them stellar scientists that have been making seminal contributions in steroids hormones and cancer. *Tom Sutter and Colin Jefcoate* were working on cytochrome P-450 lBl, particularly metabolism of estradiol at the C-4 position. *Maarten Bosland* was working in prevention of prostate cancer, especially the role of hormones in these processes. *Ercole Cavalieri* has been the pioneer in developing the concept that estrogens are like any other chemical carcinogens, and his first plan was to establish the mechanism of tumor initiation and then develop prevention strategies. His closet collaborator was *Eleanor G. Rogan*, who had begun analysis of catechol estrogen metabolites in human breast cancer samples by GC/MS; these studies also included analysis of COMT and S-transferases. *Joachim Liehr*, who died of pancreatic cancer was a pioneering figure in his work on estrogen metabolism, particularly 4-hydroxylation by cytochrome P-450 lBl and possibly other enzyme(s) in human breast and prostate tissue. He was also interested in mutations caused by estrogen-induced hydroxy radical damage of DNA. *Judy Weisz* was known for her studies on metabolic activation of estrogen to biologically reactive products and early initiating phases in normal human breast. *Bob Creveling* had been recently appointed head officer of technology development of the NIDDK, but still was collaborating with some laboratories, particularly on COMT, analyzing patient records at the Mayo Clinic with *Richard Weinchiboum* to determine whether patients with low COMT activities in red blood cells had a higher incidence of estrogen site cancers: *Hank Gardner* was the Director of the US Army Biomedical Research Laboratory in Frederick and was particularly interested in the role of oxygenated products in carcinogenesis. *Shuk-Mei Ho* was working in those days in androgen-supported estrogen promotion of prostate cancer, combined effects of estrogens and androgens to act as mitogens, inducers of oxidative stress, effects on receptors, and escape from senescence. *Leo Liu* was the Program Director, Chemical and Physical Carcinogenesis Branch at the NCI and was interested in the mechanisms of carcinogenesis, particularly in the prostate and bladder. Many of the Cube's participants have grants in their portfolio. *Krystyna Frenkel* was interested in the role of reactive oxygen species in carcinogenesis, especially as tumor promoters and biomarkers of cancer risk. *Jim Yager* had performed studies in oral contraceptives and liver tumors and at that time was interested in cell proliferation in the liver in response to levels of estrogens and the relationship between promoters and liver cell proliferation. *Deodutta Roy* was studying the influence of estrogens and estrogen-like chemicals on DNA, excision repair of DNA, and polymerase-initiated genomic instability. *Don Malins*, a member of the National Academy of Science, was working in alterations induced in DNA in human breast tumors. *Richard Santen* was mainly working on the role of anti-aromatase in breast cancer, and he was the most clinically oriented in the group. I was invited to be a part of this group for my work in breast cancer prevention, hormone modulation of proliferation and differentiation of human breast tissue and how hormones initiated breast cancer.

David Longfellow was the facilitator of the group and he indicated in that encounter that the meeting and focus group grew out of his discussions with Ercole Cavalieri and Joachin Liehr on how best to proceed rapidly with broad-based research focused on the hypothesis that activation of endogenous catechol estrogens leads to modification of DNA to initiate the process leading to cancer. The aim of this focus group was to demonstrate to the scientific community and to the National Cancer Institute leadership the opportunities for understanding the role of endogenous carcinogenesis afforded by combined efforts investigating this hypothesis, and to take advantage of the opportunity to move faster in this research arena than we could individually, and to capitalize on our intellectual and technological resources. Our mutual interests and efforts can be thought of as a *Complementary Collaborative Coalition*, which led Dr. Longfellow to name the group the "cancer Cube"(C3) on estrogen carcinogenesis. Dr. Richard Klaussner, the new Director of the NCI at that time, was promoting the idea of collaboration for furthering the research and as a focus group such as the cancer cube may serve as a new model of how to move forward.

It took almost 5 years for the group to amalgam, with encounters twice a year teaching each other and discussing how estrogen could be a carcinogen. It is difficult to forget the dinners that we enjoyed and that was due to the gourmet taste of Ercole Cavalieri to find a five-star restaurant to dine in every place around the country that we met. A real friendship resulted from all these encounters, and finally we were able to put a grant proposal together. However, from the initial group that started in 1996 a consortium was formed by only a few of us, *I* was from FCCC, *Ercole Cavalieri and Eleanor G.*

Rogan from the University of Nebraska, *Thomas Sutter* from the University of Memphis, *Richard Santen* from the University of Virginia, and *Joachim Liehr* from the University of Texas in Galveston. Dear Joachin Liehr died one day after the Breast Cancer Center of Excellence was funded by the Department of Defense in 2000. The funding of the Center of Excellence provided me with funds for extending my collaborations with Dr. Maria Luiza Mello and Dr. Benedicto Vidal from the University of Campinas, Brazil, generating information on the changes in nuclear structure of estrogen-induced cell transformation. The study on the epithelial mesenchymal transition of breast epithelial cells transformed by estrogen was performed in close collaboration with Dr. Thomas Sutter from the University of Memphis and with Dr. Daniel Tiezzi (University of Ribeiro Preito, Brazil). The epithelial mesenchymal transition of breast epithelial cells transformed by estrogen has been a part of Dr. Tiezzi's doctoral thesis. Altogether, this project has generated novel insights in the molecular basis of estrogen-induced carcinogenesis and 59 publications were generated from these studies [40, 41, 152–208].

With the resources provided by Breast Cancer Center of Excellence, funded by the Department of Defense, we were able to generate: 1) *the only model of human breast cell transformation using 17β-estradiol, 2) a new insight into the process of epithelial mesenchymal transition, and 3) a unique model of triple-negative breast cancer.*

11.6.1. *17β-estradiol induces transformation and tumorigenesis in human breast epithelial cells*

Breast cancer is a malignancy whose dependence on estrogen exposure has long been recognized, even though the mechanisms through which estrogens cause cancer are not clearly understood. This work was performed in order to determine whether 17β-estradiol (E_2), the predominant circulating ovarian steroid, is carcinogenic in human breast epithelial cells (HBECs) and whether non-receptor mechanisms are involved in the initiation of breast cancer. For this purpose, the effect of four alternating 24-hour treatment periods with 70 nM E_2

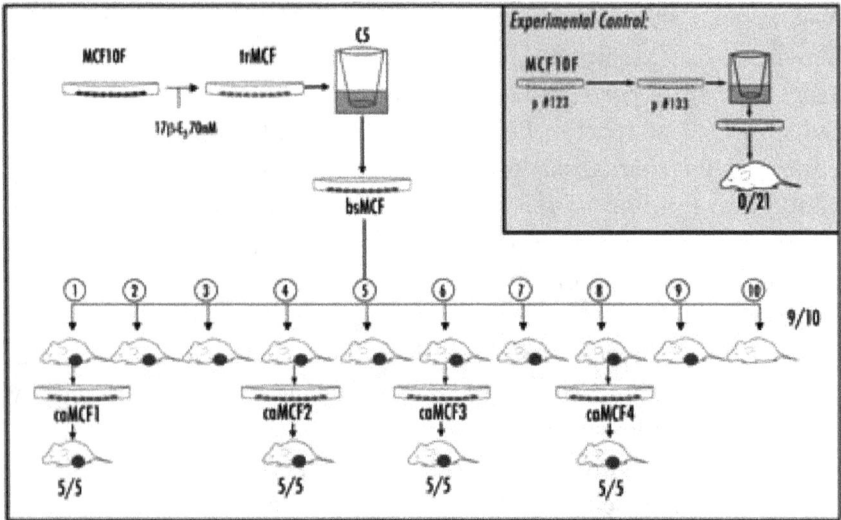

Figure 11.23: Schematic representation of the experimental protocol. MCF-10F cells were treated with 70 nM 17β-estradiol (17β-E$_2$ 70 nM) for 24-hour periods, twice a week during 2 weeks. After the last treatment, the cells were passaged 7–9 times before being tested for colony efficiency, ductulogenesis in collagen, invasion in Matrigel, and tumorigenesis in SCID mice. For the invasion assay, the cells were trypsinized and seeded in the invasion chambers at a concentration of 2.5×10^4 cells/well, incubated for 22 hours and then, the membranes of the inserts were cut and invasive cells (bsMCF) were cultured in 24 well plates. The invasive cells were expanded and evaluated for the expression of tumorigenesis in SCID mice. Here, 9 out of 10 mice injected with bsMCF developed tumors. Tumors from four of the animals were dissected in 0.5–1 mm size fragments, incubated in culture medium until confluent, generating cell lines from each tumor that were subsequently injected to 5 mice per cell line for evaluation of their tumorigenic potential. All injected animals developed tumors. All tumors and cell lines were analyzed histopathologically and immunocytochemically as well as for fingerprint and CGH analyses. None of the animals injected with MCF-10F control cells or trMCF developed tumors.

of the estrogen receptor alpha (ER-α) negative MCF-10F cell line on the *in vitro* expression of neoplastic transformation was evaluated (Figure 11.23).

E$_2$-treatment induced the expression of anchorage independent growth, loss of ductulogenesis in collagen, invasiveness in Matrigel, and loss of 9p11-13. Tumorigenesis in SCID mice was expressed only in invasive cells that in addition exhibited a deletion of 4p15.3-16. Tumors formed in SCID mice were poorly differentiated adenocarcinomas that were estrogen receptor α and progesterone receptor negative, expressed keratins, EMA and e-cadherin. Drs. Johana Vanegas and Patricia Russo in the BCRL performed a time-lapse photography in order to study the motility of MCF-10F and the effect of estrogens and its metabolites on cell motility and migratory movements. The relationship between cell motility *in vitro* and the ability of neoplastic cells to invade and metastasize *in vivo* is well known. This led us to evaluate the migratory behavior of the HBEC line MCF-10F after neoplastic transformation with 70 nM of 17β-estradiol (E_2), 4 OH estradiol (4-OH-E_2) and 2-OH estradiol (2-OH-E_2). Cells thus transformed express colony formation in agar methocel, loss of ductulogenic capacity in collagen matrix, and invasiveness in a Matrigel artificial membrane. Patricia Russo and Johana Vanegas set up a time-lapse video microscopy system to directly observe and capture the cells' images using a Nikon DXM digital camera attached to an Olympus IMT-2 microscope that was equipped with a Plexiglas incubation chamber. From each cell line a random number of cells were selected for tracking at one-hour intervals. Cell motility was evaluated by determining the speed of the tracked cell expressed in mm/min (S), the direction persistence in time (P), and the random motility coefficient (μ) that provides a measure of how fast a cell population will grow to cover a surface. Our findings were published [152] and they indicated that the transformation of HBEC by estrogen and its metabolites induce changes in cell motility *in vitro*, 4-OH-E_2 being the one inducing the most significant changes, its effect correlated to the expression of phenotypes indicative of cell transformation.

11.6.2. *Epithelial to mesenchymal transition in HBECs transformed by 17β-estradiol*

Our laboratory was one of the first to demonstrate that 17β-estradiol (E_2) induces complete neoplastic transformation of the HBECs MCF-10F. E_2-treatment of MCF-10F cells progressively induced

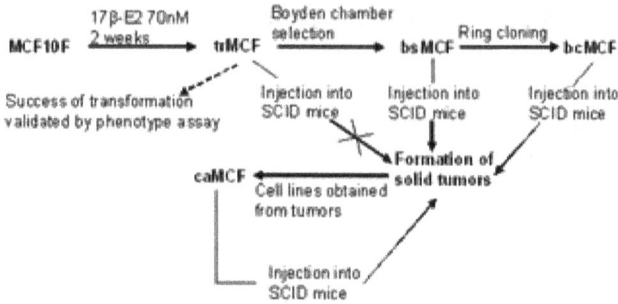

Figure 11.24: Transformation of MCF-10F cells by 17β-estradiol treatment. Experimental protocol: MCF-10F cells treated with 70 nM 17β-estradiol (E_2) that expressed high colony efficiency (CE) and loss of ductulogenic capacity in collagen-matrix were classified as transformed (trMCF). Transformed cells that were invasive in Matrigel Boyden type invasion chambers were selected (bsMCF) and plated at low density for cloning (bcMCF). MCF-10F, trMCF, bsMCF, and bcMCF were tested for carcinogenicity by injecting them into the mammary fat pad of 45-day-old female SCID mice. MCF-10F and trMCF cells did not induce tumors (cancelled arrow); bsMCF, and bcMCF formed solid tumors from which four cell lines, identified as caMCF, were derived and proven to be tumorigenic in SCID mice.

high colony efficiency and loss of ductulogenesis in early transformed (trMCF) cells, invasiveness in Matrigel invasion chambers. The cells that crossed the chamber membrane were collected and identified as bsMCF, and their subclones designated bcMCF, and the cells harvested from carcinoma formation in SCID mice designated (caMCF) (Figure 11.24). These phenotypes correlated with gene dysregulation during the progression of the transformation. The highest number of dysregulated genes was observed in caMCF cells, being slightly lower in bcMCF cells, and lowest in trMCF cells. This order was consistent with the extent of chromosome aberrations (caMCF > bcMCF >>> trMCF). Chromosomal amplifications were found in 1p36.12-pter, 5q21.1-qter, and 13q21.31-qter. Losses of the complete chromosome 4 and of 8p11.21-23.1 were found only in tumorigenic cells. In tumor-derived cell lines, additional losses were found in 3p12.1-14.1, 9p22.1-pter, and 18q11.21-qter.

Functional profiling of deregulated genes revealed progressive changes in the integrin signaling pathway, inhibition of apoptosis, acquisition of tumorigenic cell surface markers, and epithelial to mesenchymal transition. In tumorigenic cells, the levels of E-cadherin, EMA, and various keratins were low and CD44E/CD24 were negative, whereas SNAI2, vimentin, S100A4, FN1, HRAS and TGFβ1, and CD44H were high (Figure 11.25).

The phenotypic and genomic changes triggered by estrogen exposure that lead normal cells to tumorigenesis confirm the role of this steroid hormone in cancer initiation. Our work has been published in high impact journals like *International Journal of Cancer* and *Cancer Research* emphasizing the importance of being able to make a normal cell like MCF-10F neoplastically transformed by treatment with a natural hormone. More importantly, the cell is estrogen receptor negative emphasizing that the traditional pathway of action for estrogen and its receptors is not the main pathway of the neoplastic process. It is known that prolonged exposure to estrogen is a risk factor for human breast cancer, but the role of estrogen in the development of human breast cancer has been difficult to ascertain. There are three mechanisms that have been considered responsible for the carcinogenicity of estrogens: a receptor mediated hormonal activity, cytochrome P450-mediated metabolic activation, and induction of aneuploidy. The receptor-mediated hormonal activity of estrogen has generally been related to stimulation of cellular proliferation, resulting in more opportunities for accumulation of genetic damages leading to carcinogenesis. Since local synthesis of estrogen in the stromal component can increase the estrogen levels and growth rate of breast carcinoma, a paracrine mechanism is likely to account for interactions between aromatase-containing stromal cells and ER-containing breast tumor epithelial cells. More importantly, estrogen may not need to activate nuclear receptors alpha to initiate or promote breast carcinogenesis. We have evidence that ERP may also be involved in this process and that oxidative catabolism of estrogens mediated by various CYP complexes constitutes a pathway of their metabolic activation and generates reactive-free radicals and intermediate metabolites reactive

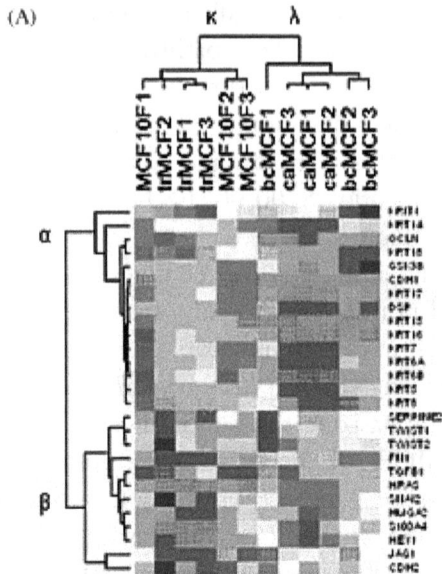

Figure 11.25: (A) A list of EMT markers and promoting genes was generated *a priori* by literature search. Hierarchical clustering of cell lines and genes was performed using dChip software. Two sample clusters (κ and λ) and two gene clusters (α and β) were identified. The red, white, and blue colors represent level above, at, and below mean expression, respectively. (B) Detection of epithelial and mesenchymal markers by immunochytochemistry: (a) Histological sections of MCF-10F cells, reacted with pre-immune mouse serum, were used as the negative control (×100); (b) MCF-10F reacted for EMA (×100); (c) MCF-10F reacted for E-Cadherin (×100); (d) MCF-10F reacted for vimentin (×100); (e) trMCF cells reacted with pre-immune mouse serum used as negative control (×100); (f), (g), (h) trMCF cells reacted for EMA, E-cadherin and vimentin, respectively (×100); (i) bsMCF cells reacted with pre-immune mouse serum as a negative control (×100); (j), (k), (l) bsMCF cells reacted for EMA, E-cadherin, and vimentin, respectively (×100); (m) caMCF tumor cell line cells reacted with pre-immune mouse serum used as negative control (×100); (n), (o), (p) caMCF tumor cell lines reacted for EMA, E-cadherin and vimentin, respectively (×100); (q), (r) invasive ductal carcinoma of the breast as positive control and immunoreacted for EMA and E-cadherin, respectively (×100); (s) histological section of an invasive adenocarcinoma immunoreacted for vimentin (×100).

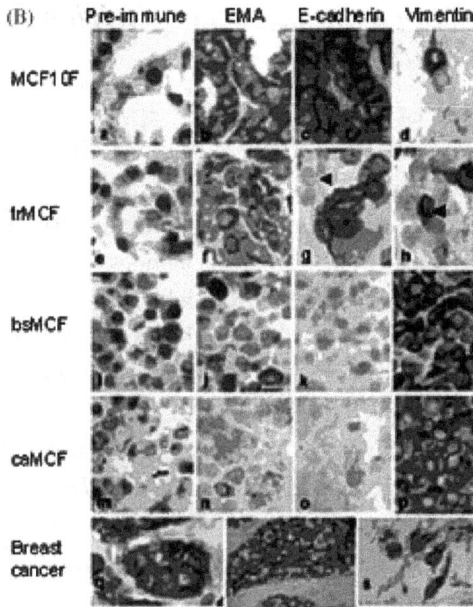

Figure 11.25: (*Continued*)

intermediates that can cause oxidative stress and genomic damage directly. Estrogen-induced genotoxic effects include increased mutation rates, MSI and LOH in chromosomes 3 and 11. A compromised DNA repair system that allows accumulation of genomic lesions is essential to estrogen-induced tumorigenesis. Metabolic biotransformation of estrogen does occur in human mammary explant culture. Increased formation of catechol estrogens as a result of elevated hydroxylation of 17β-estradiol at C-4 and C-16a positions has been observed in human breast cancer patients and in women at a higher risk of developing this disease. There is also evidence that formation of superoxide and hydrogen peroxide, as a result of the metabolism of estrogen, might also be involved in estrogen-mediated oxidative stress. In fact, a substantial increase in base lesions observed in the DNA of invasive ductal carcinoma of the breast has been postulated to result from the oxidative stress associated with metabolism of 17β-estradiol. Altogether the data thus far accumulated indicate that more than one pathway may be necessary to initiate neoplastic transformation and maintaining of the transformation phenotypes leading to tumorigenesis.

11.6.3. *Developing a unique model of triple-negative breast cancer*

Triple-negative breast cancer (TNBC) represents a heterogeneous group of cancers characterized by a lack of ER, PgR, and HER2 expression. Cluster analysis of human TNBC identified six subtypes displaying unique gene expression and ontologies [209]. Approximately 80% of TNBC show features of basal-like cancers [210]. Transcriptional profile analysis assigned 21 TNBC cell lines into three clusters: luminal, basal A, and basal B [211–213]. Basal A contains cell lines, such as BT-20, Sum149, and MDA-MB-468, which preferentially express genes such as *CK5/6*, *CK14*, and *EGFR*. Basal B includes cell lines, such as MDA-MB-231, Sum159pt, and Hs578t, which preferentially express genes, such as *CD44*, *VIM*, and *SNAI2*, and exhibit a stem cell-like profile [211]. This classification of TNBC cell lines is closely associated with cell morphology and invasive potential. Basal B cells have a more mesenchymal-like appearance and are less differentiated and much more invasive compared to the other two clusters. Analysis of the relationship between TNBC cell lines and tumor subtypes showed that most of basal A and basal B cell lines resemble basal-like tumors [211], indicating that TNBC cell lines are suitable for investigations of subtype-specific cancer cell biology.

Although there are over 20 commercially available TNBC cell lines, MDA-MB-231 is the most widely used *in vitro* and *in vivo*. In BALB/CAJCI-nu/nu mice, it took five weeks to form a xenograft around 6.5 mm in diameter with the subcutaneous injection of 5×10^6 MDA-MB-231 cells [214]. MDA-MB-468 cells had a growth speed similar to MDA-MB-231 in the same mouse strain [214].

The growth speed of MDA-MB-231 xenograft in CB17/SCID was almost the same as in nude mice, while BT-549 cells grew a little bit slower than MDA-MB-231 cells in CB17/SCID mice [215]. Sum149 and Sum159 are two highly tumorigenic cell lines; it was reported the injection of 1×10^5 cells in non-obese diabetic SCID mice could produce tumors in 3/4 and 5/6 mice, respectively [216]. But these two cell lines are mainly used for the study of inflammatory breast cancer [217, 218].

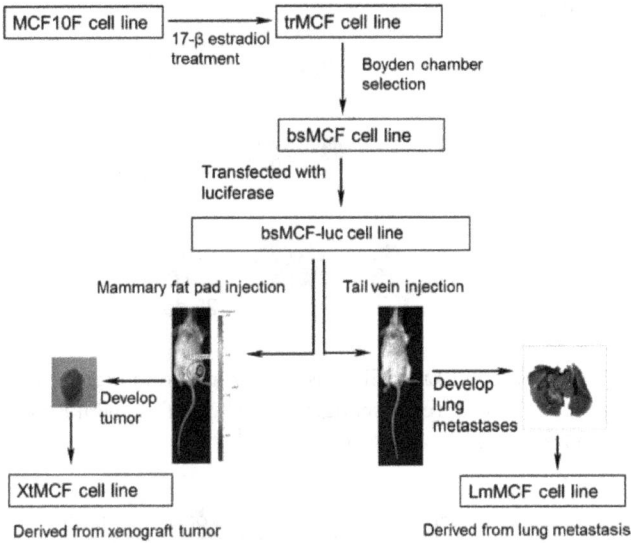

Figure 11.26:   Schematic representation of the establishment of a TNBC model.

With Dr. Yanrong Su and by support of private donation of The Flyers Wives, we have established [219] *a progressive TNBC model* (Figure 11.26) *consisting of normal MCF-10F, transformed cell line trMCF, and tumorigenic cell lines bsMCF, XtMCF and LmMCF. Compared to the other nine tumorigenic TNBC cell lines, our cell lines XtMCF and LmMCF are the most tumorigenic and metastatic.*

The expression of cytokeratin 18 (CK18) confirmed the epithelial origin of this cell model, and we observed that CK18 was down-regulated in bsMCF cell line and its derivatives. Furthermore, CK18 was lost in the lung metastases, whereas still present in the xenografts of both XtMCF and LmMCF cells, suggesting down-regulation of CK18 may be related to breast tumor progression [220]. Our study also showed that the CK5-positive cell number was inversely correlated to the clinical stage of TNBC [221, 222], suggesting that our cell model reflects features of TNBC progression.

The EMT process is not only closely related to cancer invasion and metastasis but also conferred to the generation of cancer stem cells (CSC) [223–225]. As bsMCF-luc, XtMCF, and LmMCF have

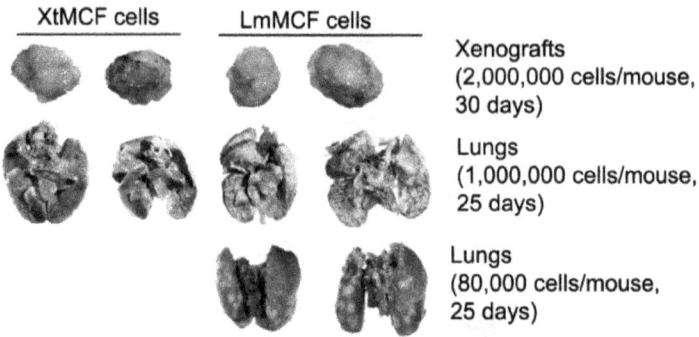

Figure 11.27: XtMCF and LmMCF cells display high tumorigenic and metastatic potential. Representative pictures of xenografts and lungs fixed with Bouin's solution. Magnification: 6.3× for xenografts. 8× for lungs.

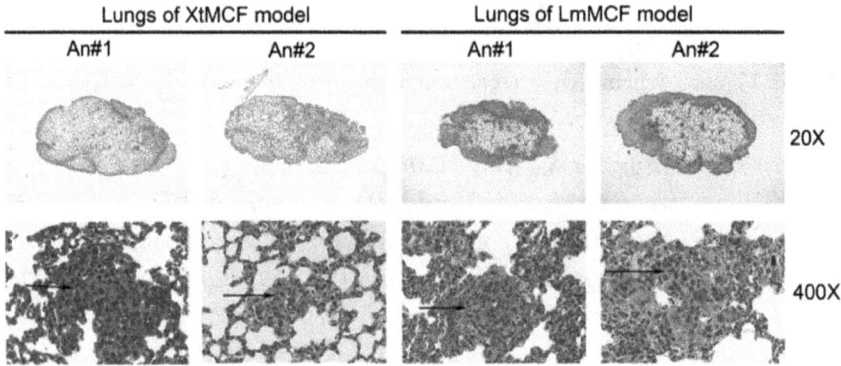

Figure 11.28: H&E staining of lungs from the injection of 1×10^6 cells into tail vein. LmMCF cells are more metastatic than XtMCF cells. Arrows indicate the metastases. Magnifications are shown in figure.

undergone EMT, we evaluated their CSC properties and the results showed that they could form tumorspheres, and the number of tumorspheres was progressively increasing from bsMCF-luc to XtMCF and LmMCF cells, consistent with *in vivo* tumorigenic and metastatic potential.

In this work [221], we postulated that the evaluation of CSC markers would give us a rationale for the high tumorigenic and metastatic potential of these two cell lines (Figures 11.27 and 11.28). Our results showed that the bsMCF-luc and XtMCF cells were

CD24^{low}/CD44$^+$, whereas LmMCF cells were CD44$^+$ with moderate CD24 expression. CD24$^{-/low}$/CD44$^+$ has been frequently used as CSC markers of breast cancers [226–228]. However, it was shown that the percentage of CD24$^{-/low}$/CD44$^+$ associates with a basal-like phenotype, not tumorigenicity, but CD24$^{-/low}$/CD44$^+$/EpCAM$^+$ cells enrich for tumorigenicity [222, 227]. EpCAM induces expressions of reprogramming factors and EMT genes, regulates EMT progression, and tumorigenesis [229]. In addition, EpCAM can be cleaved at several sites, and the nuclear translocation of cytoplasmic domain (EpCID) associates with Wnt pathway and promotes cell proliferation and tumor formation in mice [230]. One of the EpCAM cleavage sites between two arginine residues (AA80 and AA81) was detected and described in the late 1980s, but the functional consequence is still unknown [231]. Interestingly, we observed the expression of EpCAM in the cell lines we examined by immunofluorescence staining and WB, but the EGF-like domain of EpCAM was absent in mesenchymal-like cells, suggesting that the EGF-like domain might be cleaved off from the cleavage site between AA80 and AA81. This was supported by other workers [232–238]. The majority of commercial antibodies for EpCAM react with overlapped or partly overlapped epitope at EGF-like domain [239]. This may result in failing detection of EpCAM in cells which have undergone EMT. Our study indicates that the EGF-like-domain-cleaved-off EpCAM may be associated with the EMT process. Furthermore, although the total level of EpCAM is low in mesenchymal-like cells, the subcellular localization of EpCAM may be more important to the EpCAM nuclear indicating that a strong activation of Wnt signaling was observed in these cells.

The relevance of this work is the development and characterization of two highly tumorigenic and metastatic basal B TNBC cell lines, XtMCF and LmMCF. To the best of our knowledge, they are the most tumorigenic and metastatic TNBC cell lines compared to all reported cell models used for TNBC studies. In addition, the normal and early-stage counterparts of these two cell lines are also available. Altogether, these cell lines can be used to study the evolution of TNBC, investigate molecular pathways at different stages of transformation and progression in a relatively constant genetic background, and most importantly, identify new treatments for TNBC. In addition, XtMCF and LmMCF cell lines present CSC properties and can be used for developing CSC-targeted therapy. The finding that the EGF-like domain of EpCAM is cleaved off in cancer cells which have undergone EMT also provides new insights in research of EMT and CSC, two important fields in cancer biology.

11.7. My studies on epigenetic changes and breast cancer

One of the fascinating aspects of the research inquiry is how the problem of our research makes us continuously think of other mechanisms that could be different from what was previously planned. Although epigenetic changes were on my wish list for a while, it was not introduced in our research endeavor until early 2005 when Dr. Sandra Fernandez started to work in the BCRL and examined different possibilities in the action of environmental agents in HBECs and in the mechanism of cell transformation.

11.7.1. *Epigenetic control of estrogen-induced cell transformation*

The main objective with Dr. Sandra Fernandez was to determine whether the xenoestrogenic substances bisphenol A (BPA) and butyl benzyl phthalate (BBP) play a role in the initiation of human breast cancer, and if so, whether this effect was mediated by epigenetic mechanisms. The proposed study was based on the growing concern that estrogenic environmental compounds that act as endocrine disrupting chemicals might have potentially adverse effects on hormone-sensitive organs such as the breast. This concern was further fueled by evidence indicating that natural estrogens, namely 17β-estradiol (E_2), are important factors in the initiation and progression of breast cancer. Therefore, the concern that BPA and BBP, which have estrogenic properties and are widely distributed in the environment, might also be carcinogenic for the human breast was well justified. In order to accomplish these goals, we utilized our *in vitro in vivo* model, in which we demonstrated the carcinogenicity of E_2 in the HBECs MCF-10F. The use of this powerful and unique model provided us with a tool for exploring whether BPA and BBP have relevance in the initiation of breast cancer. In these studies, we found that the expression of E_2-induced transformation phenotypes were associated with hyper or hypomethylation of genes controlling branching and ductulogenesis. These findings were the basis for our postulation that the xenoestrogens BPA and BBP could induce neoplastic transformation by behaving as epigenetic modulators inducing the silencing of critical genes by hypermethylation and/or histone modification that lead to the initiation and progression of breast cancer. The results of this work were published in the literature [207, 240, 241].

11.7.2. *Epigenetic changes in breast cancer prevention*

The inhibitory effect of hCG that we have observed in both cancer initiation and progression involved the expression of differentiation markers in breast epithelial cells, including the synthesis of *inhibin, a secreted protein with tumor suppressor activity that is hypermethylated in hormone-dependent carcinomas.* We found that in HBECs *in vitro, hCG induces the synthesis of inhibin and significantly increases the levels of acetylation of histones H3 and H4.* Our observation that hCG activates the expression of tumor suppressors, such as p53 and inhibin, that it induces histones H3 and H4 acetylation, and the fact that DMBA-induced mammary tumors overexpress DNA methyltransferase, lend support to the postulate that hCG might inhibit mammary carcinogenesis by inducing re-expression of genes silenced by DNA methylation, particularly at CpG islands. Our laboratory was the first one to report that the induction of mammary gland differentiation by hCG *in vivo* and *in vitro* treatment of HBECs both stimulated the synthesis of inhibins in the mammary epithelium. Traditionally, inhibins have been considered to be gonadal hormones whose production by granulose cells is considered to be a marker of follicular responsiveness to hCG treatment in infertility treatments. Inhibins are heterodimeric glycoproteins belonging to the inhibin/ activin family that are composed of a common 18 Kd α-subunit and one of two 14 Kd β-subunits (βA or βB), thus forming the heterodimers inhibin A (α-βA), and inhibin B (α-βB), respectively. Although inhibins are known to selectively suppress the synthesis and release of the pituitary follicle stimulating hormone (FSH), they have been recognized more recently to be part of a large group of morphogenesis and differentiation-related proteins, the transforming growth factor β (TGF-β) superfamily which also includes the β-homodimer activin.

We had previously postulated that hCG induces differentiation and activation of apoptosis-related genes via activation of inhibins, which in turn might act through autocrine or paracrine mechanisms for furthering cell differentiation and inhibiting the progression of neoplastic cells. For elucidating these mechanisms, we tested the *in vitro* effect of r-hCG and inhibin β-subunit added to the culture medium of the immortalized HBECs MCF-10F. Cells were treated with 1, 10, 50, or 100 IU r-hCG or 1, 10, 100, or 1000 ng inhibin-β-subunit per ml and cells were harvested at 1, 4, 12, or 24 hours of treatment with each one of the hormones. Control cells were treated with the same volume of buffer in which the hormones were dissolved. For Western blot analysis, total cell extracts were prepared using standard procedures in our laboratory. After quantification of protein concentration, 20 mg of each extract was separated by electrophoresis in an 8% SDS-polyacrylamide gel, transferred to nitrocellulose, and probed with a 1:200 dilution of anti-acetylated histones H3 or H4 IgGs. Horseradish peroxidase-conjugated goat anti-rabbit IgG at 1:5000 dilution was used as a secondary antibody for ECL detection. Western blot analysis revealed that hCG acetylated both histones H3 and H4 at all the doses tested and the levels significantly increased at 12 and 24 hours of treatment. Inhibin β-subunit induced the accumulation of acetylated histone H3 after 4 hour treatment with 1 ng and at all time points with the higher concentrations. A slight acetylated histone H4 increase was detected in cells treated with 100 ng/ml for 12 and 24 hours. Our data indicate that both hCG and inhibin increase acetylation levels in histone H4 in the HBEC MCF-10F. It is possible to postulate that the induction of histone acetylation by hCG and inhibin plays a role in the activation and transcription of early genes, such as *c-myc* and *c-jun*, as well as the tumor suppressors, such as p53 and inhibin, previously described. The fact that DMBA-induced mammary tumors overexpress DNA methyltransferase lend support to the postulate that hCG might inhibit mammary carcinogenesis by inducing re-expression of genes silenced by DNA methylation, particularly at CpG islands.

These findings lead us to consider that in the mechanism of action of hCG in breast cancer prevention and therapy this hormone might act not only as an activator of differentiation associated genes, but might also reactivate the expression of genes transcriptionally silenced by promoter hyper methylation during the process of carcinogenesis. We generated five publications under this project [104, 106, 242–244] and more important, opened our minds to see the epigenome as another important mechanism in both cancer and prevention.

11.7.3. *Chromatin remodeling during HBEC transformation*

We have shown that treatment of the HBECs MCF-10F with 17β-estradiol (E_2) induces transformation and tumorigenesis. E_2-transformed MCF-10F cells are known to exhibit progressive loss of ductulogenesis and invasive and tumorigenic phenotypes. DNA amounts and chromatin supraorganization change in E_2-transformed MCF cells. In a collaborative study that I started with Maria Luisa Mello and Benedicto de Campos Vidal at the University of Campinas in Brazil, we showed that Feulgen-DNA content and chromatin supra organization were involved during E_2-induced transformation and tumorigenesis of the MCF-10F cells [245]. Image analysis was performed for non-transformed and E_2-transformed MCF cells, highly invasive cells (C5), and for cell lines (C5-A6-T6 and C5-A8-T8) derived from tumors generated by injection of C5 cells in SCID mice. A decrease in Feulgen-DNA amounts and nuclear sizes induced by E_2 treatment was accented with selection of the highly invasive tumorigenesis potential. However, in the tumor-derived cells, a high variability in cellular phenotypes resulted in near-polyploidy. Significant changes in textural parameters, including nuclear entropy, indicated chromatin structural remodeling with advancing tumorigenesis. An increased variability in the degree of chromatin packing states in the E_2-transformed MCF cells was followed by reduction in chromatin condensation and in contrast between condensed and non-condensed chromatin in the highly invasive C5 cells and tumor-derived cell lines.

Whereas these initial studies were not groundbreaking, they provided me, and as a consequence the whole BCRL, with a better understanding of what later on we found out could be essential for the understanding of the mechanism induced by pregnancy and hCG in the human breast.

11.7.4. *Epigenetic control of epithelial mesenchymal transition (EMT) leading to tumor invasion*

In a manuscript published in *Cancer Research* in 2007 in collaboration with the group of Thomas Sutter [165], we started to discuss the role of chromatin remodeling and epigenetic control in the transformation of HBECs. We found that a network of several signaling pathways affecting the expression and/or function of a complex hierarchical network of transcription factors (TFs) has been partially elaborated. Known signaling pathways include multiple tyrosine kinase receptors leading to Ras-mediated activation of MAPK and PI3K pathways, TGF-β, Notch and Wnt. Evidence for enhanced TGF-β and Wnt signaling pathways was found in the EMT expressing bcMCF and caMCF cells. TGF-β acting through Smad transcriptional complexes can repress expression of the Id TFs (Id1, Id2, Id3) and activate HMGA2, a DNA-binding protein important for chromatin architecture. Expression of HMGA2 is known to regulate several EMT controlling TFs including TWIST1, SNAI1, and SNAI2 (Slug) (Figure 11.29). TGF-β and Wnt signaling also affect the expression of several additional EMT-regulating TFs including ZEB1 (TCF8), TCF3 (E2A encoding E12 and E47), and LEF1. Analysis of the EMT expressing bcMCF cell line revealed the absence of expression of the secreted frizzled-related protein 1 (SFRP1), a repressor of Wnt signaling. One allele of SFRP1 was deleted in these cells, with the remaining apparently silenced by methylation, accounting for the twenty-eight-fold reduction of this

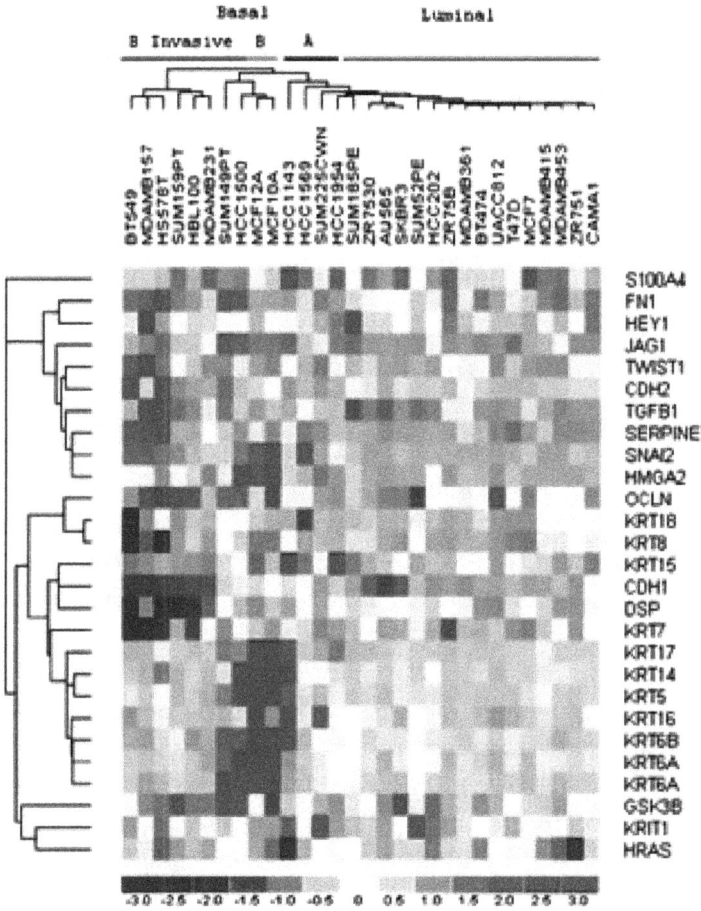

Figure 11.29: Heat map showing the EMT.

transcript. Loss and epigenetic inactivation of SFRP1 occurs often in invasive breast cancer and is associated with poor prognosis. Inspection of the SFRP1 expression levels in Basal B cell lines showed absent calls for 4 of the 8 invasive cell lines; and eight-fold decreases in another 3 invasive cell lines relative to the non-invasive MCF-10A cells (data not shown). Inspection of the expression files for bcMCF cells and the 8 invasive Basal B cell lines revealed that LEF1 was always absent, while TCF 3 and TCF 8 were expressed.

11.7.5. *Breast cancer metastasis and SATB1 as a reprogrammer of gene expression to promote breast tumor growth and metastasis*

A collaboration that was extremely enlightening was the one that I established with Terumi Kohwi-Shigematsu. I'd known her since our working together in the Chemical Pathology Study Session at the NCI, and since then we had stayed connected. She approached me to help her in a major publication she was working on with my expertise in tumor diagnosis and prognosis of breast cancer. She was working in SATB1 and demonstrated that SATB1 expression in cancer cells necessarily alters the gene expression profile to promote tumor growth and metastasis; SATB1 can serve as a sentinel indicating that cells have acquired the aggressive phenotype. The mechanism by which SATB1 globally reprograms gene expression during metastasis could be by tethering hundreds of gene loci onto its regulatory network, assembling them with chromatin modifying and transcription factors. SATB1 expression is not restricted to late clinical stages of the disease, but is also observed in a subset of primary breast tumors at early clinical stages before lymph node metastasis. The SATB1 protein levels in the nuclei of cancer cells have high prognostic significance, independent of the lymph node status ($P < 0.0001$), indicating its utility in predicting the likelihood of disease progression in patients with early-stage breast cancer. Silencing SATB1 in those tumors that are highly expressive of this protein may open a new target for cancer therapy. This was a monumental work done by Terumi, and I was honored to be a part of it. The data was published in *Nature* in 2008 [246].

11.8. Circadian rhythm and mammary gland development

As part of the UO1 grant that we have from the NIEHS, we studied the role of light as an endocrine disruptor. It has been known that light plays an important role because it synchronizes the circadian rhythm and could act as an endocrine disruptor that could influence the incidence of breast cancer, such as the increase reported in women doing shift work, including flight attendants and women working at night. A reduction in breast cancer incidence in blind women further confirms the role of light exposure on breast cancer risk. All biological processes exhibit rhythmic oscillations every 24 hours that characterize the circadian rhythms. These rhythms are centrally controlled by the master circadian clock located in the suprachiasmatic nucleus (SCN) in the anterior hypothalamus (Figure 11.30). It is in turn daily

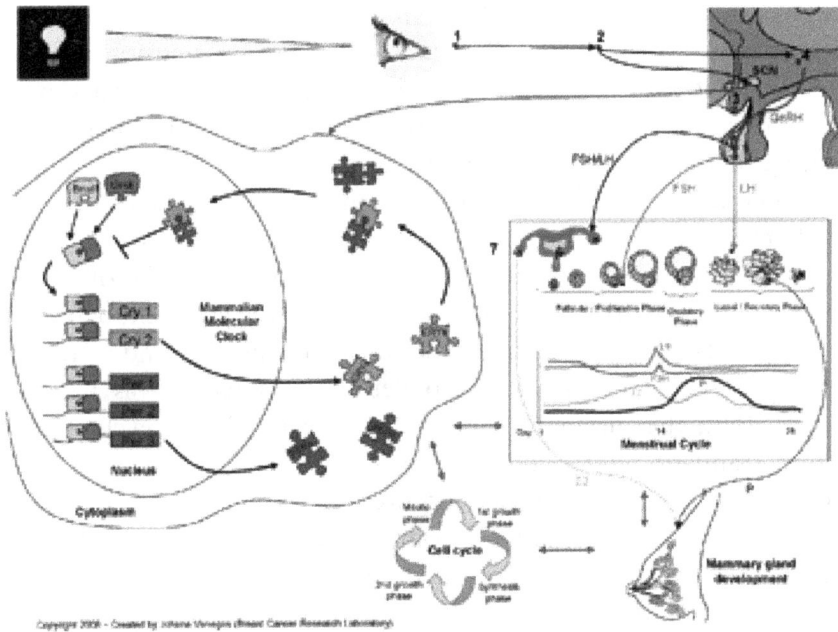

Figure 11.30: Negative-feedback loop of the molecular clock mechanism. CLOCK and BMAL1 form a heterodimer and regulate the rhythmic transcription of the mammalian Per and Cry genes. After Per and Cry translation, Cry proteins act as negative regulators by directly interacting with CLOCK and/or BMAL1 and inhibiting transcriptional activation by the BMAL1-CLOCK heterodimer. Concurrently, Per2 enhances BMAL1 transcription, which is the phase opposite to Per/Cry, and initiates the positive-feedback loop. The graphic shows the interaction between the mammalian master clock, the female reproductive hormones during the menstrual cycle, the mammary gland development, and the cell cycle. (1) Retinal rods, cones, and the intrinsically photosensitive retinal ganglion cells (ipRCCs); (2) Retino-hypothalamic tract (RHT); (3) Optic chiasm; (4) Hypothalamus; (5) Anterior pituitary gland; (6) Uterus; (7) Ovaries.

synchronized by light input from the retina. Circadian rhythms and cell division are fundamental biological systems in most organisms. There is substantial evidence that, in mammals, circadian rhythms affect the timing of cell divisions *in vivo*. The development and differentiation of the mammary gland are regulated by pituitary and ovarian hormones that are, in turn, under the control of SCN. Molecular clocks control cell-proliferation rhythms by regulating the expression of cell-cycle genes. The development and differentiation of the mammary gland are regulated in a time-dependent manner that determine the susceptibility of this organ to be transformed by environmental factors, like changes in the light patterns, which will ultimately alter the circadian rhythm and create a time of greater susceptibility to carcinogens (Figure 11.30).

In certain way, it looks unreal to come back after many years to study the circadian rhythm, and this time was at the molecular level instead of studying the mitotic activity or the amount of dried matter. This time the objective was to characterize the endogenous pattern of expression of clock genes in the mammary gland of virgin Sprague Dawley rats in order to determine whether this pattern varies along the different stages of mammary gland development under standard light conditions. For this purpose we used four groups of Sprague Dawley rats that were maintained under standard light conditions (12 light,12 hour darkness) for two weeks for collection of mammary tissues at the ages of 21, 35, 50, and 100 days. The rats from each group were euthanized every four hours, at Zeitgeber times (ZT): ZT2, ZT6, ZT10, ZT14, ZT18, ZT22 (ZT0, lights on at 6:00 hours, and ZT12, lights off at 18:00 hours). Using Real Time RT-PCR analysis, we study the expression profile of the clock genes: *Period* (*Per*) *1*, *2*, and *3*, *Cryptochrome* (*Cry*) *1* and *2*, *basic helix-loop* (*BHLHB*) *2 and 3*, brain and muscle ARNT-like protein 1 (*Bmal1*), and *Clock*. Each gene was normalized (ΔCT) using β-actin as an endogenous control gene. Analysis with two-way analysis of variance (ANOVA) showed that the mean expression level for all the genes was significantly different across age and time points as well the interaction between them, with a false discovery rate less than 1%. Since all of the interactions were found to be significant, a one-way ANOVA test was performed separately for age and time. The results obtained from the one-way ANOVA by time reveled that in the age groups 21 and 35, eight of the nine genes studied showed significant differences between the six time points observed under this study. The one-way ANOVA by age group indicated a main effect of mammary gland developmental stages on all the genes studied at certain time points. The 35-day group showed significant gene expression changes when compared with the other age groups, such as consistent lower level of expression at ZT6 and ZT10 in *Per1*, *Per2*, *BHLHB2*, and *Clock*. Of great interest was our finding that the expression of *Bmal1* in the 35-day group exhibited a significantly higher level of expression at ZT14 and ZT18 when compared to the other age groups. Our results [247–254] confirmed that the rat mammary gland expresses clock genes that cycle in response to circadian rhythms. Furthermore, these results supported the novel finding that clock genes are more greatly modified at the time of vaginal opening (puberty at 35 days of age).

The relevance of these studies was to demonstrate that since the differentiation of the mammary gland is regulated by the SCN, changes in the circadian rhythm could result in deregulation of basic developmental processes and greater susceptibility to carcinogenesis.

11.9. Reflections

It is undeniable that the period from 1991 to 2002 had been a roller coaster of scientific activity that in numerical terms was reflected in 131 peer review publications, 124 scientific abstracts, and 161 invited lectures around the world. Importantly, my personal evolution as a research scientist took place during that time. However, it is difficult to quantitatively measure that process, and the only way to express it is by citing some notes registered in my journal during those 11 years.

On November 30, 1992, I wrote:

I have received an invitation from Carlos Balaguer to participate in a gathering celebrating the twenty-five year anniversary of our medical graduation. I have answered him indicating that I will be unable to make it for the reunion but I would like him to transmit the following message:

"When I left Mendoza in 1971 I treasured each one of the faces of my classmates and experiences that we had together starting with the admissions test and our first class of Anatomy with Sanchez Guisande, through our clinical years and the diaspora after the internship. For many years I have tried to see the faces and experiences in my new environment without success, and for this reason each year I treasure the past and on December 11 when you gather together I will have all of you present in my thoughts as I remember those who started but never became physician, or those like Ramona Vila, who died in our second year of the medical school. A special regard to Jorge Fuhr, who shared my internship in the Viacava's service of Surgical Oncologyy, the sisters Gaviglio, Victor Triguy, Martha Abdala, Zoila Moran, Elsa Yáñez, Oscar Liugani, Alicia Acensio, Hugo Gil, Manuel Gutierrez, and every one that has enriched my life. Lastly I must say that during all these years I have tried to be faithful to my objectives and I wish for all of you that the dreams and objectives that inspired us to be physicians forever come to reality."

On August 20, 1993, I wrote:

Yesterday I received a very warm letter from Dr. G. Muller, thanking me for the acknowledgment of his view in hormonal carcinogenesis. It was nice coming from him and also his acknowledgment by overall perspective in the subject and in our work.

On October 12, 1997, I wrote:

There is some things that I need to solve soon regarding our work. One is the publication of the presence of ER, PgR, and Ki67 co-localization, and the other is the data of the lobular composition in the breast of women with cancer. The first topic is of importance, and I will need better acquaint myself with the publications of Clark and Anderson, who had published a similar observation. This is urgent because it is the right way to work. The second paper is also important because I am concerned that the pathologists do not see the same structures that I see. This is easily explained by the type of material that most of the pathologists observe. They see diseased breast tissue and I am looking at the normal breast.

On October 13, 1997, I wrote several entries in my journal:

I have realized that the path of inner recovery is slow. The healing from inaction and inertia is difficult to overcome. Thinking is painful because it requires a commitment to action. It is easy to dream and to believe that tomorrow it will be better, in order to keep the idleness of the present. To be tired is the easiest way to escape the action needed to be a better being.

I am conscious that my behavior and way of thinking is determined by my Christian tradition that has rooted the occidental culture. The reason why the oriental philosophies get prominence in the present time is because there is not a need of commitment. To do or not to do is the same, the creative work, the art, the music, the science are nonsense to the oriental philosophies whereas in my Christian perspective the human activity is an act of creation and reflection of the divine. Therefore the search for the cure or prevention of breast cancer has only sense in the transcendence of our immortal spirit, and without that it will be the same to do or not to do it. For example the difference with the Nirvana of the Buddhist monks is that this enlightening may be conductive to a non-creative motion. The difference between the Christian and non-Christian is the creative motion of our being as part of our transcendental needs to be co-creators of this unfinished world. Again the line is so thin that the confusion is possible. Probably the most important difference is that we as Christians are co-creators of the unfinished world, the act of research, creating art and music or literature, is part of our existential being.

I realize that a source of anxiety is the need for human recognition. How to work for the beauty of the action of creation and not because we are expecting a recompense? In retrospect my best recompenses in recognition have come when I was not expecting one. To prepare a talk, the work must be a reflection of creation, the selfishness of recognition must not be there. The urgency is only to complete the co-creative activity of our being.

On December 31, 1998, I wrote in my journal:

I have been successful in my conferences and lectures at national and international level and I do feel that they have added much to my intellectual growth. The preparation and presentation of those lectures has helped me to be more aware of the weakness in some part of our model and data.

*The book **The Monk and the Garden** describes the history of Gregory Mendel, and I have felt very touched to know more about Mendel's personality, life, and what he accomplished moved me significantly. The passages of his life when he says that he was invisible to his contemporary scientists, touch me a lot because this is the feeling that I perceive. We exist but nobody wants us to be or to recognize our work. I have the need to talk about something that could be groundbreaking in science and when I talk to an audience of people that are caring every day for cancer patients and I am talking about a promise that still we are struggling to unveil, the whole thing makes me feel very insignificant and out of place.*

I feel that I am closing a period in which all these trips to medical meetings that are outside the main focus of my research and present endeavor are reaching an end. Personally I am not interested in facing a crowd that is unresponsive because they lack the knowledge and because they have other immediate needs, like how to treat their patient the day after the meeting. The other aspect is that I do not feel that the organizers are really interested in the subject but are using the event for other reasons, like self-promotion and visibility in the community. It is not my function to judge them, but I really need to be back to the science and feel the feedback of real scientists from those that are in the field and know the intricacies of the work. This will help us in our research at the end. The worst part is the lack of response from the audience, no questions, no nothing after the talk, and I feel invisible to their eyes, to their realities in doses of chemotherapy or how much radiation to administer or what is the best of the regimens.

I remember back on my early years of the electron microscopy courses, cell biology, tissue culture, and molecular biology, and how important they were until I reached the point that those courses were not relevant for me anymore. Probably I have reached this point again. One thing is true, I feel the urge to get better in my research endeavor, our publications, and grants.

December 23, 2001:

From seven applications only an idea grant from the DOD and a subcontract will be funded. This barely solves our problem to justify keeping the people that we have in our laboratory. The DOD Spore funding seems to be in limbo, and they asked some of the applicants to attend a meeting this coming January for more specific instruction for a resubmission in sixty days. In the meantime I am preparing the NIH-SPORE and the RO1 for the NIH. In the fight for the spore grant either from the DOD or NIH I feel like a permanent contender but never a finalist or a winner. I am angry and I feel that I am walking in circle. How to overcome this feeling of being a contender among people who are the winners and my only merit is to be among the runners?

January 29, 2002:

The breast SPORE is complete and tomorrow must be via Washington to NIH. The RO1 with Gabriela on the role of DNA repair in breast cancer was signed today. The paper with Hasan has been submitted to the JNCI and the one with Gabriela to Nature Genetics. The manuscript with Xiaoshang was also submitted to Breast Cancer Research and Treatment. I am working in my own DOD spore and another one with Ercole Cavalieri. I have signed the contract for the book titled "Molecular Basis of Breast Cancer" with Springer-Verlag and is due at the end of the year.

I am centering my actions in their own intrinsic values and not in the recompense for my actions like a Pavlovian reflex looking for the prize. I am a pen in God's hand, like Mother Teresa used to say, and that I will write I will probably never know or understand, or maybe I will. I am afraid that all the hopes that these SPORE have created are a bubble that will break any minute. Should I be afraid or keep doing what I need to do and be afraid that the bubble will break any minute and with that all the human consideration, or should I keep my strength that the bubble will ascend as a rainbow full of light?

February 8, 2002:
Today we celebrate 33 years of marriage. I gave a card to Irma saying:

Dear and lovely wife, you have enlightened every minute of my life, thank you for sharing with me your body, your mind, and your soul. Pray together, lovely wife that we may do what we need to do even though we are afraid that the bubble will break any minute and with that all the human consideration. Pray together, dear wife that we keep the faith that the bubble will ascend as a rainbow full of light.

March 21, 2002:

Today I have received the notification from the NIH that our grant application Genomic Basis of Reproductive History is in the 10.1 percentile. I called and they tell me that it will be funded. This isextraordinary news. The significance of the NIH award, cannot be overstated. The idea we proposed to develop in this application is the epitome of our research work. To demonstrate that pregnancy induces in the breast a genomic signature that is responsible for the protective effect against carcinogenesis. We are presenting again the DOD spore and a new one. If the pre-proposal is viable, then a final application could emerge.

March 24, 2002:

Thanks God, because I am still alive on my sixtieth birthday. The birthday card from Irma is beautiful and It reads as follows:

For my husband

Do you know why I love you?
Let me tell you why I fell in love with you . . . Because you were the man I had always dreamed of because you were not all what I expected, because I looked into your eyes and saw my soul's companion.

I fell in love with you because I heard your voice and knew I'd found my heart's desire, because you could make me laugh and kiss away my tears, because you were strong but didn't need to prove it.

I fell in love with you because you were wise beyond your years, but would always be a little boy, because I wanted to understand you, but you would always remain a mystery.

I fell in love with you in one moment. I married you because I needed a lifetime to tell you why.

References

[1] Kreeger, K. America's First Cancer Center Celebrates Centennial. *J. Natl. Cancer Inst.* 96: 171–172, 2004.

[2] Kurzrock, R., Kantarjian, H. M., Druker, B. J. and Talpaz, M. Philadelphia chromosome-positive leukemias: From basic mechanisms to molecular therapeutics. *Ann. Intern. Med.* 138: 819–830, 2003.

[3] Melo, J. V. The molecular biology of chronic myeloid leukemia. *Leukemia* 10: 751–756, 1996.

[4] Fox Chase Cancer Center. 50th Anniversary of the Discovery of the Philadelphia Chromosome.

[5] Nowell, P. and Hungerford, D. A minute chromosome in chronic granulocytic leukemia . *Science* 132: 1497, 1960.

[6] *Hepatitis B. The Hunt for a Killer Virus*, Princeton University Press. 2010.

[7] Blumberg, B. S. Polymorphisms of the serum proteins and the development of isopreciptins in transfused patients. *Bull. NY Acad. Med.* 40: 377–386, 1964.

[8] Obituary: Barry Blumberg, *The Economist*, 30 April 2011, p. 92.

[9] Knudson, A. Mutation and cancer: statistical study of retinoblastoma. *Proc. Natl. Acad. Sci. USA* 68: 820–823, 1971.

[10] Lewis, E. B. A tribute to Alfred G. Knudson. *Genes Chromosomes Cancer* 38: 292–293, 2003.

[11] www.foxchase.org. Retrieved 11 July 2016.

[12] Knudson, A. G. and Strong, L. C. Mutation and cancer: a model for Wilms' tumor of the kidney. *J. Natl. Cancer Inst.* 48: 313–324, 1972.

[13] Russo, J. Differentiation and Pathogenesis of breast cancer. *Women and Cancer* 1: 14–21, 1998.

[14] Zekri, A-R., Bahnassi, A. A., Bove, B., Huang, Y., Russo, I. H., Rogatko, A., Shaarawy, A., Shawki, O. A., Hamza, M-R., Omer, S., Khaled H. M. and

Russo, J. Allelic instability as a predictor of survival in breast cancer patients. *Int. J. Oncol.* 15:757–767, 1999.

[15] Bahnassy, A. A., Zekri, A. R., Bove, B., Raafat, A., El-Bolkainy, M. N., Ali, N. M., Omar, S. and Russo, J. The role of allelic imbalance at chromosome 2p16 in breast cancer progression. *J. Egypt. Natl. Cancer Inst.* 12: 211–220, 2000.

[16] Fuqua, S. A. W., Russo, J., Shackney, S. E. and Stearns, M. E. Estrogen, Estrogen Receptors and Selective Estrogen Receptor Modulators in Human Breast Cancer. *J. Womens Cancer* 2: 21–32, 2000.

[17] Fuqua, S. A., Russo, J., Shackney, S. E. and Stearns, M. E. Selective estrogen receptor modulators. An aid in unraveling the links between estrogen and breast cancer. *Postgrad. Med.* Spec No: 3–10, 2001.

[18] Glass, A. G., Donis-Keller, H., Mies, C., Russo, J., Zehnbauer, B., Taube, S. and Aamodt, R. The cooperative breast cancer tissue resource: Archival Tissue for the investigation of tumor markers. *Clin. Cancer Res.* 7: 1843–1849, 2001.

[19] Meyer, J. S., Alvarez, C., Lister, K., Milikowski, C., Olson, N., Russo, I. H., Russo, J., Zehnbauer, B., Glass, A. and Parwaresch, R. Breast carcinoma malignancy grading by Bloom-Richardson system vs proliferation index: reproducibility of grade and advantages of proliferation index. *Mod. Pathol.* 18: 1067–1078, 2005.

[20] Gutiérrez Diez, P. J., Su, Y. and Russo, J. Immunocytochemical stem cell markers can predict clinical stage of breast cancer. *Oncol. Rep.* 38: 1507–1516, 2017.

[21] Moral, R., Wang, R., Russo, I. H., Pereira, J. S., Lamartiniere, C. A. and Russo, J. Prepubertal exposure to bisphenol A changes the gene expression profile of rat mammary gland. *J. Endocrinol.*, 2008.

[22] Moral, R., Wang, R., Pereira, J. S., Russo, I. H., Lamartiniere, C. A. and Russo, J. In utero exposure to butyl benzyl phthalate induces morphological, proliferative and genomic modifications in the rat mammary gland. *BMC Genomics.* 8: 453–460, 2007.

[23] Jenkins, S., Rowell, C., Wang, J. and Lamartiniere, C. Prenatal TCDD Exposure Predisposes for Mammary Cancer in Rats. *Reproductive Toxicol.* 23: 391–396, 2007.

[24] Rowell, C., Carpenter, D. M. and Lamartiniere, C. A. Chemoprevention of Breast Cancer, Proteomic Discovery of Genistein Action in the Rat Mammary Gland. *J. Nutrition Sci.* 135: 2953S–2959S, 2005.

[25] Rowell, C., Carpenter, D. M. and Lamartiniere, C. A. Modeling Biological Variability in 2-D gel Proteomic Carcinogenesis Experiments. *J. Proteome Res.* 4: 1619–1627, 2005.

[26] Wetmur, J. G., Kumar, M., Zhang, L., Palomeque, C., Wallenstein, S. and Chen, J. Molecular haplotyping by linking emulsion PCR: Analysis of PON1 haplotypes and phenotypes. *Nucleic Acids Res.* 33: 2615–2619, 2005.

[27] Wolff, M. S., Britton, J. A. and Russo, J. TCDD and Puberty in Girls. *Environ. Health Perspect.* 113: A17, 2005.

[28] Wallenstein, S., Chan, J. and Wetmur, J. G. Comparison of statistical models for analyzing genotype, inferred haplotype and molecular haplotype data. *Mol. Genet. Metab.* 89: 270–273, 2006.

[29] Wetmur, J. G. and Chen, J. An emulsion of PCR-based method for molecular haplotyping. Methods in Molecular Biology. In: Martin, C., (ed), *Environmental Genomics*, Humana Press, Totowa, NJ. 2008. *Methods Mol. Biol.* 410: 351–361, 2008.

[30] Wolff, M. S., Teitelbaum, S. L., Windham, G., Pinney, S. M., Britton, J. A., Chelimo, C., Godbold, J., Biro, F., Kushi, L. H., Pfeiffer, C. M. and Calafat, A. M. Pilot Study of Urinary Biomarkers of Phytoestrogens, Phthalates, and Phenols in Girls. *Environ. Health. Perspect.* 115: 116–121, 2007.

[31] Teitelbaum, S. L., Britton, J. A., Calafat, A. M., Ye, X., Silva, M. J., Reidy, J. A., Galvez, M. P., Brenner, B. L. and Wolff, M. S. Temporal variability in urinary concentrations of phthalate metabolites, phytoestrogens and phenols among minority children in the United States. 106: 257–269, 2007.

[32] Galvez, M. P., Hong, L., Choi, E., Liao, L., Godbold, J. and Brenner, B. Childhood obesity and neighborhood food-store availability in an inner-city community. *Acad. Pediatr.* 9: 339–343, 2009.

[33] Claudio, L. Translation: Breast Cancer Takes Center Stage. *Environ. Health Perspect.* 112: A92–A94, 2004.

[34] Claudio, L. Making progress on breast cancer. *Environ. Health Perspect.* 114: A98–A99, 2006.

[35] Claudio, L. RTP leaders unite to advance environmental health. *Environ. Health Perspect.* 114: A524–A525, 2006.

[36] Glass, R. I., Bridbord, K., Rosenthal, J. and Claudio, L. Global perspective on environmental health. *Environ. Health Perspect.* 114: A454–A455, 2006.

[37] Claudio, L. Centered on Breast Cancer. *Environ. Health Perspect.* 115: A132–A133, 2007.

[38] Jenkins, S., Raghuraman, N., Eltoum, I., Carpenter, M., Russo, J. and Lamartiniere, C. A. Oral Exposure to Bisphenol A Increases Dimethylbenzanthracene-Induced Mammary Cancer in Rats. *Environ. Health Perspect.* 117: 910–915, 2009.

[39] Chen, J-Q., Brown, T. R. and Russo, J. Regulation of Energy Metabolism Pathways by Estrogens and Estrogenic Chemicals and Potential Implications

in Obesity Associated with Increased Exposure to Endocrine Disruptors. *Biochim. Biophys. Acta.* 1793: 1128–1143, 2009.

[40] Fernandez, S. V. and Russo, J. Estrogen and Xenoestrogens in Breast Cancer. *Toxicol. Pathol.* 38: 110–122, 2010.

[41] Hsu, P-Y., Hsu, H. K., Singer, G. A. C., Yan, P. S., Rodriguez, B. A. T., Liu, J. C., Weng, Y-I., Deatherage, D. E., Chen, Z., Pereira, J. S., Lopez, R., Russo, J., Wang, Q., Lamartiniere, C. A., Nephew, K. P. and Huang, T. H-M. Estrogen-mediated epigenetic repression of large chromosomal regions through DNA looping. *Genome Res.* 20: 733–744, 2010.

[42] Betancourt, A. M., Mobley, J., Russo, J. and Lamartiniere, C. A. Proteomic Analysis in Mammary Glands of Rat Offspring Exposed In Utero to Bisphenol A. *J. Proteomics* 73: 1241–1253, 2010.

[43] Lamartiniere, C. A., Jenkins, S., Betancourt, A. M., Wang, J. and Russo, J. Exposure to the Endocrine Disruptor Bisphenol A Alters Susceptibility for Mammary Cancer. *Horm. Mol. Biol. Clin. Invest.* 5: 46–52, 2011.

[44] Russo, I. H. and Russo, J. In search of the optimal experimental model. In: Russo, J., (ed), *Environment and breast cancer*, Springer, NY. 2011, 43–54, 2011.

[45] Lopez de Cico, R., Santucci-Pereira, J., Moral R., Peri, S., Slifker, M., Russo, I. H., Russo, P. A.,Wang, R. and Russo, J. Endocrine disruptors affect the genomic profile of the rat mammary gland at different developmental stages. In: Russo, J., (ed), *Environment and breast cancer,* Springer, NY. 2011, 69101.

[46] Fernandez, S. V., Huang, Y., Snider, K. E., Zhow, Y., Pogash, T. J. and Russo, J. Expression and DNA methylation changes in human breast epithelial cells after bisphenol A exposure. *Int. J. Oncol.* 41: 369–377, 2012.

[47] Betancourt, A. M., Wang, J., Jenkins, S., Mobley, J., Russo, J. and Lamartiniere, C. A. Altered carcinogenesis and proteome in mammary glands of rats after prepubertal exposures to the hormonally active chemicals bisphenol a and genistein. *J. Nutr.* 142, 2012.

[48] Betancourt, A., Mobley, J. A., Wang, J., Jenkins, S., Chen, D. Q., Kojima, K., Russo, J. and Lamartiniere, C. A. Alterations in the Rat Serum Proteome Induced by Prepubertal Exposure to Bisphenol A and Genistein. *J. Proteome Res.* 13: 1502–1514, 2014.

[49] Russo, J. Significance of Rodent Mammary Tumors for Human Risk Assessment. *Toxicol. Pathol.* XX: 1–26, 2014.

[50] Wang, R., Balogh G. A., Russo I. H. and Russo, J. Use of Laser Capture Microdissection for Study Genomic Expression in Rat Mammary Gland. *Proceeding of the Emerging Topics in Breast Cancer and the Environment Research Meeting*, November 4–6, 2004, Princeton, NJ.

[51] Moral, R., Russo, I. H., Sheriff, F., Fernbaugh, R., Lamartiniere, C. and Russo, J. Proliferative Index in the Rat Mammary Gland as a Marker of Neonatal/Prepubertal Estrogenic Xenobiotic Exposure. *Proceeding of the Emerging Topics in Breast Cancer and the Environment Research Meeting*, November 4–6, 2004, Princeton, NJ.

[52] Moral, R., Balogh, G. A., Mailo, D., Russo, I. H., Ochs, M., Lamartiniere, C. and Russo, J. Differential Gene Expression in the Mammary Gland of Rats exposed to Xenobiotic Agent. *Proceeding of the Emerging Topics in Breast Cancer and the Environment Research Meeting*, November 4–6, 2004, Princeton, NJ.

[53] Moral, R., Russo, I. H., Sheriff, F., Fernbaugh, R., Lamartiniere, C. and Russo, J. Neonatal/Prepubertal Exposure to Estrogenic Xenobiotics Alters the Pattern of Mammary Gland Differentiation in Rats. *Proceeding of the Emerging Topics in Breast Cancer and the Environment Research Meeting*, November 4–6, 2004, Princeton, NJ.

[54] Balogh, G. A., Russo, I. H. and Russo J. Selection of the Best Platform for Determination of Genomic Signature in the Rat Mammary Gland. *Proceeding of the Emerging Topics in Breast Cancer and the Environment Research Meeting*, November 4–6, 2004, Princeton, NJ.

[55] Russo, I. H., Wang, R., Moral, R., Fernbaugh, R. and Russo, J. Basic definitions for the morphological evaluation of the effect of environmental factors on the development and differentiation of the rodent mammary gland. *Proceeding of the Emerging Topics in Breast Cancer and the Environment Research Meeting*, November 4–6, 2004, Princeton, NJ.

[56] Moral, R., Balogh, G. A., Mailo, D., Russo, I. H., Lamartiniere, C. and Russo, J. Effect of the Contaminant Bisphenol A (BPA) on the Genomic Signature of the Rat Mammary Gland. *Proc. Am. Assoc. Cancer Res.* 46: 2099a, 2005.

[57] Moral, R., Balogh, G. A., Mailo, D., Russo, I. H., Lamartiniere, C. and Russo, J. Influence of Prepubertal Exposure to Benzyl Butyl Phthalate (BBP) on the Genomic Signature of the Rat Mammary Gland. *Proc. Am. Assoc. Cancer Res.* 46: 2100a, 2005.

[58] Moral, R., Balogh G. A., Mailo, S. A., Russo, I. H., Lamartiniere, C. A. and Russo, J. Neonatal and Prepubertal Exposure to the Estrogenic Xenobiotic N-Butyl Benzyl Phthalate (BBP) Alters the Gene Expression Pattern of the Rat Mammary Gland. *Proceeding of the Emerging Topics in Breast Cancer and the Environment Research Meeting*, November 10–11, 2005, Lansing, MI.

[59] Moral, R., Balogh G. A., Mailo, S. A., Russo, I. H., Lamartiniere, C. A. and Russo, J. Changes in Gene Expression Profile in the Rat Mammary Gland

after Neonatal and Prepubertal Exposure to the Xenoestrogen Bisphenol A (BPA). *Proceeding of the Emerging Topics in Breast Cancer and the Environment Research Meeting*, November 10–11, 2005, Lansing, MI.

[60] Wang, R., Moral, R., Sheriff, F. S., Fernbaugh, R. L., Lamartiniere, C., Russo, I. H. and Russo, J. Prenatal Exposure to the Xenoestrogens Bisphenol A (BPA) and N-Butyl Benzyl Phthalate (BBP) Alter the Pattern of Rat Mammary Gland Development. *Proceeding of the Emerging Topics in Breast Cancer and the Environment Research Meeting*, November 10–11, 2005, Lansing, MI.

[61] Russo, I. H., Wang, R., Moral, R. and Russo, J. The Expression of Clock Genes in the Rat Mammary is Regulated by the Circadian Rhythm. *Proc. Am. Assoc. Cancer Res.* 47: 1071, 2006.

[62] Moral, R., Wang, R., Mailo, D. A., Russo, I. H., Lamartiniere, C. A. and Russo, J. Prepubertal exposure to endocrine disruptor Bisphenol A but not to Benzyl Butyl Phthalate alters the expression of immune surveillance genes in the rat mammary gland. *Proc. Am. Assoc. Cancer Res.* 47: 1899a, 2006.

[63] Chace, R. Growing up healthy in East Harlem and the Bronx, New York. *The Ribbon* 12: 9–12, 2007.

[64] Pereira, J. S., Wang, R., Moral, R., Russo, I. H., Lamartiniere, C. A. and Russo, J. Prenatal exposure of 2,3,7,8 Tetrachlorodibenzo-p-dioxin (TCDD) affects the morphology and genomic profile of the mammary glands. *Proc. Am. Assoc. Cancer Res.* 2007.

[65] Vanegas, J. E., Moral, R., Russo, I. H., Wang, R. and Russo, J. Clock genes in the rat mammary gland. *Proc. Am. Assoc. Cancer Res.* 2007.

[66] Pereira, J. S., Medvedovic, M., Moral, R., Russo, I. H., Lamartiniere, C. and Russo, J. Exposure to bisphenol A (BPA) during the prenatal or prepubertal period induces a similar genomic signature at the time of high susceptibility of mammary carcinogenesis. *Proceeding of the Emerging Topics in Breast Cancer and the Environment Research Meeting*, November 8–9, 2007, Cincinnati, OH.

[67] Vanegas, J. E., Rea, M. S., Figueiro, M. G., Bullough, J. D., Possidente, B. P., Moral, R., Pereira, J. S., Russo, J. and Russo, I. H. The clock gene ARNT (Bmal1) and estrogen receptor alpha are influenced by circadian disruption in rat mammary gland. *Proceeding of the Emerging Topics in Breast Cancer and the Environment Research Meeting*, November 8–9, 2007, Cincinnati, OH.

[68] Pereira, J. S., Medvedovic, M., Moral, R., Russo, I. H., Lamartiniere, C. and Russo, J. Prenatal and prepubertal exposures to bisphenol A (BPA) induce genomic alterations in the rat mammary gland during the window of high

susceptibility to carcinogenesis. *Proceedings of the 99th Annual Meeting of the American Association for Cancer Research*, 49: 3155a, Apr 12–16, 2008, San Diego, CA.

[69] López, R., Russo, P., Pereira, J. S., Lamartiniere, C. and Russo, J. Optimal Protocol for RNA Purification from Rat Mammary Gland, Whole Blood, and Buccal Mucosa for Microarray Analyses. *Proceeding of the GEI Exposure Biology*, Organized by the NIEHS, Hyatt Regency Hotel, January 24–25, 2008, Bethesda, MS.

[70] Lopez, R., Russo, P., Pereira, J. S., Lamartiniere, C., Biro, F. and Russo, J. RNA Purification from Human Whole Blood and Buccal Mucosa for Microarray Analyses. *Proceeding of the GEI Exposure Biology*, Organized by the NIEHS, Hyatt Regency Hotel, January 24–25, 2008, Bethesda, MS.

[71] Lamartiniere, C., Biro, F. and Russo, J. Genomic and Proteomic Biomarkers of Biological Responses to Exposure (1U01ES016003-01). *Proceeding of the GEI Exposure Biology*, Organized by the NIEHS, Hyatt Regency Hotel, January 24–25, 2008, Bethesda, MS.

[72] Lopez, R., Pereira, J. S., Peri, S., Slifker, M., Russo, I. H., Lamartiniere, C. and Russo, J. The effect of exposure to BPA, BBP or TCDD on rat mammary gland fatty acid and lipid metabolism. *Proceeding of the 5th annual Early Environmental Exposures Meeting*, November 13–14, 2008, Birmingham, AL.

[73] Russo, J. Early exposure to environmental xenoestrogens alters the genomic profile of the mammary gland. *Proceeding of the 5th annual Early Environmental Exposures Meeting*, November 13–14, 2008, Birmingham, AL.

[74] Lopes, E., Pereira, J. S., Lopez, R., Sheriff, F., Snider, K. and Russo, J. The effect of pre-pubertal exposure of Benzyl Butyl Phthalate (BBP) on the rat mammary gland. *Proceeding of the 5th annual Early Environmental Exposures Meeting*, November 13–14, 2008, Birmingham, AL.

[75] Pereira, J. S., Lopez, R., Medvedovic, M., Russo, I. H., Lamartiniere, C. and Russo, J. Notch and wnt/β-catenin signaling pathways in the mammary gland are dysregulated by prepubertal but not by prenatal exposure to BPA and are determinant of the increase susceptibility to DMBA-induced carcinogenesis. *Proceeding of the 5th annual Early Environmental Exposures Meeting*, November 13–14, 2008, Birmingham, AL.

[76] Pereira, J. S., Moral, R., Wang, R., Russo, I. H., Lamartiniere, C. and Russo, J. Prenatal exposure to 2,3,7,8-tetrachlorodibenzo-p-dioxin significantly affect the expression of immune response genes in the adult rat's mammary gland. *Proceeding of the 5th annual Early Environmental Exposures Meeting*, November 13–14, 2008, Birmingham, AL.

[77] Pereira, J. S., Lopez, R., Slifker, M., Peri, S., Russo, I. H., Lamartiniere, C. and Russo, J. Global gene expression changes induced in the mammary gland of animals exposed to BPA, BBP, and TCDD at different developmental stage. *Proceeding of the 5th annual Early Environmental Exposures Meeting*, November 13–14, 2008, Birmingham, AL.

[78] López, R., Pereira, J. S., Medvedovic, M., Russo, P., Lamartiniere, C. and Russo, J. Gene expression changes induced by DEHP (diethyl hexyl phthalate) in mammary gland, blood and buccal mucosa of 35 days old rats. *Proceeding of the 5th annual Early Environmental Exposures Meeting*, November 13–14, 2008, Birmingham, AL.

[79] Lopez, R., Pereira, J. S., Wolff, M., Wetmur, J., Ambrosone, C., Voho, A., Teitelbaum, S., Davis, W., Hong, C., Windham, G., Lamartiniere, C., Hiatt, R., Russo, I. H., Kushi, L. and Russo, J. Comparison between SNPs found in prepubertal girls exposed to BBP and gene expression profile of BBP exposed rats during prepubertal period. *Proceeding of the 5th annual Early Environmental Exposures Meeting*, November 13–14, 2008, Birmingham, AL.

[80] Wu, S., Pereira, J. S., Lopez, R., Sheriff, F., Snider, K. and Russo, J. The effect of prepubertal 2,3,7,8-tetrachlorodibenzo-p-dioxin exposure on the rat mammary gland. *Proceeding of the 5th annual Early Environmental Exposures Meeting*, November 13–14, 2008, Birmingham, AL.

[81] Rotter, Z., Pereira, J. S., Lopez, R., Sheriff, F., Snider, K. and Russo, J. The effect of prepubertal exposure to Bisphenol A on rat mammary gland morphology and gene expression. *Proceeding of the 5th annual Early Environmental Exposures Meeting*, November 13–14, 2008, Birmingham, AL.

[82] Pereira, J. S., Slifker, M., Peri, S., Wang, R., Russo, I. H., Lamartiniere, C. A. and Russo, J. In utero and lactational exposure to 2,3,7,8-tetrachlorodibenzo-p-dioxin (TCDD) affects the proliferation and gene expression of the rat mammary gland during postnatal development. *Proceeding of the 6th annual Early Environmental Exposures Meeting*, November 18–20, 2009, Cavallo Point, Sausalito, CA.

[83] Ansari, F., Fishstein, T. T., Vanegas, J., Bidinotto, L. T., Sheriff, F., Snider, K. Pereira, J. S., Lamartiniere, C. A. and Russo, J. Prepubertal exposure to Bisphenol A (BPA) and 2,3,7,8 tetrachlorodibenzo-p-dioxin (TCDD) affects the architecture and proliferative compartment of the rat mammary gland. *Proceeding of the 6th annual Early Environmental Exposures Meeting*, November 18–20, 2009, Cavallo Point, Sausalito, CA.

[84] López de Cicco, R., Yan, B., Russo, P. A., Pereira, J. S., Pinney, S. M., Biro, F., Lamartiniere, C., Medvedovic, M. and Russo, J. Comparison of gene

expression changes induced by BPA and BBP in blood of pubertal girls and 35 days old rats. *Proceeding of the Annual Meeting of the NIEHS-Breast Cancer and the Environment Research Program,* November 17–18, 2011, Cincinnati, OH.

[85] Russo, J. The windows of susceptibility in breast cancer and its prevention. *Proceeding of the Annual Meeting of the NIEHS-Breast Cancer and the Environment Research Program,* November 17–18, 2011, Cincinnati, OH.

[86] López de Cicco, R., Yan, B., Russo, P. A., Pereira, J. S., Pinney, S. M., Biro, F., Lamartiniere, C., Medvedovic, M., Russo, I. H. and Russo, J. Comparison of gene expression changes induced by BPA and BBP in blood of pubertal girls and 35 days old rats. *Proceeding of the Annual Meeting of the NIEHS-Breast Cancer and the Environment Research Program,* November 17–18, 2011, Cincinnati, OH.

[87] Lamartiniere, C., Russo, J., Pinney, S. and Biro, F. Combinational Environmental Chemical Exposure in Prepubertal Rats and Adolescent Girls. *Proceeding of the Interim Meeting of the WOS NIEHS,* July, 2013.

[88] Russo, J., (ed). *Environment and Breast Cancer,* Springer, New York. 2011.

[89] Russo, J., Balogh, G. A., Russo, I. H. and the Fox Chase Cancer Center Hospital Network Participants. Full-term Pregnancy Induces a Specific Genomic Signature in the Human Breast. *Cancer Epidemiol. Biomarkers Prev.* 17: 51–66, 2008.

[90] Russo, J., Balogh, B. A., Heulings, R., Mailo, D. A., Moral, R., Russo, P. A., Sheriff, F., Vanegas, J. and Russo, I. H. Molecular basis of pregnancy induced breast cancer protection. *Eur. J. Cancer Prev.* 15: 306–342, 2006.

[91] Russo, J., Mailo, D., Hu, Y-F., Balogh, G. A., Sheriff, F. and Russo, I. H. Breast differentiation and its implication in cancer prevention. *Clin. Cancer Res.* 11: 931s–936s, 2005.

[92] Russo, J., Moral, R., Balogh, G. A., Mailo, D. A. and Russo, I. H. The Protective role of pregnancy in breast cancer. *Breast Cancer Res. J.* 7: 131–142, 2005.

[93] Balogh, G. A. Heulings, R., Mailo, D. A., Russo, P. A., Sheriff, F., Russo, I. H., Moral, R. and Russo, J. Genomic Signature Induced by Pregnancy in the Human Breast. *Int. J. Oncol.* 28: 399–410, 2006.

[94] Russo, J., Balogh, G., Mailo, D., Russo, P. A., Heulings, R. and Russo, I. H. The genomic signature of breast cancer prevention. In: Senn, H-J., Kapp, U., (eds), *Cancer Prevention,* Springer, Heidelberg. 2007, 111–150.

[95] Maglietta, R., *et al.* Statistical assessment of functional categories of genes deregulated in pathological conditions by using microarray data. *Bioinformatics* 23: 2063–2072, 2007.

[96] Russo, J., Balogh, G. and Russo, I. H. Breast Cancer Prevention. *Climacteric* 10(2): 47–53, 2007.

[97] Balogh, G. A., Russo, I. H., Spittle, C., Heulings, R. and Russo, J. Immune surveillance and programmed cell death related genes are significantly over expressed in the normal breast epithelium of postmenopausal parous women. *Int. J. Oncol.* 31:303–312, 2007.

[98] Balogh, G. A., Russo, J., Mailo, D. A., Heulings, R., Russo, P. A., Morrison, P., Sheriff, F. and Russo, I. H. The breast of parous women without cancer has a different genomic profile than those with cancer. *Int. J. Oncol.* 31: 1165–1175, 2007.

[99] Santucci-Pereira, J., Zeleniuch-Jacquotte, A., Afanasyeva, Y., Zhong, H., Peri, S., Ross, E. A., Slifker, M., López de Cicco, R., Zhai, Y., Russo, I. H., Sheriff, F., Nguyen, T., Arslan, A. A., Bordas, P., Lenner, P., Åhman, J., Landström, A. S., Johansson, E. R., Hallmans, G., Toniolo, P. and Russo, J. Gene expression profile induced by pregnancy in the breast of premenopausal women. *Proc. Am. Assoc. Cancer Res.* 2360a, 2014.

[100] Russo, J. and Russo, I. H. Toward a physiological approach to breast cancer prevention. *J. Cancer Epidemiol. Biomarkers Prev.* 3: 353–364, 1994.

[101] Russo, J. and Russo, I. H. *Role of Transcriptome in Breast Cancer Prevention*, Springer, New York. 2013.

[102] Russo, I. H., Koszalka, M. and Russo, J. Human chorionic gonadotropin and rat mammary cancer prevention. *J. Natl. Cancer Inst.* 82: 1286–1289, 1990.

[103] Srivastava, P., Russo, J. and Russo, I. H. Chorionic gonadotropin inhibits rat mammary carcinogenesis through activation of programmed cell death. *Carcinogenesis* 18: 1799–1808, 1997.

[104] Alvarado, M. E., Alvarado, N. E., Russo, J. and Russo, I. H. Human chorionic gonadotropin inhibits proliferation and induces expression of inhibin in human breast epithelial cells in vitro. *In Vitro* 30A: 4–8, 1994.

[105] Alvarado, M. V., Russo, J. and Russo, I. H. Immunolocalization of inhibin in the mammary gland of rats treated with hCG. *J. Histochem. Cytochem.* 41: 29–34, 1993.

[106] Russo, I. H. and Russo, J. Role of hCG and inhibin in breast cancer (review). *Int. J. Oncol.* 4: 297–306, 1994.

[107] Meunier, H., Rivier, C., Evans, R. and Vale, W. Gonadal and extragonadal expression of inhibin a-, bA-, and bB-subunits in various tissues predicts diverse functions. *Proc. Natl. Acad. Sci. USA* 85: 247–251, 1988.

[108] Srivastava, P., Russo, J., Estrada, S. and Russo, I. H. P53 and cyclins A and D regulate the inhibition of tumor progression induced by chorionic gonadotropin. *Proc. Am. Assoc. Cancer Res.* 37: 2a, 1996.

[109] Kliesch, S., Behre, H. M. and Nieschlag, E. High efficacy of gonadotropin or pulsatile gonadotropin-releasing hormone treatment in hypogonadotropic hypogonadal men. *Eur. J. Endocrinol.* 131: 347–354, 1994.

[110] Kauschansky, A., Frydman, M., Nussinovitch, M. and Varsano, I. Evaluation of human chorionic gonadotropin stimulation tests in prepubertal and early pubertal boys. *Eur. J. Pediatr.* 154: 890–892, 1995.

[111] Quenby, M. B. and Farquharson, R. G. Human chorionic gonadotropin supplementation in recurring pregnancy loss: a controlled trial. *Fertil. Steril.* 62: 708–710, 1994.

[112] Chen. C., Jones, W. R., Fern, B. and Forde, C. Monitoring embryos after in vitro fertilization using early pregnancy factor. In: Seppala, M., Edwards, R. G., (eds), *In vitro fertilization and embryo transfer. Ann. NY Acad. Sci.* 442: 428, 1985.

[113] Bernstein, L., Hanisch, R., Sullivan-Halley, J. and Ross, R. K. Treatment with human chorionic gonadotropin and risk of breast cancer. *Cancer Epidemiol. Biomarkers Prev.* 4: 437–440, 1995.

[114] Gill, P. S., McLaughlin, T., Espina, B. M., Tulpule, A., Louie, S., Lunardi-Iskandar, Y. and Gallo, R. C. Phase I study of human chorionic gonadotropin given subcutaneously to patients with acquired immunodeficiency syndrome related mucocutaneous Kaposi's sarcoma. *J. Natl. Cancer Inst.* 89: 1797–1802, 1997.

[115] Gill, P. S., Lunardi-Iskandar, Y., Louie, S., Tulpule, A., Zheng, T., Espina, B. M., Besnier, J. M, Herman, P., Levine, A. M., Bryant, J. L. and Gallo, R. C. The effect of preparations of human chorionic gonadotropin on AIDS-related Kaposi's sarcoma. *N. Engl. J. Med.* 335: 1261–1269, 1996.

[116] Harris, P. J. Human chorionic gonadotropin hormone is antiviral. *Med. Hypotheses* 47: 71–72, 1996.

[117] Russo, J., Tay, L. K. and Russo, I. H. Differentiation of the mammary gland and susceptibility to carcinogenesis. *Breast Cancer Res. Treat.* 2: 5–73, 1982.

[118] Lambe, M., Hsieh, C-C., Chan, H-W., Ekbom, A., Trichopoulos, D. and Adami, H. O. Parity, age at first and last birth, and risk of breast cancer: a population-based study in Sweden. *Breast Cancer Res. Treat.* 38: 305–311, 1996.

[119] Janssens, J. Ph., Russo, J., Russo, I. H., Michiels, L., Donders, G., Verjans, M., Riphagen, I., Van den Bossche, T., Deleu, M. and Sieprath, P. Human Chorionic Gonadotropin (hCG) and prevention of breast cancer. *Mol. Cell. Endocrinol.* 269: 93–98, 2007.

[120] Therasse, P., *et al.* New guidelines to evaluate the response to treatment in solid tumors. *J. Natl. Cancer Inst.* 92: 205–216, 2000.

[121] World Health Organization. *WHO Handbook for Reporting Results of Cancer Treatment,* WHO, Geneva. 1979.

[122] Russo, J. and Russo, I. H. A new paradigm in breast cancer prevention. *Med. Hypotheses Res.* 1: 11–22, 2004.

[123] Russo, J., Balogh, G. A., Chen, J., Fernandez, S. V., Fernbaugh, R., Heulings, R., Mailo, D. A., Moral, R., Russo, P. A., Sheriff, F. A, Vanegas, J. E., Wang, R. and Russo, I. H. The concept of stem cell in the mammary gland and its implication in morphogenesis, cancer and prevention. *Front. Biosci.* 11: 151–172, 2006.

[124] Russo, I. H. and Russo, J. Primary prevention of breast cancer by hormone-induced differentiation. In: Senn, H-J, Kapp, U., (eds), *Cancer Prevention,* Springer, Heidelberg. 2007, 111–130.

[125] Russo, I. H. and Russo, J. The Use of Human Chorionic Gonadotropin in the Prevention of Breast Cancer. *Women Health* 4(1): 1–5, 2008.

[126] Kocdor, H. l., Kocdor, M. A., Russo, J., Snider, K. E., Vanegas, J, E., Russo, I. H. and Fernandez, S. V. Human Chorionic Gonadotropin (hCG) Prevents the Transformed Phenotypes Induced by 17 β-estradiol in Human Breast Epithelial Cells. *Cell Biol.Int.* 33: 1135–1143, 2009.

[127] Russo, J., Vanegas, J. E. and Russo, I. H. Prevención del Cancer de Mama. CÁNCER DE MAMA EN EL 2010. Estado actual del diagnóstico y tratamiento 2011, 45–56.

[128] Noronha, S. M. R., Correa-Noronha, S. A. A., Russo, I. H., Lopez de Cicco, R., Santucci-Pereira, J. and Russo, J. hCG and a 15aa peptide of the hormone induce down-regulation of CXCR1 gene in normal breast epithelial cells. *Horm. Mol. Biol. Clin. Investig.* 6: 241–245, 2011.

[129] Santucci-Pereira, J., George, C., Armiss, D., Russo, I. H., Vanegas, J. E., Sheriff, F., Lopez de Cicco, R., Su, Y., Russo, P. A., Bidinotto, L. T. and Russo, J. Mimicking Pregnancy as a Strategy for Breast Cancer Prevention. *Breast Cancer Manag.* 2: 283–294, 2013.

[130] Russo, J. Prevention of Breast Cancer Could be a Consequence of pregnancy: A Review. *J. Gen. Pract.* 2(4): 1–7, 2014.

[131] Russo, J., Lareef, M. H., Russo, I. H. and Jiang, X. Modulation of Hox gene expression in human breast epithelial cells by human chorionic gonadotropin. *Proc. Am. Assoc. Cancer Res.* 42: 2649a, 2001.

[132] Guo, S., Russo, I. H., Hu, Y. F. and Russo, J. Comparative analysis of gene expression between epithelial cells from undifferentiated and differentiated lobular structures of the human breast. *Proc. Am. Assoc. Cancer Res.* 43: 2002.

[133] Mailo, D., Russo, J., Sheriff, F., Hu, Y. F., Tahin, Q., Mihaila, D., Balogh, G. and Russo, I. H. Genomic signature induced my differentiation in the rat mammary gland. 43: 5368a, 2002.

[134] Russo, I. H., Mailo, D., Srivastava, P. and Russo, J. Human chorionic gonadotropin (hCG) induces in the virgin rat mammary gland the same genomic signature that is induced by pregnancy. *Proc. Am. Assoc. Cancer Res.* 44: 3588a, 2003.

[135] Russo, J. and Russo I. H. A new paradigm in the prevention of breast cancer. *J. Mol. Med.* 12(1): 146a, 2003.

[136] Mailo, D., Balogh, G. V., Russo, I. H. and Russo, J. Human chorionic gonadotropin induces differential expression of genes controlling multiple DNA repair pathways in human breast epithelial cells. *Proc. Am. Assoc. Cancer Res.* 45: 1550a, 2004.

[137] Wang, R., Russo, J., Balogh, G. A., Mailo, D., Sheriff, F. S., Fernbaugh, R., Russo, P. A., Moral, R. and Russo, I. H. The mammary cancer preventive effect of hCG is associated with a specific genomic signature in the rat mammary gland. *Proc. Am. Assoc. Cancer Res.* 46: 1578a, 2005.

[138] Mailo, D., Russo, J., Sheriff, F., Balogh, G., Heulings, R. and Russo, I. H. Specificity of the Genomic Signature of Human Chorionic Gonadotropin in its Preventive Effect on Mammary Carcinogenesis. *Proc. Am. Assoc. Cancer Res.* 46: 5202a, 2005.

[139] Russo, J. and Russo, I. H. The genomic Profile of the Postmenopausal Nulliparous and Parous Breast. *Climacteric* 8(2): 24–104, 2005.

[140] Mailo, D. A., Russo, P. A., Balogh, G. A., Russo, I. H., Sheriff, F. S., Appt, S. A., Blair, R. M., Cline, J. M. and Russo, J. Human Chorionic Gonadotropin (hCG) Induces Specific Molecular Pathway of Cell Differentiation in the Mammary Gland of *Macaca fascicularis. Proc. Am. Assoc. Cancer Res.* 47: 1424a, 2006.

[141] Russo, I. H., Mufei, L., Fernandez, S. V. and Russo, J. Methylation of the estrogen receptor alpha by pregnancy and human chorionic gonadotropin. *Proc. Am. Assoc. Cancer Res.* 47: 1595a, 2006.

[142] Mailo, D. A., Russo, P. A., Balogh, G. A., Russo, I. H., Sheriff, F. S., Appt, S. A., Blair, R. M., Cline, J. M. and Russo, J. Human Chorionic Gonadotropin (hCG) Induces Specific Molecular Pathway of Cell Differentiation in the Mammary Gland of *Macaca fascicularis.* Proc. Cancer Prev. 4: 49, 2006.

[143] Liu, M., Fernandez, S. V., Russo, J. and Russo, I. H. Estrogen receptor alpha (ERα) Downregulation by Pregnancy and Human Chorionic Gonadotropin (hCG) Treatment is mediated by Methylation. *Proc. Endocrine Soc.* 2006.

[144] Vanegas, J. E., Kocdor, M., Pereira, S. J., Kocdor, H., Russo, J., Snider, K., Sheriff, F. and Russo, I. H. Preventive effect of hCG on rat mammary carcinogenesis. Proc. Int. Conf. Gonadotropins and Receptor. 2008.

[145] Kocdor, H., Kocdor, M. A., Russo, J., Vanegas, J. E., Snider, K., Sheriff, F., Russo, I. H. and Fernandez, S. V. Human chorionic Gonadotropin (r-hCG) Prevents the Neoplastic Transformation of Human Breast Epithelial Cells by 17 Beta Estradiol. Proc. International Conference on Gonadotropins and Receptor. 2008.

[146] Russo, I. H. and Russo, J. Use of hCG in the prevention of breast cancer in young nulliparous women. Proc. International Conference on Gonadotropins and Receptor. 2008.

[147] Vanegas, J. E., Kocdor, M. A., Pereira, J. S., Kocdor, H., Russo, J., Snider, K., Sheriff, F. and Russo, I. H. Preventive effect of hCG on rat mammary. Carcinogenesis. *Proc. Am. Assoc. Cancer Res.* 50: 2059a, 2009.

[148] Kocdor, H., Kocdor, M. A., Russo, J., Snider, K., Vanegas, J. V., Russo, I. H. and Fernandez, S. Human chorionic gonadotropin (hCG) prevents the tarsnfromation phenotypes induced by 17 beta estradiol in human breast epithelial cells. *Proc. Am. Assoc. Cancer Res.* 50: 5a, 2009.

[149] Pereira, J., Vanegas, J. V., Moral, R., Russo, J., Wang, R. and Russo, I. H. Restortaion of rodent reproductive capabilities after human gonadotropin treatment. *Proc. Am. Assoc. Cancer Res.* 50: 2097a, 2009.

[150] Santucci-Pereira, J., Lopez de Cicco, R., Russo, P. A., Pfeiler, G., Daly, M., Masny, A., Russo, I. H., Sheriff, F. A. and Russo, J. The use of r-hCG changes the transcriptome profile of nulliparous women carrying BRCA1 mutation. *Proc. Am. Assoc. Cancer Res.* 2011.

[151] Russo, J. and Russo, I. H. The transcriptome of breast cancer prevention. *Proceeding of the Rat Genome and Models in the Cold Spring Harbor Symposium*, December 7–10, 2011.

[152] Russo, J., Lareef M. H., Balogh, G., Guo, S. and Russo I. H. Estrogen and its metabolites are carcinogenic in human breast epithelial cells. *J. Steroid Biochem. Mol. Biol.* 87: 1–25, 2003.

[153] Soares, R., Guo, S., Gartner, F., Schmitt, F. C. and Russo, J. estradiol-mediated vessel assembly and stabilization in tumor angiogenesis-b17 and EGFR crosstalk *Angiogenesis* 6: 271–281, 2003.

[154] Russo, J. and Russo, I. H. Genotoxicity of Steroidal Estrogens. *Trends Endocrinol. Metab.* 15: 211–214, 2004.

[155] Soares, R., Balogh, G., Guo, S., Gartner, G. F., Russo J. and Schmitt, F. Evidence for the notch signaling pathway on the role of estrogen and angiogenesis. *Mol. Endocrinol.* 18: 1–10, 2004.

[156] Lareef, M. H., Garber, J., Russo, P. A., Russo, I. H., Heulings, R. and Russo, J. The estrogen antagonist ICI-182-780 does not inhibit the transformation phenotypes induced by -estradiol and 4-OH estradiol in human breast epithelial cells. *Int. J. Oncol.* 26: 423–429, 2005.

[157] Fernandez, S. V., Russo, I. H., Lareef, M. H., Balsara, B. and Russo, J. Comparative Genomic Hybridization of Human Breast Epithelial Cells Transformed by Estrogen and its Metabolites. *Int. J. Oncol.* 26(3): 691–695, 2005.

[158] Chen, J-Q, Yager, J. D. and Russo, J. Regulation of mitochondrial respiratory chain structure and function by estrogens/estrogen receptors and potential physiological/pathophysiological implications: Review. *Biochim. Biophys. Acta* XX: 1–17, 2005.

[159] Fernandez, S. V., Lareef, M. H., Russo, I. H., Balsara, B. R., Testa, J. R. and Russo, J. Estrogen and its metabolites 4-Hydroxy-estradiol induce mutations in TP53 and LOH in chromosome 13q12.3 near BRCA2 in human breast epithelial cells. *Int. J. Cancer* 118(8): 1862–1868, 2006.

[160] Cavalieri, E., Chakravarti, D., Guttenplan, J., Hart, E., Ingle, J., Jankowiak, R., Muti, P., Rogan, E., Russo, J., Santen, R. and Sutter, T. Catechol Estrogen Quinones as Initiators of Breast and Other Human Cancers. Implications for Biomarkers of Susceptibility and Cancer Prevention. Review. *Biochim. Biophys. Acta* 1766: 63–78, 2006.

[161] Russo, J., Fernandez, S. V., Russo, P. A., Fernbaugh, R., Sheriff, F. S., Lareef, H. M., Garber, J. and Russo, I. H. 17 beta estradiol induces transformation and tumorigenesis in human breast epithelial cells. *FASEB J.* 20: 1622–1634, 2006.

[162] Russo, J. and Russo, I. H. The role of estrogen in the initiation of breast cancer. *J. Steroid Biochem. Mol. Biol.* 102: 89–96, 2006.

[163] Mello, M. L., Vidal, B. C., Lareef, M. H., Russo, I. H. and Russo, J. DNA content and estradiol chromatin Texture of Human breast epithelial cells treated with 17- and the estrogen antagonist ICI 182,780 as assessed by Image Analysis. *Mutation Res.* 617: 1–7, 2007.

[164] Tiezzi, D. G., Fernandez, S. V. and Russo, J. Epithelial to Mesenchymal transition during breast cancer progression. *Int. J Oncol.* 31: 823–827, 2007.

[165] Huang, Y., Fernandez, S. V., Goodwin, S., Russo, P. A., Russo, I. H., Sutter, T. and Russo, J. Epithelial to Mesenchymal Transition in Human Breast Epithelial Cells Transformed by 17- beta- Estradiol. *Cancer Res.* 67: 11147–11157, 2007.

[166] Harvey, J. A., Santen, R. J., Petroni, G. R., Bovbjerg, V., Smolkin, M. A., Sheriff, F. and Russo, J. Histology changes in the breast with menopausal

hormone therapy use: correlation with breast density, ER, PgR, and proliferation indices. *Menopause* 15(1): 2008.

[167] Russo, J. and Russo, I. H. Estradiol. In: Schwab, M., (ed), *Encyclopedia of Cancer,* 2nd ed., Springer, Heidelberg. 2007.

[168] Chen, J-Q., Russo, P. A., Cooke, C., Russo, I. H. and Russo, J. ERβ shifts from the mitochondria to the nucleus during 17β estradiol induced neoplastic transformation of human breast epithelial cells and is involved in E2 induced synthesis of mitochondrial chain proteins. *Biochim. Biophys. Acta* 1773: 1732–1746, 2007.

[169] Chen, J-Q. and Russo, J. Mitochondrial estrogen receptors and their potential implications in estrogen carcinogenesis in human breast cancer. *J. Nutritional Environ. Med.* 17: 76–89, 2008.

[170] Mello, M. L., Russo, P. A., Russo, J. and Vidal, B. C. Benedicto C. 17-β-estradiol affects nuclear image properties in MCF-10F human breast epithelial cells with tumorigenesis. *Oncol. Rep.* 18: 1475–1481, 2007.

[171] Saeed, M., Rogan, E., Fernandez, S. V., Sheriff, F., Russo, J. and Cavalieri, E. Formation of depurinating N3Adenine and N7Guanine adducts by MCF-10F cells cultured in the presence of 4-hydroxyestradiol. *Int. J. Cancer* 120: 1821–1824, 2007.

[172] Rahman, M., Lax, S. F., Sutter, C. H., Emmert, G. L., Russo, J., Miller, R., Santen, S. and Sutter, T. S. CYP1B1 is not a major determinant of the disposition of aromatase inhibitors in epithelial cells of invasive ductal carcinoma of the breast. *Drug Metab. Dispos.* 36: 963–970, 2008.

[173] Russo, J. and Russo, I. H. Breast development, hormones and cancer. In: *Innovative Endocrinology of Cancer,* Springer-Verlag, Berlin, Heidelberger, Germany. 2008, 52–56.

[174] Santen, R., Cavalieri, E., Rogan, E., Russo, J., Guttenplan, J., Ingle, J. and Yue, W. Estrogen mediation of breast tumor formation involves estrogen receptor-dependent, as well as independent, genotoxic effects. *Ann. NY Acad. Sci.* 1155:132–140, 2009.

[175] Chen, J-Q., Brown, T. R. and Russo, J. Regulation of Energy Metabolism Pathways by Estrogens and Estrogenic Chemicals and Potential Implications in Obesity Associated with Increased Exposure to Endocrine Disruptors. *Biochim. Biophys. Acta* 1793: 1128–1143, 2009.

[176] Mello, M. L. S., Russo, P., Russo, J. and Vidal, B. C. Entropy of Feulgen-stained 17-beta-estradiol-transformed human breast epithelial cells as assessed by restriction enzymes and image analysis. *Oncol. Rep.* 21(6): 1483–1487, 2009.

[177] Chen, J-Q. and Russo, J. ERα-Negative and Triple Negative Breast Cancer: Molecular Features and Potential Therapeutic Approaches. *Biochim. Biophys. Acta Rev. Cancer* 1796: 162–175, 2009.

[178] Russo, J., Pereira. J., Snider, K. and Russo, I. H. Estrogen induced breast cancer is the result in the disruption of the asymmetric cell division of the stem cell. *Horm. Mol. Biol. Clin. Investig.* 1: 53–65, 2010.

[179] Russo, J., Santen, R. and Russo, I. H. Hormonal control of the breast development. In: DeGroot, L. J., Jameson, J. L., (eds), *Endocrinology*, 5th ed, Chapter 123, W.B. Elsevier. 2009.

[180] Fernandez, S. V., Snider, K. E., Wu, Y. Z., Russo, I. H., Plass, C. and Russo, J. DNA methylation changes in a human cell model of breast cancer progression. *Mutat. Res. Fund. Mol. Mech. Mut.* 688: 28–35, 2010.

[181] Chen, J-Q. and Russo, J. Potential Roles of ERβ, GPCP-30/EGFR, and ERR in Pathogenesis of ERα-Negative and Triple-Negative Breast Cancer. *Eur. J. Clin. Med. Oncol.* 22: 11–34, 2010.

[182] Gargon, V., Fernandez, S. V., Goin, M., Giulianelli, S., Russo, J. and Lanari, C. L. M. Hypermethylation of the progesterone receptor A in constitutive anti progestin resistant mouse. *Breast Cancer Res. Treat.* 126: 319–332, 2011.

[183] Lareef, M. H., Russo, I. H., Slater, C. M., Rogatko, A. and Russo, J. Estrogen induces transformation phenotypes in the estrogen receptor negative MCF10F cells. *Proc. Am. Assoc. Cancer Res.* 42: 4743a, 2001.

[184] Lareef, M. H., Russo I. H., Sheriff, F., Slater, C. and Russo, J. Estrogen and its metabolites are carcinogenic in the human breast epithelial cells. *Proc. Am. Assoc. Cancer Res.* 43: 2002.

[185] Lareef, M. H., Russo, I. H., Sheriff, F., Tahin, Q. and Russo, J. Estrogen-receptor independent induction of loss of heterozygosity in human breast epithelial cells by estrogen and its metabolites. *Breast Cancer Res. Treat.* 76(1): 383a, 2002.

[186] Lareef, H. M., Russo, I. H., Sheriff, F., Tahin, Q. and Russo, J. Genomic Changes induced by Estrogens in human breast epithelial cells (HBEC). *Proc. Am. Assoc. Cancer Res.* 44: 904a, 2003.

[187] Russo, J., Lareef, H. M., Balogh, G. and Russo, I. H. Estrogen is a carcinogenic agent in the human breast. *Int. J. Mol. Med.* 12(1): 147a, 2003.

[188] Fernandez, S. V., Lareef, M. H., Russo, I. H., Balsara, B. B., Testa, J. and Russo, J. Estrogen and its metabolite 4-OH-E2 induce LOH at 13q12.3, at a locus 0.8cM from the BRCA2 gene in human breast epithelial cells. *Proc. Am. Assoc. Cancer Res.* 45: 7a, 2004.

[189] Russo, P. A., Balogh, G. V., Russo, I. H. and Russo, J. Estrogen-induced transformation of human breast epithelial cells involves mutations in mismatch repair genes. *Proc. Am. Assoc. Cancer Res.* 45: 2629a, 2004.

[190] Lareef, M. H., Heulings, R., Russo, P. A., Garber, J., Russo, I. H. and Russo, J. The estrogen antagonist ICI-182-270 does not inhibit the proliferative activity and invasiveness induced in human breast epithelial cells by estradiol and its metabolite 4-OH-Estradiol. *Proc. Am. Assoc. Cancer Res.* 45: 11a, 2004.

[191] Mello, M. L., Vidal, B. C., Lareef, M. H. and Russo, J. Image analysis of 17--estradiol-treated human breast epithelial cells. *Proc. Am. Assoc. Cancer Res.* 45: 8a, 2004.

[192] Harvey, J. A., *et al.* Histology findings of Mammographically Dense Breast Tissue in Postmenopausal Women with and without Hormone Replacement Therapy. *Breast Cancer Res. Treat.* 88(1): 5008a, 2004.

[193] Vanegas, J., Russo, P. A., Russo, I. H. and Russo, J. Estrogen-Transformed Human Breast Epithelial Cells Exhibit an Altered Migratory Behavior *in Vitro. Proc. Am. Assoc. Cancer Res.* 46: 2005.

[194] Fernandez, S. V., Russo, I. H. and Russo, J. Estrogen and its metabolites 4-hydroxy-estradiol and 2-hydroxy-estradiol induce mutation of p53 and LOH in a gene located 0.8cM of BCR2 in human breast epithelial cells. *Proc. Am. Assoc. Cancer Res.*46: 2098a, 2005.

[195] Russo, P. A., Lareef, M. H., Garber, J., Russo, I. H., Fernandez, S., Fernbaugh, R., Balsara, B. R., Sheriff, F., Balogh, G. A., Mailo, D., Heulings, R. and Russo, J. An in Vitro-in Vivo Model of Estrogen Induced Human Breast Carcinogenesis. *Proc. Am. Assoc. Cancer Res.* 46: 2097a, 2005.

[196] Russo, J. Estrogens as carcinogens in the human breast. *Proc. Am. Assoc. Cancer Res.* 46:14–1, 2005.

[197] Vanegas, J. E., Russo, P. A., Russo, I. H. and Russo, J. Estrogen and its metabolites alter the migratory behavior of human breast epithelial cells. *Proc. Era of Hope*, June, 2005.

[198] Russo, P. A., Lareef, M. H., Garber, J., Russo, I. H., Fernandez, S. V., Fernbaugh, R., Balsara, B., Sheriff, F., Balogh, G., Mailo, D., Heulings, R. and Russo, J. A model of estrogen induced human breast carcinogenesis. *Proc. Era of Hope*, June, 2005.

[199] Fernandez, S. V., Russo, I. H. and Russo, J. Estrogen and its metabolites 4-Hydroxy estradiol and 2-Hydrox-yestradiol induce mutations in human breast epithelial cells. *Proc. Era of Hope*, June, 2005.

[200] Chen, J. Q., Russo, P., Russo, I. H. and Russo, J. ER shifts from mitochondria to nucleus during 17-estradiol induced neoplastic transformation of human breast epithelial cells. *Proc. Am. Assoc. Cancer Res.* 47: 2932a, 2006.

[201] Huang, Y., Fernandez, S., Goodwin, S., Russo, P. A., Sutter, T. R. and Russo, J. Genomic profile of the estrogen induced neoplastic transformation of the human breast epithelial cell MCF10F. *Proc. Am. Assoc. Cancer Res.* 47: 149a, 2006.

[202] Fernandez, S. V., Wu, Y-Z., Russo, I. H., Plass, C. and Russo, J. The role of DNA methylation in estrogen-induced transformation of human breast epithelial cells. *Proc. Am. Assoc. Cancer Res.* 47: 1590a, 2006.

[203] Saeed, M., Rogan, E., Cavalieri, E., Sheriff, F., Fernandez, S. V. and Russo, J. Formation of the DNA depurinating N3Ade and N7Gua adducts of 4-Hydroxyestradiol by MCF10F cells cultured with the carcinogenic estrogen metabolite 4-Hydroxyestradiol. *Proc. Am. Assoc. Cancer Res.* 47: 1895a, 2006.

[204] Chen, J. Q., Russo, P. A., Russo, I. H. and Russo, J. Mitochondria-to-nucleus shift of the estrogen receptor beta during estrogen-induced transformation of human breast epithelial cells. *Proc. Endocrine Soc.* 2006.

[205] Tiezzi, D. G., Fernandez, S. V., Huang, Y., Sutter, T. and Russo, J. Epithelial-mesenchymal transition during breast cancer progression. *Proc. Am. Assoc. Cancer Res.* 2007.

[206] Chen, J-Q., Tiezzi, D., Russo, I. H. and Russo, J. Estrogen receptor beta is directly involved in 17-estradiol (E2)-induced synthesis of mitochondrial DNA (mtDNA)-encoded mitochondrial respiratory chain proteins. *Proc. Am. Assoc. Cancer Res.* 2007.

[207] Fernandez, S. V., Russo, I. H. and Russo, J. Role of DNA-methylation in the branching pattern of Estrogen-Transformed Human Breast Epithelial Cells. *Proc. Am. Assoc. Cancer Res.* 2007.

[208] Mello, M. L. S., Russo, P. A., Russo, J. and Vidal, B. C. DNA content and chromatin supra organization change in estrogen-transformed human breast epithelial cells. Amsterdam meeting 2007.

[209] Lehmann, B. D., *et al.* Identification of human triple-negative breast cancer subtypes and preclinical models for selection of targeted therapies. *J. Clin. Investig.* 121: 2750–2767, 2011.

[210] Tan, D. S., *et al.* Triple negative breast cancer: molecular profiling and prognostic impact in adjuvant anthracycline-treated patients. *Breast Cancer Res. Treat.* 111: 27–44, 2008.

[211] Kao, J., *et al.* Molecular profiling of breast cancer cell lines defines relevant tumor models and provides a resource for cancer gene discovery. *PLoS ONE* 4: e6146, 2009.

[212] Neve, R. M., *et al.* A collection of breast cancer cell lines for the study of functionally distinct cancer subtypes. *Cancer Cell* 10: 515–527, 2006.

[213] Grigoriadis, A., *et al.* Molecular characterisation of cell line models for triple-negative breast cancers. *BMC Genom.* 13: 619, 2012.

[214] Yunokawa, M., *et al.* Efficacy of everolimus, a novel mTOR inhibitor, against basal-like triple-negative breast cancer cells. *Cancer Sci.* 103: 1665–1671, 2012.

[215] Tate, C. R., *et al.* Targeting triple-negative breast cancer cells with the histone deacetylase inhibitor panobinostat. *Breast Cancer Res.* 14: R79, 2012.

[216] Fillmore, C. M. and Kuperwasser, C. Human breast cancer cell lines contain stem-like cells that self-renew, give rise to phenotypically diverse progeny and survive chemotherapy. *Breast Cancer Res.* 10: R25, 2008.

[217] Flanagan, L., Van Weelden, K., Ammerman, C., Ethier, S. P. and Welsh, J. SUM-159PT cells: a novel estrogen independent human breast cancer model system. *Breast Cancer Res. Treat.* 58: 193–204, 1999.

[218] Zhang, D., *et al.* Epidermal growth factor receptor tyrosine kinase inhibitor reverses mesenchymal to epithelial phenotype and inhibits metastasis in inflammatory breast cancer. *Clin. Cancer Res.* 15: 6639–6648, 2009.

[219] Su, Y., Pogash, T. J., Nguyen, T. D. and Russo, J. Development and characterization of two human triple-negative breast cancer cell lines with highly tumorigenic and metastatic capabilities. *Cancer Med.* 5: 558–573, 2016.

[220] Woelfle, U., Sauter, G., Santjer, S., Brakenhoff, R. and Pantel, K. Down-regulated expression of cytokeratin 18 promotes progression of human breast cancer. *Clin. Cancer Res.* 10: 2670–2674, 2004.

[221] Su, Y., Gutiérrez-Diez, P. J., Santucci-Pereira, J., Russo, I. H. and Russo, J. In Situ methods for identifying the stem cell of the normal and cancerous breast. In: Russo, J., Russo, I. H., (eds), *Techniques and methodological approaches in breast cancer research*, 1st ed, Springer, New York. 2014, 151–182.

[222] Aguiar, F. N., Mendes, H. N., Cirqueira, C. S., Bacchi, C. E. and Carvalho, F. M. Basal cytokeratin as a potential marker of low risk of invasion in ductal carcinoma in situ. *Clinics* 68: 638–643, 2013.

[223] Morel, A. P., Lièvre, M., Thomas, C., Hinkal, G., Ansieau, S. and Puisieux, A. Generation of breast cancer stem cells through epithelial-mesenchymal transition. *PLoS ONE* 3: e28882008.

[224] Mani, S. A., *et al.* The epithelial-mesenchymal transition generates cells with properties of stem cells. *Cell* 133: 704–715, 2008.

[225] Xue, C., Plieth, D., Venkov, C., Xu, C. and Neilson, E. G. The gatekeeper effect of epithelial-mesenchymal transition regulates the frequency of breast cancer metastasis. *Cancer Res.* 63: 3386–3394, 2003.

[226] Al-Hajj, M., Wicha, M. S., Benito-Hernandez, A., Morrison, S. J. and Clarke, M. F. Prospective identification of tumorigenic breast cancer cells. *Proc. Natl. Acad. Sci.* 100: 3983–3988, 2003.

[227] Sheridan, C., *et al.* CD44+/CD24-breast cancer cells exhibit enhanced invasive properties: an early step necessary for metastasis. *Breast Cancer Res.* 8: R59, 2006.

[228] Wright, M. H., Calcagno, A. M., Salcido, C. D., Carlson, M. D., Ambudkar, S. V. and Varticovski, L. Brca1 breast tumors contain distinct CD44+/CD24- and CD133+ cells with cancer stem cell characteristics. *Breast Cancer Res.* 10: R10, 2008.

[229] Lin, C.-W., Liao, M.-Y., Lin, W.-W., Wang, Y.-P., Lu, T.-Y. and Wu, H.-C. Epithelial cell adhesion molecule regulates tumor initiation and tumorigenesis via activating reprogramming factors and epithelial-mesenchymal transition gene expression in colon cancer. *J. Biol. Chem.* 287: 39449–39459, 2012.

[230] Maetzel, D., *et al.* Nuclear signalling by tumour-associated antigen EpCAM. *Nat. Cell Biol.* 11: 162–171, 2009.

[231] Thampoe, I. J., Ng, J. S. and Lloyd, K. O. Biochemical analysis of a human epithelial surface antigen: differential cell expression and processing. *Arch. Biochem. Biophys.* 267: 342–352, 1988.

[232] Keller, P. J., *et al.* Mapping the cellular and molecular heterogeneity of normal and malignant breast tissues and cultured cell lines. *Breast Cancer Res.* 12: R87, 2010.

[233] Gorges, T. M., *et al.* Circulating tumour cells escape from EpCAM-based detection due to epithelial-to-mesenchymal transition. *BMC Cancer* 12: 178, 2012.

[234] Mego, M., *et al.* Characterization of metastatic breast cancer patients with nondetectable circulating tumor cells. *Int. J. Cancer* 129: 417–423, 2011.

[235] Sieuwerts, A. M., *et al.* Anti-epithelial cell adhesion molecule antibodies and the detection of circulating normal-like breast tumor cells. *J. Natl Cancer Inst.* 101: 61–66, 2009.

[236] Hayes, D. F. C. M. Anti-epithelial cell adhesion molecule antibodies and the detection of circulating normal-like breast tumor cells. *J. Natl. Cancer Inst.* 101: 894–895, 2009.

[237] Van Laere, S. J., Elst, H., Peeters, D., Benoy, I., Vermeulen, P. B. and Dirix, L. Y. Re: anti-epithelial cell adhesion molecule antibodies and the detection of circulating normal-like breast tumor cells. *J. Natl. Cancer Inst.* 101: 895–896, 2009.

[238] Connelly, M., Wang, Y., Doyle, G. V., Terstappen, L. and McCormack, R. Re: anti-epithelial cell adhesion molecule antibodies and the detection of

circulating normal-like breast tumor cells. *J. Natl. Cancer Inst.* 101: 895, 2009.

[239] Balzar, M., *et al.* Epidermal growth factor-like repeats mediate lateral and reciprocal interactions of Ep-CAM molecules in homophilic adhesions. *Mol. Cell. Biol.* 21: 2570–2580, 2001.

[240] Fernandez, S. V., Wu, Y.-Z., Russo, I. H., Plass, C. and Russo, J. DNA Methylation in Human Breast Epithelial Cells transformed by estradiol. *Proc. Endocrine Soc.* 2006.

[241] Fernandez, S. V., Russo, I. H., Snider, K. E. and Russo, J. Estrogen induces Transformation of Breast Epithelial Cells by Epigenetic Gene Silencing. *Proc. Endocrine Soc.* 2008.

[242] Jiang, X., Russo, I. H. and Russo, J. Human chorionic gonadotropin and inhibin induce histone acetylation in human breast cancer cells. *Int. J. Oncol.* 20: 77–79, 2002.

[243] Alvarado, M. V., Ho, T-Y., Russo, J. and Russo, I. H. Human chorionic gonadotropin regulates the synthesis of inhibin in the ovary and the mammary gland of rats. *Endocrine* 2: 1–10, 1994.

[244] Srivastava, P., Russo, J. and Russo, I. H. Inhibition of rat mammary tumorigenesis by human chorionic gonadotropin is associated with increased expression of inhibin. *Mol. Carcinog.* 26: 10–19, 1999.

[245] Mello, M. L., Russo, P. A., Russo, J. and Vidal, B. C. 17-β-estradiol affects nuclear image properties in MCF-10Fhuman breast epithelial cells with tumorigenesis. *Oncol. Rep.* 18: 1475–1481, 2007.

[246] Han, H. J., Russo, J., Kohwi, Y. and Kohwi-Shigematsu, T. SATB1 reprograms gene expression to promote breast cancer metastasis. *Nature* 452: 187–193. 2008.

[247] Vanegas, J. E., Russo, I. H., Moral, R., Pereira, J. S., Wang, R. and Russo, J. Influence of age on the circadian rhythm of clock gene expression in the rat mammary gland. *American Association for Cancer Research (AACR) Annual meeting,* April, 2007, San Diego, CA.

[248] Vanegas, J. E., Rea, M. S., Figueiro, M. G., Bullough, J. D., Possidente, B. P., Moral, R., Pereira, J. S., Russo, J. and Russo, I. H. The clock gene ARNT (Bmal1) and the estrogen receptor alpha are influenced by circadian disruption in the rat mammary gland. *4th Annual Breast Cancer and the Environment Research Center (BCERC) symposium,* November, 2007, Cincinnati, OH.

[249] Vanegas, J. E., Moral, R., Russo, I. H., Pereira, J., Wang, R. and Russo, J. Expression of circadian rhythm related genes during the Sprague Dawley rat

mammary gland development. *Future Research on Endocrine Disruption: Translation of Basic and Animal Research to Understand Human Disease,* August, 2007, Durham, NC.

[250] Russo, I. H., Vanegas, J. E., Anderson, L. E., Morris, J. E., Russo, J. and Stevens, R. G. Circadian rhythm alterations induce age-dependent changes in mammary gland development and in cell proliferation. *Hormone action in development and cancer —Gordon Research Conference (GRC),* July, 2007, New London, NH.

[251] Vanegas, J. E., Moral, R., Russo, I. H., Pereira, J., Wang, R. and Russo, J. Clock genes in the rat mammary gland. *Hormone action in development and cancer — Gordon Research Conference (GRC),* July, 2007, New London, NH.

[252] Vanegas, J. E., Moral, R., Russo, I. H., Wang, R. and Russo, J. Clock genes in the rat mammary gland at 35 and 100 days of age. *AACR annual meeting,* April, 2007, Los Angeles, CA.

[253] Vanegas, J. E., Moral, R., Russo, I. H., Wang, R. and Russo, J. Clock genes in the rat mammary gland at 50 and 100 days of age. *3rd Annual BCERC Symposium,* November, 2006, Berkeley, CA.

[254] Bullough, J. D., Possidente, B. P., Figueiro, M. G., Rea, M. S, Russo I. H., Wang, R., Moral, R., Vanegas, J. E. and Russo, J. Lighting-induced circadian disruption: simultaneous effects on mammary and liver clock gene expression. *10th Biennial Meeting of the Society for Research on Biological Rhythms,* Organized by the Society for Research on Biological Rhythms, May, 2006, Sandestin, FL.

Chapter 12

Accomplishments, Sickness, and Death

12.1. Facing a new reality

There is never a single unique landmark that defines a particular period in world history but rather several successive events that define one period in relation to another. For example, the end of the Middle Ages could be traced to 1492, when Christopher Columbus reached the New World. But there were other events too, like the 1494 signing of the Treaty of Tordesilla by Spain and Portugal, agreeing to divide the world outside of Europe between themselves, or in 1497 when Vasco da Gama began his first voyage from Europe to India and back, and finally in 1499 when the Ottoman fleet defeated the Venetians at the Battle of Zonchio, the first naval battle that used cannons on ships. All of these events clearly define the end of the Middle Ages and the beginning of the modern ages [1].

But in the life of an individual human being, the events heralding turning points are easier to single out. In my case, the period from 2003 to 2013 was a special time in my life, because in the middle of major research successes and as I stood professionally in the main theater of events in cancer research, sickness and death entered in my life in a way that I never expected.

In the early 2000s, I was a part of the action for major events; I was invited to important scientific meetings as a plenary or keynote speaker, and I also organized major conferences like the first meeting

508 Memoirs of a Cancer Researcher

of the NIEHS Breast Cancer and the Environment Research Center (BCERC) and chaired the 2011 Hormone Action in Development and Cancer Gordon Research Conference (GRC). The first conference of the BCERC was held in Princeton, New Jersey, in 2004, and we discussed all the emerging topics in breast cancer and the research environment, and it was the conference that set the pace for the entire program. The GRC was held at Bryant University, in Smithfield, Rhode Island, from July 31 to August 5, 2011. At that conference, we discussed the forefront of research in developmental biology, hormone action, and cancer that are crucial topics in modern science. This GRC was the convergence of three intertwined fields that all address the inner core of the biological system. We discussed the recent advances in our understanding of hormone action on gene expression, development, and physiology, as well as how these pathways can be manipulated by mutations, endocrine disruptors, diet, and lifestyle, which can all lead to cancer and other major pandemics. We also focused on the hormonal control of metabolism, and the reciprocal roles of newly discovered metabolic hormones on development, biological clocks, behavior, and disease. While many important conferences were held that year, these were two particularly significant scientific gatherings that touched the lives of hundreds of people.

During this decade, I also received important grant awards and produced a vital set of data that has sealed my contribution to science. Paradoxically, in the middle of all this professional success, I faced my own illness and Irma's death. These events not only touched me but they shook my whole existence.

12.2. In the center stage

The Department of Defense (DOD) Breast Cancer Center of Excellence Award that I presented with Ercole Cavalieri was funded, but not the one that I presented alone. The most disgusting part was that my score was better than the one that I got with Ercole but it was simply not funded and no further explanation was offered, something which was difficult to digest. After reviewing the scores and critiques, I decided the lack of logic was so rampant that I would appeal. I was supported by Dr. Robert Young, President of the FCCC, and the members of the board, which intervened in this motion. Even a Pennsylvania congressman was involved in the process, and the final decision was clear and simple, it was "not appealing." The DOD funding was well known for these kinds of decisions, in which the funding was determined not by the Study Session that evaluated the grant and gave the quality and funding scores but by the Integration Panel, the final group of individuals that decide who is or is not funded. This is a significant difference from the funding provided by the NIH in which the Study Session score determines the funding; in the DOD, the Study Session is acting as an advisor to the Integration Panel, which makes the final decision based on the agenda that the advocates, those lobbying the government for the funds, believe is the priority of things that need to be done in breast cancer research. The fiasco with the DOD Cancer Center of Excellence caused me to write in my journal on *April 24, 2003*:

> *There are several things difficult to understand, one is the fact that the coalition and lobbying in the DOD is for prevention, and I have not been funded for the idea that we considered and everybody praised as important and innovative.*

Although my Cancer Center of Excellence from the DOD was not funded, the influx of funding in 2003 was very good due to the approval of other grants that we had with Irma making the institution interested in us by approving the renewal of new equipment in the BCRL and putting forward the idea of moving us to larger quarters in the building where the nuclear magnetic resonance (NMR) laboratory was located. At the end, only the funds for renewal of equipment were granted, and the move to a new laboratory was not effective until the new Prevention Pavilion was finished in 2012 when Dr. Michael Seiden was the President and CEO of the FCCC. I must admit that I was very enthusiastic about the idea of moving to new facilities, but in retrospect I needed to accept that the space from the NMR required significant remodeling and that waiting for the completion of the new Prevention Pavilion, where I am presently located, was worthwhile.

While this was happening, I presented my application for the Breast Cancer Center for Environmental Research; it was the largest one I had ever done, with an 11 million dollar budget for a period of 7 years (see Chapter 11). Also in June of that year, I visited my father in Mendoza and I met with Mr. Raul Massone and Dr. Emilio Sojo and established a relationship that helped me obtain funding for a research project using urinary hCG, the main pharmaceutical product of Massone. In that month, I also attended a meeting of the Cancer Cube in Washington, DC. The organization was at this time losing strength due to the funding from the DOD Breast Cancer Center of Excellence and also because of the recent death of Joachim Liehr. A few days later, I returned to Washington, DC, to participate in the congressional briefing on Breast Cancer and the Environment. On *June 4, 2003,* I wrote in my journal:

> *This morning we have a briefing on breast cancer in the Rayburn Office Building for the staff of an Ohio congressman. I was the third speaker and explained in less than ten minutes the idea of the pubertal growth of the breast and its importance in developing breast cancer. I did well, and the audience was young women very motivated to know more on this subject. . . . The four speakers were Michael Gallo, Cheryl Walker, Susan Gelfinger, and myself; we were all applicants to the RFA from the NIEHS. It has been an interesting experience and the dinner last night was congenial and friendly. Marshall Anderson, the director of the NIEHS, was also there from Cincinnati.*

Of the four speakers, only Susan Gelfinger, who was working with Marshall Anderson, and I received funding in answer to the RFA.

In the middle of 2003, I was practically everywhere the action was taking place. I was working on the idea of the NIH breast cancer SPORE, which had been in the back of my mind for several months, and I decided to network with the researchers of the University of Pennsylvania medical school (Penn Med). I succeeded in making them a part of the SPORE. The application was a strong one and received a very good to excellent score but was not funded. However, the critiques were answerable, and in a second attempt, we thought the chances were excellent to be funded.

I was also in charge of organizing the FCCC Disparity Office by request of Dr. Robert Young; it was badly needed to comply with the renewal of the NIH core grant. This introduced me to a new series of obligations, among them to meet and know the movers and shakers of the Black, Latino, and Oriental communities in Philadelphia. Ms. Michelle Jones was the person who helped me organize the Disparity Office at the FCCC, and her significant knowledge of the Philadelphia community opened more than one door for me. At the national level, I participated in a Washington, DC, meeting organized by the NIH to discuss the health issue disparities in this country, and in August on another meeting in Chicago organized by the NIH on health disparities. I became an advisory member of several boards and, palpating the real problem of cancer disparity, I was involved in these activities for almost 3 years. It was a rewarding and rich personal experience.

On *August 26, 2003,* I wrote several impressions in my journal:

> *The Center of Breast Cancer Tissue Resource or CBCTR and the R21 that I presented to NIH will be funded, but I am uncertain about the Breast Cancer and the Environment Research Center, or BCERC, from the NIEHS.*
>
> *The aging of our parents, the loss of people who were around us, the aging and weakness of a body that wants to stay in idleness and not pursue further, the aging of all of our surroundings and the expense necessary to keep them functioning, like the house, the car, the lab, all of our paraphernalia, and possessions, starts to weigh too much.*
>
> *My awareness of the disparity issues in our society made me feel the need to overcome the burden by increasing my creativity and work and to finish the tasks ahead of me, to better understand the process of the disease that is affecting so many. To be in the world but not be possessed, to understand and love and to see beyond the appearance.*
>
> *I am mortified by my inability to deeply understand the mechanism of prevention by the hCG and pregnancy and how to do the clinical trial.*

On August 28 of that year, I was in Chicago at a meeting on health disparity organized by the NCI when I met Dr. Edward Trepido. I'd known him when he was a part of the Miami group of the CBCTR project, and now he was working in the NCI. Dr. Trepido told me that my grant application for the Breast Cancer and the Environment Research Center was in the first position for funding. This shattered my sense of déjà vu after the experience with the DOD Center for Excellence Application. On September 16, I received a call from the NIEHS telling me that the Center for Breast Cancer Research and the Environment would be funded in full (11 million dollars) with some additional funding for bioinformatics and data management. This was great news because it was a positive conclusion to the anticipation and wondering about the final outcome.

On *September 19*, I wrote:

> *Dr. Gwen Colman calls me and the center is now a fact. She congratulated me for that, and they requested my presence in Washington and in Marin County, California, for a press release.*

All of this was happening at the same time that my prostate cancer was discovered (see Section 12.5). The official announcement of the Cancer Centers was done in Marin County on October 14, 2003. I needed to be there and make a short presentation regarding the center. In my journal, I wrote:

> *This trip to California adds an extra leg to the trip to Greta, Lisbon, and San Antonio. I was invited to San Antonio by the Institute of Biotechnology of the University of Texas. I will talk about the paradigm of breast cancer prevention.*

On *October 12, 2003*, I transcribed in my journal a copy of the FCCC's press release.

National Institutes of Health Announce Funding of New Breast Cancer and the Environmental Research Center at Fox Chase Cancer Center

Fox Chase Cancer Center is One of Four Newly Named Centers in the United States.

Fox Chase Cancer Center has been selected as one site for the National Institutes of Health's newly developed Breast Cancer and Environmental Research Center that will probe early environmental exposures that may predispose women to breast cancer.

Fox Chase is one of four sites chosen for the Centers. The Centers are funded jointly by the National Institute of Environmental Health Sciences and the National Cancer Institute, both agencies of the National Institutes of Health, at $5 million a year over seven years for a total of $35 million. The other Centers will be located at University of Cincinnati, University of California, San Francisco, and Michigan State University.

The strength of these Centers is that all will work collaboratively towards the common goal of clarifying whether exposures to environmental agents affect early development of the breast and its subsequent cancer risk. The studies will be carried out through the analysis of the effects of specific environmental agents on the development of mammary tissue in animals, and observing breast development in different ethnic groups of young girls to study their exposures to environmental agents as they go through puberty.

"These four centers will work in close cooperation, bringing all of their expertise to bear upon these questions," said NIEHS director Kenneth Olden. "This will be a united effort among the Centers, not four centers working in isolation."

Fox Chase breast cancer researcher Jose Russo, M.D., is the lead investigator for the Fox Chase Breast Cancer and Environmental Research Center. While the four Centers will network and interact as a single program, each Center will specialize in a particular area of research.

"These multidisciplinary research Centers were specifically designed to fill essential gaps in our knowledge on how environmental exposures impact the development of the breast during puberty and ultimately affect a woman's lifetime breast cancer risk," explained Russo. "This effort represents a bold and innovative concept that takes advantage of the most recent genetic, molecular, endocrinological, and technological advances to address breast cancer prevention."

"*Fox Chase Cancer Center is well-known for the quality of its cancer research,*" said Cong. "*Dr. Russo and his collaborators have developed strong research goals for this project and I'm confident his findings will make significant contributions to our knowledge about breast cancer.*"

"*An excellent and dedicated team of co-investigators, including Dr. Irma Russo at Fox Chase Cancer Center, Dr. Coral Lamartiniere from the University of Alabama, Birmingham, and Drs. Mary Wolff and Luz Claudio from Mount Sinai School of Medicine in New York, are the main collaborators in this Center,*" said Russo.

The Fox Chase Center will work to understand how exposures to estrogenically-active chemicals during early critical periods of development will alter predisposition for breast cancer.

Dr. Coral Lamartiniere and his colleagues at the University of Alabama will investigate the potential of chemicals present in our environment, such as TCDD, bisphenol A, butyl benzyl phthalate and diethylstilbestrol, which are known to disrupt the endocrine system, and genistein, a nutritional agent that has been demonstrated to protect against breast cancer, to affect the development and differentiation of the mammary gland. His team, in collaboration with Dr. Russo's group, will also characterize the changes they induce on the genes and protein profiles of the mammary gland.

"*This research should provide clues about the pathways that are responsible for modulating the susceptibility or resistance of the mammary tissue to carcinogenesis,*" explained Russo.

"*Dr. Mary Wolff and her colleagues at Mount Sinai will investigate risk factors for pubertal milestones in young African American and Hispanic girls, specifically for age at first breast development, age at menarche, and tempo (duration of puberty, or time from breast development to menarche).*"

"*The aim of this work is to verify whether premenopausal breast cancer, that is more common in African-American women, is related to their earlier age at menarche,*" Russo said. "*Therefore, a better understanding of factors affecting pubertal development will contribute essential knowledge on breast cancer predisposition.*"

"A strongly emphasized component of the Fox Chase Center is community outreach. Dr. Luz Claudio at Mount Sinai will lead the effort to establish a bi-directional communication between Mount Sinai and the East Harlem community through a community outreach program. This will provide for communication between researchers of the Center and community members who participate in the study. The study will also draw from the cultural richness of the community to support activities that enhance the experience of the young girls participating in the study and their parents."

"We will develop and coordinate on-site educational workshops and activities for the young girls and their parents who are interested in helping with the study," said Russo. "One of the ways in which this sharing of information will occur is through The East Harlem Girl Power News, a newsletter directed by Dr. Claudio's group that will be distributed to the young girls, their parents, researchers, and local policy makers. We expect that the activities of the outreach program will enhance the overall project by providing innovative activities in which the young girls can engage as a group to learn about issues related to their growth and development."

"The Bioinformatics facility of the Fox Chase Cancer Center under the direction of Dr. Robert Beck has also been selected as the core that will serve all the Centers," Russo said.

NCI director Andrew von Eschenbach explained how past research has contributed significantly to cancer prevention efforts. "The discovery that most lung cancer was caused by tobacco smoke gave us a way to prevent that cancer. Similarly, the banning of certain industrial chemicals has helped prevent bladder and other cancers. If we can also find environmental causes for breast cancer, we will be on our way to preventing many of these cases."

Russo concluded, "I am confident that the knowledge created through these studies will enrich us intellectually and at the same time will allow us to implement general and public measures for protecting our population from environmental factors that affect the breast during the most vulnerable phases of its development, thus contributing to a definitive reduction in the burden of breast cancer."

This is a copy of what I said at the meeting in Marin County FCCC Breast Cancer Center.

October 14, 2003

Marin County, San Raphael, California

It is a real honor for me to be here today and to share with all of you this important moment that for many years we have been waiting for.

The initiative of the National Institute of Environmental Health Sciences and the National Cancer Institute to join efforts for creating a multidisciplinary network of research centers specifically designed to fill important gaps in our knowledge on how environmental exposures impact the development of the mammary gland and ultimately a woman's lifetime breast cancer risk is unprecedented.

For fully understand my personal excitement caused by this event it is necessary that I share with you what happened twenty-eight years ago.

It was the spring of 1975 when Irma, my wife and colleague for more than thirty years, and I were celebrating that our paper on mammary carcinogenesis was accepted for publication in the Journal National Cancer Institute. Our excitement was because in that paper we proposed for the first time that the susceptibility to develop cancer was dependent on the stage of development and differentiation of the mammary gland.

It was not clear at that moment, but in retrospection, to demonstrate this single biological principle has been the quest that brought me here. We envisioned that the most effective approach for eradicating breast cancer is its prevention by modifying or preventing the interaction between the etiologic agents that are present in the environment and the growing breast before it becomes damaged.

When Dr. Ken Olden and Dr. Gwen Collman were gestating this program, and finally announced in the fall of 2002, we knew that this could be the great opportunity to solve many of the questions posed by us and other groups around the country about the importance of the environment on mammary gland development and its effect on cancer. We knew that it would not be easy to fulfill all the requirements of the request for grant application issued by the NCI and the NIEHS, but in our case it was something that emerged almost simultaneously from a call of Dr. Coral Lamartiniere from Alabama and of Dr. Mary Wolff from New York that we must join efforts and present a multi-institutional and multidisciplinary application.

What do we want to accomplish?

In our center we are aiming at understanding how exposure to estrogenically-active chemicals alone, and in combination, during early critical periods of development will alter predisposition for breast cancer.

With Dr. Lamartiniere we propose to investigate the potential of environmental chemicals, such as TCDD, bisphenol A, and butyl benzyl phthalate, which are known endocrine disruptors present in our environment, as well as genistein, a nutritional agent that has been demonstrated to protect against breast cancer.

We will define how each of these chemicals affects the development and differentiation of the mammary gland, and will characterize the changes they induce on the genes and protein profiles of the mammary gland. This study should provide clues on the pathways that are responsible for modulating the susceptibility or resistance of the mammary tissue to carcinogenesis.

We will also build a bridge for translating what we found in the experimental animal system to the human population. The partnership with Dr. Mary Wolff from Mount Sinai School of Medicine in New York will allow us to investigate risk factors for pubertal milestones, specifically for age at first breast development, age at menarche, and tempo (duration of puberty, or time from breast development to menarche).

These studies will allow us to verify whether premenopausal breast cancer, that is more common in Black women, is related to their earlier age at menarche. Therefore, a better understanding of factors affecting pubertal development will contribute essential knowledge on breast cancer predisposition.

We will study a prospective cohort study of Black and Latina girls in East Harlem, New York City, will examine the effect of environmental exposures on pubertal milestones. Of primary interest are specific xenoestrogens, such as phenols and phthalates, the same ones that we are studying in the animal system, dietary constituents, such as phytoestrogens, fiber, fat, and antioxidants, physical activity, and family-environment stress.

Any study in the community requires a strong leadership and presence. The partnership with Dr. Luz Claudio will allow us to establish a bi-directional communication between Mount Sinai and the East Harlem community through the Community Outreach Program. This will provide a vehicle for communication between scientists conducting the research components of this center and community members who participate in the study.

The study will also draw from the cultural richness of the community to support activities that enhance the experience of children participating in the study and their parents. We will develop and coordinate on-site educational workshops and activities for study participants at the community-based clinical recruitment sites. Conversely, there is a need for study participants and other community members to communicate with researchers about many of the issues that may arise through the conduct of the project.

I am confident that the knowledge created through these studies will enrich us intellectually and at the same time will allow us to implement general and public measures for protecting our population from environmental factors that affect the breast during the most vulnerable phases of its development, and thus contributing to a definitive reduction in the burden of breast cancer.

Thank you for allowing me to be here and sharing this historical moment.

My travel schedule was very steady during this 10-year period, and I made a log of all my trips. In 2006, I registered 18 trips covering 94,000 miles, as depicted in Figure 12.1. The same pattern was maintained from 2003 until 2013, meaning that I had an average of 14–20 travel engagements a year.

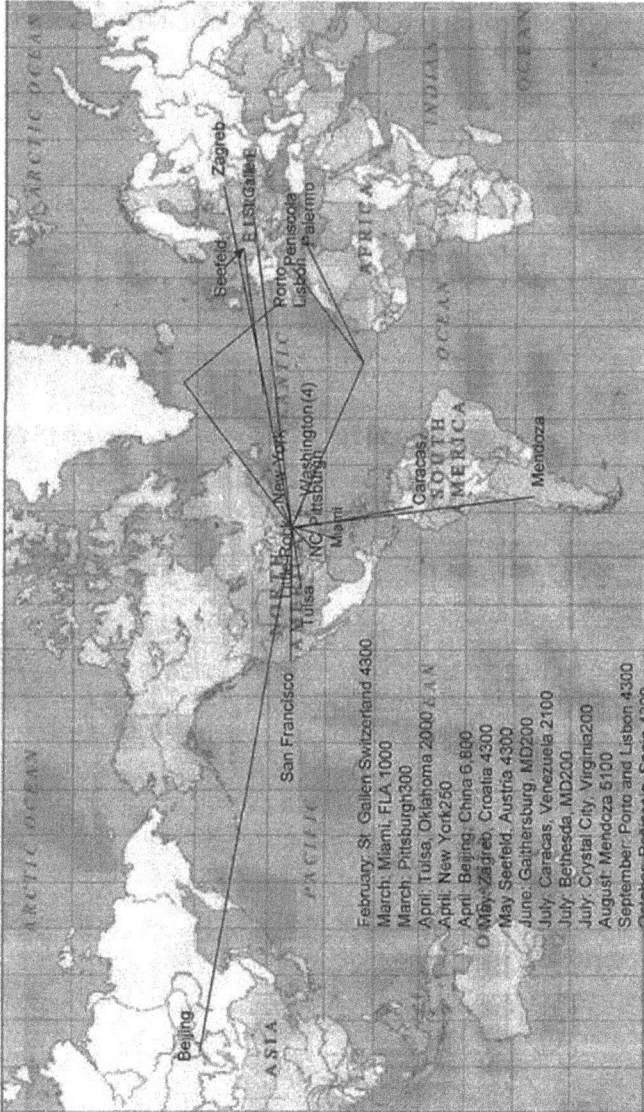

2006 Travel Engagements

February: St. Gallen Switzerland 4300
March: Miami, FLA 1000
March: Pittsburgh300
April: Tulsa, Oklahoma 2000
April: New York250
April: Beijing China 6,800
May: Zagreb, Croatia 4300
May: Seefeld, Austria 4300
June: Gaithersburg, MD200
July: Caracas, Venezuela 2100
July: Bethesda MD200
July: Crystal City, Virginia200
August: Mendoza 5100
September: Porto and Lisbon 4300
October: Penisola; Spain 4300
October: San Francisco 2500
November: Palermo, Italy4300
December: Chapel Hill, NC300
December: Little Rock Arkansas100

18 travel engagements
Approximately 94,000 miles

Figure 12.1: My traveling itinerary from 2006.

12.3. My adventure with the SPORE on breast cancer

On *March 30, 2004,* I wrote:

> *I received the information on Craig Jordan's coming to the FCCC, and it was good news to have somebody of his reputation at the FCCC. Robert Ozols, the vice president of the medical division at the FCCC and my superior, called me few days ago to tell me that I will no longer be the PI for the Breast SPORE to the NCI and that Craig Jordan will be the next PI of the Breast Specialized Programs of Research Excellence, or SPORE application. Dr Jordan wanted to be the PI of the SPORE as part of the package that he received. This is an unexpected blow to my leadership of a project that I have been nurturing for the last three years. However, looking at this in the big picture, I must admit to myself that although I have been working and doing my duty to make this program successful, I was not happy and comfortable because the requirements of the SPORE were so numerous that to make everybody happy I had to do a little bit of everything to comply with the program, so that the real accomplishment was difficult to see. Analyzing the major success of the SPOREs around the country did not leave me impressed by their achievements. Now that Craig Jordan is the PI I am released of this burden. The only thing that I need to do now is to keep myself in one piece and not despair about looking like a loser and a destitute person.*

In the same journal entry, I wrote:

> *Tomorrow Craig Jordan is coming to talk with me, and I already indicated by mail to him that Irma and I decided not to be part of the SPORE. The reality is that I have lost my interest and I feel tired and in great* need to recover *myself from this physical ordeal of my prostate surgery (see Section 12.5).*

A note of interest for this memoir is that the SPORE grant application presented by Craig Jordan as PI received a poorer score than the one that I presented, and his was never funded. This was not a reflection on Craig Jordan but of multiple factors and one of them was that the main players of Penn Med had dropped other projects since they were not as strong as they were before.

12.4. My literary work

On *October 1, 2003,* I wrote:

> *In front of me I have the outline of the new book that I am planning to write. Its tentative title is A Handbook for the Apprentice of a Research Scientist. It contains twelve chapters based in areas that involve what is the research scientist, the research ideas, and how to organize a protocol book. Although the idea of the book is less than twenty-four hours old, the concept has been in my mind since 1996, when I presented some of these ideas to my research team in order to give them a few guidelines in cancer research. I feel enthusiastic about the idea of writing this book.*

The book was published by World Scientific in 2011 and the final title is *The Handbook for the Apprentice of Biomedical Research: The Tools of Science* (Figure 12.2) [2]. The final book contained only 10 chapters and was aimed at providing useful tips for the understanding of scientific research processes and practical advice for people engaged in this field. It was a reflection of my more than 40 years of experience in medical and cancer research, and was written in a colloquial style to reach not only the young readers who are considering devoting their lives to biomedical research, but also to those who are already engaged in this field. I emphasize the unique traits and qualifications required for performing scientific research and also I describe the different modalities which can be performed in our actual scientific environment. I provided numerous practical advices, such as guidelines on writing a grant proposal and the first peer-reviewed manuscript, the selection criteria of the training laboratory and mentors, as well as experimental record. I also provided my insight on the personal inner drive and motivation critical for conducting scientific research, as well as the importance of working on a problem without losing the human perspective of this

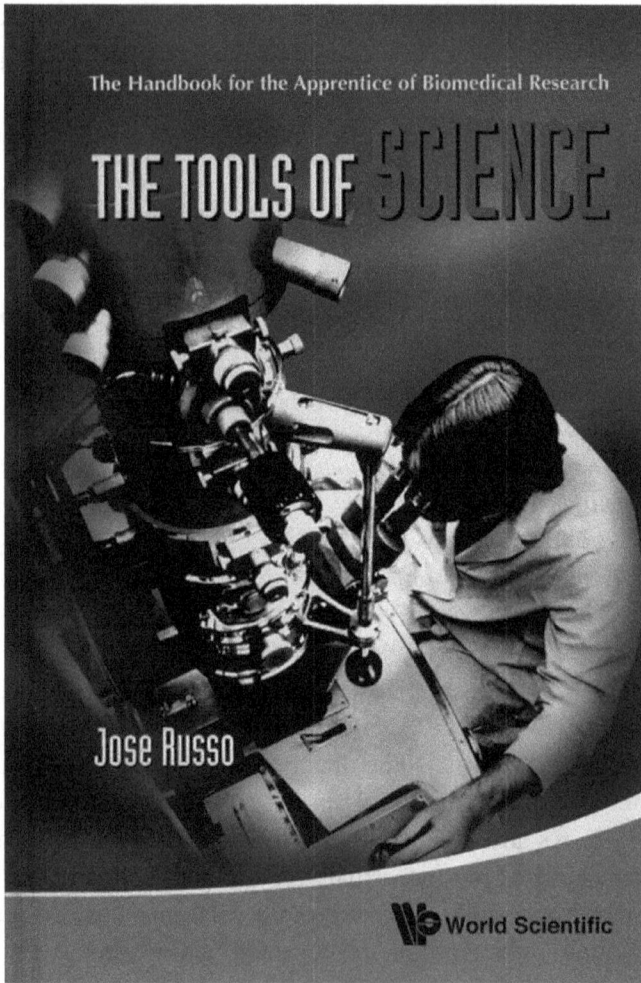

Figure 12.2: Cover of the book *The Tools of Science*, published in 2011.

specific and unique human endeavor. This was my sixth book [3–7] and 10 more came after that one [8–17], the importance of this book for me is that was my first solo literature piece. I received many compliments about this book but the two that I appreciated the most came from Dr. Jonathan Chernoff, at that time the Scientific Director of the FCCC, and the other from Dr. Josiah Ochieng, professor in biochemistry and cancer biology at Meharry Medical College.

Chernoff wrote:

I have read this book from cover to cover and of all the books I have read in my academic life, this one is at the top. My only regret is that this book was not available twenty-five years ago when I entered the PhD program. Clearly this is an exceptional road map for a budding scientist. Since it may take a lifetime for an average person to know all the intrigues in scientific research, it is not too late for most of us who are already established to take a refresher course from this book. I therefore recommend it for all scientists including those like me who are contemplating an early retirement from our beloved vocation.

Ochieng wrote:

In this book Dr. Russo emphasizes to the reader the joy of persevering in science. It is indeed a calling and if you do the right things and follow the recommendations in this book you can avoid the pitfalls and frustrations that have followed many scientists. Such as inability to attract research funds, inability to publish in high impact journals, and frankly the inability to convince others that you have a story. I wish for as many young people as possible to enter this vocation but with their eyes fully open to see the horizon. To think outside the box and become discoverers rather than those who simply tie the loose ends after the "discoverers" have done their jobs.

12.5. Facing cancer

On *September 13, 2003,* I wrote in my journal:

I went to see Dr. S. Samaha, the urologist that treated me for my kidney stone, because I have been bothered for quite a while with pain and all the symptoms of a lithiasis, and interestingly associated with increase in my blood pressure. The latter is probably the one that bother me the most. . . . He detected a hard nodule in my prostate and after a PSA, X-rays, and a scan I will need to go for a biopsy. The excitement of the NIEHS award for seven years of funding and an eleven-million-dollar budget

is clouded by this uncertainty about my prostate and my kidney. I feel
pain in the right flank and for a moment it gets very strong; my mind
is oscillating in a benign process or the announcement of a metastasis.
It is true that in retrospect this pain has been there for quite a while but
my mind is cloudy. The CT-SCAN did not show stones in the right side
but in the left and no other abnormalities, like evident metastasis were
observed. The PSA was 5.4, higher than the 4.00 values considered as
threshold warranting that the biopsy must follow.

In those days, I could not admit that I must stop my schedule of
trips and research activities. To be sick was for me something to
endure as part of my daily routine, however, this call of my mortality
made me feel uneasy. On *October 16, 2003*, I wrote in my journal:

I am in Athens waiting for my flight to Heraklion. This is the last leg
of this trip. I feel the sensation that I do not know if I belong here; I feel
that I am extraneous to all of this. The fight for the grants and for the
everyday activities in the BCRL has produced a feeling that coming to
meetings and traveling is foreign and far away from me. The feeling
of sickness and that I do not know what will happen to me also distances
me in one way or another from everything. The feeling of ageing
among a new generation of men and women makes me feel also far
away. I do not know why I am writing all these things in this particular
moment in the middle of a semi-deserted waiting room in Athens on
my way to a meeting. Probably the excitement and the importance of
going places and giving talks is fading. Probably because the real
importance is in solid publications and grants? I do not know. But
what I feel is the need of more transcendental and meaningful work.

All these reflections did not stop me from taking my next trip to
a Lisbon meeting organized by *Maturitas, a Journal of the Menopause*
Society. The meeting took place in the Pestana Palace in Lisbon, and
I wrote in my journal:

The palace is a construction of the 1904 designated Palacio Valle Flor
and a national monument now run by Carlton. In the middle of this

my health, clouded by a cancer, made me realize even more that I need to work harder to accomplish the work that I need to do and I must separate myself from the need for human recognition. As Cristian Larson said: "To use all my time on my personal improvement means that there is not place or time to criticize the other ones."

Around *October 30, 2003*, at Abington Hospital, I had a prostate biopsy, which turned out to be more painful and discomforting than I was expecting. The following day I went to Sacramento to the meeting organized by Robert Cardiff. This meeting was the rebumped International Cancer Research Association that used to be run by Marvin Rich. The diagnosis of my biopsy was carcinoma, and Irma started doing the arrangements to go to John Hopkins (JH) for treatment. After gathering the X-ray, CT scan, and slides, we met Dr. Su at JH, and he advised me to do a laparoscopic prostatectomy. I was in anguish and afraid to die, to leave Patricia and Irma and all the work incomplete. During this ordeal, I attended the first meeting of the BCERC in North Carolina, and the trip to Boston was organized by the SPORE groups. Also I had been in contact with Robert Bryant from Wake Forest University about testing hCG in monkeys. Although this could be an important piece of work, there were intrinsic difficulties working with monkeys that made a collaboration impossible. Among them were the impossibility of establishing the precise age and pregnancy history of the monkeys and also the limitations in biopsying the mammary glands. At the same time, this door closed and I received the call from Paolo Toniolo indicating that parous women with cancer have lower levels of hCG than those without breast cancer. This epidemiological data confirmed our work.

On November 26, I had an appointment for a bone scan that resulted normal. This was very important because it indicated that the cancer was localized, as far as we knew, to the prostate. Irma found that the surgery could be done on December 24 and insisted on it. Because we had some days left before that date, we went to Somerset Medical Center in New Jersey to attend a conference for the medical staff; we wanted to see if there was a possibility of recruiting more cases for our genomic studies. I drove the Jaguar that we bought with the unexpected royalties check for the book *Molecular Basis of Breast Cancer,* published by Springer [7]. The check paid for almost all the price of the 2004 Jaguar XJ8. I asked myself if this purchase was an act of faith for the unknown. Or a gratification for something well done? Independent of the reason, the Jaguar is a beautiful driving machine and the book provided the scientific basis of a new paradigm according to which breast cancer prevention and treatment should be developed. We described the developmental pattern of the breast in rodents and humans. We emphasized the biological law that we had discovered indicating that the susceptibility of the breast to carcinogenesis is determined by the degree of differentiation of the gland. The application of this law was supposed to have a repercussion on the way that strategic tools for prevention and treatment of breast cancer must be developed [7].

On *December 23, 2003,* I wrote:

We are in Baltimore at the Marriott hotel. This morning we arrived on time to make all the preoperative analysis and examination. I must be on the surgical floor tomorrow at six a.m. We are tired because we woke up very early. Thus far only Irma, Patricia, and I know about this surgical procedure. I am afraid to die in the process or that I'll wake up impaired in my functions; that the cancer is more advanced and I cannot recover from the whole thing. I am afraid that doing the surgery at JHSM was a mistake. Doubts and anxiety cloud my spirit. . . . So suddenly life and every marvelous thing in it seem to be so fragile, so weak, and we are so insignificant when the disease cripples all our plans and ambitions.

On *January 1, 2004,* I wrote:

I am slowly recovering from the surgery last week. It has been painful and uncomfortable but at least I AM ALIVE. In a couple of hours we are going back to Bayview for a cintigraphy and removal of the catheter. I am not so sure yet what the data on LN status is. . . . The removal of the Foley catheter was followed by urinary retention that resulted in my admission to the emergency room at Abington

Memorial. The catheter was reinstalled by urology resident from Temple University.

Tomorrow, January 2, 2004, I am expecting to go back to work. We are rehearsing with Irma to show a good face and give no indication that I am still have the catheter draining in a bag on my right leg. The surgical report indicated that the tumor involved both lobules and was invading the seminal vesicles. The LNs were negatives. The Gleeson score was 6. In three months I need to have a PSA again and follow up.

Although my recovery was not complete, I made the decision to go to Madrid to see my sister. Araceli and Pedro, and to Porto for the thesis of Raquel Soares. Was it a heroic or a stupid decision? Probably both because my Foley catheter was still in place and attached to it was the plastic bag strapped to my right leg, and in this condition I traveled to Spain and Portugal enduring all these inconveniences to avoid breaking a promise to be there for Raquel's doctoral dissertation and to visit my family in Valladolid. Not to go was to tell the reason and admit that I'd had surgery for prostate cancer. In retrospection, it was a stupid decision of pride but the trip was rewarding to see Raquel making a beautiful dissertation and to be part of the tradition of the Porto University with my toga and cap, listening the presentation and giving her support. With my relatives, we had a good time and even visited Salamanca; they never suspected my true physical condition during that trip.

On *March 24, 2004,* I wrote:

I am today sixty-two years old. The PSA is undetectable meaning that up to now there is no evidence of residual prostate cancer. We had been in San Juan, Puerto Rico, for a meeting organized for the publishers of biomedicine, and followed by a Cancer Center meeting in Bethesda. I am preparing part of the report of the work that we are doing and after my birthday I am going with Irma to Miami and Orlando for the CBCTR and the AACR meeting respectively. In the latter we are presenting ten papers, two of them Patricia is an author. The more I think about the trip to Peru, the less interested I am in going. I am more pressured by the immediate issues of my health and my need to accomplish something beyond these main tasks. I AM AFRAID TO GET LOST IN THE DAILY Activities AND FORGET the IMPORTANT ISSUES.

On *May 2, 2004,* I wrote:

This evening I am flying to Birmingham, Alabama, as a part of the External Advisory Board for the Center of Genetic and Nutrient Interaction directed by Barnes. I am still recovering from my kidney stone colic that started on April 22 with severe pain in my left flank with nausea and vomiting, resulting in an admission to Abington Hospital. The attending physician inserted a stem to keep my stone to obstruct my already hydronephrotic kidney. I was released from the hospital Saturday morning April 24 and this was followed by a lithotripsy four days later. I have been recovering since. In the meantime we had the Breast Cancer for Environment Research Center meeting that was a positive one, and I have finished the IDEA grant for the DOD, and working with Irma in the mathematic approach of prevention. . . . From this period until the end of June I was working with Irma to review the manuscript that we had written with Gabriela. It was not accepted by Genes, Chromosomes and Cancer. Irma suggested that we send it to the International Journal of Cancer. Irma amassments me for her analytical power and to read beyond the appearance. I admire her and love her and I treasure all the minutes of our life together.

On *December 24, 2004,* I wrote in my journal:

I am in Mendoza and this is my third day here. Yesterday Papa experienced an apparent recovery since my arrival.

My father was not doing well and did not recognize me. Mary, the person taking care of him, was the only one who could obtain some response. His face was emaciated and his green-brown eyes looked at me but he could not register me in his brain. He responded to my sister Pitty's voice but mostly he responded to Mary and gave her a kiss of appreciation. Any kind of movement triggered pain and discomfort. My father died on January 5, 2005. His funeral was a small one and only the family was there. All those that had known him were not present. It was a sad day in the suffocating heat of Mendoza's summer. I still feel the pain and sadness of his death. With the death of my father, I felt that my last link to my birthplace was finally cut.

12.6. Irma's sickness and death

It is difficult to pinpoint when the beginning of the end starts. Our life was interrupted by my prostate cancer in 2003, and we overcame that and kept up a frantic research agenda until the middle of 2009. Irma and I felt that we were in the midst of the action. On January 19 of that year, we were in Brussels attending a meeting of the European Cancer Prevention Organization where Irma and I received the Hill Memorial Prize for our work in breast cancer prevention. Two days later, on January 21, I was going to Washington, DC, to chair a DOD Study Session and the same day Barack Obama assumed the position of President of the United States. Almost two weeks later Carmen died; the loss of my dear mother-in-law who had been with us since Patricia was born left an empty space in our hearts. But our life continued, and we went to Miami for the Avon Forum, where the data of the genomic signature of pregnancy were presented. After that I went to New York by invitation of the Population Council to deliver a lecture on breast cancer prevention. On March 24, I reached 67 years of age and planned a trip to North Carolina for a site visit at Duke University. At the same time, I was preparing two grant applications and expecting the results on the RO1. I was also planning an R21 and RO1 for June and expecting the verdict of the innovation grant from the DOD. In April of 2009, I went to the AACR in Denver, and one week later Irma and I went to Lausanne, Switzerland, for a meeting with the Pregnancy Group that we had formed with Paolo Toniolo. We presented the data of Avon showing that the discovery phase illustrates differences in the genomic expression in the parous versus nulliparous women and this was a good set of solid data. We were full speed in our research plans and with our life and on *June 21, 2009*, I wrote in my journal:

> *Today is the beginning of the summer and the garden is blooming and full of life, however for me there is only sadness reflecting my profound pain. Irma is sick, and she has been diagnosed with an ovarian cancer that is taking the pelvis and has ascites. She must go to surgery soon because her breathing is difficult. Only God knows what is going on inside of me. I am crying and cannot stand the idea of losing Irma. I love her so much and I cannot conceive living without her. I need to go to Washington to present a lecture at the meeting of Toxicology Pathology but everything looks so stupid and ludicrously empty.*

On *Sunday, June 28*, of the same year I wrote:

> *Last Friday Irma was scheduled for surgery with Dr. Elin Sigurdsson, but it was postponed until tomorrow. The paracentesis obtained five liters of fluid containing neoplastic cells. I pray incessantly that the surgery goes well and without complication, asking for her life and helping her to recover and that this process not be an irreversible one. I asked God that she live to see Patricia married with children and realized as a woman also I asked God to guide everyone who will be involved in her treatment and care.*
>
> *The blackest thoughts and apprehension cover my hours. I cry and I do not know what to do but to ask God for help and protection. . . . The surgery confirmed an ovarian cancer disseminated to the peritoneum and neighbor organs. It was also invading the cecum and resection was needed. It was not LN involvement and if it is maintained localized it will be better for therapeutic response.*
>
> *In the meantime I continued with my research work, and I went to New York for a meeting with the Avon Group and few days later I went to Research Triangle for a meeting of the BCERC. Estela Irma's sister is with us.*

Irma's recovery was slow and before my trip to Izmir, Turkey, for a conference by an invitation from Hilal and Mehmet Kocdor, Irma started the chemotherapy. This cycle ended in November 8, and she resumed her work in the BCRL. We went together to Piscataway where the environmental agency from the Wood Johnson is located. This lecture was by invitation of Michael Gallo and the trip to Rutgers was very good and the conference was well received. A few days later, Irma and I flew to San Francisco to a meeting organized by Susan Fenton from the NIEHS and Silent Spring and that same week we started the meeting of the BCERC.

In March of 2010, I was full of silent pain and anguish. I wrote several entries in my journal saying:

My spirit is in pain and feels bad for not being able to carry my cross and control this pain and crying desperation. The pain of thinking of losing her, that she might have a recurrence of her cancer, that I must stay alone and face every single day of my life without her is unbearable. Deep in me I feel that I am going down, that our research will be stopped any minute, for lack of funding that I will lose the lab and I will be relegated to a corner without project or idea and everything in failure and disarray.

This dark picture of desolation and misery deprives my soul of any light or hope that it will be different. In every single incident I see as a harbinger of the future I have received bad news and rejections of the grant applications that I presented.

I feel so miserable, so empty, so full of nothing. I pray to God, but He knows that I am unable to see or to have hope because I feel desolate and worst nothing. I pray for forgiveness and to have the peace and strength to see the path and understand what I must do.

On *April 23, 2010*, I wrote:

It is two-thirty in the morning and I cannot sleep. Yesterday I noticed that our work was cited in the news section of the JNCI. This is good for our projects. The final application for Avon was mailed out. If this project is funded it will be together with the other project newly funded by the Komen, a solid basis for continuing the research on the prevention issues.

We are extending the R21 trial on the use of r-hcg in women at high risk. Irma has been instrumental in asking the help of the Avon army of women for recruitment. We have received only one response but it could be a good way to reach the target population for achieving our enrollment aim. With the budget still left in this project we are extending the subcontract with the University of Texas and the Mayo Clinic.

Irma is a source of solace in my sea of desperation. Talking with her, listening to her, and seeing her enlighten my heart and a tremendous unbearable pain comes to me when I think or perceive that I can lose her.

On Monday, *August 2, 2010,* I wrote in my journal:

This week we are moving the BCRL to the Women's Cancer Center in the new building of the FCCC that is part of the Prevention Pavilion. There is excitement in the lab about this and we have been planning this event for almost a year.

On *September 12, 2010,* I wrote:

Tomorrow I am going to the DOD Integration Panel and on my way back, I will give a conference at the National Academy. This latter meeting is organized by an environmental group sponsored by the Komen for the cure.

Irma is doing fine, and she is helping to put the manuscript of the genomic signature of pregnancy together. This is our main task. There are consistent data, and I believe that we have a new discovery and a mechanism by which pregnancy modulates protection. Our idea is to publish the work in the Proceedings of the NAS. There is a pressure to finish this work because on October 14 we must present the data of the Genomic Signature of Pregnancy (GSP) in NY in front of the board of the Avon foundation; this could be decisive moment for the funding that we have requested.

We started the Komen promise grant project under Experiment 896. Almost the whole lab is working in the in vitro and in vivo part of it. We are fully installed in the new BCRL and it is impressive compared with the old one, there are small details but overall it is a good location and environment.

On *October 8, 2010,* I wrote:

I am in the airport of Santo Domingo waiting for my flight to Miami that has been delayed. I am anxious to be at home, and I feel very tired. The journey to this place has been good and I feel that I have provided useful information and a blueprint on how to proceed. My lecture on Wednesday went very well and smart questions were aroused, and also last night I was well received. The First Lady was there, and she personally thanked me for my participation, and we were having dinner together with other members of her staff and the physician interested in implementing a National Tumor Registry. The First Lady of this country is a very smart and warm person with a great vision to help her people and the health situation of the country. [Unfortunately I never received feedback on whether the project planned in that meeting was successful or not.]

I made several entries in my journal:

Today, October 20, I am going to Montreal to a meeting at McGill University to talk about cell transformation. I have been invited to be part of the Environmental Health Committee of the NIEHS. On November 8 I am traveling to San Diego for an expert consultation with Arena Pharmaceutical. This will be done through the Pathology Consultation Services, or PCS, that I have established as a for-profit company that helped me to provide consultation on my area of expertise and support and receive the benefits of my books' publication hoping to help our shackled domestic economy. Arena required my expert opinion at a hearing that they had with the FDA in DC.

On *November 16, 2010,* I was in Palermo, Italy, for the Amazon project. The meeting was a good one, however, I do not know how my lecture impacted the people in the audience, which was very diverse. It was organized by the Amazon Group, and it is difficult to know what they are really looking for. Meetings like this shake my confidence in the way that I present the data, and I wrote in my journal:

> *I would like to be home with Irma, without her I feel so empty. I am so afraid to be alone, without her, without her love, without her joy, her spirit and wittiness.*

On *December 15, 2010*:

> *Irma went for a PET scan to determine if the masses or cysts detected under the liver are active disease. We have received the grant for Avon; it is one million for us over two years. We'd requested one and a half million but it is okay, we will manage and it is a blessing.... The book: The Tools of Science [2] was published and the Avon grant allowed us to continue with the project genomic signature of pregnancy for a two-year period. Patricia was still working with us and had finished her second master's. The entrance to Penn for her PhD was truncated by the accident of Ron in early October.*

On *January 2, 2011*, I entered in my journal:

> *Irma was doing fine after one year of chemotherapy but she was hiding from me the diagnosis that she got before Christmas. Her tumor has recurred in two visible masses that have been localized with the PET scan; one is in the surface of the liver and the other near the spleen. These last two weeks have been a roller coaster of emotions and turmoil in my spirit. We still do not know what to do, the physicians at FCCC are not very resourceful and the only thing that they suggest is waiting and having another course of chemo. The suggestion of laparoscopic resection or focal radiation has not been encouraged by them, but there is some alignment among the attendants in recommending her the same. We talked with Michael Seiden and he promised to study the case. I want to pursue and see outside of FCCC for a qualified second opinion. I feel my chest oppressed by the anguish and pain. I do not*

know how to ask your blessing and miracle for her life. I feel so in pain because everything that I do with her comes to my mind as the last time that I will see her do it. Although she is feeling and looking fine, the idea that something is killing her inside is unbearable. I am questioning all our knowledge and advances, and they look to me as we are walking in a nonsense situation. I feel a sense of a catastrophic event going on in my life, it is like something terrible or unexpected will strike my life, and a feeling of disaster and pain is all inside me. One thing I know is that I want to interiorize this pain and not show this unbearable feeling to Irma. I wish to sanctify myself in this suffering to be better and to concentrate on what you, God, want from me.

On *February 24, 2011,* I wrote:

We are going to the Memorial Sloan Kettering Cancer Center (MSKCC) in New York for a consultation for Irma's tumor. Dr. Chi is a young but experienced surgeon and he agrees and suggests that Irma go through a tumorectomy for the two lesions in the liver and spleen. He is very confident and that scares me. The surgery is scheduled for March 25. We must go for a pre-surgical check out on March 22 for her scheduled surgery on Friday the 25, after that her recovery and chemo.

On *March 24, 2011,* I wrote:

"I am sixty-nine years old. Thanks for every minute of the life that you gave me. We are going with Irma to NY, first to the Affinia Gardens Hotel and tomorrow morning Irma will be admitted at the MSKCC for surgery.

Irma was released from the hospital on April 1, and she recovered from her surgery.

On *May 22, 2011,* I have several notes in my journal:

I feel suspended in time and I need to find a way to get back to the original point of departure in these recurrent dreams of mine. It seems that an eternity has passed from the trips to NY and Irma's surgery and coming back to my journal and I'm focused on how what is going on will help me to overcome this feeling of awaking from a dream mixed with nightmares and insomnia. Irma is doing better, and she feels fine. We do not have the last CT scan results yet but thus far the C125 is low and the results of the path report showed only two foci of serous adenocarcinomas that were removed at surgery.

"Drs Yamrong Su and Bin Yan have been incorporated into the lab and we are still waiting for Julia to clear her visa papers. Theresa Nguyen will be hired this coming July and Dr. Sandra Fernandez has found a job with Dr. Massimo Cristofanilli. The Komen Promise grant that we presented with Massimo will not be funded as well as the Mary Kay grant. The supplementary grant from Avon for the hCG trial that was supposed to be presented by Paolo Toniolo was not done, and I am upset about his behavior and lack of response to my persistent requests on the matter. There is, however, some hope that the contract with Arena will be effective and also is promising the interest of Dompe to finance our studies on epithelial mesenchymal transition or EMT. If these contracts are approved it will give resources to maintain the lab, hire another technician, and replace some equipment.

The experiments are starting to shape up, mainly Experiment 896, which carries the proposal of the Komen Promise grant. The in vivo data showed thus far that hCG is still the most powerful differentiating agent in the 15aa peptides tested. The carcinogenicity study is not finished yet but they are going in the same direction. Experiment 901 is basically that the phase 2 of the Avon project with the new fundings are starting but we are having problems with the amount of tissue. Probably it will require a larger core biopsy.

The book Environment and Breast Cancer, published by Springer [8], is in press and probably will see the light in August of this year. The book Evolution of Mathematics in Cancer Research [9] will be delayed due to Pedro's new responsibilities as director of the Santa Cruz College in Valladolid. Finally the book Breast Cancer Prevention [12] is in progress but I have not put any fire or energy into it.

I was invited to be part of a panel on environment risk by the University of Utrecht and after saying yes I changed my mind.

I found it irrelevant, like so many other things that I am doing, like the trip to NY tomorrow to discuss the data on the Phase II of the Avon project.

On *August 2, 2011,* I wrote:

Irma's presence seems so ethereal and distant and this continuous consciousness that she can die of her disease and that I will be alone in this world that seems each day so complicated and full of emptiness that it makes my sadness even more profound. I cannot ventilate this emotion but I know that even without talking or in my slightest remark I am projecting all this torment that is going on inside of me. I feel so empty about a conference that I have organized and that I feel that I do not have anything to say, I am the instrument in other people's hands, and I am not writing my message and not allowing that you be my inspiration and I be the pen in your hands like Mother Teresa said. I have organized this GRC, and my presence is unremarkable because I feel empty and that I do not have anything to say.

We are expecting Irma's CT SCAN and although the C125 is extremely low there still could be residual disease. We pray for no recurrence and in September 20 we are going back to the MSKCC in NY for another checkup. I feel so apprehensive that my spirit for moments is bleak and full of anxiety and pain. The emptiness and darkness invade my soul. The worst part is that it seems so bleak that I am losing hope and faith and everything is becoming unbearable. Jesus Lord, help me to understand what you want from me, to have the energy to keep creating and researching without losing faith and hope that we will make it. Protect Irma's life and Patricia, and do not separate them from me. Lord Jesus, forgive me for my weaknesses and for not understanding what you are asking me.

On *August 30, 2011,* I wrote:

Now that Irma's cancer has returned, I am demolished.

Next week we are seeing the oncologist, Dr. L. Martin, to reinitiate the chemotherapy. You have cured the leper, made the blind see and the deaf hear, save Irma and stop her cancer, you are the only one that can do it.

On September 13, Irma started the first cycle out of the four weekly chemo regimens. *On October 7,* I wrote:

I cannot sleep. It is past midnight and I cannot reconcile my sleep, and my brain is on full speed with all my memories running at the same time, with all my windows open. Irma has received this week her fourth course of chemo and more are coming. The paper that we submitted to the International Journal of Cancer has been accepted but we are struggling to get all the authors to sign the conflict of interest form. I am trying to put together two RO1 for the middle of November, and there are some experiments that are not coming clear to me how to execute them. There is some funding pending but there is no clear response if they will be granted or not. One is from Dompe and the other is from Novartis. We are working full speed to complete the Arena contract and other experiments that are crucial for our future research grants.

On *December 18*:

Irma and I are traveling to Spain. We will stay in Araceli's house and we have been invited to give a talk in the Santa Cruz College and in the medical school.

On that trip, we received the distinction of becoming members of the Santa Cruz College. During the following year, 2012, our scientific activity was mixed with Irma's chemotherapy sessions. In February, Irma and I attended the SPORE study session of the NIH. In February, I went to San Diego for the Arena consultation. In April, I was working in the LOI for the DOD Transformative Vision application, and at the same time, on May 8 I went to WDC for a meeting with the FDA regarding the Arena contract. On *June 6, 2012,* Irma and I went to Virginia to participate in a DOD Study Session, and Irma completed her 22nd round of chemo, I had the sense that everything could be finished, and desolation and loneliness shadowed my spirit. In the middle of this, I submitted the entire book *The Transcriptome of Breast Cancer Prevention* to Springer [10]. We resubmitted the genomic signature of pregnancy to BMC Medical Genomics but there was no feedback yet. We submitted the RO1 to NCI, that is a corrected version of our previous NCI RO1 provocative questions and also we submitted a manuscript dealing with EMT in estrogen transformed cells. I presented two book proposals to Springer. One was *Methodological Approaches to Breast Cancer Research* [11], and the second was *The Future of Cancer Research*. The first proposal was accepted but not the second one. This resulted later on in the book that World Scientific published for me with the title *The Training of Cancer Researchers* [14]. I was glad to write this book because it was better crafted than the proposal to Springer. On *August 10,* I wrote: *"Irma completed the twenty-fifth round of chemo, and they are debating whether to continue with further treatment."*

On *November 13, 2012,* I wrote in my journal:

> *Many months and weeks and days have passed since August 20 when I was admitted to Abington Hospital for a subdural hematoma followed by admission to Penn and Temple hospital. Death was near me, and now I am counting my blessing and still not understanding what my whole family including myself have been going through.*

From my own recollection and my family's experiences, what happened was that I started to have severe headaches of a migraine type that did not abate with even high doses of Tylenol. This brought me to the emergency room of Abington Hospital where they diagnosed a subdural hematoma. I was admitted and then I do not have any recollection except that Irma took me to Penn hospital because I did not improve. I was admitted and I was in a coma for a week until I woke up in a room in the Temple Hospital, where they recovered me from the excess of surgery performed in the hospital of Penn. I noticed then that my walk was unbalanced, my speech was blurry, and my handwriting was gone.

After two weeks in the Temple Hospital, I was released and a recovery phase started at home very slowly. Only on *November 13,* was I well enough to write in my journal again.

Today Irma and I are going to San Francisco for a meeting of the BCERC or Windows of Susceptibility program from the NIEHS, I have been invited to give a talk and I will present our latest data that finally have been published in the International Journal of Cancer and BBG Medical Genomics.

Sadness surrounds us including Irma; she still has the tumor and the recurrence, although small, is still there. No official treatment but only phase 1 clinical trials. I see her very down lately and I feel the same way. Sadness covers my soul.

"We are resubmitting the R21 and presenting the application to Komen that the LOI was accepted for full application. Also we are presenting a special grant for the tobacco funds through PA care".

On *January 11, 2013,* I wrote:

This is my first entry in my journal for this year, and one of the few of the last months. It is almost three in the morning and I cannot sleep. Irma is in the hospital receiving her second round of isophosphamide that requires hospitalization for four nights. I am in turmoil, scared, sad, and sick. Irma's sickness is bringing me every day to the edge of my mortality, fears of being alone, to die and be forgotten.

My subdural hematoma on August 20 of the last year put me in the bergs of a catastrophic event in which all my cognitive and physical functions were severely damaged. I recovered, and during the last two weeks, the headache is coming back as a reminder of the beginning of my previous accident. My blood pressure has increased and I am controlling it with higher doses of Norvac and Tylenol. This regimen more or less keeps in check the symptoms. I am taking sleeping pills to rest during the night. Last night I did not take any one, and the insomnia is hunting me again. To be alone in the house makes me feel more vulnerable, and lacking the continuous presence and support of Irma makes me feel weaker. In this physical reality, my spirit is troubled by a sense that I have lost my way, that at the end of the road I found emptiness in my work. The grants are still my main concerns and the papers are residents in a corner, like nothing good will comes from all the experiments. The FCCC has merged with Temple, and yesterday the president, Dr. Michael Seiden, was fired. This created more uncertainties, because at least he knows us. He has provided us with better laboratories when we were in a pit in the old building, encouraged and gave us moral support when Irma received the diagnosis of ovarian cancer in 2009, and helped Irma taken me out of Penn Hospital to Temple where they stabilize my disease. Although I was completely unconscious during what happened to me in those days, it is Irma's accounts that brought all these events to my attention.

On *March 24, 2013*, I wrote in my journal:

I am seventy-one years old today. I feel more vulnerable than ever and the life of Irma is in the equation. It seems that she is tolerating and subjectively responding to the new chemo. We are looking for additional alternatives with cytoreduction surgery at the University of Pittsburgh, but we are postponing until the third week of May when we have a better evaluation of the present treatment.

In April, Irma was not feeling well, her tumor was growing, and our only hope was surgery. We went to the Pittsburgh Cancer Center by recommendation of Dr. Elin Sigurdsson to see Dr. Ping Pack who had agreed that surgery was the only way to alleviate the compression that the two tumor masses were inflicting on the stomach, liver, kidney, and duodenum. Irma was vomiting and experiencing significant discomfort. I had not seen her like that since the surgery in 2009. On April 23, Irma was in the ICU, after a nine hour long surgical procedure in which 20% of the liver was removed, the right kidney, an adrenal, plus part of the stomach and duodenum, with part of the colon. In the ICU, she was conscious, tired, and connected to a respirator that was extremely uncomfortable. The tumors were removed, and we waited for her recovery. It took almost a week for her to start a semisolid diet but a few days later she developed a fistula in her wound that brought her to surgery again to improve the drainage of her wound, and on *May 7* I entered in my journal: *"I see her life floating away."* She was connected to the saline, antibiotic, and two drainage, and received parenteral food 16 hours a day. On May 12, 2013, we celebrated Mother's Day; it was her third week in the hospital. She was slowly recovering, and Dr. Ping Pack advised us to start making the arrangements to take her home and continue with home care and with Patricia and Estela, who were with us all the time. We took care of making the arrangements to take her back home on May 15. The home care worked fine until I noted that she was developing fevers, and after talking with Dr. Elin Sigurdsson, we decided to bring her to FCCC. On *May 21,* I wrote:

> *They found liquid in the pleura and abdomen. They removed and put a drain in the left side of the abdomen for drainage. In the left side of the lung they removed 600cc. That could explain her fatigue, malaise, and fever. Today she is more alert and the physician is planning to go to the right lung where also liquid accumulation has been found.*

On *Thursday, May 23, 2013,* I wrote:

> *Irma is stable but I found her very confused. She cannot complete the sentences and find the right words. I have my heart broken, and I would like to be more optimistic but I do not know the outcome of this ordeal for her. Honestly I do not see that the situation will clear completely in the days ahead. I do not know the final outcome; she was seat in the bed today but her strength for mobility on her own is very limited. I cry and release my pain but I am so afraid for her life, for the inexorable end.*

On *Tuesday, May 28, 2013,* I wrote:

> *Irma is going through another tag in the pleura. The CRT scan of the abdomen looks like abscesses, or tumors, and she is not improving. Today I feel that is the beginning of the end. Lord help Irma to survive this ordeal. My heart is broken thinking of her, and I pray with all my being that she recovers, that she can be reestablished back home, physically, spiritually, and mentally sound and can walk the rest of our life*

together. I am so sad seeing her suffering and so afraid that this is the beginning of the end. I never knew that to love a person was so painful.

On *May 30, 2013*, I wrote:

Irma has developed a Vancomyn Resistant Infection and probably this plus the abscess in the abdomen is the source of all the damage.

On *June 3*, I wrote:

Irma is doing better but still has difficulty completing sentences and ideas. I feel so much pain in my heart seeing her so defenseless in bed. The pleural effusion last night seems to be in check, and the antibiotics seem to start working. On June 4 I talked with Dr. Unger, the pulmonologist, and he believes there is a neoplastic growth in the pleura. However no malignant cells are in the pleural effusion. "Irma is connected with me but she does not coordinate who is around her. . . . I don't know how to quench my anguish, and crying aloud in the car or in the house when I am alone discharges my emotions but it is a basal status that churns my inner being and does not allow me to have a moment of quietness . When I think that she cannot be any longer with us, that I will lost her, the pain is unbearable, and everything get cloudy and without sense."

On *June 19*, I wrote:

The pain is unbearable. Irma has spiked a fever and gram negative infection is showing up again. Every hour each drop of hope is fading away. It is three-thirty p.m., and I saw the CT scan. The tumor is spreading fast in the lung and in the liver plus multiple abscesses that are difficult to reach even for a diagnosis.

On *Tuesday, June 25, 2013*, I wrote:

Today Irma died after three days in agony. Patty, Estela, and Ron were there. I had left the room thirty minutes earlier, and Estela called me to the room and Irma was there without life and gone forever until the end of time when we will meet again if my soul is pure enough to see her again. I embraced her dead body and told her how much I love her and that I hoped she forgave me for my weakness and all the suffering that I caused her, for my rush and anxiety.

Oh Lord, forgive me for this unbearable pain and anxiety, loneliness and despair. **Dear Lord, embrace her soul because she was the essence of good and give her a place in your home and help me to fill this loneliness and pain in faith and hope.**

References

[1] Durant, W. and Durant, A. *The Story of Civilization*, The Easton Press, Norwalk. 1992.

[2] Russo, J. *The Apprentice of Science: A Handbook for the Budding Biomedical Researchers*, World Scientific, Singapore. 2011.

[3] Russo, J. *Immunocytochemistry in Tumor Diagnosis*, M. Nijhoff Publishing, Boston. 1985.

[4] Russo, J. and Sommers, S. C. *Tumor Diagnosis by Electron Microscopy*, Field, Wood and Associates, Inc., New York. 1986.

[5] Russo, J. and Sommers, S. C. *Tumor Diagnosis by Electron Microscopy*, Vol. 2, Field and Wood, Inc., New York. 1988.

[6] Russo, J. and Sommers, S. C. *Tumor Diagnosis by Electron Microscopy*, Vol. 3, Field and Wood, Inc., New York. 1989.

[7] Russo, J. and Russo, I. H. *Biological and Molecular Basis of Breast Cancer*, Springer, Heidelberg, Germany. 2004.

[8] Russo, J. *Breast Cancer and the Environment*, Springer, NY. 2011.

[9] Gutierrez, P., Russo, I. H. and Russo, J. *The Evolution of the use of Mathematics in Cancer Research*, Springer, New York. 2012.

[10] Russo, J. and Russo, I. H. *Role of the Transcriptome in Breast Cancer Prevention*, Springer, New York. 2012.

[11] Russo, J. and Russo, I. H. *Methodological Approaches to Breast Cancer Research*, Springer, New York. 2014.

[12] Russo, J. *Trend in Breast Cancer Prevention*, Springer, New York. 2016.

[13] Russo, J. *The Pathobiology of Breast Cancer*, Springer, New York. 2016.

[14] Russo, J. *The Training of Cancer Researchers*, World Scientific, Singapore. 2017.

[15] Russo, J., Su, Y. and Pereira, J. *Chromatin Remodeling*, Springer, New York. 2018.

[16] Russo, J., Barton, M. and Pereira, J. *Long non coding RNA*, Springer, New York. 2019.

[17] Russo, J. *Memoirs of a Cancer Researcher*, World Scientific, Singapore. 2018.

Chapter 13

Rebuilding My Life

13.1. My feelings after Irma's death

I could not find consolation after Irma's death. I wanted to see her again, to hear her voice, and to feel her near me, but the loneliness and devastation was so great that I could not contain my tears and cried aloud until I did not know what else to do. I felt empty and without a future; it was the feeling that I was walking without life or aspiration for anything. The pain was mortal and the feeling of nonsense was even worse. I could not erase from my mind watching her fade from my life.

I organized the best that I could the papers that Irma left, her notes, her scribbling, her writings, everything that she had touched, and I boxed it as memorabilia. I collected all the mail and cards that we received, and the love that she had left and the sparseness around everything that she had touched. Maybe someday Patricia or her descendants will put Irma's memories together. Everything that she did to help me avoid this turbulence in my soul that I could not quench made me feel even sadder and more mortified.

The pain was intense, and the realization that Irma was not coming back made my days more difficult. All those who came to present their condolences made me feel even sadder, and thinking about her so much weakened my existence without objective, nothing could fill this tremendous vacuum.

I followed the routine every day and desperately tried to create and keep working, and then I realized that she was not there to share my work or my comments or for listening and talking, her voice full of tender care. The images of her suffering and remembering how she faded away before her death haunted me.

In *September of 2013*, I wrote in my journal:

I have been in Westfield, Chantilly, Virginia, to chair a Study Session of the DOD. For moments I wanted to be back home but then realized that I do not have Irma any longer and the sadness invades my soul. When I arrived at the Union Station, Kevin, the driver who has taken care of me for the last fifteen years, was waiting for me, and he knew about Irma and it was difficult to keep myself composed.

The days are passing and my pain persists, I cry most of the time remembering Irma and seeing my future without her. This is the part that I cannot reconcile in me.

September 7 Patricia and Ron had their wedding in our home, friends and family were with us. It was a day of light in the middle of my darkness.

I have been attending the bereavement group organized by the FCCC. It was a roller coaster of emotions by all the attendees. The pain for the lost one is excruciating, and my pain is not unique. . . . The grief meeting is helping me to realize that all the ones who are in my situation have the same feelings and some of them protract the pain for years.

On *September 23, 2013*, I wrote:

I want to cry in my loneliness. I feel so sad. I am missing Irma so much that I have the impression there is no future for me. The emptiness that I am experiencing is desolating. My only consolation is to speak a few words with Patty in the evening, but after that is nothing. Every day I am more aware of how lonely I am and there is no hope for me to improve it. Who could replace Irma? Then I realize that I need to get used to this life, to this situation, and that I must continue as long as God allows me to live. I know that are so many people like me, alone, sick, and without anybody who can love them, and it is selfish on my part to feel the way that I feel.

I remember Irma's face in death and the sadness invades me, I remember vividly her death, a sound so terrible that she is gone, that I will return home, and she is not there to share my thoughts, my experiences, and points of view.

The minutes and hours are passing so slowly that it is a source of anxiety to find myself waiting or expecting without expectation.

On *September 25, 2013,* I wrote:

Today at this time of the day makes three months since Irma passed away. The pain is still with me and the sadness is part of my daily life. Crying is a consolation that discharges all my emotions and cleans up my soul. For moments it seems impossible that she is not here anymore.

I am facing everyday tasks, trying to solve all the problems that she used to do for me. It makes me feel good to know that I can do it and it is like she is helping me. I am working on several projects and thinking of another book. This makes me feel good, to be extremely busy and thinking that she is near me when I am working hard.

On *October 12, 2013,* I entered in my journal:

If my father was alive he would be 101 years old today. I have been going through the motions to do everything that we were doing, Irma and I together.

I have removed some clothes from the closet, arranged the foyer and kitchen closet, and in the motion I found the Modado watch that I gave her for her birthday, and that I was sure had been lost in the hospital. I cannot stop crying; my pain and desolation is so intense, it is difficult to find a sense and purpose, when I feel like this moment I am empty without any purpose. I feel so lonely and insecure about my future, which looks so bleak and without purpose. Patty has called me twice to be sure that I am okay but how can I tell her how I feel and produce in her more pain?

On *October 25*, I transcribe in my journal a letter that I sent to my sister:

Today is four months since Irma's death. The scientific director of the FCCC told me that there will be a special meeting in honor of Irma and her name will be given to the Breast Cancer Research Laboratory that from now on it will be called: The Irma H. Russo, MD, Breast Cancer Research Laboratory of the FCCC-Temple Health. Several speakers have been invited, and one of them is Dr. Leena Hilakivi-Clarke from Georgetown University. The meeting will be on December 18. This is a great recognition in her memory, for somebody like Irma that has been so generous with everybody.

On *November 4, 2013*, I wrote:

I feel pain, anxiety, and anguish, and I do not know how to quench these feelings. I feel lonely and standing alone in the middle of this big world and that the company of others is not enough to heal the emptiness that I am living.

On *November 26, 2013*, I wrote:

Tomorrow I am going to surgery for repairing an inguinal hernia that was produced working in the lower garden. It has been bothering me and I am afraid that it will get strangulated. Dr. Frankel from Abington will do the surgery at noon. The memory of Irma and all her suffering comes to my mind like slashes that make me feel desperate and sad. I miss her so much and it is so difficult to overcome this feeling of desolation and emptiness. I do not know how to keep myself together. The prospective surgery and this feeling of weakness accentuate even more my anxiety and sadness.

The sadness surrounds me like a blanket that suffocates my spirit and purpose. These slashes of memories and feelings of her are for a moment unbearable, and tears and crying are the only natural reaction to these storms that come and wane like the wind. Last Sunday

I visited her tomb in Laurel Hill and everything was so empty and cold that the desolation broke my spirit.

On December 18 will be the dedication of the BCRL to Irma's name. This is a way to honor her memory at the FCCC, but all the searching through photos and preparing the brochure that will be distributed that day make me feel even more sad to remember her beauty, her tenderness and love when she was alive.

13.2. The Irma H. Russo, MD, Breast Cancer Research Laboratory

On *December 18, 2013,* I wrote: *Today the Breast Cancer Research Laboratory has been named and dedicated to Irma and it will be: "The Irma H. Russo, MD, Breast Cancer Research Laboratory at FCCC"* (Figure 13.1).

I created the brochure that was distributed during this special event. Figure 13.2 depicts the terminal end buds that she pointed out for the first time disappear during pregnancy, and she was the one that originated the whole concept of differentiation of the mammary

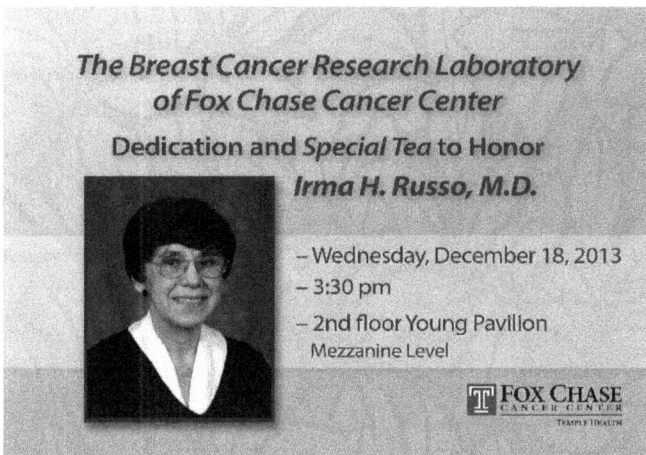

The Breast Cancer Research Laboratory of Fox Chase Cancer Center

Dedication and *Special Tea* to Honor
Irma H. Russo, M.D.

– Wednesday, December 18, 2013
– 3:30 pm
– 2nd floor Young Pavilion
Mezzanine Level

FOX CHASE CANCER CENTER
TEMPLE HEALTH

Figure 13.1: Announcement that was distributed to the FCCC.

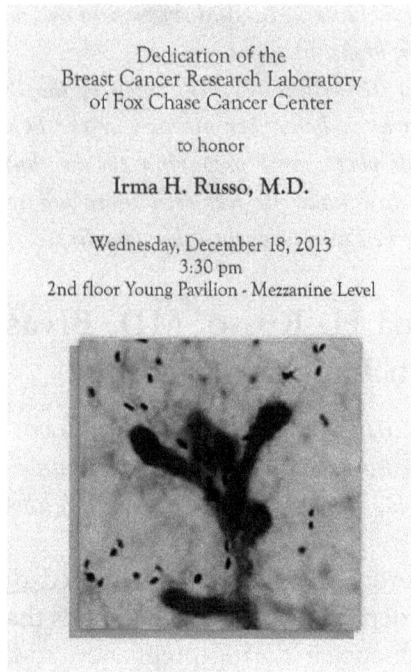

Figure 13.2:   First page of the program.

gland during pregnancy. The second page of the program (Figure 13.3) contained a favorite portrait of her with brief biographical data. On the third page was a summary of her accomplishments and the last photo that we took with her in the BCRL on February 25, 2013 (Figure 13.4). The last page of the program (Figure 13.5) is the roster of all the speakers that honored her on that day.

In Figure 13.6 is a photograph of the speakers that honored her. I sent a personal letter to each of the speakers.

To Jonathan Chernoff I wrote:

Dear Jonathan;

Patricia and I deeply appreciate your words at Irma's dedication to the Breast Cancer Research Laboratory in the ceremony that took place

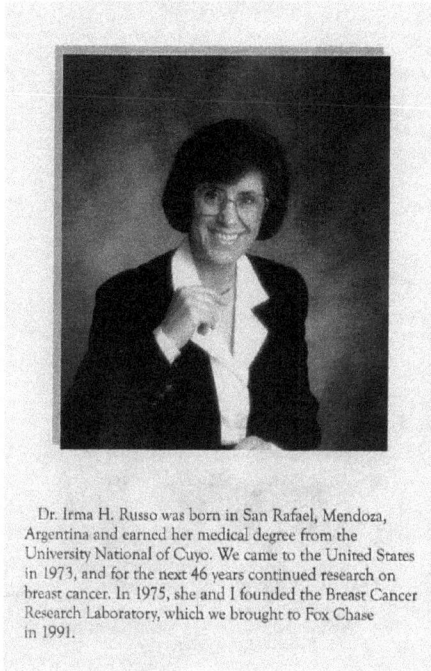

Dr. Irma H. Russo was born in San Rafael, Mendoza, Argentina and earned her medical degree from the University National of Cuyo. We came to the United States in 1973, and for the next 46 years continued research on breast cancer. In 1975, she and I founded the Breast Cancer Research Laboratory, which we brought to Fox Chase in 1991.

Figure 13.3: Portrait of Irma H. Russo, MD.

yesterday, December 18. Thanks for all the efforts that you and your team have done to make that moment a memorable one. Irma's wish on the legacy of the BCRL has been put at rest.

Jose

To Leena, a good friend of Irma's for many years, I wrote:

Dear Leena;

Patricia and I deeply appreciate your words at Irma's dedication to the Breast Cancer Research Laboratory in the ceremony that took place yesterday, December 18.

Thanks for all the efforts that you and Robert have done to make that moment a memorable one.

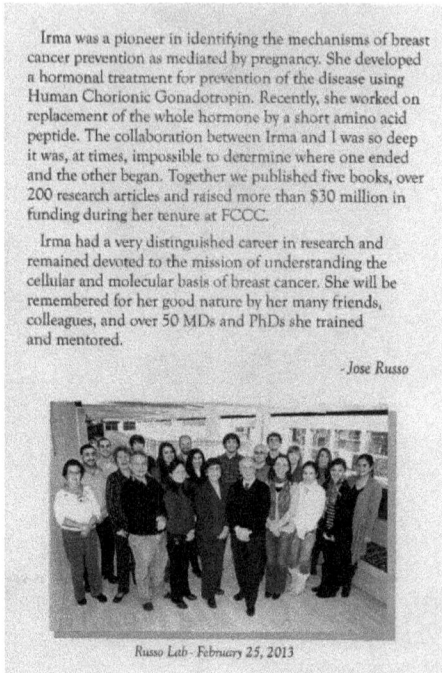

Irma was a pioneer in identifying the mechanisms of breast cancer prevention as mediated by pregnancy. She developed a hormonal treatment for prevention of the disease using Human Chorionic Gonadotropin. Recently, she worked on replacement of the whole hormone by a short amino acid peptide. The collaboration between Irma and I was so deep it was, at times, impossible to determine where one ended and the other began. Together we published five books, over 200 research articles and raised more than $30 million in funding during her tenure at FCCC.

Irma had a very distinguished career in research and remained devoted to the mission of understanding the cellular and molecular basis of breast cancer. She will be remembered for her good nature by her many friends, colleagues, and over 50 MDs and PhDs she trained and mentored.

                                                              -*Jose Russo*

Russo Lab - February 25, 2013

Figure 13.4:   Accomplishments of Irma H. Russo, MD, and the last photo that she posed for with the members of the BCRL in February 25, 2013.

> *You described Irma's character of love, dedication, and devotion to helping others extremely well, and we will keep the warm friendship that you had with her very close to our heart and memories.*
> *Irma's wish on the legacy of the BCRL has been put at rest.*

Jose

Answer from Leena, December 19, 2013:

Dear Jose,

Thank you for asking me to attend the ceremony. It was such an honor to speak about Irma and her importance for the breast cancer research community around the world. Robert also was deeply moved by the ceremony, and really wanted to attend to remember and honor Irma.

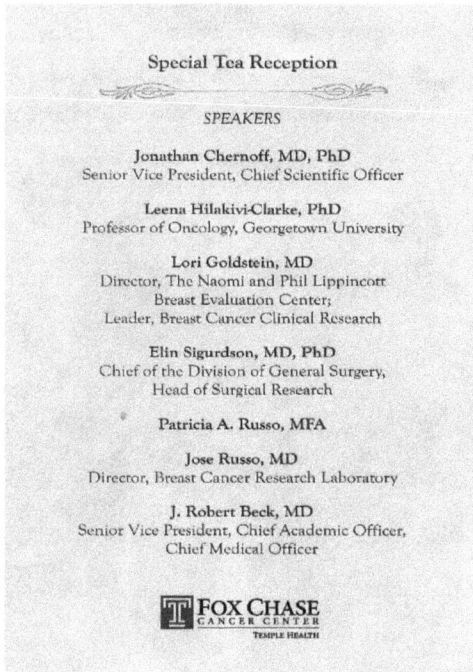

Figure 13.5:   Roster of the speakers that honored her.

To continue to do research without her must be hard for you, but it is important that you do so to fulfill her legacy and yours. Your work is so, so very important. When I was speaking with the students and postdocs in your laboratory yesterday I realized that your and my research have many similar interests, and if you ever need help regarding interacting with your students, I am happy to do so. I am saying this because loosing Irma understandably is taking a lot of your energy and you need time to continue to grieve. Although you will never stop missing her, please trust me, life will get better but it will take time. If you ever feel overwhelmed by having to look after your students, I am more than happy to help any way I can.

Please have a peaceful Christmas in Spain.

Love, Leena and Robert

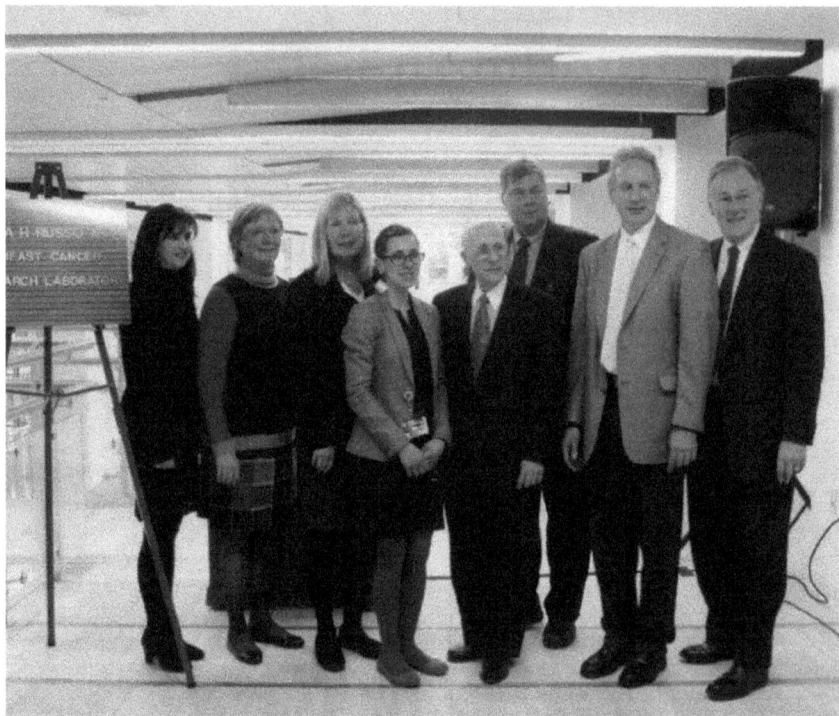

Figure 13.6: Photographs of the speakers, taken after the ceremony. From left to right: Drs. Lori Goldstein, Elin Sigurdsson, Leena Ivaliki-Clarke, Patricia A. Russo, Jose Russo, Robert Beck, Jonathan Chernoff, and Robert Fisher.

To Robert Beck, I wrote:

Dear Bob;

I deeply appreciate your words at Irma's dedication to the Breast Cancer Research Laboratory in the ceremony that took place yesterday, December 18. I also want to thank you for your initiative that she be named professor posthumously. This will be a great recognition. When she was in the process of filling the papers for the promotion she realized that she would not have five or ten year plans because she knew that she was near the end and so desisted of the idea.

   Whatever you can do to recognize her is deeply appreciated.

   Thanks for your friendship and warms words.

Jose

On *January 3, 2014,* I opened my email and read:

Jose:

Irma was a remarkable woman, a dear colleague and friend, an outstanding scientist and pathologist. I was fortunate to consider her a close and dear friend. I want to share with you an email Irma sent to me a little over two years ago (see below). When I read this, it brought a tear to my eyes. I have saved this email and cherish it very much.

Harry Cooper

From: *Russo, Irma*
Sent: *Wednesday, September 21, 2011 2:04 PM*
To: *Cooper, M.D., Harry*
Subject: *Thank you for the coffee!*

Dear Harry,

I enjoyed our brief meeting yesterday and even more your kind invitation to coffee. I consider you a dear and trusted friend that has given me support and affection through these past two years of tribulations. I will never forget your beautiful flowers in my surgery room and your kind words of encouragement.

I am thankful for having met you and wish that you will obtain all the happiness and success that you deserve just by being you.
Sincerely,
Irma

13.3. Reorganizing my life

After Irma's death Patricia came to live with me, and Ron joined us during the weekends. She cooked and organized the meals, and it was a great discovery for me to see her at home showing all the abilities of a grown-up woman who was completely different than the girl who left for college so many years ago. Patricia went back to her home after her wedding on September 7, 2013. We had arranged to dine together at least twice a week and mainly during the weekends. She calls me three times every single day, and our line of communication is open and Irma is in our midst all the time.

The winter of 2013 was cold with many icy storms that made the days longer; although they were passing the pain, sadness of Irma's absence was not gone. It was there when I recognized that I still was alive and that I must keep my life together by creating a series of activities to help me to quench my isolation and loneliness and increase my personal development. I faced this period like a general developing a logistic plan of attack. First, I started to attend the cultural events organized on the campus of the Pennsylvania State University (PSU), which was in my neighborhood, basically across the street from my home. PSU offers a series of educational activities to the community and one of them is the Abington Reading Book group chaired by Dr. Karen Weekes, an Associate Professor of English at PSU. I started attending these gatherings in 2014, and they are now part of my monthly activities. Four books are discussed a year, and most of the attendees are women, the number of men rarely reaches four. However, I have not been intimidated by this and learned instead to appreciate the insights of these women that come from very different backgrounds. Altogether it has been a pleasant and stimulating gathering formed by people who basically like to read books. For me, it has been good because the group has introduced me to literary pieces that I never imagined existed, like *The Storied Life of A. J. Fikry*, a book written by Gabrielle Zevin. However, not all the books were interesting to me such as *The Sympathizer*, by Viet Thanh Nguyen, or *Between the World and Me*, by Ta-Nehisi Coates, or *The Luminaries*, by Eleanor Catton. I did not like *Fun Home: A Family Tragicomic* by Alison Bechdel. This particular one was shocking to me because it is written as a comic strip and made me reminiscence on my childhood and the concept that those people who read this comic strip were not intellectually fitted. However, this book was interesting and not for the intellectually unfitted people but the cartoons interrupting the prose were extremely distracting. I enjoyed *The Vegetarian*, by Han Kang, a terrific book on a typical case of schizophrenia, and *The Revenant*, by Michael Punke. This latter one was a good book based on the real history of Hugh Glass, and it was a compelling one for the powerful instinct of survival. Also, I liked *Purple Hibiscus* by Chimamanda Ngozi Adichie, and

I considered that this was a good murder story. My observations on the writing style as well as the interpretation of the message of the books did not always agree with the most talkative and opinionated participants, but overall my presence and comments are welcomed and expected. Therefore, spending one hour a month discussing literature and writing style is rewarding and enjoyable.

At PSU, I also started to attend the movie discussion that is moderated by Dr. Maylan C. Mills, professor emeritus of integrative arts. One of the films that was extremely impacting for me was *The Homesman*. The story is about a pious woman, Mary Bee Cuddy, taking three women, driven mad by life on the Western frontier, back East with the help of a disreputable drifter played by Tommy Lee Jones. The movie haunted me for days. I really like movies because of the art and the message behind them. I realized that compared with all the other attendees I was an illiterate, and Dr. Mills got my attention for *being* a very good analyst of the content as well as the performer/s in the movie.

At the same time that I started the Abington reading group, I reinitiated my tennis playing. I have tried to be a part of a group that plays regularly but I have been unsuccessful in being accepted, probably because nobody wants to have an old man in their team that could slow them down. However, I wanted to continue practicing tennis so I acquired a tennis ball machine. This one is programmable to mimic an opponent player, and although it sounds tragicomic the machine keeps me in shape by practicing at least once a week and being ready to play with my nephew, Pedro, during his annual summer visit to Rydal.

As a part of my plan, I decided to be more active in our parish by attending the meetings of the Holy Name Society. The parish, Our Lady Help of Christians, has Pastor Anthony W. Janton, a very active, energetic, and more important, an excellent priest. Among the multiple groups in the parish that are covering the needs of the parishioners is the Holy Name Society, a group of 28 Catholic men. The mission of this group is to help Father Janton with the parish activities. I was welcomed into the group, and I really was impressed by the dedication and faith of these men. The meetings were structured around activities in the parish, and I found that the spiritual reflection that should be the core of the gathering was weak. I was not too happy about that because I was looking for more discussion around relevant spiritual matters. I was ready to leave the group but I loved those men for their dedication and efforts to keep the parish running, so I concluded that what was needed was to give them a sample of what I was thinking about, and I offered to give a reflection on *The meaning of prayer in the Gospel*. I prepared a handout summarizing the concept, in reality a little essay on praying based on the Gospel and also what St. Thomas Aquinas had said about praying in the *Summa Theologica*. In each part of the *Summa*, Thomas wrote several questions; in the case of prayer is Question 83, which has 17 articles, and I focused on Article 1, whether or not prayer is an act of the appetitive power. And in Article 13, whether or not attention is a necessary condition of prayer. Probably it was overwhelming for some of them when I showed up to the meeting with the volume of the *Summa* and two additional reference books and the Bible and started my reflection on praying. God only knows that I was not just showing up but that I also wanted to deliver a message. My next move was to suggest an agenda of topics to discuss that might help to turn the things around.

In my journal on *February 14, 2016*, I wrote:

> *My suggestion of an agenda of themes for the reflections in the monthly meeting, elicited a positive response and most important, was welcomed by many of the members who indicated that it was badly needed. In reality I expected neither that response nor the comments that everybody enjoyed my previous reflection.*

On *March 26, 2016* I wrote:

> *The idea to develop an agenda for the reflections in the Holy Name Society was consolidated in a meeting that we had on March 15,* and on **November 20, 2016**, I wrote: *In the Holy Name Society meetings my contribution to discussing the reflections is germinating and the last two ones given by Ray and Thomas were deep and elicited a positive response from the group.*

Ray talked on "The Experiences of the Men of the Holy Name Society in the Administration of the Sacraments to the Sick" and Thomas discussed "Advent as an Instrument of Renaissance in Our Spiritual Life." The topics to be presented in the Reflections part of each meeting are now a part of the agenda.

On *July 12, 2014,* I wrote:

> *Dr. Lou Welsh approached and invited me to be part of "The Oldie Doctors Group." This is a group of physicians, most of them retired but some of them still very active, that meets from September to June on the third Saturday of each month at the Huntington Country Club. I was happy to be invited to be part of this group that Irma was well acquainted with because she was invited and gave a talk years before. It was through Irma that I met Dr. Welsh and knowing that I was alone he invited me to his group.*

From the first meeting I felt comfortable with them, and I have given two conferences: one referring to my research project on breast cancer prevention and a second on the mechanism of cancer metastasis. One of the attractions of this group is that physicians are caring people with a significant amount of interests, from politics to art, and some of them are involved in more than one. Three of them also are painting and showing their work. It is this genuine curiosity and interest in both medical and non-medical issues that made me feel good among this group. In the last Christmas luncheon on December 17, 2016, they asked me to deliver the Thanksgiving prayer, and I said:

> *On this special day I want that we join ourselves in a common prayer of thanksgiving to our God for being alive, and for celebrating Christmas that is the birth of Jesus Christ that was a Jew born from the line of Davis. This means that this day touches all of us because Christmas is the convergence of Judaism and Christianity.*
>
> *Christmas is the celebration of birth, of our new rebirth in hope, love and faith for the life in front of us; it's thanking God for all the benefits that we have received and also for being together and sharing our love and understanding for each other.*

We ask our Lord to bless us in our interactions and our daily lives and that give eternal life and peace for those that are not physically with us but they are present in our hearts and thoughts.
Amen.

My last topic that I presented to them was *The Enterprise of Cancer Research,* on February 10, 2018, based on my book *Memoirs of a Cancer Researcher,* which was published in 2017 and also will be one of the chapters in the book that I signed with Springer titled *The Future of Breast Cancer Research.*

I also became a member of the Philadelphia Photographic Society, the Philadelphia Museum of Art, the Barnes Foundation, and the Philadelphia Academy of Fine Arts (PAFA). These were important frontiers that I'd wanted to cross for many years but I postponed until the end of 2013 when I decided to join them. I found that I needed to break the isolation, and whereas those groups were not the best for meeting and socializing with people they provided instead the material and the venues that I needed to work more in my photography and painting.

The Photographic Society of Philadelphia is the oldest society of this type in the world and I joined them on May 20, 2015.

I wrote in my journal my impression of the first meeting:

Last night I attended my first meeting of the Photographic Society of Philadelphia. I must say that the environment was pleasant and better than I expected it to be. There were some professional photographers but most of the attendants were like me, enthusiastic and amateur photographers. I sent an email today to Eileen Ekstein, the president of the society, congratulating and thanking her for the meeting. I asked her to include me in the roster for presenting some of my works. This will be a way to measure how good I am in this art that I have been cultivating for so long.

I had been participating regularly in these meeting, and on September 15, 2015, I made my first presentation on: *Three Folders: I am Part of What I Met, The Universe of Microscopic Details, and The People That I Met* (Figure 13.7).

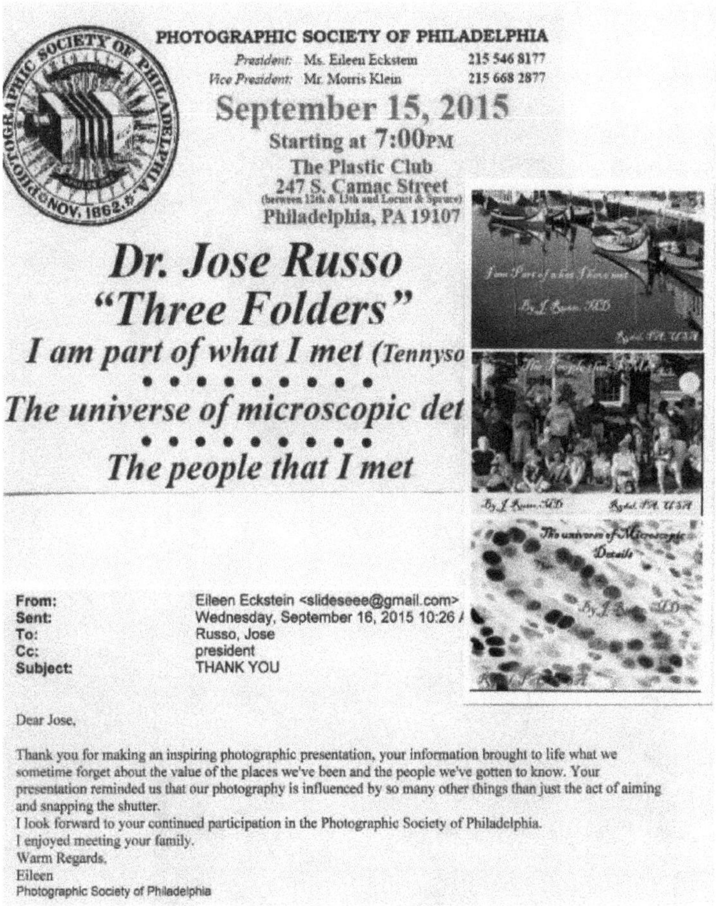

PHOTOGRAPHIC SOCIETY OF PHILADELPHIA

President: Ms. Eileen Eckstein 215 546 8177

Vice President: Mr. Morris Klein 215 668 2877

September 15, 2015

Starting at 7:00PM

The Plastic Club

247 S. Camac Street

(between 12th & 13th and Locust & Spruce)

Philadelphia, PA 19107

Dr. Jose Russo

"Three Folders"

I am part of what I met (*Tennyso*

• • • • • • • • • •

The universe of microscopic det

• • • • • • • • • •

The people that I met

From: Eileen Eckstein <slideseee@gmail.com>
Sent: Wednesday, September 16, 2015 10:26 /
To: Russo, Jose
Cc: president
Subject: THANK YOU

Dear Jose,

Thank you for making an inspiring photographic presentation, your information brought to life what we sometime forget about the value of the places we've been and the people we've gotten to know. Your presentation reminded us that our photography is influenced by so many other things than just the act of aiming and snapping the shutter.
I look forward to your continued participation in the Photographic Society of Philadelphia.
I enjoyed meeting your family.
Warm Regards,
Eileen
Photographic Society of Philadelphia

Figure 13.7: Presentation to the Photographic Society of Philadelphia.

The society also organized the Photographic Salon of the Photographic Society of Philadelphia as a commemoration of writing with light for 154 years. The exhibit was on July of 2016, and I presented two macro-photographies. One of the photos depicts the claws of the *musca domestica*, or housefly, showing the adhesive pads, or pulvilli. I called it: "*I can walk on the ceiling*" (Figure 13.8), and the other one "*I detect you*" (Figure 13.9). This latter one shows the olfactory receptors located in the antenna of the May bug, or

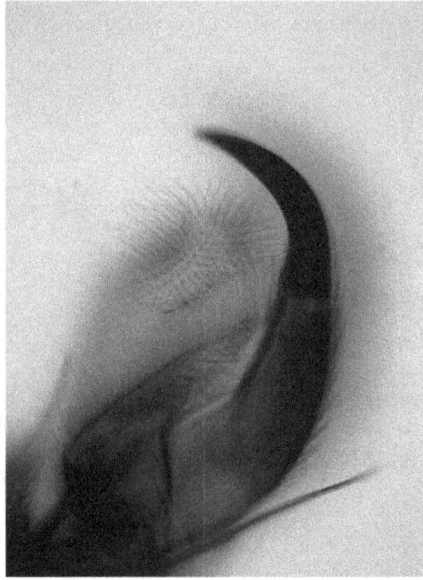

Figure 13.8:   Claw of the *musca domestica*.

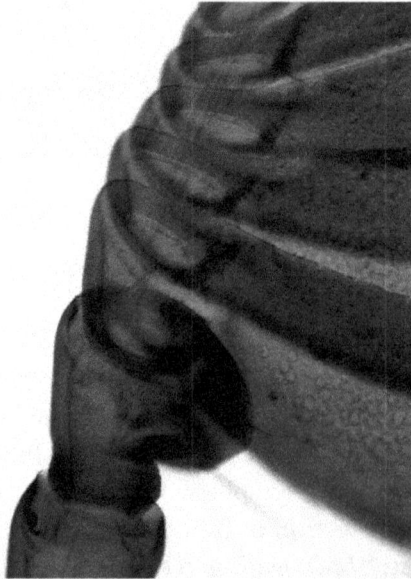

Figure 13.9:   Olfactory receptors located in the antenna of the May bug, or cockchafer.

cockchafer. Because the male has 50,000 of these receptors, that is superior to the number in the female species that is 8,000, allowing the male to detect the presence of the female because they cannot see her but rather smell her presence. This was my first exposure in the world of high amateurs and professional photographers. I put the price of 250 dollars for each piece and none of them were sold. As a consolation, of the 150 photos that were displayed only two were sold.

After the BCRL was dedicated to Irma, I realized that my pain for the loss must not be an excuse to retract myself from scientific activity at the FCCC. There are my colleagues and the one who helped create the environment of what the FCCC is. Therefore, I started to participate more in the conferences that FCCC was offering at least twice a week and being more attentive to the meeting of the Cancer Biology Program, attending all the gatherings that the FCCC invited me to, and in other words breaking the isolation and seeking the presence of other human beings.

On *January 1, 2015, I wrote:*

I am making a conscious effort to be more visible at the FCCC conferences and meetings. This effort at increasing my visibility is good for my integration, and I've noticed that they noticed me. I have been invited for the first time in years to talk of my work in the Cancer Biology Program in September of this year, and on **May 20** I wrote: *This evening there is a faculty meeting in the Knowlton Mansion in Verree Road, where are presented all the promotions at the FCCC, and Irma was included in promotion posthumously as professor in the FCCC, this make me very happy because it was the result or response to my talk with Beck and Chernoff a few weeks ago.*

13.4. Patty in medical school

Irma and I saw in Patty the qualifications for going into the biomedical sciences because even as a young child in elementary and, later on, high school she was doing naturally well in all the biology related subjects. We noticed her attention to detail in the medical subjects and her curiosity of the photographs that she saw us taking under the microscope. Although she had that natural ability to understand biological concepts, she was reluctant to consider science or even medicine as a subject of her interest.

On *Wednesday, April 2, 2014,* I entered in my journal:

Patty revealed to me that she wants to go medical school and has already presented applications for the pre-med to Jefferson, Temple, and Penn. If any of them do not accept her, she will already start a program by herself to take the pre-med examination. This has been extremely revealing for me, and I am very happy to hear that she is really considering going to medical school.

On April 23, Patricia was accepted in the pre-med program at Jefferson Medical School, and I was so excited and happy for her. She resigned from the AACR (American Association for Cancer Research) where she was working as an editorial assistant and had under her responsibility the new journal *Cancer Discovery.* She dealt with the authors' compliances as well as the reviewers of the original manuscripts. I offered my help in covering the salary gap and with that and some freelance work that she did for Elsevier Publishing Co., she completed the 18 months before her final admission to the medical school. Before starting the pre-med program, she approved and passed the three tests to be certified as an emergency technician, and she applied to volunteer at the ambulance service in Willow Grove. She had done an outstanding job, but she was critical enough to realize that there was a long way to go and she needed to retrain herself on how to study and learn, retaining things in her memory basic until they became a part of her. It is a process that needed her to go alone and that I walked with her, making me the happiest man on earth. In *March of 2015,* Patricia asked me in the name of her pre-med course at Jefferson to deliver a short talk on the research work that I was doing, and I saw pride in her eyes.

On *February 14, 2016,* I wrote in my journal:

Patty was accepted to the Rowan Osteopathic Medical School in New Jersey. I am extremely happy that she was accepted and that she will stay in the area.

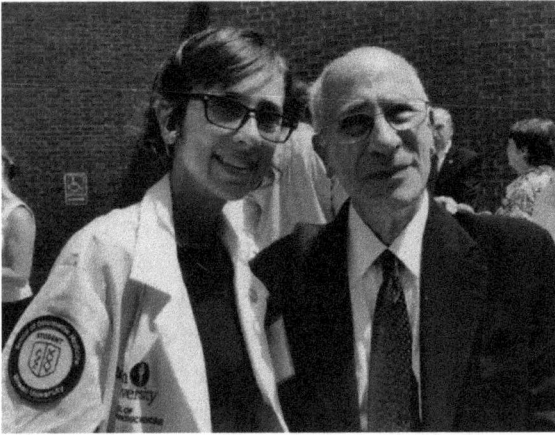

Figure 13.10: White coat ceremony on July 31, 2016.

On *July 31, 2016*, I attended the white coat ceremony that took place on the campus of Rowen University (Figure 13.10) and gave her a card containing the following note:

Dear Patty,

I am so happy to watch how you have evolved from being an artist to wanting to be a physician, a healer, because there is no more noble profession than to help alleviate the pain of others.

Today you have in front of you a white canvas in which you first will trace the knowledge that you will acquire in the next four and subsequent years, but the real painting will emerge to your eyes and to the eyes of others when you add the color, the transparency and the vibrancy provided by your own experience as a physician. At the end you will find out that you have created a masterpiece.

Be a hummingbird carrying hopes for love, joy and easiness to those that suffer, be aware that beauty is everywhere and that every personal connection every time that you touch someone as a physician has a special meaning.

As your dad I would like to see before the end of my life your painting taking shape and hope that I can help to add the life, the bright and spiritual value in it.

Your Father with love

July 31, 2016

13.5. My painting and drawing

At the end of 2013, after almost 40 years without touching a brush, I started to paint again. My first attempts as a painter was in 1972 when I painted a flying geese using China ink in different dilutions like an aquarelle on tracing paper. But what I wanted to do was oil painting, and my objective was to make portraits but after my first attempt, a clown, I realized that I needed to start with something simpler, like still life. After that came a *Dog in the Forest, A Flower Vase*, which I copied from a Rembrandt reproduction, and three landscapes inspired by the Michigan winter [1] (Figure 13.11).

From 2013 to 2015, my painting area was in my study at Rydal. My first oil portrait was *The Girl with the Red Hair* at the beginning of 2014, and on April of that year I started taking formal classes with Frederick Kaplan at the Philadelphia Academy of Fine Arts (PAFA) for oil painting of human figures. Kaplan's course was intended to capture general forms and details of light and shadows and that was the most valuable experience. However, he was not concerned with

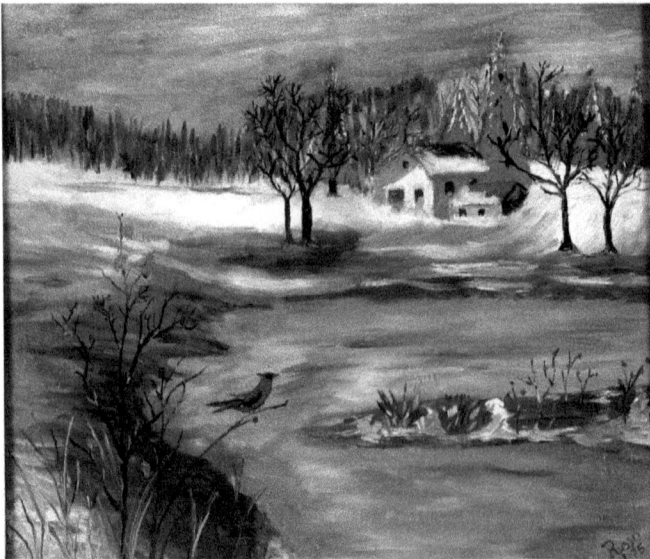

Figure 13.11:   *Winter landscape.* Oil on canvas, Ann Arbor, Michigan, 1974.

the details of portrait paintings. Kaplan insisted, *"Try not to dismay in the period of apprenticeship; before everybody call him 'Maestro Leonardo' he was called 'Leo do this,' 'Leo do that.'"* He also said: *"In the process of painting we will find our own style and that will take place after many trials and errors."*

Two important people that encouraged me in that period were Patricia and Ron; they indicated the good and the errors in each painting. They emphasized the advances and details on the new paintings versus the old ones. Their delicate spirit was a balsam that helped me to navigate from one painting to another. Patricia and Ron never laughed at my work, even though I recognized in retrospect that many of them were bad and infantile portraits. However, at the end of 2014, I had completed 76 portraits from which 66 were decent enough to display.

I wrote in my journal on *January 1, 2015:*

I am improving my painting since I started in March of 2014. I am trying to master the glassing, which is one important technique in portraiture painting. Patricia and Ron are my best critics and advisers in the process, and I not only welcome and gladly receive their suggestions but also I value them because they are excellent ones. I painted several portraits of Irma from different periods of her life, taking from photographs most of them in black and white and only in one have I captured her beauty and freshness, that is the photo that was taken in front of my house in Guaymallen, Mendoza, when she was eighteen years old by Pages, a photographer that left. He was also the one that taught me photo processing when I started in my second year of medical school working in the Experimental Pathology Institute.

During the year 2015, my objective was to provide a tridimensional perspective on the canvas by managing the shadows and protuberances. In the process, I wanted to provide a distinctive likeliness with the subject and try to capture their personality. During that year, the quality of my painting was improving but not yet where I wanted it to be. I had been reading and practicing new techniques and better understanding the process. I was studying each project in advance and had a better handling of shapes and shades. Probably the most important growth was that I knew when something did not look right. I moved my paintings to a room of the house that was underutilized, and I decided to hang the old and new portraits to see and compare my evolution in the process of painting. I call this place "my atelier." I was oblivious to the critiques of some members of my family that I should get rid of the old ones.

The competition was with me and not with anybody else. Being acquaintance with PAFA inspired me to make incursions in their permanent collections of portrait paintings, and I discovered Sully, Peele, and Eakins. More important, I found T. Xaros, a teacher of good reputation in PAFA but he did not admit students unless they at least knew how to draw. This made me reconsider the whole project and I started from the beginning, meaning I took classes and learned how to draw.

In the winter and spring of 2016, I took additional training in drawing in PAFA. The instructor was Phyllis Gellmin Laver. Phyllis was the right person to canalize my motivations, and she started with our small group of five moving from the most elemental to the final portrait drawings. In those six months, I was determined to learn how to draw from scratch and Phyllis's guidance was masterfully done. In addition to this six-month course, I obsessively completed all the exercises of portrait drawing from 10 oil-painting books that Ron gave me as a gift. I also completed the 36 lessons of David Brody given in the great courses. Figure 13.12 is a photo of my studio in those days. I learned drawing in perspective and composition and made hundreds of studios of faces and gestures. In March of 2016, my atelier looked as is shown in Figure 13.13.

Phyllis G. Laver was encouraging me to take additional classes. I expressed to her my interest in concentrating in oil painting portraits with T. Xaros, and she indicated that he was starting a course in the summer. In July 2016, I was admitted to the classes of T. Xaros at PAFA. With Xaros, everything started to fall in place. He was an excellent human being, humble and a master in portraiture painting. My color palette was reduced from 60 colors to only six (white, burnt sienna, light red, ultramarine blue, burnt amber, and yellow ochre). I started using

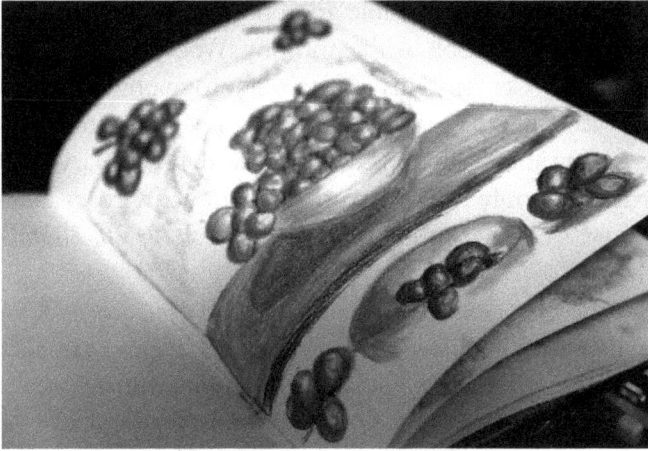

Figure 13.12: Studios of my drawings in 2016.

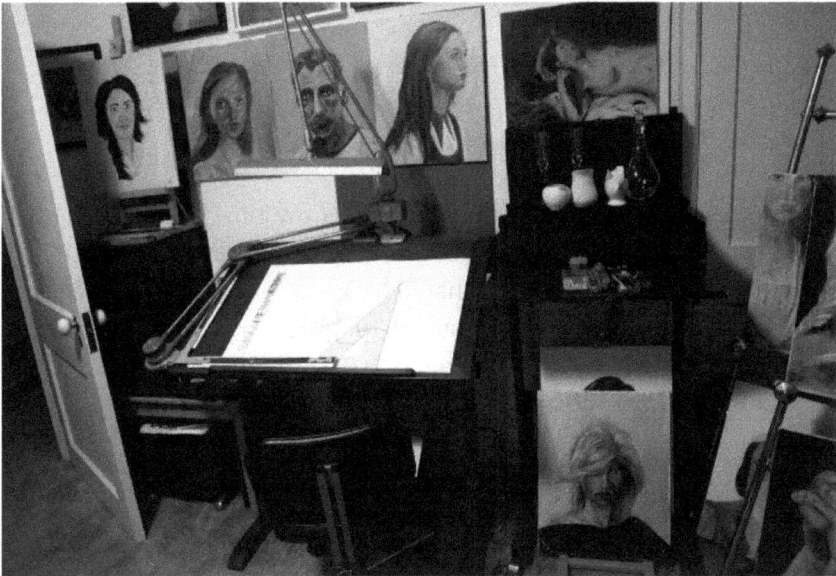

Figure 13.13: Atelier in March of 2016.

live models and where not possible good portrait photos that I mastered with a course that I took with Anthony Wood at the Philadelphia Photography Art Center. This portrait photography course was also hammered with eight classes of "Photoshop for Photographic Portrait" also given by Anthony Wood in the same place in February of 2017.

I learned not only how to paint but also how to evaluate other paintings, and I entered in my journal on *January 20, 2016:*

> *Last Sunday we went with Patty and Ron to the Philadelphia Museum of Art, and I saw a painting of Henry Ossawa Tanner that make me cry of emotion. The painting is called "The Annunciation" painted in 1898. It is a powerful painting of the Virgin Mary as a poor Jewish young woman receiving the request of Gabriel to be the mother of Jesus. Her expression transcends the human and divine.*

On *November 20, 2016,* I wrote:

> *Two weeks ago I attended to an art exhibit organized by Phyllis Gellmin Laver. She was happy to see me, and I sent my latest drawings and she has positive comments on them.*

I am drawing and painting as much as my time allows me and I have compiled and published in *Drawings* (Figure 13.14) and *100 Works of Art* (Figure 13.15) what I have accomplished until March 2017 that is 3 years after I started oil painting in 2014. Putting together drawings in graphite, charcoal, and oil paintings, I have created more than 350 pieces.

13.6. My books and literary work

I wanted to transform my pain and loneliness into creative work and to use all these inner feelings to fuel: (1) my research initiatives, (2) being a portrait oil painter, and (3) to transform myself into a writer. These three objectives were the basic pillars of my HEALING BALSAM. Of course the research initiatives were my primary and more important responsibility for building my legacy as a cancer

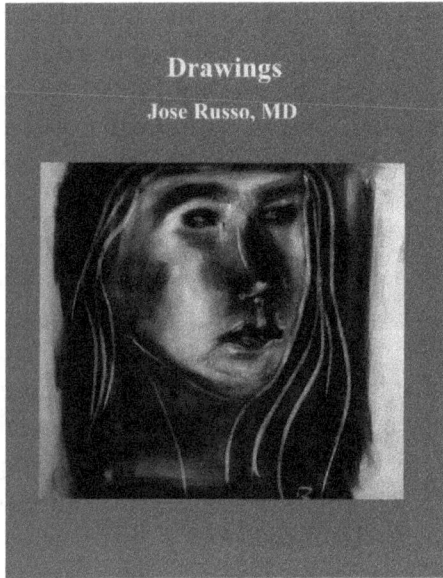

Figure 13.14: Drawings published in 2017.

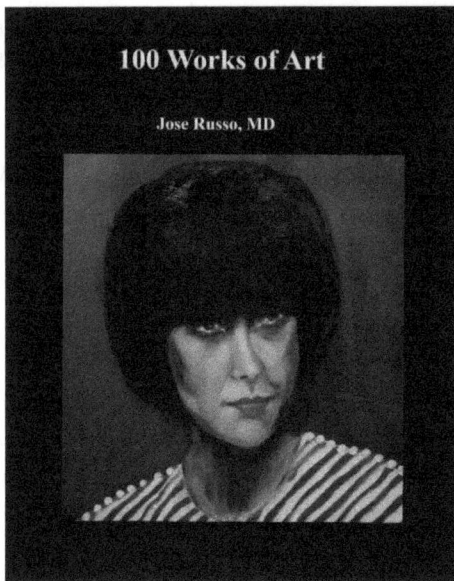

Figure 13.15: 100 Works of Art published in 2017.

researcher. My love for the beauty of forms and colors was imprinted in my wish to capture the human face as portraiture, and in addition it was another component of my being that was there like a seed without germinating or a bud of a flower that was still showing up, and it was to be a writer. Of course all my life I have been writing scientific articles, grant proposals, reports, essays, and scientific books because they are a part of my trade as a scientist, and during the period from 2013 to 2017, I wrote biomedical books like *Technical and Methodological Approaches in Breast Cancer Research, The Pathobiology of Breast Cancer,* and *The Trend in Breast Cancer Prevention.* I have signed a new contract with Springer to write a book on chromatin remodeling that is due in December of 2018.

But I needed to write for all the people, giving a message to scientists and non-scientists to create a permanent record of what has been my life and what I am thinking of it. In the middle of July of 2015, I received a letter from World Scientific Publishing in Singapore that published my book *The Tools of Science* in 2011, inviting me to write a book on *The Training of Cancer Researchers.* This book was a special challenge for me because it was a literary piece that must follow the first book *The Tools of Science.* The contract was not signed until the fall of 2015, but I was eager to work on this book. This book contained most of the material that I started compiling for a few years with the title *The Future of Science,* but Springer was not interested in a book of this nature. Therefore, it was a challenge for me when World Scientific asked me to write a book on *The Training of Cancer Researchers.* It was the opportunity that I had been waiting for.

In the *summer of 2015* I wrote in my journal:

> *I have finished the final draft of the first chapter in* The Training of Cancer Researchers *to be published by World Scientific Publishing Company. It has been more time-consuming that I expected. The reason is that it is a new set of ideas and themes that I only have a slight notion of but I never went in depth. It has been a good exercise, and I am pleased with the outcome. It needs to be reviewed several times before I'll consider it finished, but it is a good start.* In January of 2016 I wrote: The

Training of Cancer Researchers *is in progress, and although ten chapters have been written, they need to be revised and reedited before being considered finished.*

The book was finally published in the spring of 2017 (Figure 13.16), and it was well received. Dr. Richard Fisher, the President and CEO of the FCCC-Temple Health, wrote the following comment:

I wanted to congratulate you on your excellent book which I was finally able to read. It is carefully thought out and provides useful insights for future scientists. Once again thanks for a job well done.

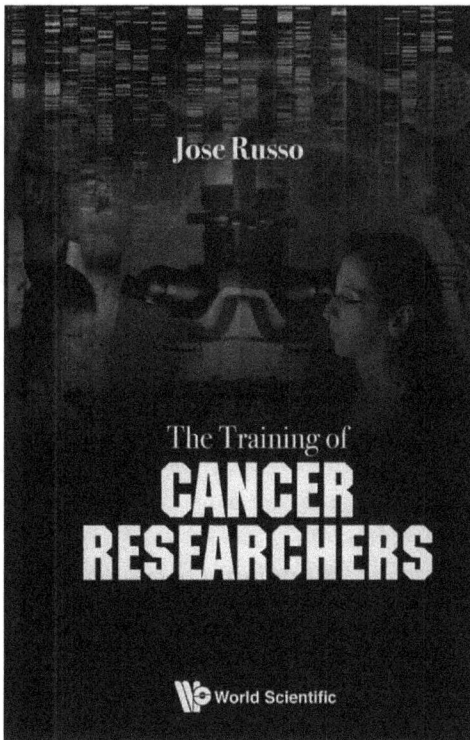

Figure 13.16: Cover of the book *The Training of Cancer Researchers.*

On *September 8, 2016,* I entered in my journal:

I am planning to start a new book on My Memoirs as a Cancer Researcher. *I have asked World Scientific Publishing if they could be interested in publishing the book. They sent me the application, and I will complete and return it to them. They requested a sample chapter, and I sent Chapter 7 dealing with my first three years at the Michigan Cancer Foundation when I was working in the search for a viral particle in the etiology of breast cancer. The contract was signed during the fall of 2016 and the manuscripts will be ready in June of 2018.*

13.7. Facing cancer again

During the year 2014, I was managing my life like a general maneuvering his army, overcoming my feeling of loneliness and sadness, and keeping my body healthy as I thought should be done. I was managing my life in a chronometric way including the care of my body. However, like all diseases they started insidiously until the real cause of the problem start to emerge. Around the middle of May 2015, I began to have a persistent diarrhea that at the beginning was attributed to some antibiotic medications I took for a bronchitis that I developed during one of my trips to the West Coast to be part of the Study Session of the California Cancer Coalition during the last week of April.

On *May 20,* I entered in my journal:

My intestines are a little more stable probably because all the anti-histaminic drugs that I am taking made me feel better and that could indicate that probably an allergy to some meal is the main cause of my symptoms. If they come back I will need to seek medical attention.

On June 4, I consulted Dr. Jilani, my family doctor, and she requested a series of tests.

On *June 12, 2015,* I wrote in my journal:

I feel worried about the possibility that my symptoms are an indication of a neoplastic process with surgery and all the treatments that follow

that diagnosis. Today I talked with Dr. Jilani and the CT scan shows a
mass in the duodenum and a thickening in the colon wall. I requested
an appointment with Dr. E. Sigurdsson to ask her opinion on how to
proceed, and if she can take care of me. The important thing now is to
proceed without damaging my health even more, and that I do not
interrupt Patricia's plan and activities.

Dr. Elaine Sigurdsson was nice and expeditious, and on June 19 I was admitted as a patient at the FCCC. The worst part of the colonoscopy and endoscopy was the liquid diet. The results were not good. I had a tumor mass in the pylorus that was protruding or fungating in the duodenum. And the colon was affected by numerous polyps and a tumor that was near the rectum. Dr. John Hoffman was brought to the consultation, and he and Sigurdsson did the surgery on July 7. They maintained the ascending colon and anastomosed with the rectum. Hoffman also removed a portion of the stomach that contained the fungating mass. My stay in the hospital was not easy, and I finally went home on July 25. The surprise was the discovery that I was a carrier of a genetic mutation in the MSH2 gene that was consistent with Lynch syndrome. When I met Henry Lynch in 1994, I never imagined that I was carrying a mutation holding his name. Henry Lynch was brought to our midst because Irma invited him to one of the meetings that she organized under LOWAC and from there a collaboration that lasted many years emerged. Through his network of surgeons, he provided the breast tissue of women who went for subcutaneous prophylactic mastectomies after discovering that they were carriers of BRCA1/2 mutation. The results of this collaboration were two publications [1, 2]. The first publication was in 1997 showing that environmental chemical carcinogens induced transformation of the breast epithelial cells obtained from those women that were carriers of genetic mutation [1]. The second publication in 2001 was the study of the breast architecture of the women carriers of the BRCA1/2 mutations and the factor that increases their susceptibility to cancer [2].

The recovery from my surgery was also aggravated by a sciatic pain that persisted for many months. I lost almost 40 pounds and went from a 38-inch waist to a 32-inch one, making all my wardrobe obsolete. To this ordeal, a kidney stone was added on New Year's Eve and I was admitted to the Abington Hospital for three days.

I am a cancer survivor, and every three months I have a checkup of my markers and every year a colonoscopy. I had considered myself a strategist, a logistic planner, and I realize that my life can be finished in any moment by those cancer cells that I try to understand and fight.

13.8. Rebuilding my research endeavor

After Irma's death, my research endeavor was my blood line that gave me a purpose to be vertical every day.

On *February 5, 2014*, I wrote:

> *Several original articles are submitted in addition to the invited reviews. There are one grant and two LOIs that I am expecting for an answer. I am working on two ideas for RO1 that I am aiming for June, because I need to think and ask for help in the meantime. I am working with Julia on the manuscript to collect all the data of the Avon study and that also requires significant acumen on my part.*

Although I was working without pause, nothing was funded and the Pioneer grant application that I was so sure would be scored did not pass either. I was facing no new funding for the BCRL, and the pressure from the FCCC was mounting that I was in a deficit for 2015 jeopardizing the salary of the people who work with me. The rejections that I'd had during the last years bothered me significantly because I started to feel that it was my fault and not the economic situation. On May 18, I was ready to present new grant applications and requested the opinions of reviewers inside and outside of the FCCC to be sure that I was not missing some vital information that made me outdated. I even agreed to be a part of the Study Session for the NCI on June 24, to have a better feeling of how the review process was at that moment. Even though these measurements and even my external and internal reviewers did not find anything wrong or weakness, the applications were scored insufficiently low for funding. Some of the critiques were so ridiculous that they leveled up with incompetence. However, I kept pounding and on *July 5, 2014,* I wrote in my journal:

> *Three applications for the NCI have been submitted this past month and now I am working on the progress report for the PA health that contains all the data on the epigenetic control of cancer metastasis. . . . The main objective is not only to continue working in the mechanism of the genomic signature of pregnancy but also to publish the data that we have been generating during the last three years. This also will help me to prepare the conferences for Mendoza, Las Vegas, Athens, and Belgium. The preparation of these lectures is forcing me to review several basic concepts of cancer biology.*

On *September 15, 2014,* I wrote in my journal:

> *Chernoff asked me to empty Irma's office and also the one that was occupied by Su and Maria. This has opened a torrent of feelings and sentiments of sadness. Day after day I accept my reality that I am alone and that I do not have any idea how my future will be. Realities like retirement and fixed resources are starting to be part of my readings and planning. The death of Irma has washed my soul leaving a sense of no expectation.*

On *October 24, 2014,* I wrote:

> *Yesterday I opened the email of the NIH era of common and found that I was notified that my RO1 application on the effect of hCG in chromatin remodeling will not be funded. It was not discussed, meaning that the priority score was very low. I do not know if funding will be available to keep the core of the lab, or if the FCCC gently decided to retire me. I do not know. **What I really know is that I must keep working.***
>
> *The ideas and methodology that I present in my grant applications are matching with the complexity of the science of today. However, when I listen to the new generation of scientists and the intricacy of the data presented and the complexity of them, I found that the core of their*

research is not original, all of them are cookie cutter of the same principle. Ergo who will honor those papers that are known for the past generation of scientists and now they are in the oblivion? It is true that the gestalt of my hypothesis could be good but I have so many things to prove that without funding everything looks senseless. I should quit and stay in a corner? Or been truthful with myself to honestly verbalize what I know is correct and help and participate positively in the common good? I think that the latter is the way to go.

At difference of other moments of my life, I do not feel desperation or even anguish for this realization and by the contrary I want to catch up, to do better in everything that I do and excel in quality. I do not know if I will have the time, I will work to enjoy the work that I do and aiming for perfection in my art and intellectual work.... I realized how the love of Irma changed my way of thinking because when every day I face a problem or a situation, I try to act and think how she would do it — by putting compassion, love, and attention for the other and the task in front of me.

On *December 2, 2014*, I wrote:

My trip to Europe last month was successful. The course at the University of Valladolid was well received and the talk at the College Santa Cruz, feminine site was outstandingly received with a previous TV interview in Channel 6/8 from Castilla y Leon. We made a good team with Pedro, and I even received honorarium that I had not expected to have. The possibility of collaboration with a biomathematics group at the University of Valladolid for further analysis of the data on the genomic signature of pregnancy was also an unexpected outcome. The excess of euros that I received I have distributed among my sister, Araceli, and Pedro with some money left for Ariel, Paola, and Julieta for Christmas gifts.

The trip from Valladolid to Brussels was also very good. Magda Janssens was expecting me with a friend in the airport and Jaak and the rest of his family were extremely nice with me. The meeting was excellent, and my conference was well received with the tangible possibility of developing a clinical trial with hCG. Coral and DD

Lamartiniere were there as well as Andrea Mani and his wife and Brian Czerniecki. I also mingled with other accountancies and the formal invitation to go to Jerusalem at the end of April for a conference in breast cancer. If the group of Halsted with Jaak as a head are able to procure funding, the hCG trial will be a real possibility and complete the idea that we were pursuing for so long. I also met Drs. Magda Johanna Vandeloo who was working with Jaak and showed interest in our work, and I extended her the invitation to visit me in Philadelphia.

On *January 1, 2015,* I wrote:

In this New Year I have several tasks in front of me. One of them is to construct my part of the UO1 grant application that I am developing with the Harvard group lead by Karin Michel. She approached to me few weeks ago about working in collaboration in an RFA that was originated by the NIEHS and the NCI for studying the windows of breast cancer susceptibility. This UO1 is in certain way a continuation of the BCERC that I have been working first as a PI and later on with Coral Lamartiniere. Karin indicated that my contribution to the experimental part will be extremely important for the whole application.

I am also presenting a LOI for Avon in which I will push again for the hCG trial this time backed by Jaak Janssens and Herman Depypere in Belgium, who are interested in doing all the clinical parts, meaning the recruitment of the volunteers. I am not so sure if the Avon will accept the LOI for a final application, but it is a door that is opened and I would like to see how feasible it is to obtain the funds.

It is also in the plan for this year to present a rebuttal of the R21 on the study of the lncRNAs in the parous and nulliparous women. At least this application has been in the 20 percent of funding. It will be difficult to see whether it will go through, but at least we will fight in the second round.

My main concern for this year is to keep the basic structure of the BCRL that now is formed by Julia, Su, Theresa, Maria, and Joseph. The last two are graduate students. Besides some funds that I have received from donations, I will need considerable help and support from the FCCC to keep this basic group together.

I have three books in progress, two international meetings one, in Bolzano and other in Madrid, and also chairing an internet meeting on breast cancer. This latter is a new experience. I have also been invited to be part of the NCI SPORE study session and to chair the Pathobiology Study Session of the DOD. The Pharmacy Group Eisai would like to have my advice on the previous work that I have done for them and Arena on Lorcaserine.

I am keeping active the Coop group that Irma started and some of the interns have provided new insights and rewarding experiences.

On *March 20, 2015,* I wrote:

I have been preparing my small talk for March 24, the day that the Flyers wives are visiting the FCCC, and I am giving a short presentation and thanking them for the two hundred thousand dollar donation that they made to the BCRL. This donation, divided over a two-year period, will help to cover my shortage of funding for the 2016 budget.

On *April 2, 2015,* I wrote in my journal:

It is almost three p.m., and my talk with Robert Beck was rescheduled earlier. My talk with him was not related directly to this year's budget, but to my lack of extramural support and for how long I want to keep the lab running. I indicated to him that I am not planning to retire, that it is my intention to continue asking for extramural support and that is my main concern. I also indicated to him that I am physically and mentally eager to keep going until something impairs me, and what I want is to consolidate my research to accomplish the objectives that are now clearer than ever. He indicated that they cannot do anything legally until 2017 to push me out, meaning that seventy-five years of age will be the critical point. Their concern is the same as mine: not having enough grants to keep the lab running. Seven days later in my talk with Beck on April 9 of the same year, I received a letter from him and I wrote in my journal: *The letter of Beck is clear and it is a formal notification that if I do not have extramural support for*

sustaining the research projects my laboratory will be closed on July 1,
2016, and I will be kept in my position until July 2017. At this time
I must retire and my scientific endeavor is finished.

This was not the letter that I expected but every time that
somebody wants to push me back I remember the Russian dolls that
have a round base and when you push back they spring forward to the
original position therefore that is what I did. I started working on
another grant in response to an RFA on early factor in cancer
development. We were proposing to study the effect of cigarette
smoke and electronic cigars in the development and susceptibility of
the mammary gland to early exposure. We were introducing the idea
that exposure to cigarette smoke and e-cigarette may be noxious
factors on the mammary gland that may trigger the development of
cancer later on in life.

All of these things were happening during my recovery from my
colon cancer surgery that was at the end of July of 2015. This was a
sad demonstration by the FCCC that I was as good as the amount of
external funding I brought to the institution, after all for every dollar
that I bring they charge the federal government 86 cents for
administering that dollar; in technical terms that is called indirect
cost. I have discussed this point in detail in my book *The Training of*
Cancer Researchers. On September 27, 2015, I received the good
news that the UO1 was funded and this was a real break for
maintaining the BCRL. This award also abrogated the threatening
letter of Robert Beck, and I wrote an email to him indicating that
with this new grant the term of his letter was not in effect any longer.
He agreed on that.

During the middle of the fall of that year and after the award of
the UO1, I signed and prepared the contract with Colgate Palmolive
for the meeting of the advisory panel for the coming November. The
assignment was not completely laid out until the meeting got closer
but the contract was to study a bacteriostatic compound called
"triclosan" that has been considered an environmental hazard. I felt
good about this assignment mainly because it gave me a sense of being
back in the arena and my conclusions given to the panel were warning

signs of the possible estrogenic effect of this compound. However, I will never know the final decision that the panel provided to the firm.

During this time, I received an invitation from the Kimmel Cancer Center at Jefferson to nominate myself for the position of Director of the Breast Oncology Section in the Department of Oncology. I was curious and I answered the invitation indicating that I was interested to know more and that definitely I would like to know what I could contribute with my experience to the goals of Jefferson Medical School. I talked with one of the committee members, Ms. Pam Lisle, and the talk was very general and the decision was that they would establish another meeting in person but I did not receive a call from them until weeks later indicating that they wanted to convene a meeting. This time I disregarded any further interest in this offer and later on I found out that this was the same position held by Dr. Massimo Cristofanilli, and that he resigned to take a position at Northwestern University. It seemed that this position has been a musical chair for years, and it was good that I did not spend too much energy on them.

The rest of 2016 and 2017 was full of activity, and I had been engaged with the NCI and the DOD Study Session review panels, honoring speaking invitations such as the one from De Sales University and Dr. Alfredo Barros to go to the meeting in San Paulo, Brazil. All of them were rich experiences and the most important was that I started to enjoy the journey and not only the finished tasks.

In the lecture in De Sale University, I reviewed how the MCF-7 and MCF-10 were developed and the main contributions that those cells paved into our present understanding of cancer. Almost 46 years of my life was in the review so that, in one way or another, I was a part of the story. I also gave a lecture on the meeting of Family Nursing that took place in the Double Tree Hotel in Philadelphia on breast cancer prevention and the lecture was well received and the nurses asked meaningful and engaging questions. I organized a brainstorming meeting to discuss a potential PO1 with Dr. Jeffrey Peterson, and it was better than expected but I reached the conclusion that it was not wise to pursue further.

After too much pain from Irma's death, my life had returned to writing papers, grant applications, reading and catching up with the growing literature, revising manuscripts, and reviewing grants. The joy of planning experiments, analyzing data, and talking with my younger staff about the data and new approaches has not gone from me. The only cloud that is all the time on the horizon is the funding of my research.

13.9. Finding Johanna

We cannot predict the future, we can only trace from the past our present situation and from there vaguely try to plan the days ahead of us. After Irma's death, every day was about surviving the pain of her loss and learning to live alone. Every day was a struggle to transform my pain, sadness, and weakness into creative energy that I desperately wanted to see in my writing, in my photography, in my drawing and painting, and more importantly in my research endeavor. This could be called a surviving strategy. But this mental attitude allowed me to keep going and not think that I would be alone for the rest of my life. The idea of developing feelings for another woman was basically out of the question; it seemed ludicrous that I could feel something for any other woman or that I could awake in another woman feelings of love for me. Basically, it was impossible for me to think that I could feel love again.

It was in this frame of mind that I lived until March 18, 2017, the day that I discovered Magda Johanna Alfons Maria Vandeloo, the woman who helped me to find love again. How I met her and how our understanding of each other and love developed will be the story of my next book titled *Finding Love Again in the Autumn of My Life*.

References

[1]   Hu, Y. F., Russo, I. H., Zalipsky, U., Lynch, H. T. and Russo, J. Environmental chemical carcinogens induce transformation of breast epithelial cells from women with familial history of breast cancer. *In vitro Cell. Dev. Biol.* 33: 495–498, 1997.

[2]   Russo, J., Lynch, H. and Russo, I. H. Mammary gland architecture as a determining factor in the susceptibility of the human breast to cancer. *Breast J.* 7: 278–291, 2001.

Chapter 14

My Legacy

14.1. Defining my legacy

The word *legacy* has many uses in the English language, but the one that applies for this chapter is Merriam-Webster's definition: *"something transmitted by or received from an ancestor or predecessor or from the past."* Therefore, my legacy as a cancer researcher is showing another way to prevent breast cancer using a physiological concept of how early pregnancy differentiates the gland and makes it refractory to cancer. Based on this premise, the final goal is to mimic pregnancy without pregnancy by using a hormone that remodels the chromatin of the breast cells.

In my book *The Tools of Science,* published in 2011, I wrote, *"Finding the research question to solve is one of the most important steps in the life of a scientist and could define the work for the rest of his or her life."* The driving force for me has been to answer two questions: One, what is the mechanism that makes normal cells into cancer ones, and second, why parity produces protection against breast cancer. In answering my first question, I have produced original work showing how a normal cell can be transformed by known chemical carcinogens and also by the natural hormone 17-β-estradiol (See Chapters 10 and 11). I will continue working in this subject for all the years that I am able, because from the first day that I started working on this topic I have been fascinated by the intricacy of normal cells becoming malignant, and how to stop that process is the holy grail of cancer research. However, I feel that my contribution, or my legacy, to future generations will not be in that specific field but instead in the developing of a strategy for breast cancer prevention. The idea is simple: *If I understand the biological process by which early pregnancy protects a woman against breast cancer then I will have a way to develop a preventive mechanism against the disease.* The reason this will be our legacy is because Irma and I were the first ones to develop a rational explanation using an experimental model to illustrate why an early first pregnancy protects a woman for life against developing breast cancer; this was outlined in our seminal work published in the *Journal National Cancer Institute* in 1978 [1, 2]. From these publications up to the present, I have continued hammering at this idea.

Breast differentiation is a very delicate mechanism played by several components at the same time, like gene repression and activation, and all of them interlaced in changing the chromatin pattern, remodeling it, mimicking what happens with early development during the process of organogenesis. Pregnancy completes the process of breast differentiation as the organ is not fully developed until this event takes place. From the understanding that differentiation of the target organ is what makes it refractory to the cancer emerged, the concept of the need to mimic pregnancy arose. We identified that the natural hormone produced by the placenta, human chorionic gonadotropin (hCG), could be the one involved in this process, and our data show how the hormone remodels the chromatin and explain what we have observed in our experimental rat model. The full proof of the concept is to demonstrate that when we use this hormone we can remodel the chromatin of the breast of young women making them refractory to cancer.

At the time of writing these memoirs, the clinical trial for testing this idea is ongoing, and if we succeed with the collaboration of physician scientists like Dr. Herman Depypere and Dr. Jaak Jannsens, at the University of Ghent (Belgium) and the European Cancer Prevention Organization, respectively, and Dr. Yanrong Su at the Irma H. Russo MD Breast Cancer Research Laboratory in Philadelphia, my legacy will be complete.

In the following sections of this chapter, I will describe how we have been unveiling this process and my tribulations and successes in developing a clinical trial to translate the research idea to the clinical practice.

14.2. Breast cancer prevention

Breast cancer is a heterogeneous and complex disease resulting from the uncontrolled growth of cells that are unique and specific to the breast. The occurrence of cancer of the breast has long been known, as documented in the Edwin Smith surgical papyrus, written between 3000 and 1500 BC (Table 14.1). A common denominator for the risk of developing breast cancer has been found to be a reproductive history. Increased breast cancer incidence and mortality were associated with nulliparity as early as the 1700s, as reported by Bernardino Ramazzini, who attributed the phenomenon to the childlessness of nuns in Italian convents (Table 14.1).

Epidemiological data from various parts of the world have consistently shown that early full-term pregnancy and multiparity are associated with breast cancer risk reduction in postmenopausal women [3–5], whereas late pregnancy and nulliparity are associated with increased risk [6]. It has been postulated that the mechanism of pregnancy-induced protection is mediated by changes in environmental

Table 14.1:   Landmarks in the history of breast cancer.

Year	Landmark discovery or observation	Reference
3000–1500 BC	Edwin Smith surgical papyrus describes eight cases of breast cancer in women	[119]
1700	Bernardino Ramazzini attributed the high incidence of breast cancer in nuns to their childlessness.	[120]
1970	MacMahon *et al.* reported that pregnancy exerted a protective effect in women whose first child was bore from early teens to the middle 20s.	[6]
1978	Russo and Russo established the concept that the mammary gland differentiation induced by full-term pregnancy is the mechanism behind the protective effect against breast cancer.	[1, 2]

settings [7], and/or alterations in the immunological profile of the host [8]. Our studies on the differentiation of the breast [9–11] under the influence of the complex hormonal milieu created by two newly formed endocrine organs, the placenta and the fetus [12], have unraveled the morphological, functional, genomic, and transcriptomic changes that ultimately result in the induction of a permanent and specific profile that serves as an indicator of reduced cancer risk [13, 14]. My laboratory has provided evidence supporting the concept that the degree of differentiation acquired through an early pregnancy changes the genomic signature that differentiates the lobular structures of the parous breast from those of the nulliparous one [1, 2, 13].

14.2.1. *Transcriptomic differences*

During the last 25 years we have been working on characterizing the molecular basis underlying the mechanism of pregnancy-induced protection that resulted in hundreds of publications, however, those published in 2011 and 2012 are the ones that finally demonstrated in humans that our hypothesis developed in the experimental system is correct [15–17].

14.2.1.1. *Our approach to studying transcriptomic differences*

Chapter 9 (Figure 9.12) described that the predominant structure in the human breast, as long as a woman does not become pregnant, is Lob 1. Lob 1, or terminal ductal lobular unit, is the site of the main type of ductal carcinoma of the human breast. With pregnancy and lactation, the mammary parenchyma reaches the final stage of secretory lobule type 4 (Lob 4) that forms by the end of the repro- ductive process and remains present during lactation until they involute to Lob 1 in postmenopausal years (Figure 9.12 in Chapter 9). Therefore, we postulated that the protection conferred by an early pregnancy is mediated by the induction of differentiation that we defined as the coordinated and sequential series of events induced in the breast by the hormonal milieu of pregnancy, or pregnancy-like conditions (such as hCG administration), which culminate in the activation of genes controlling ductal and lobular development inducing a unique genomic signature. This genomic signature is induced by the process of lobular differentiation that takes place when the Lob 1 differentiates in Lob 2 and then in Lobs 3 and 4. Therefore, the Lob 1 of the involuted breast of parous women, although it looks morphologically similar to the Lob 1 of nulliparous women, is different because the latter has undergone the process of full differentiation where the genomic changes have been imprinted (Figure 9.12 in Chapter 9).

Therefore, it was crucial for our research to determine if the genomic signature induced by pregnancy was different in the parous breast compared with the nulliparous one. One way to assess whether a specific genomic fingerprint is permanently imprinted in the breast by a full-term pregnancy (FTP) is to compare the transcriptomic profiles of breasts from parous and nulliparous women. For this purpose, we decided to use a genome-wide approach to identify long-term genomic changes associated with FTP by studying breast core needle biopsies (CNBs) obtained from healthy pre- and postmenopausal volunteers.

14.2.1.2. *The consortium*

The difficulty posed by this study was that we needed to obtain normal breast tissues from asymptomatic women, meaning women without sign of disease. Not only must they agree to a core biopsy, but we also wanted to be sure that we had enough volunteers to have statistical power when comparing pre- and postmenopausal women who were nulliparous or parous at the time of the procurement of the sample.

I already described in Chapter 9 the case control study supported by an NCI-RO1 and published in *Cancer Epidemiol Biomarkers Prevention* in 2008 [5] showing that parous women have a different genomic signature not only from nulliparous with and without breast cancer but also from parous with breast cancer. Although the publication did not become a landmark, it provided the basis for a larger study that was possible by a consortium created between my laboratory at the FCCC, New York University, and the University of Umea in Sweden and financed with a grant that we obtained from Avon Foundation (Avon Foundation for Women Breast Cancer Research Program grant (02-2010-117)).

The history of this consortium was initiated by an invitation that I received from Paolo Toniolo to a meeting on "Women's Health" that he organized in Camogli, Italy, in October of 2005 as part of the "Nordic Cohort" study that was sponsored by the NCI (Figure 14.1). In that meeting, I presented my data in a talk on "The Biological and Molecular Basis of Hormone-Induced Breast Cancer Prevention." It was at this opportunity that I was introduced to Toniolo's group from New York University and his collaborators at the Umea University in Sweden and Tampere University in Finland. It was a powerhouse meeting in which I felt invigorated because I knew this was the right group to collaborate with. The New York

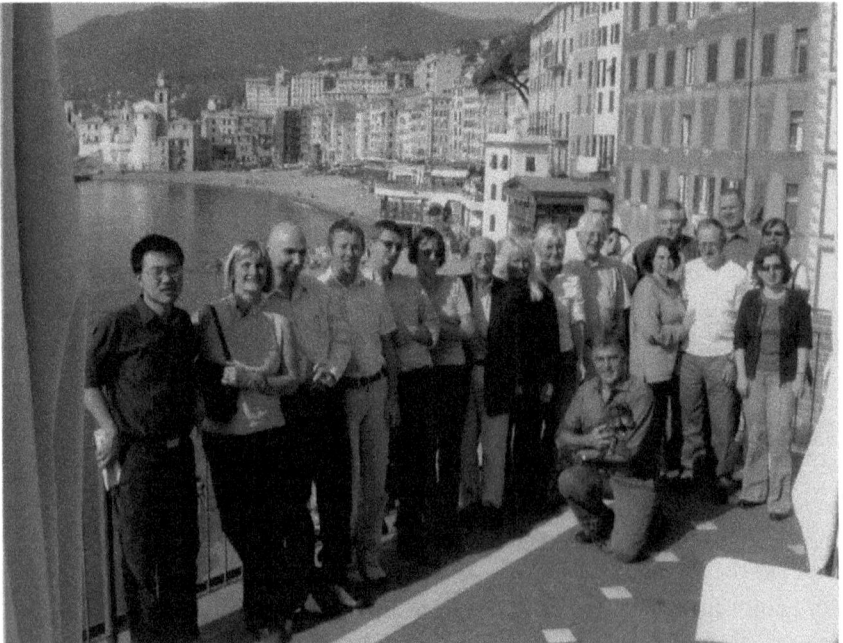

Figure 14.1: Photo of the group that would later integrate into the consortium to study the genomic signature of pregnancy. Camogli, Italy, October of 2015.

group was represented by Paolo Toniolo, Anne Zeleniuch-Jacquotte, and Alan Arslan, the Umea group was represented by Goran Hallmans and Per Lenner, and the Finland group was represented by Mattis Lehtinen and Aero Pukkala. My presentation was well received and generated significant brainstorming, spurring my predictable reaction to pursue a clinical trial by using hCG in young women. Aero Pukkala made a convincing presentation on how in Finland they have achieved significant reduction in diabetes and cardiovascular diseases by a proactive preventive program that led Matti Lehtinen, who was working on developing a clinical trial of human papillomavirus vaccine, to propose that we should start a clinical trial using hCG in young women. The basic idea was to use our data and preventive use of hCG in the animal system for developing a clinical trial using the infrastructure of Finland and Sweden. This was the most exciting moment that I had had in years, to see somebody verbalizing my wish, and moreover coming from a person of the caliber of Lehtinen. However, the enthusiasm to pursue a clinical trial using hCG was not unanimous. The New York group was cautious about the idea of a clinical trial, and Anne Zeleniuch-Jacquotte felt we did not have strong data on the genomic signature of pregnancy because the data published in *Cancer Epidemiol Biomarkers Prevention* in 2008 [5] were not statistically powerful enough. Alan Arslan was more enthusiastic on the hCG trial proposed by Lehtinen, and Paolo Toniolo supported the point that a trial was a premature thing to do. The group from Umea University, mainly Per Lenner, felt a trial was not feasible and it would not pass the ethical committee. My take-home message from that meeting was that only researchers like Matti Lehtinen would be able to help me push the idea of a clinical trial in young women. I was right, and it took me 9 years to find the right group of physician scientists who could help me execute the clinical trial.

Almost 18 month after the meeting in Comogli, in May of 2007, I was invited again by Paolo Toniolo to the International Consortium on Pregnancy and Health, in Monterotondo di Gavi, Italy, where I spoke on "Development of Signature Markers of Exposure to Pregnancy and hCG." The Finland group was not present at that meeting, and I saw clearly that the idea of an hCG clinical trial was diluting and difficult to bring back to the group's focus. The third meeting was at the Centre Hospitalier Universitaire Vaudois, University of Lausanne, in Switzerland on April of 2009. Here I presented the data recently published in *Cancer Epidemiology Biomarkers* and *Prevention* in 2008 and spoke on "A New Perspective in Breast Cancer Prevention." Although the hCG trial was not on the agenda, it was in this meeting that we clearly hammered out a consortium to study and establish the presence or not of a definitive genomic signature of pregnancy (GSP), and this in itself was an important achievement. Another contributing factor was that Avon had shown interest in funding a proposal of this nature. As a consortium, we wrote a successful grant application to the Avon Foundation for Women Breast Cancer Research Program; it was funded in 2010 for 4 years to study the genomic signature of the parous and nulliparous pre- and postmenopausal breast. On March 1, 2011, I presented the data that we had obtained to the Avon Breast Cancer Program in New York by talking on the "Characterization and Validation of a Genomic Signature of Pregnancy." *We published three seminal papers on the data obtained* [15–17] and in the last meeting of this consortium, which took place in Umea, Sweden, in May of 2013, I presented the "Biological Considerations of the Genomic Signature of the Premenopausal Breast," and it was agreed that Dr. Julia Pereira would write the manuscript on the GSP of the premenopausal breast.

We kept in touch, and different members of the group discussed areas of common interest and future collaborative work, but we were unable to reproduce the invigorating teamwork that we had accomplished in previous years. This could be due to many factors, among them Avon was no longer interested in funding our ideas; the retirement of Paolo Toniolo, Goran Hallmans, and Per Lenner; the death of Irma; and the change in interests of many other members of the group. Paolo Toniolo played an important role in this group, and his idea to be the leader of an international group based in Lausanne, Switzerland, was no longer appealing to those who had supported him at New York University.

The fact that needs to be recognized by our peers is that we were the only group that studied the normal breast of nulliparous and parous pre- and postmenopausal women providing a unique set of genomic data that explained a 300-year-old observation that pregnancy is a protective factor in breast cancer.

14.2.1.3. *How we did it*

The breast tissue of nulliparous and parous pre- and postmenopausal women was collected from healthy women volunteers residing in Norrbotten County, Sweden, an ethnically homogeneous population of Swedish or Finnish ancestry [15] (Figure 14.2).

The samples were collected from those women who fulfilled the eligibility criteria and signed an informed consent to participate in the study and donate breast tissue in the form of core needle biopsies (CNB). It was important to separate the samples according to their

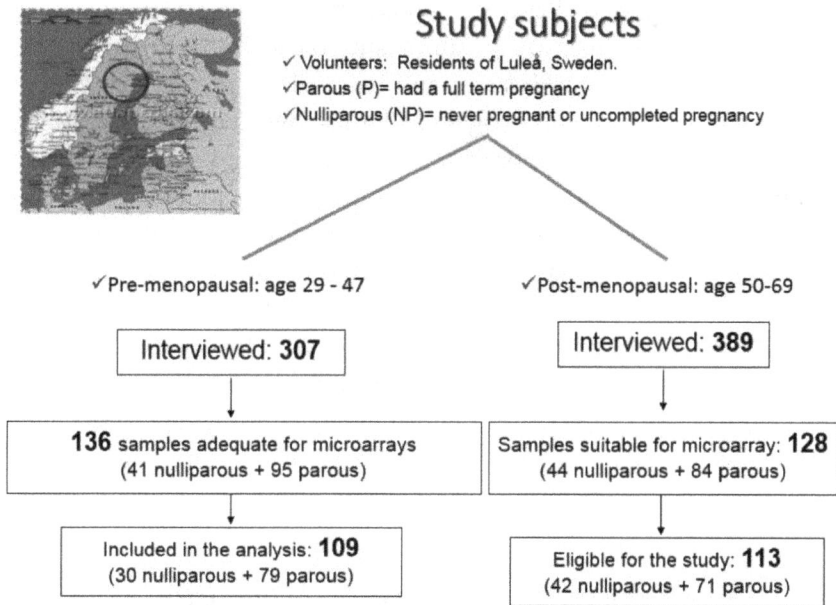

Figure 14.2: Diagram of the study subjects' distribution in pre- and postmenopausal women and parity history.

reproductive histories, and eligible subjects were categorized as either parous or nulliparous. The parous group (P) included all women who had been pregnant (gravida) one or more times and had delivered (parous) one or more live children. The nulliparous group (NP) included both nulligravida women who had never become pregnant and therefore never had a full-term delivery, and women who had become pregnant one or more times (G ≥ 1) but never completed a full-term pregnancy (FTP), identified as nulligravida nulliparous (NN) and gravida nulliparous (GN), respectively. Both NN and GN women were considered as a single group (NP) for most analyses.

I need to emphasize that this work would not have been possible without the synchronized work of the three different players in the consortium, the University of Umea in Sweden, New York University, and our laboratory at the FCCC. The publications generated from this project [15–17] list all the contributors to this study, and each one played a unique role (Figure 14.2). Suffice it to say that in my laboratory Dr. Julia Pereira and the support of the bioinformatics department, mainly S. Peri, M. Slifker, and E. Ross, were pivotal in the analysis of these data. An important role was played by Dr. Pal Bordas from Sunderby Hospital and the Lulea and the Norrbotten Mammography Screening Progam in Umea, Sweden, which obtained the core biopsies of these precious biological samples. A supporting group of other doctors, nurses, and logistical personnel from both Lulea and Umea in Sweden made it possible for the samples to arrive in Philadelphia in perfect condition. A unique role was also played by the New York University team, directed by Dr. Paulo Toniolo, that designed the questionnaire administered to each participant and identified the samples in such a way that all the studies were performed in a blinded fashion. It was a real joy to work with these colleagues who were so rigorous in the collection of epidemiological data making our data unbiased.

14.3. The genomic signature of prevention (GSP)

In the BCRL working with Dr. Julia Pereira, we used the Affymetrix oligonucleotide arrays that were top of the line in 2010 and allowed

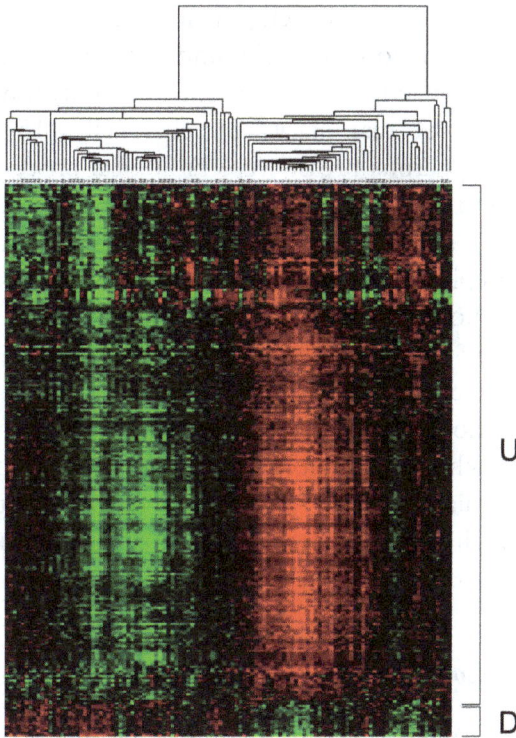

Figure 14.3:   Hierarchical clustering of differentially expressed probesets in parous and nulliparous women. Red represents expression values above the median across all samples, and green represents values below the median. In the two top-level clusters of samples, the right cluster is composed mainly of parous samples and the left cluster is composed mainly of nulliparous samples. U represents the intensity of up-regulated probesets among parous samples whereas D represents the intensity of down-regulated probesets. N represents nulliparous and Y represents parous. A chi-square test of independence on parity status and subtree membership resulted in a p-value of 0.001 [16].

us to identify 305 differentially expressed probesets (corresponding to 208 distinct genes) between P and NP women. Of these, 267 were up-regulated and 38 were down-regulated (Figure 14.3). To understand the biological theme of the observed gene expression differences, we carried out bioinformatics-based analysis of microarray data. Gene ontology (GO) enrichment analysis revealed biological processes that were categorized into groups including RNA metabolic processes, differentiation and development of epidermis and ectoderm, and cell-substrate junction assembly, findings that are in agreement with existing knowledge that pregnancy hormones promote the differentiation of mammary epithelial cells [15–17]. Highly represented in the parous breast were biological processes involving both mRNA and RNA metabolic processes and RNA splicing machinery. Biological processes such as differentiation and development of epithelial and ectodermal cells as well as genes which are pivotal in anchoring of epithelial cells to the basement membrane, hemidesmosome, and cell-substrate junction assembly were up-regulated in the P group.

Among the down-regulated genes, insulin-like growth factor 1 (IGF-1) was enriched in 19 biological processes that comprised cell proliferation, regulation of IGF-like growth factor receptor signaling, somatic stem cell maintenance, muscle cell differentiation, and apoptosis, among others [16, 17].

14.3.1. *Spliceosomes in the GSP*

One of the most exciting parts of this study was identifying the genes that were up- and down-regulated by an early pregnancy and, most important, how they cluster together and deciphering the possible mechanism of its action. It is in this way that we discovered the complex molecular machine found in the speckles of the nuclei were associated with the splicing mechanism of the eukaryotic cells [18].

The whole molecular complex is called spliceosome with the primary function of removing introns from a transcribed pre-mRNA, a type of primary transcript; this process is generally referred to as splicing. The main components of the spliceosome machinery, including RNA and proteins that undergo dynamic changes during the splicing reaction, were up-regulated in the parous breast. Among them were the heterogeneous nuclear ribonucleoproteins (HNRPs) that include HNRPA3, HNRPA2B1, HNRPD, and HNRPU [19], which are implicated in the regulation of mRNA stability, as well as other functions, such as mammary gland involution [20], negative regulation of telomere length maintenance [21], and regulation of mRNA trafficking from the nucleus to distal processes in neural cells [22]. We postulated that spliceosome-related genes may play an important regulatory function as transcriptional regulators. In addition, post-transcriptional methylation of internal adenosine residues in eukaryotic mRNAs by METTL3 (methyltransferase like 3), which was up-regulated in the parous breast, could play a role in the efficiency of mRNA splicing, transport, or translation in the differentiated breast epithelium. Other members of the spliceosome complex were the proteins encoded by the genes SF3B1, SFRS2, SFRS7, SFRS8, SFRS14, SFRS16, SNRP70, SNRPB, SNRPA1, PRF3, and PHF5A, all of which were overexpressed in the parous breast. In the case of the small nuclear ribonucleoproteins (snRNPs), there is evidence that they suppress tumor cell growth and may have major implications as cancer therapeutic targets (Figure 14.4).

The pre-mRNA splicing factors are enriched in nuclear domains termed interchromatin granule clusters or nuclear speckles. Among the members of the splicing factor compartment are CCNL1 and CCNL2, which participate in the pre-mRNA splicing process and are located in the nuclear speckles [23, 24]. CCNL1 and CCNL2 are up-regulated in the parous breast and the protein of the latter is also

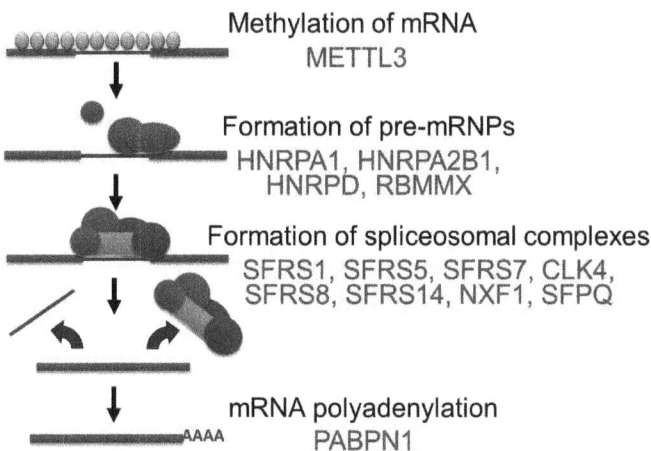

Methylation of mRNA
METTL3

Formation of pre-mRNPs
HNRPA1, HNRPA2B1,
HNRPD, RBMMX

Formation of spliceosomal complexes
SFRS1, SFRS5, SFRS7, CLK4,
SFRS8, SFRS14, NXF1, SFPQ

mRNA polyadenylation
PABPN1

Figure 14.4: Scheme of RNA processing pathway and up-regulated genes in parous breast tissue [26].

overexpressed in the nucleus of breast epithelial cells [16]. CCNL1 and CCNL2 are transcriptional regulators [23, 24] that modulate the expression of critical factors leading to cell apoptosis, possibly through the Wnt signal transduction pathway [25], a signaling pathway that is enriched by down-regulated genes in the parous breast.

In our previously published preclinical and clinical studies [5, 9, 11, 13], we have reported that pregnancy confers protection from breast cancer development by inducing gland differentiation, which imprints a specific and permanent genomic signature in this organ. To re-emphasize this concept, I compared the study reported by us in 2008 [5], a case control study of transcriptomic analysis of normal breast tissues obtained from parous and nulliparous women free of breast pathology, and parous and nulliparous women with a history of breast cancer who served as controls and cases, respectively, with the study that we performed several years later with another population of women and reported in 2012 [17]. The relevance of this comparison is that when we applied GO enrichment analysis to the gene lists generated from both studies it was found that in both studies the processes involved in RNA metabolism and RNA processing were similar. This uniqueness of the data pushed us forward to study, with Julia Pereira, this mechanism in more detail, and for that reason we performed RNA-sequencing P and NP breast biopsies from postmenopausal women free of disease. Alternative splicing events were identified through the Multivariate Alternative Transcript Splicing Software (MATS) and considered statistically significant when the FDR (false discovery rate) was less than 5%. We evaluated the differences between P and NP of five types of splicing: mutually exclusive exon, alternative 5′ splice site, alternative 3′ splice site, skipped exon, and *retained intron*. The last type, the retained intron, had the higher number of statistically significant events different between P and NP. From 95 retained intron (RI) events, P women had 21 events, while in the NP we found 74 RI events. *Retained intron (RI) events were selected for further examination because these events can either be splicing errors or a form of gene expression regulation, which indicated that they have lower expression and/or they produce lower quantities of functional proteins.*

Several of the genes containing RI belong to PI3K-Akt signaling and spliceosome pathways. GO analysis revealed that those genes with higher levels of RI in the NP breast enriched mainly GO terms related to RNA processing and splicing. This is in agreement with our previous gene expression results, in which genes involved in RNA processing and splicing were down-regulated in the NP women. *The relevance of this data is that alternative splicing is disproportionately affecting important pathways such as PI3K-Akt, spliceosome, and other genes involved in mRNA processing in NP women which may explain their higher risk for breast cancer.* These data led us to suggest that post-transcriptional regulation is a key element in the differences between the breasts of parous and nulliparous women and their lifetime breast cancer risk. We reported this data in 2015 [26], and we are still actively working on this subject.

14.3.2. *The role of long non-coding RNA in the GSP*

In our study of the genes displayed with the Affymetrix oligonucleotide arrays, we were able to see few sequences identified as long non-coding RNA. This data opened our minds to a new set of mechanisms that had never been explored as relevant since non-coding RNAs were once thought of as the "dark matter" of the genome, but it is becoming increasingly clear that they play major roles in gene regulation as 98% of the human genome is non-protein-coding material. Non-coding RNAs are transcripts of RNA that do not code for a protein and can be classified as short non-coding RNA (for example, miRNA; between 18–22 nucleotides in length) and long non-coding RNA (lncRNA; equal or greater than 200 nucleotides in length). Long non-coding RNAs have diverse gene expression regulatory functions including transcriptional regulation, post-transcriptional regulation, or direct regulation of proteins, and they may act as tumor suppressors while others act as oncogenes.

The non-coding RNAs that include XIST, MALAT-1 (also called NEAT2) and NEAT1 are up-regulated in the parous breast. XIST, which inactivates X chromosome as an early developmental process, plays an essential role in female mammals by providing dosage equivalence between males and females. Up-regulation of XIST occurs upon differentiation, whereas failure to express XIST is often seen in malignancies and in early embryogenesis [27]. Our findings are supported by reports in the literature suggesting that XIST is expressed in adult well-differentiated cells in order to maintain gene repression [27–30].

Oxytocin, a neurotransmitter that acts through its specific receptor OXTR and is overexpressed during lactation, up-regulates the expression of MALAT-1, a highly conserved non-coding RNA [31–34]. Interestingly, both MALAT1 and OXTR remain overexpressed in the breast of postmenopausal parous women.

NEAT1 and NEAT2 localize to the periphery and to the interior spliceosome assembly factor SC35 domains, or speckles. Our observation [16] that in breast epithelial cells CCNL2 is highly enriched in nuclear speckles indicates that CCNL2 might co-localize with NEAT1 and NEAT2. The down-regulation of NEAT1, NEAT2, and XIST in the breast of nulliparous women, in whom this organ never reached a stage of complete differentiation similar to that achieved after completion of pregnancy and lactation [16, 7], suggests that the undifferentiated breast is not actively involved in the RNA metabolism that is necessary for maintaining a state of differentiation.

At the beginning of 2011, our findings of the lncRNA introduced a new line of research in our laboratory, and I knew that was important but I did not have the manpower for tackling this important subject. Then in May of 2011 I received a letter from Maria Barton, a recent MS graduate under Dr. Robert Silverman at the Cleveland Clinic, indicating that she was interested in getting her PhD from Temple University and she asked if I could mentor her. I have been a professor of biochemistry at Temple University since 2009, and therefore I was qualified to be her mentor. I met Maria for the first time in July of 2011, and she started her graduate studies at Temple University in August of that year. The research project that I assigned to Maria was to work in the role of lncRNA in the mechanism of breast cancer prevention. She started to work on this research project in January 2012 and on August 30, 2016, she had all the data for her thesis dissertation, which she defended in May of 2017. Although her thesis was confined to only two lncRNA, EPCAM and Lnc-BHLHE41, she was able to demonstrate that both lncRNAs are regulators of breast cancer and prevention, respectively [35].

The first experiment that we designed with Maria Barton and with the significant input of Julia Pereira was to expand our knowledge on the expression of the lncRNA in nulliparous and parous women by using RNA sequencing utilizing the Illumina HiSeq 2000 sequencer that had been incorporated in our laboratory a year earlier. The technique is a laborious one because after RNA extraction from breast tissue biopsies from parous (P) and nulliparous (NP) women without history of breast cancer, poly A tail RNA was obtained using poly (T) oligos covalently attached to magnetic beads. This RNA was then reverse transcribed to obtain cDNA. The cDNA template is fragmented into 200–300 nucleotides prior to sequencing to avoid secondary structure formation that could interfere with the reading during RNAseq. The high-throughput sequencing technology generates millions of short reads (50 base-pair long; paired end) from the prepared RNA library. The characterization of gene expression in the P versus NP tissue via measurement of RNA levels was performed to determine how the transcriptional machinery of the breast is affected by full-term pregnancy that occurred in the past, when the woman was in her mid-twenties to early thirties, and as a consequence how the breast tissue has been imprinted by this unique physiological process and maintained until the postmenopausal age as a specific transcriptome signature. Basically, we found 42 lncRNAs differentially expressed between the two groups (Figure 14.5).

As exciting as it was to have so much inspected differences, we started first to search the literature to identify lncRNAs involved in mammary gland development and/or disease and no literature was found detailing any of our specific lncRNAs (except for lncEPCAM which was vaguely described as BC200), so we determined that these were all novel lncRNAs in our system. We further tried to determine if some of these regions may have aliases depending on the lncRNA database used and for this purpose we used LNCipedia (https://www.ncbi.nlm.nih.gov/pubmed/23042674), which is a comprehensive compendium of human lncRNAs. We next analyzed the coverage of

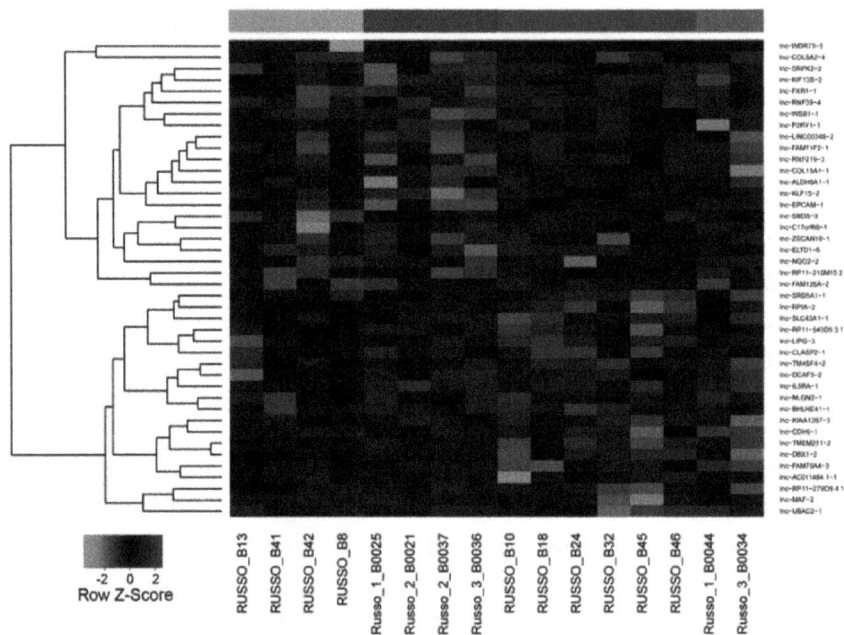

Figure 14.5: Heatmap representing differentially expressed lncRNAs between parous and nulliparous women. Up-regulated lncRNAs are represented in red and down-regulated lncRNAs are represented in green. Light and dark blue colors under parous represent two different batches of samples. Both batches were determined to be comparable and thus samples were grouped under "parous." Idem for dark and bright red under nulliparous [35].

earlier sequencing with the software tool called Integrated Genomics Viewer (IGV) (https://www.ncbi.nlm.nih.gov/pmc/articles/PMC3346182/) in order to ensure that custom probes and primers to be used in RT-qPCR would be specific to the region of interest. We follow our studies by using the Local Alignment Search Tool (BLAST) in order to check for sequence specificity. Each sequence was run through Nucleotide BLAST and searched versus the human genomic for highly similar sequences. Sequences which returned multiple matches in any assembly searched by the query were discarded as potential candidates for further study due to the possibility of generating reagents that may have off-target effects. After the list was narrowed down, Applied Biosystems (ABI) was selected to create custom primers and probes for each lncRNA. All remaining candidates were then run through ABI's software available through their Custom TaqMan® Assay Design Tool. ABI detected that 13 sequences were adequate for primer/probe specific design (Table 14.2). More details of this part of our work has been described in Maria's Thesis [35]. In summary, from all the ranking shown in Table 14.2, obtained after careful consideration of all 42 lncRNAs differentially expressed between parous and nulliparous, we determined that lnc-BHLHE41 and lnc-EPCAM were top of the list candidates for further study. Based on these two lncRNA, Maria's thesis was produced. I will not detail here all the experiments that are described in her thesis [35] but I like to conclude that her data clearly has shown that lncBHLHE41 behaves as a tumor suppressor gene and can be responsible for the

Table 14.2: LncRNAs ranked by RNAseq coverage and BLAST. All 13 lncRNAs were analyzed by IGV to determine quality of coverage during RNAseq and were then BLASTed to determine potentiality of off-target effects during primer design.

Rank	Name
1	lnc-BHLHE41
2	lnc-EPCAM
3	lnc-NLGN2
4	lnc-COL15A1
5	lnc-DCAF5
6	lnc-KLF 15
7	lnc-WSB1
8	lnc-CDH5
9	lnc-ALDH9A 1
10	lnc-P2RY1
11	lnc-KIAA1267
12	lnc-GPBP1
13	lnc-THSD4

preventive effect of pregnancy in due that is highly expressed in this group of women whereas the lncEPCAM/BC200 that is down-regulated in parous and up-regulated in nulliparous breast behaves as an oncogene.

Studies on the lncRNA are ongoing in our laboratory and is the seed for new grants development.

14.3.3. *Estrogen receptor pathway*

We did not observe differential expression in estrogen receptor between parous and nulliparous breasts [16], several genes that are directly or indirectly regulated by estrogen receptor were up- or down-regulated in the parous breast and were found to be enriched in the breast cancer estrogen signaling gene set [16, 17]. Among them, GATA3, an important component of this gene set, is crucial to mammary gland morphogenesis and differentiation of progenitor cells. GATA3 has been suggested to be a tumor suppressor [36], a fact supported by the observations that induction of its expression in GATA3-negative undifferentiated carcinoma cells is sufficient to induce tumor differentiation and inhibition of tumor dissemination [37–39]. The down-regulation of RASD1 (RAS, dexamethasone-induced 1), a potential miR-375 target that negatively regulates ER alpha expression in breast cancer further confirms that the genes involved in the estrogen receptor regulated pathways could be under permanent transcriptional modification as a manifestation of a higher degree of cell differentiation of the parous breast, in spite of the lack of transcriptomic differences in the levels of the receptor between parous and nulliparous breast tissues [16, 17].

14.3.4. *Cell communication*

Cell communication, which is a key element in the process of cell and organ differentiation, is well represented in the breasts of parous women. The parous breast exhibits up-regulation of desmocollin (DSC3), a calcium-dependent glycoprotein that is a member of the desmocollin subfamily of the cadherin superfamily. Members of this desmosomal family, along with the desmogleins, are found primarily in epithelial cells where they constitute the adhesive proteins of the desmosome cell–cell junction and are required for cell adhesion and desmosome formation. In addition, the up-regulation of matrix Gla proteins (MGP), laminins (LAMA3 and LAMC2), and keratin 5 (KRT5) in the parous breast reflected the greater differentiated state of the breast epithelial cells [40]. This concept is supported by the observation that the loss of Matrix Gla protein expression may be associated with tumor progression and metastasis [41].

14.3.5. *Down-regulated genes*

Our findings that insulin-like growth factor 1 (IGF-1) is down-regulated in the parous breast [16, 17] is consistent with published data reporting overall lower levels of IGF-1 in parous than in nulliparous women [42] and support the association of IGF-1 with increased breast cancer risk [43]. It is known that IGF-1 stimulates mitosis and inhibits apoptosis, playing a significant role in signaling pathways involved in the pathogenesis of breast cancer. The down-regulation of IGF-1 in the parous breast, in association with the significant down-regulation of SOX6, EBF1 (early B-cell factor 1), ABHD5, RASD1, a potential miR-375 target that negatively regulates ER alpha expression in breast cancer [44], and RALGAPA2, could represent a significant driving force in the reduction of breast cancer risk conferred by pregnancy.

14.3.6. *Relevance of the genomic signature in the postmenopausal breast*

The demonstration that differentiation of the breast induced by an early pregnancy imprints a specific genomic signature [15–17] that can be detected in postmenopausal women was used to identify enriched biological processes and pathways such as RNA related processes, differentiation, and development of epidermis and ectoderm, and cell-substrate junction assembly; whereas in the case of down-regulated genes, the biological processes that were enriched included IGF-like growth factor signaling, somatic stem cell maintenance, and apoptosis. Pathways that were enriched by up-regulated genes included breast cancer estrogen signaling, cell communication, and mRNA processing machinery. Numerous pathways were enriched by down-regulated genes; the most significant ones were the insulin, Wnt and integrins signaling pathways, MAPK, cytokine–cytokine receptor interaction, tight junction, and focal adhesion, all representing proteins that are highly expressed in malignancies.

A very novel contribution was to demonstrate that the genomic signature suggests that the differentiation process of breast cells is centered in the mRNA processing reactome, which emerges as an important regulatory pathway induced by pregnancy [16, 17]. The biological importance of the differential expression of genes that control the spliceosome could be an indication of a safeguard mechanism at post-transcriptional level that maintains the fidelity of the transcriptional process. *In addition, the critical regulatory pre-mRNA splicing mechanism could also regulate the expression of specific genes controlling estrogen signaling pathways, cell communication, and differentiation, as well as pathways related to chromatin remodeling, altogether resulting in control of cell differentiation and breast cancer prevention* [16, 17].

14.4. Genomic signature of the premenopausal breast

The differences in gene expression between parous and nulliparous women were also studied in premenopausal women [44] (Figure 14.2). We analyzed the gene expression profile of breast tissue from 30 nulliparous and 79 parous premenopausal volunteers between the ages of 30 and 47 years of age, who were free of breast pathology at the moment of biopsy. Because of the known transient increase in breast cancer risk preceding the long-term protective effect of FTP, we examined gene expression differences in parous versus nulliparous women as a function of time since last FTP. The results show 286 genes differentially expressed comparing all parous versus all nulliparous, and/or, parous women whose last FTP was less than five years before biopsy versus all nulliparous women. Among these, 238 genes were up-regulated, and 48 genes were down-regulated in parous compared to nulliparous breast.

Of interest is that the up-regulated genes presented three expression patterns: (1) *transient:* genes up-regulated after FTP but whose expression levels rapidly returned to nulliparous levels. These genes were mainly related to immune response; (2) *long-term changing:* genes up-regulated following FTP, whose expression levels decreased with increasing time since last FTP but did not return to nulliparous levels. These genes included genes related to immune response and development; (3) *long-term constant:* genes that remained up-regulated in the parous compared to nulliparous breast, independent of time since last FTP (Figure 14.6).

The *long-term constant* genes were mainly involved in developmental processes, cell differentiation, and chromatin remodeling (Figure 14.6). The importance of these findings is that an FTP induces long-term expression of genes that are detected after the

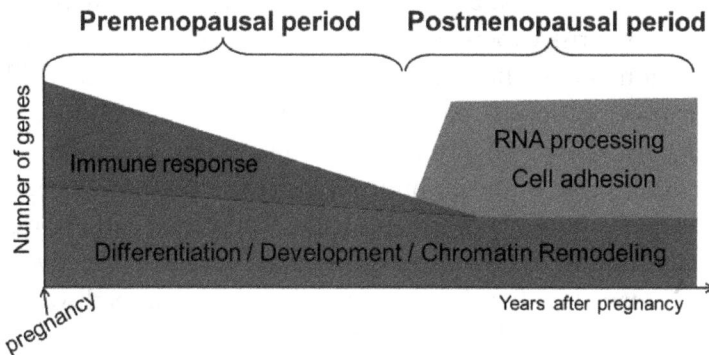

Figure 14.6: Genes related to development, differentiation, and chromatin remodeling are up-regulated after pregnancy and remain up-regulated in pre- and postmenopausal women.

end of pregnancy [44] and are still observed in the parous postmenopausal breast [15–17, 45].

It was not surprising that during the first 5 years after FTP, activation of several genes related to immune response were observed. Growth factors, hormonal signaling and cytokines/chemokines are known to participate in mammary gland differentiation and lactation [46]. However, these transiently activated genes may play a role in the short-term increase of breast cancer risk following FTP [44]. Some of these genes showed large differences in expression among the parous women, and that could be one of the explanations why some women develop breast cancer soon after their FTP. Rotunno *et al.* [47] studied the gene expression between parous and nulliparous, including premenopausal women (mean age = 37), and observed a significant amount of genes associated with immunity, inflammation, and wound responses.

The inflammatory microenvironment as well as the wound response genes could contribute to the development of breast cancer in certain women [46–48]. What is important is that the genomic profile of nulliparous and parous women in the premenopausal and postmenopausal period have shown that some groups of genes are only activated during the first years after FTP [44], while others are a part of a long-lasting signature [15–17, 45]. Genes that are only activated during the first 5 years after pregnancy [44], may contribute to the increased risk experienced by some women after pregnancy. My interpretation is that the transient genes up-regulated after FTP but whose expression levels rapidly returned to nulliparous levels were genes mainly related to immune response (CCL5, CD48, IL7R). Among other genes of the immune response that are also up-regulated are those controlling dendritic cells and T killer cells, and Figure 14.7 is an interpretation of how these transcripts could be protective in the parous women, but for those women in which the pathway is not activated, like those who have cancer during the first 5 years after pregnancy, could well explain their increased risk by an absence of immune response mechanisms that eliminate the transformed cells. On the contrary, the long-lasting signature induced by the FTP observed in the pre- and postmenopausal women explains pregnancy's

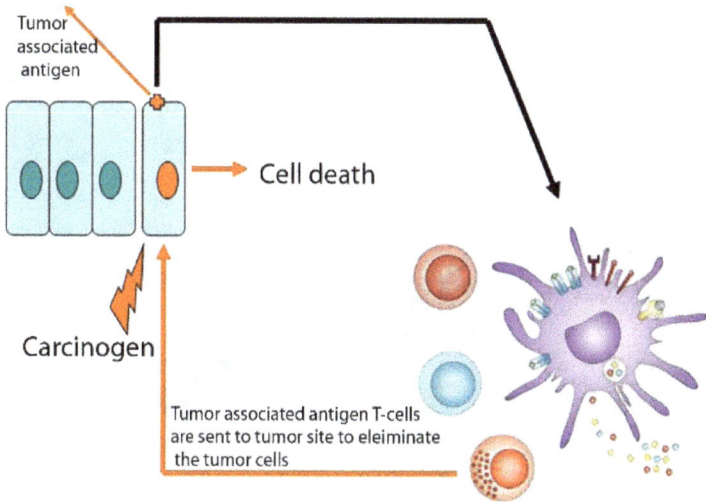

Figure 14.7: Among the genes of the immune response that are activated during the first 5 years post pregnancy in the premenopausal women are those controlling dendritic cells and T killer cells. These transcripts could be protective in the parous women, but in those women in which the pathway is not activated, like those that have cancer during the first 5 years after pregnancy, it could well explain their increased risk by an absence of immune response mechanisms that eliminate the transformed cells.

preventive effect. Evidence points toward chromatin remodeling being the major molecular mechanism that explains pregnancy's preventive effect [16, 45] (Figure 14.8).

14.5. Epigenomic signature of breast cancer prevention

Our observations that during the postmenopausal years the breast of both parous and nulliparous women contains preponderantly Lob 1, and the fact that nulliparous women are at a higher risk of developing breast cancer than parous women indicate that Lob 1 in these two groups of women differ biologically and exhibit different susceptibility to carcinogenesis [5].

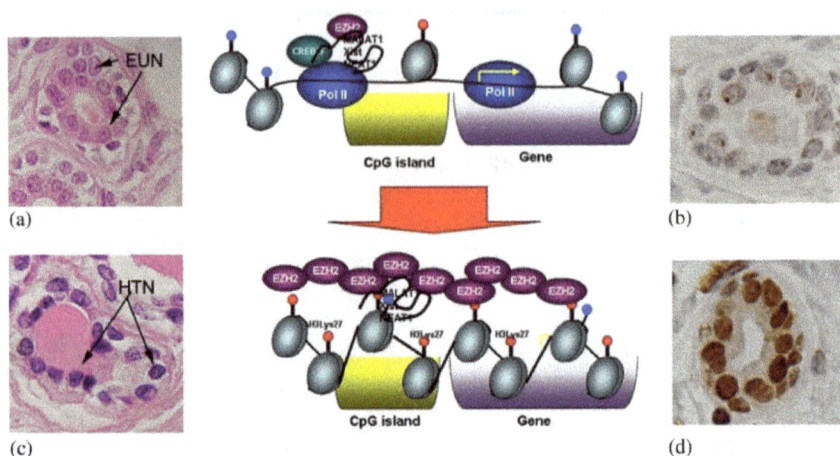

Figure 14.8: Transcriptionally active chromatin is predominantly expressed in the EUN of the nulliparous women's breast (A, B). Transcriptionally inactive chromatin is more frequently found in the heterochromatin rich nuclei (HTN) of the parous breast (C, D); its presence is associated with histone 3methylation at lysines 9 and 27, and transcriptional silencing in heterochromatin complexes [16].

The breast tissues of the P and NP women contained ducts and Lob 1 [13, 14]. The microscopic analysis of the breast tissue revealed that the population of luminal cells lining ducts and Lob 1 was composed of cells that were characterized by their nuclear appearance into two types: one that contained large and palely stained nuclei with prominent nucleoli and another consisting of small hyper chromatic nuclei [16]. The pale staining of the large former nuclei is a feature indicative of a high content of non-condensed euchromatin; these nuclei were called euchromatin-rich nuclei (EUN) (Figure 14.8). The hyperchromasia observed in the latter nuclei was indicative of chromatin condensation and high content of heterochromatin; these nuclei were identified as heterochromatin-rich nucleus (HTN) (Figure 14.8). The analysis of the distribution of HTN and EUN cells in histological sections of the breast core biopsies revealed that EUN were more abundant in the NP than in the P breast tissues, whereas the inverse was true for the HTN; these differences were statistically significant [16].

In collaboration with Dr. Maria Luiza S. Mello and Dr. Benedicto C. Vidal from the Institute of Biology, University of Campinas in Sao Paulo, Brazil, we have confirmed the differences between the HTN and EUN using a quantitative image analysis system [16]. The nuclear size (diameter, area, and perimeter) of the EUN as a whole was significantly higher ($p < 0.05$) than that of the HTN in both nulliparous and parous women. Differences were also found to be statistically significant ($p < 0.05$) regarding the nuclear shape (nuclear feret ratio) in the breasts of nulliparous women, indicating that in these breasts the nuclei of the HTN had a more elongated ellipsoidal shape than the EUN. The light absorbance (mean gray values/nucleus) was always greater for EUN than for HTN of both NP and P breasts, either considered as two groups or individually, an indication that under densitometric terms HTN were always more densely stained than EUN. Comparison of the EUN of nulliparous versus parous breasts revealed significant differences in nuclear size, stainability, and densitometric energy, leading us to conclude that epithelial cell nuclei were larger, less stainable, and with smaller regions with uniform densitometric intensity in nulliparous breasts.

Comparison of the HTN of nulliparous versus parous breasts revealed significant differences in nuclear diameter, perimeter, shape, and stainability; cell nuclei showed larger contours and more elongated ellipsoidal shape, and they were more stainable in nulliparous breasts. These observations indicated that a shift of the EUN cell population to a more densely packed chromatin cell (HTN) had occurred in association with the history of pregnancy as a distinctive pattern of the postmenopausal parous breast [16] (Figure 14.8).

Since chromatin condensation is part of the process of chromatin remodeling toward gene silencing that is highly regulated by methylation of histones, we verified this phenomenon by immunohistochemistry (IHC) incubating NP and P breast tissues with antibodies against histone 3 dimethylated at lysine 9 (H3K9me2) and trimethylated at lysine 27 (H3K27me3) [16] (Figure 14.9). The IHC stain revealed that methylation of H3 at

(a)

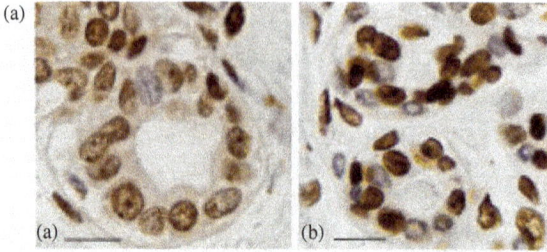

(b)

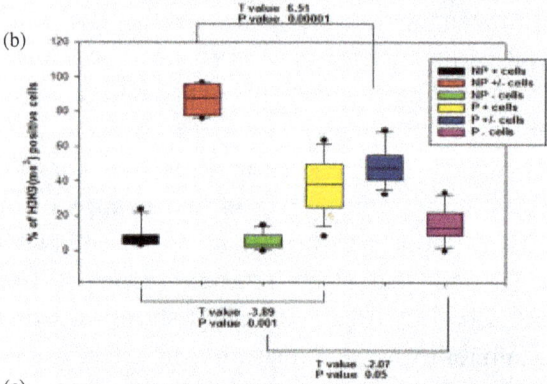

(c)

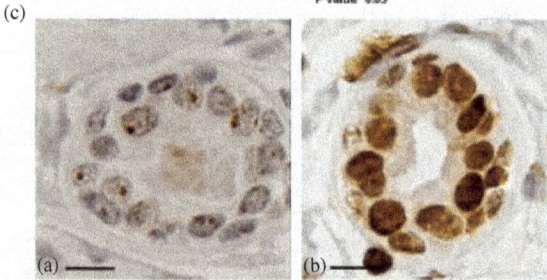

(d)

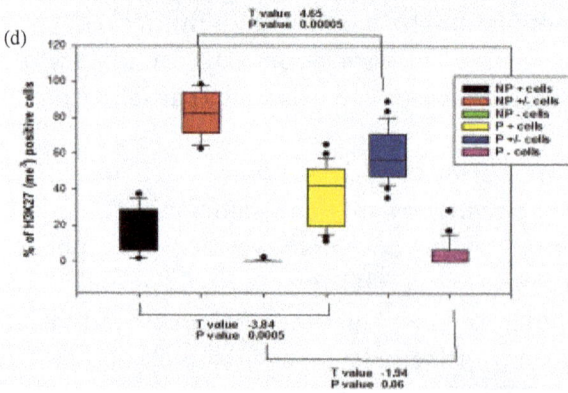

←

Figure 14.9: (Figure on facing page) (a) The H3K9(me²) IHC staining is of higher (+) intensity in the nuclei of the P (b′) breast than in NP breast (a′); a moderately diffuse (±) stain predominates in most of the NP breast. SSP-HRP/ DAB and Hematoxylin counter stain; magnification bar: 100 μm. (b) Box plot shows a significantly higher number of strongly positive cells (+) in P than in NP breasts (p < 0.001); moderately positive (±) cells predominate in the NP tissues (p < 0.00001), and negative cells are more numerous in the P cells (p < 0.05). (c) IHC reaction of H3K27(me³) is of higher (+) intensity in the nuclei of the P (b′) breast than in NP breast (a′), in which the nuclear stain is faint and finely granular, being mostly circumscribed to the nucleoli. SSP-HRP/DAB and H counter stain; magnification bar: 100 μm. (d) Box plot shows a significantly higher number of strongly positive cells (+) in P than in NP breasts (p < 0.0005); weakly to moderately positive (±) cells predominate in the NP tissues (p < 0.00005); negative cells are more numerous in the P than in the NP breast cells (p < 0.06) [16].

both lysine 9 and 27 was increased in the heterochromatin condensed nuclei of epithelial cells of the parous breast when compared to the euchromatin rich nuclei of the nulliparous breast. In the nulliparous breast, the reactivity in individual cells was less intense and the number of positive cells was significantly lower. These variations in chromatin reorganization were supported by the upregulation of CBX3, CHD2, L3MBTL, and EZH2 genes controlling this process [16] (Figure 14.10).

Our data clearly indicate that there are morphological indications of chromatin remodeling in the parous breast, such as the increase in the number of epithelial cells with condensed chromatin and increased reactivity with anti-H3K9me2 and H3K27me3 antibodies. Histone methylation is a major determinant for the formation of active and inactive regions of the genome and is crucial for the proper programming of the genome during development [34,49]. In the parous breast, there is up-regulation of transcription factors and chromatin remodeling genes such as CHD2 or chromodomain helicase DNA-binding protein 2 and the CBX3 or Chromobox homolog 3, whose products are required for controlling recruitment of protein–protein or DNA–protein interactions.

CBX3 is involved in transcriptional silencing in heterochromatin-like complexes, and recognizes and binds H3 tails methylated at lysine 9,

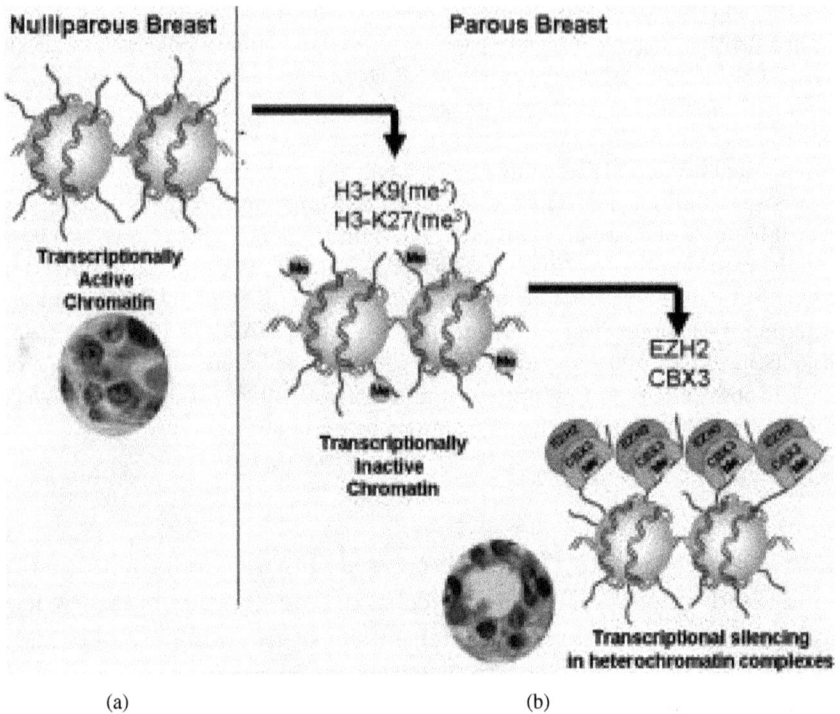

Figure 14.10: (a) Transcriptionally active chromatin is predominantly expressed in the euchromatin-rich nuclei (EUN) of the nulliparous woman's breast. (b) Transcriptionally inactive chromatin is more frequently found in the heterochromatin-rich nuclei (HTN) of the parous breast; its presence is associated with histone 3 methylation at lysines 9 and 27 and transcriptional silencing in heterochromatin complexes [16].

leading to epigenetic repression. Two other important genes related to the polycomb group (PcG) protein that are up-regulated in the parous breast are the L3MBTL gene or l(3)mbt-like and the histone-lysine N-methyltransferase, or EZH2. Members of the PcG form multimeric protein complexes that maintain the transcriptional repressive state of genes over successive cell generations. EZH2 is an enzyme that acts mainly as a gene silencer, performing this role by the addition of three methyl groups to lysine 27 of histone 3, a modification that leads to chromatin condensation [49–51].

14.5.1. *Methylation changes in the DNA of parous women are part of chromatin remodeling and the genomic signature of pregnancy*

The chromatin remodeling process is demonstrated not only by the shifting of the EUN to the HTN cells, but also confirmed by the increase in methylation of histones H3K9me2 and H3K27me3. This is an indication that methylation of other genes could also be involved in the process. For this purpose we went one step further and using the DNA from nulliparous and parous breast core biopsies and applying the MBD-cap sequencing methodology [51], we identified 583 genes showing different levels of methylation between the parous and nulliparous breasts. From the 583 genes, 455 were hypermethylated in the parous while 128 were hypermethylated in the nulliparous breast, *confirming the reprogramming of the chromatin to a more silenced or resting stage in the parous breast.* To get a better understanding of the methylation profile of the 583 genes, we used a software called Integrative Genomics Viewer (IGV) [45, 52, 53]. The IGV allowed us to identify the distinct areas, throughout the entire gene, where the methylation levels differed between the sample groups. The identification of these areas, known as differentially methylated regions (DMRs), was important because they were more likely to affect gene expression as has been shown in the literature [54]. With Julia Pereira and Irma Russo, we performed the comparison between the nulliparous and parous methylation profiles against the human reference genome "hg 18" and against each other [45]. We found that, for example, the gene COBRA 1, which is the cofactor of BRCA1 and has been shown to work in its regulatory pathway [55], was hypermethylated in the nulliparous breast. The methylation levels for each sample at each base pair showed an area of higher methylation occurring in at least four of the samples of one group as compared to all members of the opposing group, that area was defined as a (DMR) (Figures 14.11 and 14.12). COBRA 1 had a DMR near the end of the gene, which was marked in Figure 14.11 using the IGV's marking tool. When a differentially methylated area is found and marked, hovering over the red marker at the top of the

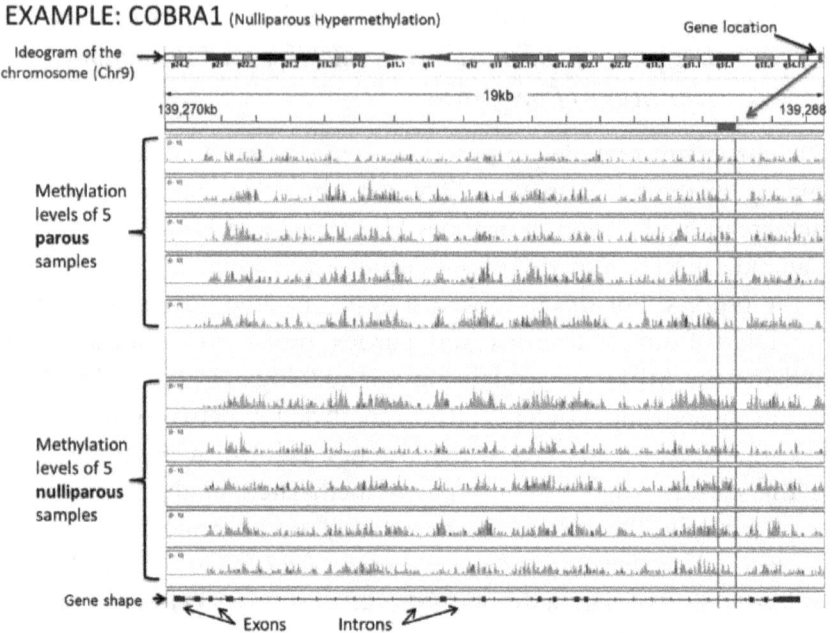

Figure 14.11: Overview of how the DNA methylation levels appear in the integrative genomics viewer (IGV). At the top of the figure is the ideogram of the chromosome given by IGV, with the area currently being examined marked in red. At the bottom is the overall shape of the gene containing exons and introns. Exons are shown as thicker blue sections on the overall gene. The gray bars represent the methylation levels of each volunteer at each base pair. They are created by combining each read resulting from the sequencing done on the samples. The higher they are, the higher the percentage of methylation is at any given base pair. When there was an area of higher methylation occurring in at least four of the members of one parity group as compared to all members of the opposing group, that area was defined as a differentially methylated region (DMR) [45].

sample area gives the exact chromosomal location. Every gene within the 583 gene list was closely examined for DMRs and the chromosomal locations at which these DMRs were found and marked were published by us [45].

After analysis of the 583 genes using the IGV, we have identified the DMRs of 53 genes. Of the 455 parous hypermethylated genes, 41 had DMRs. The exact locations of these DMRs were published in the

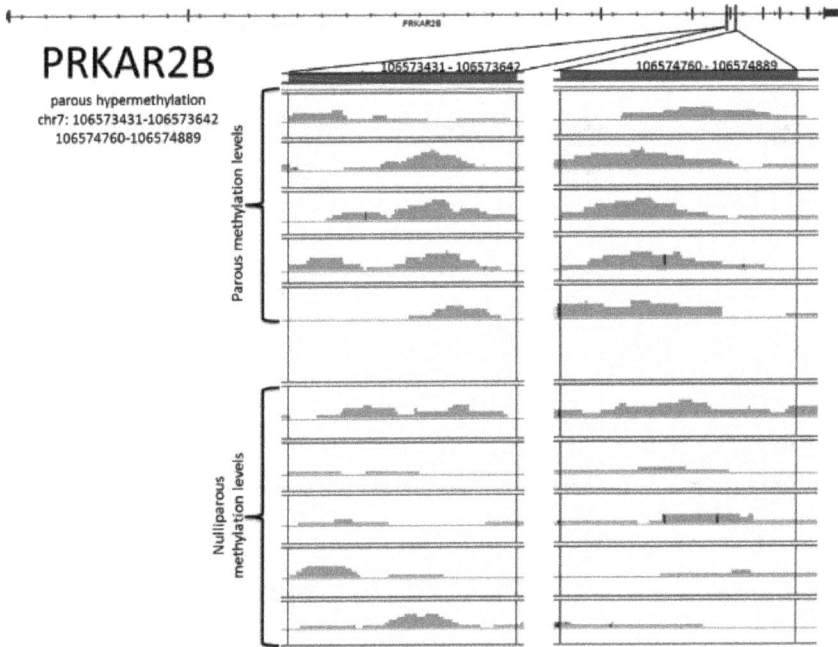

Figure 14.12: DMRs for PRKAR2B. At the top, we see the gene shape, with the red marked DMRs. Any colored locations within the gray bars indicate a nucleotide read which is different from the reference genome [45].

journal *Genes* in 2014 [45]. Of the 128 nulliparous hypermethylated genes, 12 had DMRs [45].

Analysis and research into the functions of these 53 genes identified seven which interacted with each other in either the Wnt signaling pathway or its controlling PI3K/AKT/mTOR pathways. An overview of the involvement in the canonical Wnt pathway is shown in Figure 14.13. The interworking of these genes with each other and with other genes within the statistically methylated 583 can be seen in Figure 14.14 [45].

Of the seven genes with DMRs which we have shown to work together in the Wnt pathway or its controllers, three worked directly in canonical Wnt signaling. Interestingly, when we analyzed the genes differentially expressed between parous and nulliparous [17, 45], we

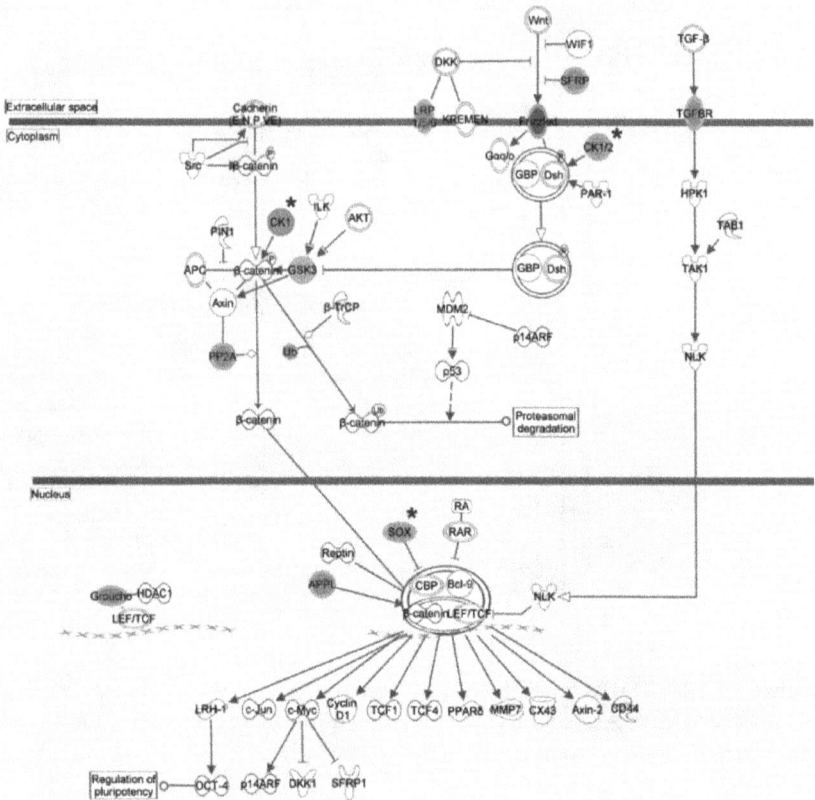

Figure 14.13: Canonical WNT/β-catenin signaling genes marked in green are hypermethylated in parous women (suggesting down-regulation of the gene in parous women). Genes in red are hypermethylated within nulliparous women. Genes marked with an asterisk (*) were observed differentially expressed the microarray data. This canonical pathway was generated through the use of IPA (Ingenuity® Pathway Analysis. 18030641. Available online: http://www.ingenuity.com) [45].

found genes that also participate in the Wnt pathway, such as CSNK1A1 and SOX family (Figure 14.13). FZD1, which is hypermethylated in the nulliparous breast, codes for the Frizzled receptor. When activated, this receptor directly activates Disheveled (Dsh) in the cytosol to begin the Wnt signaling cascade [56]. GSK3B, which also contains DMRs hypermethylated in the nulliparous

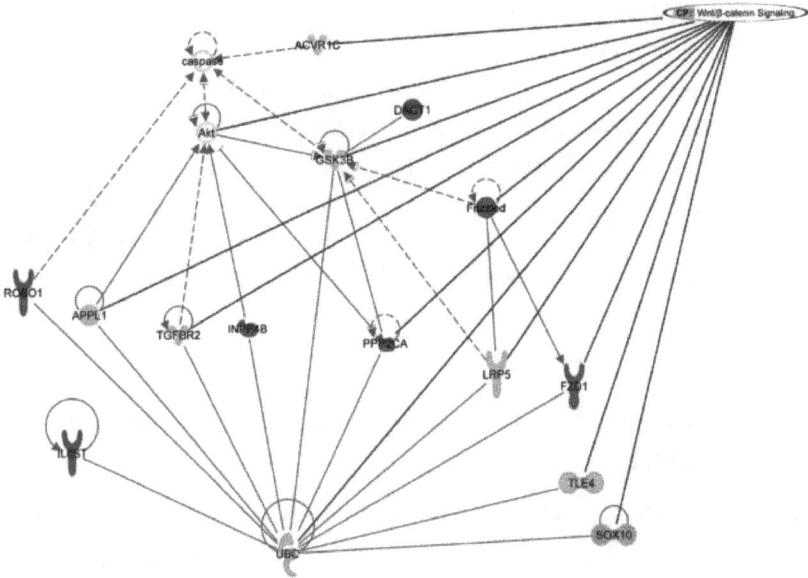

Figure 14.14: Interaction of target genes in Wnt/β-catenin signaling. The green genes are statistically parous hypermethylated, while the red ones are statistically nulliparous hypermethylated. The darker genes have recorded DMRs, and this is to the exception of GSK3B, which was first found statistically significant hypermethylated in the parous breast, but its DMR is hypermethylated in the nulliparous samples. This network was generated through the use of IPA (Ingenuity® Pathway Analysis. 18030641. Available online: http://www.ingenuity.com) [45].

women, has as main rule to decrease beta-catenin levels in the Wnt signaling pathway [57]. PPP2CA (PP2A) is suggested to work both upstream and downstream of beta-catenin to assist in its stabilization [58, 59]. DACT1 assists in Wnt signaling by up-regulating GSK3B [58, 59]. ROBO1, INPP4B, and IL6ST genes are active in PI3K-dependent AKT signaling [60–61].

The potential significance of the Wnt signaling pathway is rooted in an experiment performed in 1982 to find which genes would mutate in mice injected with mouse mammary tumor virus locating int1, a proto-oncogene [63, 64]. Int1 was soon found to be highly conserved across multiple species, including drosophila and humans. Int1 was discovered to be the mammalian homologue of the drosophila Wingless (Wg), a gene previously found to be a segment polarity gene in embryonic development. The Wnt signaling pathway was given its name from the combination of Wg and int1, and has always had a close relationship to both differentiation and breast cancer. We have discussed the potential role of Wnt in the preventive effect of pregnancy in our previous publication [45], and I will not go into detail here but only indicate that we are pursuing more mechanistic studies to understand the role of methylation in the Wnt signaling pathway.

14.5.2. *Relevance of gene methylation in breast cancer prevention*

Our work [15–17, 45] has clearly demonstrated that the breast of parous pre- and postmenopausal women exhibits a specific signature that has been induced by a full-term pregnancy. This signature reveals for the first time that the differentiation process is centered in chromatin remodeling by epigenetic changes induced by methylation of specific genes that are important regulatory pathways induced by pregnancy.

14.6. Manipulating chromatin remodeling

In 2011, Dr. Yanrong Su joined the BCRL and with her a new expertise in cell and molecular biology was introduced in our group. She was the right person to work at both sides of the spectrum when asking mechanistic questions. Together with Julia Pereira, Dr. Su formed the right team to keep moving forward. When Yanrong joined my laboratory, we already knew that in the postmenopausal years the breast of both parous and nulliparous women contains preponderantly morphologically similar lobules type 1; they differ in exhibiting different susceptibility to developing cancer, and in their genomic profile which includes up-regulation of long non-coding RNAs such as XIST and chromatin remodeling genes, as well as in the presence of histone H3 methylation on lysine 27 (H3K27me3) and 9

(H3K9me2) in epithelial cells [16, 45]. Mimicking pregnancy by using r-hCG in rats induces the differentiation of the mammary gland and gains the same protection against developing mammary tumors [11]. hCG may play an important role in the protection induced by pregnancy. In supporting this concept, Toniolo *et al.* reported that maternal breast cancer risk decreased with increasing hCG levels especially for pregnancies before 25 years of age [65]. Furthermore, women with a maximum body mass index (BMI) < 27.5 exhibited a significant protective effect against breast cancer after r-hCG use [66], suggesting r-hCG is able to remodel mammary epithelial cells, leading to a new cell state that is resistant to malignancy.

With Dr. Lee K. Tay in the early 1980s [10, 67], we have shown that the parous rat has a more efficient DNA repair capacity in mammary epithelial cells, suggesting the difference in DNA damage response is related to the parity-induced protection. In support of this data, p53, the tumor suppressor gene that has many mechanisms of anticancer, was observed in 1997 by Dr. Pramod Srivastava and Dr. Irma Russo that was up-regulated in parous and r-hCG-treated rats [68]. It was further demonstrated that p53 is required for hormone-mediated protection of mammary tumorigenesis [69]. Interestingly, the analysis of transcriptome of the parous and nulliparous postmenopausal breast showed the changes of long non-coding RNA and chromatin remodeling genes. XIST, the long non-coding RNA gene responsible for the initiation of X chromosome inactivation, is up-regulated in parous breast [16].

Based on this previous research, we embarked with Dr. Yanrong Su on further exploring the mechanism underlying the protection induced by r-hCG that in turn would help us to reveal how early FTP has an important consequence on breast cancer protection later in life, and provide the basis for the use of r-hCG as a preventive strategy for breast cancer. I obtained donations from Joseph and Barbara Breitman and the Flyers Wives to study in more detail the role of r-hCG in triple-negative breast cancer, and from those studies we demonstrated with Yanrong that r-hCG-treated MCF-10F cells increased XIST expression. Consistent with the up-regulation of XIST, which is important for the inactivation of X chromosome, HDAC8, an

X-linked gene is down-regulated in the parous breast [15–17]. Inhibition of HDAC8 remarkably enhances p53 acetylation and p53 protein in leukemia stem cells [70, 71]. HDAC6, another X-linked gene, also has similar effect on regulating p53, HDAC6 inhibition differentially modulates p53 by up-regulating wild-type p53 [72]. *Therefore, we concluded that up-regulation of XIST by r-hCG regulates p53 through epigenetic regulation of X-linked regulatory genes.* These findings were supported by data in the literature indicating that X-linked genes differentially expressed between mammary tumors of mouse model and normal mammary glands are predominantly related to chromatin remodeling, chromosome segregation, and translational control [73].

Loss of X chromosome inactivation is a common phenomenon in breast cancers [74], and there are publications supporting this idea, X-linked genes HUWE1 [75], RbAp46 [76], and BRCC36 [77] are shown to be involved in BRCA1 regulation. BRCA1 is the best-known breast cancer susceptibility protein linked to breast cancer risk, one of its functions is to repair cell damage. Although the association between XIST and BRCA1 is controversial, *we postulated with Yanrong Su that not only BRCA1 can regulate XIST, but also XIST regulates BRCA1 through epigenetic control of regulatory genes on X chromosome.* In addition, increased global H3K27me3 and H3K9me2 modifications were consistently observed in parous breast epithelium and r-hCG-treated MCF-10F cells. Histone lysine methylation is a major determinant for the formation of active or inactive chromatin and is crucial for the proper programming of the genome during development [78]. The chromatin remodeling genes such as EZH2, CHD2, CBX3, AEBP2, and L3MBTL were up-regulated in the parous breast [16]. EZH2 is a key regulator in controlling cellular differentiation. EZH2 catalyzes the tri-methylation of histone H3 on Lys 27 (H3K27me3) to generate epigenetic mark [79]. The study that explored H3K27me3 marks in different breast cancer subtypes showed H3K27me3 is inversely associated with tumor grade, and is the least abundant in triple-negative and HER2 tumors [80]. Consistently, Yan *et al.* reported that H3K27me3 activation by inhibiting demethylases JMJD3 and UTX leads to inhibition of breast cancer stem cells and self-renewal, as well as global level of stemness factors [81]. These observations lead us to postulate that the histone modification is also involved in the protection induced by pregnancy and r-hCG by regulating a subset of genes.

The relevance of this line of research germanes from the fact that r-hCG mimics pregnancy. The mechanism of this protection is that long non-coding RNA XIST is up-regulated in parous breast and in r-hCG-treated MCF-10F cells and that the X-linked genes are associated with the regulation of breast and ovarian cancer susceptibility protein BRCA1 and p53. The hCG receptor is predominantly found in breast and ovary, and early full-term pregnancy decreases the risk of developing breast cancer and ovarian cancer; and lastly increased histone H3 methylation on lysine 27 and lysine 9 are consistently observed in the parous breast and r-hCG-treated MCF-10F cells. All of these lead us to postulate that increase XIST and H3K27me3 induced by parity and r-hCG treatment regulate the expression and function of genes (especially BRCA1 and p53) involved in cell differentiation, DNA repair, and prevention of neoplastic transformation, thus providing protection against breast cancer.

This work has clinical translation implications, given the fact that modern society is changing our lives, more and more women choose to have their first child later in life, and at that time the environment or other exposures in their early lives may have already caused the changes in the mammary gland genome and abrogated the protection offered by pregnancy. The understanding of how early pregnancy and hCG induce protection provides the possibility to use r-hCG in early life as a preventative strategy against breast cancer. In addition, the panel of genes differentially expressed by hCG treatment may have the potential to be biomarkers to predict the protection against breast cancer. Moreover, for those women at high risk, such as women with BRCA1/BRCA2 mutation and women with strong family history, if we demonstrate in our clinical trial that r-hCG is able to induce protection against breast cancer through epigenetic control of p53, BRCA1, and other genes, it would be greatly helpful as nowadays the only way to reduce their risk is bilateral prophylactic mastectomy.

14.7. Developing new peptides that could be used in replacing the whole molecule of hCG

The well-proven role of hCG in inducing molecular changes resulting in a lifetime reduction in breast cancer incidence is hampered when we translate this to the clinical situation by the need to administer the hormone every two days, either subcutaneously or intramuscularly due to its large size and its inactivation when given orally. Therefore, it was important for us to investigate the possibility of activating the hCG receptor by the use of small peptides with an end to confer the same protective effects against breast cancer that the whole hormone does. Our first experiment was to use the peptide encompassing hCG residues 81-95, which has been shown to compete with the hormone for binding to the receptor [82, 83]. We have shown that both hCG and this peptide decrease cell proliferation of human breast epithelial cells [84]. These also up-regulate the gene expression of hCG receptor (CG/LH-R), while decreasing the expression of CXCR1 (cytokine IL-8 receptor) [36], found up-regulated in breast carcinomas [85, 86]. To test the ability of hCG and its peptide to induce differentiation, we have evaluated the capacity of these compounds to induce branching formation of breast epithelial cells *in vitro*. The human breast epithelial cells MCF-10F reproduce the normal processes of ductulogenesis and branching, mimicking the architectural pattern of the normal breast when seeded in a 3D collagen matrix. The cells grow along hollow branches forming ductules lined by a monolayer of epithelial cells. These normal-appearing ductules become disarrayed when the cells are treated with chemical carcinogens [87] or with E_2 [88–91], forming instead spherical structures, named solid masses, with a multilayered epithelium that exhibits marked atypia, similar to that observed in atypical hyperplasia and *in situ* carcinomas reported in primary breast lesions. The recombinant-hCG treatment of MCF-10F and E_2-transformed MCF-10F cells (E_2 cells) increases the number of secondary and tertiary branching in the ductular structures, a phenomenon that characterizes the differentiating properties of r-hCG. Treatment of E_2 with 2.5 mcg/mL r-hCG resulted in a significant decrease in the number of solid masses in comparison to the controls. For invasion evaluation, normal-like MCF-10F, transformed E_2, tumorigenic E2-T4 cells and breast cancer cell lines MCF-7 and MDA-MB-435 were tested using Boyden chambers. We observe that r-hCG and its peptide inhibit invasion and that the 81-95 peptide was more efficient than r-hCG in modulating these processes.

The hCG receptor is a member of the subfamily of glycoprotein hormone receptors within the superfamily of G protein-coupled receptors (GPCR). The hormone-binding domain has been localized to exons 1–7 in the extracellular (EC) domain/region of the receptor, which contains several leucine rich repeats. High-affinity binding of hCG and LHR causes secondary hormone or receptor contacts to be established with regions of the EC loop/transmembrane module that initiate signal transduction. CG/LH-R coupling functions are exerted primarily through cAMP/protein kinase A-mediated events in the gonads [92, 93]. For verifying the presence and functionality of the receptor in normal and transformed MCF-10F cells, we used the monoclonal antibody (mAb) 20C3 raised against the human LHR-transfected Chinese hamster ovary (CHO-LHR) cells, which was kindly provided by Drs. A. Funaro and F. Malavasi, from the Department of Genetics, Biology and Biochemistry at the University of Torino, Italy. MCF-10F and E2-transformed cells exhibited punctuate positive reaction along the plasma membrane, in a distribution similar to that seen in the positive control MA-10A cells. For testing the functional capacity of hCG and the 81-95 peptide, MA-10 and MCF-10F cells were treated with 2.5 µg r-hCG/ml or 20 µM 81-95 peptide by measuring their effect on intracellular cAMP production. Both treatments induced in MA-10 and MCF-10F cells a time-dependent increase in intracellular cAMP production, indicating that the expressed human LH/hCG-R functionally couples with endogenous adenylyl cyclase.

A step forward in this research was to work in close collaboration with Dr. Mark Andrake from the Molecular Modeling Facility at the FCCC, and we constructed a model of hCG bound to the CG/LH-R, based on the Protein Data Bank (PDB) structure 1XWD [94]. *Our final goal is to obtain an effective preventive agent that would be a small-molecular-mass mimic of the receptor ligand, which would be economical to manufacture and could get to the site of action through more efficient delivery, stability and potency.* For this purpose, we have designed an improved model of hCG bound to the CG/LH-R. The sequences of hCG and CG/LH-R have been aligned to their respective homolog chains in these template structures using the program Biological Assembly Modeller [94–97], which simultaneously models several proteins in a complex while allowing all side chains to move in both hormone and receptor. The structural details of this model have revealed several aspects of the functional specificity conferred by both the α and β chains of the hormone. We are working on developing smaller portions of the hormone that can be used to target the CG/LH-R for activation, and we propose to develop small peptides that will mimic the native hormone activation.

We also reasoned that a chimeric peptide combining residues from the Cys knot region of hCG-β chain (residues 91–107) with 16 residues from the α chain (residues 40–56) will serve for testing the hypothesis that a stable chimeric peptide agonist comprised of residues from both chains that make contact with the receptor (Figure 14.15)

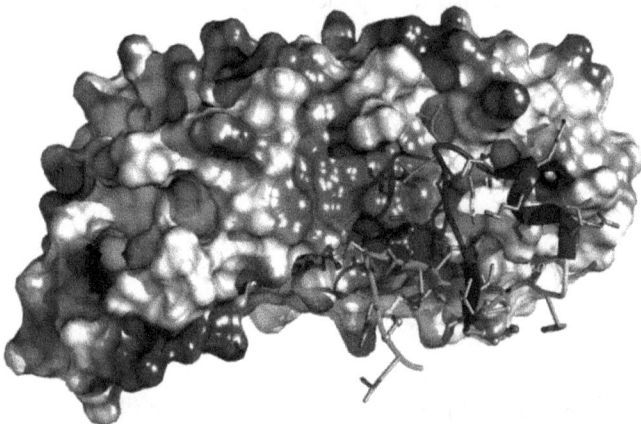

Figure 14.15:   Model of LHR-hCG-chimeric peptide complex. LHR is shown as electrostatic surface representation (red acidic residues), and the designed chimeric peptide comprised of β-chain residues (green ribbon and ball-and-stick residues) and α-chain (blue ribbon). Both chains contribute significantly to the hormone–receptor interface.

will be a more effective hormone mimic. The importance of these studies is that given the evident limitations of current strategies for breast cancer prevention [97–111], it is of significance to develop a new approach capitalizing on the preventive effect of hCG [112], on hormonally-induced differentiation, on the ability to identify specific genomic signatures [15–17, 45] that allow us to predict risk reduction, and on the novel findings that specific oligopeptides can be tailored to target pathways.

Our objective is to demonstrate that the use of small peptides derived from hCG will allow the development of an efficacious innovative strategy for breast cancer prevention and that using this approach we can target undruggable molecular pathways that are controlling chromatin remodeling. Mimicking pregnancy by using small hCG peptides could result in a new mechanism whereby nulliparous women or BRCA1/2 mutation carriers could gain the same protection against breast cancer that occurs in parous women, which would result in a dramatic decline in mammary cancer incidence. This research project is presently ongoing in our laboratory.

14.8. The clinical trial

14.8.1. *Our first attempt at developing a clinical trial using r-hCG*

In 2008, Irma and I were awarded an R21 CA124522 for studying the *Genomic Markers of Breast Cancer Prevention Induced by hCG in Women at High Risk*. The primary objective of this study was to establish the proof of the principle that treatment of asymptomatic nulliparous women carriers of BRCA1 germline mutations with recombinant human chorionic gonadotropin will change their breast epithelium's genomic profile to one similar to that identified in women with a history of early full first-term pregnancy. This was to demonstrate that the r-hCG can induce the same genomic signature that we have described in the parous women as we have described in the same year in the publications *Cancer Epidemiology Biomarkers* and *Prevention* [5]. The ultimate goal of this study was "primary prevention," i.e., reduction of cancer mortality via reduction in the incidence of breast cancer. Suffice to say that this R21 was an important award and in a certain way was an iconic moment for Irma and me, that the National Cancer Institute gave us the resources to carry on this pilot clinical trial. Irma was incredible at developing all the documents for the Internal Review Board; they were approved, and we were ready to start in July of that year. The work proposed consisted of the characterization of the genomic profile of breast epithelial cells obtained from 18 asymptomatic high breast cancer risk nulliparous premenopausal women carriers of BRCA1 deleterious mutations. An important part of this project, and probably one of the main reasons because it was awarded was because we have recruited the association with researchers that have access to these women and that will be able to ask them to enter in the study. They were the crucial part of the feasibility of the entire project. This is the way that we did it: We asked Dr. Mary Daly, MD, Senior Vice President of Population Science at the FCCC and the Director of the Risk Assessment Clinic at the FCCC, and Dr. Richard Bleichert, MD, a newly recruited Breast Surgeon in the Department of Surgery at the FCCC to be the Co Investigators of this project. They were in the budget like the responsible nurse working under Dr. Daly, Ms. Agnes Masny, who was in charge of handling the practical part of the trial at the FCCC. Other co-investigators in this project were Dr. David M. Euhus, at that time an Associate Professor in the Department of Surgery at University of Texas Southwestern Medical Center in Dallas; Dr. Sandhya Pruthi, MD, who was the Director of the Breast Diagnostic Clinic; Dr. Amy Degnim, MD, an Assistant Professor of surgery, and Dr. James Ingle, MD, who was Professor of oncology and co-leader of the Women's Cancer Program. Three of them were from the Mayo Clinic College of Medicine in Rochester, Minnesota. In addition, I recruited Dr. Georg Pfeiler, MD, from the Universitaetsklinik fuer Frauenheilkunde in Vienna, Austria. All these co-investigators had in common a family risk assessment program similar to the one presently available at the FCCC directed by Dr. Mary Daly, and all the institutions had applied for matching IRS approval for clinical protocols and ancillary forms and questionnaires. In addition, we got in contact with the director of Avon's Women Cancer Program and he directed us to contact the PI of the program funded by them called "The One Million Army of Women" that were supposed to be able to provide assistance in this project. The trial was posted in the https://clinicaltrials.gov/beta/ with the Clinical Trials Gov Identifier: NCT00700778. The logistics and planning of all these collaborators network was first class at least in papers for making this project a reality.

All eligible women accrued to this study will weekly receive three injections of 250 micrograms r-hCG for a total of 12 weeks. Normal breast tissue specimens will be collected by FNA at the beginning (0 day) and at the end of treatment and at six months post treatment, FNA specimens will be primarily utilized for analysis of genomic expression by cDNA microarray. In addition, a series of surrogate intermediate markers such as cytomorphologic evaluation and cell proliferation index will be analyzed. Based on recommendations of the FCCC IRB, the following schema was designed:

Childless Women who are at Increased Risk of Breast Cancer because of Inheritance of BRCA1 Mutation

⇩

Fine needle aspiration (FNA)

⇩

R-hCG (Ovid rei®, Serono) sc (250 micrograms/day) three times per week for 12 weeks

⇩

FNA at the end of treatment

⇩

24-week drug holiday after end of treatment — FNA for genomic analysis and cell banking

The epilogue of this trial was that only two women were recruited and finished the protocol as planned in the term of four years. One woman from Israel that saw the website of this trial in the https://clinicaltrials.gov/beta/ and covered her expenses of traveling and hosting during the three months treatment, and the second volunteer was recruited by Dr. Georg Pfeifer from the Universitaetsklinik fuer Frauenheilkunde in Vienna, Austria. These two volunteers were enrolled in the first year and were not the type to complain of negative outcome of the trial. As a matter of fact the women felt extremely well, more energetic and mostly invigorated with no other physical or laboratory testing indicating an adverse effect. This was a very good news although we had expected this from previous data obtained in women with primary and metastatic breast cancer treated with r-hCG; they felt extremely well with the treatment [113].

The bitterest reality of that R21 was that we did not recruite any woman in FCCC, none in Texas, none in the Mayo Clinic and none from the One Million Army of Women. We have been pondering the multiple reasons for this failure. Was there not enough financial reward for the co-investigators? Was the protocol too cumbersome? The list of possible explanations is too long but the bottom line is that we still cannot have a rational explanation from all the collaborators who cover three states in the USA, and of one million possible donors why were no women recruited. There is also the distinct possibility that the generation of young women in the period of 2008–2012 were less socially motivated to find a solution to their problem, and if that was the case we started a clinical trial at the wrong time of history.

Saying all of the above, I want to express in these memoir how desperate my situation was in those years because I saw the resources that we had received from the NCI draining month after month and no recruitment at all. I felt defeated and any other intention to get things for this project was tainted by failure. We presented a similar but more robust project to the Department of Defense, the Komen Cause for the Cure, and the Avon Foundation, and we even presented an application to the NCI Prevent that is basically proposing the idea and them that could be taking by anybody, but none of them succeeded. We closed the project in 2012 when I got sick and after Irma's death. I felt that even talking about the r-hCG trial was a futile exercise until, at a meeting in November of 2014 in Genk, Belgium organized by the European Cancer Prevention Organization, I raised the issue again of the need of a trial.

14.8.2. *The clinical r-hCG trial at Ghent University*

In November of 2014 I was invited to the annual meeting of the European Cancer Prevention Organization in Genk, Belgium. In that meeting, I was the plenary speaker and the title of my talk was: "The Molecular Mechanisms of the Dual Effect of Pregnancy in Risk and Prevention of Breast Cancer." I presented the data that we had collected in the GSP project in both pre- and postmenopausal nulliparous and parous women and how based on these data we were interested in developing a prevention trial. In the talk, I also presented our data on the recent experiment done in the BCRL showing that small 15 aminoacids peptide of hCG may also produce some of the effects observed by the whole molecule. The conference was well received with numerous questions from the audience. All these were very rewarding but the most important surprise was when Dr. Jaak Jannsens from the European Cancer Prevention Organization and Dr. Herman Depypere, a Professor from Ghent's university, came to see me because they were interested in organizing a clinical trial in the use of r-hCG in women carriers of the BRCA1 and/or 2 mutation. After this no time was wasted and Herman Depypere and Jaak Janssens were the new collaborators in this enterprise. Jaak has been pivotal in procuring the funds from the European Cancer Prevention Organization and the Think Pink of Belgium to support the clinical studies, and I was able to obtain a donation from the Flyers Wives to provide support for the laboratory studies.

An important difference of this trial is that instead of using the fine needle aspirate that was recommended by all our previous clinical associates, we used the Spirotome that had been developed by Jaak Janssens. This instrument allows us to acquire high quality soft tissues like breast and it comes in a ready-to-use kit containing a trocar, receiving needle with helix, cutting cannula, and release element.

The other improvement in the protocol was that we increased the number of samples from 19 to 36, and the fact that we were able to get more breast tissue, up to four fragments 2 cm in length by 1 mm in thickness, gave us more material for performing RNA, DNA, and protein studies, and in addition probing better morphological

parameters and immucytochemcial studies. The obtention of blood at
different points not only would allow us to determine the hormone
levels, such as estrogen, progesterone, and hCG, but also to use the
serum for a new project that is the isolation of exosomes to determine
if the changes observed in the breast tissue can also be detected in the
circulating exosomes.

The main objective of this trial was still to evaluate the genomic
profile of breast epithelial cells obtained from core biopsies specimens
performed in 36 high-risk women and treated for 90 days with r-hCG.
The comparison of the RNA sequence profiles before and after
treatment with r-hCG, both at 90 and 270 days, are of particular
importance in determining the duration of the hCG effect on the
transcription profile. The women will receive three weekly injections
of 250 µg r-hCG for a total of 12 weeks. Normal breast tissue
specimens will be collected by Spirotome core needle biopsies at the
beginning (0 day) and at the end of treatment (90 days), and at six
months post treatment (270 days). High breast cancer risk women
carriers of BRCA1 and BRCA2 mutations will be invited to participate
in this study and the inclusion criteria are: (1) premenopausal women
between the ages of 18–29 years of age; (2) having normal menstrual
cycles and intact ovaries; (3) nulliparous, never pregnant (G0P0);
(4) carriers of a deleterious mutation on the BRCA1/2 gene, as
determined by testing in a CLIA-certified clinical genetics laboratory;
(5) not pregnant and not on oral contraceptives or hormone replacement
therapy; (6) currently not participating in a chemopreventive trial for
breast cancer; (7) currently not taking tamoxifen for chemoprevention;
(8) no previous diagnosis of breast or ovarian cancer; (9) normal
ovarian size report from pelvic ultrasound; (10) eligible candidates
should not be taking oral contraceptives, and if taking them, stopping
six weeks prior to the initiation of treatment and the performance of
the first CNB and blood drawing; (11) willingness to self-administer
r-hCG for three months and to return for two repeat CNBs. *Among
the exclusion criteria are:* (1) prior hypersensitivity to hCG preparations
or one of its excipients; (2) prior history of ovarian cancer; (3) ovarian
enlargement of undetermined origin at the time of admission;
(4) ovarian cysts larger than 2 cm; (5) microcystic ovaries, which have

been reported to predispose to the development of ovarian hyperstimulation syndrome (OHSS) under treatment with FSH for assisted reproduction techniques; (6) history of prior cancer other than non-melanoma skin cancer; (7) ever pregnant; (8) taking medications that could interfere with the study protocol such as hormonal contraceptives, androgens, prednisone, thyroid hormones, and insulin; (9) severe cognitive deficit; and (10) unable to give informed consent.

Four CNB samples will be collected at 0, 90, and 270 days of treatment during the progestational phase of the menstrual cycle. At the time of each CNB, 45 ml of blood is collected by venipuncture. The study drug, r-hCG (Ovidrel, Serono) is an analog of luteinizing hormone (LH) and binds to the LH/hCG receptor of the granulose and theca cells of the ovary. In rodents, hCG obtained from the urine of pregnant women as well as r-hCG act mainly as LH, inducing the ovulation of already existing ovarian follicles and maintaining their respective corpora lutea in a pseudo pregnancy condition in which there is no further ovulation or risk of pregnancy. After cessation of treatment the corpora lutea regress, and the ovaries return to their normal size, with maturation of new follicles for resuming their cyclic activity. HCG has been used clinically for many years for the treatment of male and female infertility, corpus luteum insufficiency, habitual or threatened abortion, hypogonadism and cryptorchidism in the male, and weight reduction [114]. R-hCG has been approved by FDA for its use as a subcutaneous injection and for patient self-administration in assisted reproductive technologies (ART) [115]. The hormone is well tolerated without significant toxicities [113, 116–118]. Due to the direct effect of hCG on the ovarian follicle, it is recommended to monitor women receiving follitropin, a recombinant preparation of follicle-stimulating hormone (FSH) prior to the administration of r-hCG in ART for ovarian hyperstimulation syndrome (OHSS). In our knowledge, there is no report in the literature that r-hCG per se induces OHSS. Nevertheless, in this protocol, ovarian size is monitored by ultrasound, as it is recommended for the combined FSH/rhCG treatments for ovulation induction in ART as a precautionary measure. In addition, the r-hCG is administered in the progestational phase (16–20 of her menstrual cycle — day 1 is the first day of bleeding) to avoid interference with the ovulation process.

At the time of writing these memoirs, all the samples of the 36 volunteers have been collected and the study of the genomic RNA sequence is on its way. Although we do not have the final outcome of this trial, the fact that we have been able to recruit the 36 volunteers, followed the protocol with 100% retention and without any secondary or adverse effect in the collection of the samples and the administration of the r-hCG are in itself a success.

14.9. My legacy as a mentor

The BCRL has been a continuous training environment for graduate and undergraduate students by developing projects that allowed the mentee to express individual personality and needs and recognizing that each mentee using their strengths and even their weaknesses to develop short- and long-term goals and helps them figure out how to get where they want to go. I have been able to train students from different races and nationalities and help them in their adjustment to the new surroundings provided by the American culture. My approach has been that the students embrace and develop new ideas and not to be afraid to be pioneers in opening new fields of engagement.

As a mentor, I have provided my mentees with a broad view of the research endeavor by instilling the concept that the researchers are co-creators of this universe that is in our hands. I also have been clear with my mentees about my position against termination of life and the respect of each human being as a unique invaluable entity and avoiding the word *evolution* as in the atheistic view that we humans are an accident in the process of living. It is in this deep belief in the power of the human being as such that I rejected discrimination and any xenophobic position. All the members of my laboratory easily show the faces of a multicultural and multiethnic participation.

Science is constituted by scientists who are human and therefore the humaneness of science never can be forgotten. I believe that our technical advances can create artificial intelligence that may accomplish marvelous tasks, even overpowering our brain capabilities, but I strongly support that these technological advances must be in the realm of our humaneness in which passion and compassion not be eliminated as well as our ability as humans to have the freedom to believe in God.

I have been against the misconception that one group of human beings is smarter and better than another and believe that most important is how we communicate with each other and respect the unique essence of each of us. I believe that we humans are the same but with differences and the important thing is to understand our differences and work around them to communicate with the other person who is also another human being.

Although poverty is an important root for our human problems, lack of education is the original cause of our social problems. Therefore, to educate people is to empower them to solve all the main problems of our human race, and each of us has a role in this aim.

References

[1] Russo, I. H. and Russo, J. Developmental stage of the rat mammary gland as determinant of its susceptibility to 7, 12-dimethylbenz (a) anthracene. *J. Natl. Cancer Inst.* 61: 1439–1449, 1978.

[2] Russo, J. and Russo, I. H. DNA labeling index and structure of the rat mammary gland as determinant of its susceptibility to carcinogenesis. *J. Natl. Cancer Inst.* 61: 1451–1459, 1978.

[3] Clarke, C. A., Purdie, D. M. and Glaser, S. L. Population attributable risk of breast cancer in white women associated with immediately modifiable risk factors. *BMC Cancer* 6: 170, 2006.

[4] Jemal, A., Siegel, R., Ward, E., Murray, T., Xu, J. and Thun, M. J. Cancer statistics, 2007. *CA Cancer J. Clin.* 57: 43–66, 2007.

[5] Russo, J., Balogh, G. A. and Russo, I. H. Full-term pregnancy induces a specific genomic signature in the human breast. *Cancer Epidemiol. Biomarkers Prev.* 17: 51–66, 2008.

[6] MacMahon, B., Cole, P., Lin, T. M., Lowe, C. R., Mirra, A. P., Ravnihar, B., Salber, E. J., Valaoras, V. G. and Yuasa, S. Age at first birth and breast cancer risk. *Bull. World Health Organ.* 43: 209–221, 1970.

[7] Thordarson, G., Jin, E., Guzman, R. C., Swanson, S. M., Nandi, S. and Talamantes, F. Refractoriness to mammary tumorigenesis in parous rats: is it caused by persistent changes in the hormonal environment or permanent biochemical alterations in the mammary epithelia? *Carcinogenesis* 16: 2847–2853, 1995.

[8] Sinha, D. K., Pazik, J. E. and Dao, T. L. Prevention of mammary carcinogenesis in rats by pregnancy: effect of full-term and interrupted pregnancy. *Br. J. Cancer* 57: 390–394, 1988.

[9] Russo, J. and Russo, I. H. Influence of differentiation and cell kinetics on the susceptibility of the rat mammary gland to carcinogenesis. *Cancer Res.* 40: 2677–2687, 1980.

[10] Tay, L. K. and Russo, J. Formation and removal of 7, 12-dimethylbenz[a] anthracene–nucleic acid adducts in rat mammary epithelial cells with different susceptibility to carcinogenesis. *Carcinogenesis.* 2: 1327–1333, 1981.

[11] Russo, I. H., Koszalka, M. and Russo, J. Comparative study of the influence of pregnancy and hormonal treatment on mammary carcinogenesis. *Br. J. Cancer* 64: 481–484, 1991.

[12] Fisher, D. A. Fetal and neonatal endocrinology. In: DeGroot, L. J., Jameson, J. L., (eds), *Endocrinology*, Elsevier Saunders, Philadelphia, PA. 2006.

[13] Russo, J., Moral, R., Balogh, G. A., Mailo, D. and Russo, I. H. The protective role of pregnancy in breast cancer. *Breast Cancer Res.* 7: 131–142, 2005.

[14] Russo, J. and Russo, I. H. Role of differentiation in the pathogenesis and prevention of breast cancer. *Endocr. Relat. Cancer* 4: 7–21, 1997.

[15] Belitskaya-Levy, I., Zeleniuch-Jacquotte, A., Russo, J., Russo, I. H., Bordas, P., Ahman, J., Afanasyeva, Y., Johansson, R., Lenner, P., Li, X., de Cicco, R. L., Peri, S., Ross, E., Russo, P. A., Santucci-Pereira, J., Sheriff, F. S., Slifker, M., Hallmans, G., Toniolo, P. and Arslan, A. A. Characterization of a genomic signature of pregnancy identified in the breast. *Cancer Prev. Res.* 4: 1457–1464, 2011.

[16] Russo, J., Santucci-Pereira, J., de Cicco, R. L., Sheriff, F., Russo, P. A., Peri, S., Slifker, M., Ross, E., Mello, M. L., Vidal, B. C., Belitskaya-Levy, I., Arslan, A., Zeleniuch-Jacquotte, A., Bordas, P., Lenner, P., Ahman, J., Afanasyeva, Y., Hallmans, G., Toniolo, P. and Russo, I. H. Pregnancy-induced chromatin remodeling in the breast of postmenopausal women. *Int. J. Cancer* 131: 1059–1070, 2012.

[17] Peri, S., *et al.* Defining the genomic signature of the parous breast. *BMC Med. Genomics* 5: 46–57, 2012.

[18] Herrmann, A., Fleischer, K., Czajkowska, H., Müller-Newen, G. and Becker, W. Characterization of cyclin L1 as an immobile component of the splicing factor compartment. *FASEB J.* 21: 3142–3152, 2007.

[19] Wahl, M. C., Will, C. L. and Luhrmann, R. The spliceosome: design principles of a dynamic RNP machine. *Cell* 136: 701–718, 2009.

[20] Taga, Y., Miyoshi, M., Okajima, T., Matsuda, T. and Nadano, D. Identification of heterogeneous nuclear ribonucleoprotein A/B as a cytoplasmic mRNA-binding protein in early involution of the mouse mammary gland. *Cell Biochem. Funct.* 28: 321–328, 2010.

[21] Huang, P. R., Hung, S. C. and Wang, T. C. Telomeric DNA-binding activities of heterogeneous nuclear ribonucleoprotein A3 in vitro and in vivo. *Biochim. Biophys. Acta* 1803: 1164–1174, 2010.

[22] Han, S. P., Friend, L. R., Carson, J. H., Korza, G., Barbarese, E., Maggipinto, M., Hatfield, J. T., Rothnagel, J. A. and Smith, R. Differential subcellular distributions and trafficking functions of hnRNP A2/B1 spliceoforms. *Traffic* 11: 886–898, 2010.

[23] Loyer, P., Trembley, J. H., Grenet, J. A., Busson, A., Corlu, A., Zhao, W., Kocak, M., Kidd, V. J. and Lahti, J. M. Characterization of cyclin L1 and L2 interactions with CDK11 and splicing factors: influence of cyclin L isoforms on splice site selection. *J. Biol. Chem.* 283: 7721–7732, 2008.

[24] Li, H. L., Wang, T. S., Li, X. Y., Li, N., Huang, D. Z., Chen, Q. and Ba, Y. Overexpression of cyclin L2 induces apoptosis and cell-cycle arrest in human lung cancer cells. *Chin. Med. J. (Engl.)* 120: 905–909, 2007.

[25] Zhuo, L., Gong, J., Yang, R., Sheng, Y., Zhou, L., Kong, X. and Cao, K. Inhibition of proliferation and differentiation and promotion of apoptosis by cyclin L2 in mouse embryonic carcinoma P19 cells. *Biochem. Biophys. Res. Commun.* 390: 451–457, 2009.

[26] Santucci-Pereira, J., Weng, S., Slifker, M. and Russo, J. RNA splicing events are related to breast cancer prevention. *Proc. Am. Assoc. Cancer Res.* 2015

[27] Erwin, J. A. and Lee, J. T. Characterization of X-chromosome inactivation status in human pluripotent stem cells. *Curr. Protoc. Stem Cell Biol.* Chapter 1: Unit 1B.6, 2010.

[28] Vincent-Salomon, A., Ganem-Elbaz, C., Manie, E., Raynal, V., Sastre-Garau, X., Stoppa-Lyonnet, D., Stern, M. H. and Heard, E. X inactive-specific transcript RNA coating and genetic instability of the X chromosome in BRCA1 breast tumors. *Cancer Res.* 67: 5134–5140, 2007.

[29] Xiao, C., Sharp, J. A., Kawahara, M., Davalos, A. R., Difilippantonio, M. J., Hu, Y., Li, W., Cao, L., Buetow, K., Ried, T., Chadwick, B. P., Deng, C. X. Panning B: The XIST noncoding RNA functions independently of BRCA1 in X inactivation. *Cell* 28: 977–989, 2007.

[30] Silver, D. P., Dimitrov, S. D., Feunteun, J., Gelman, R., Drapkin, R., Lu, S. D., Shestakova, E., Velmurugan, S., Denunzio, N., Dragomir, S., Mar, J., Liu,

X., Rottenberg, S., Jonkers, J., Ganesan, S. and Livingston, D. M. Further evidence for BRCA1 communication with the inactive X chromosome. *Cell* 128: 991–1002, 2007.

[31] Breton, C., Di Scala-Guenot, D. and Zingg, H. H. Oxytocin receptor gene expression in rat mammary gland: structural characterization and regulation. *J. Mol. Endocrinol.* 27: 175–189, 2001.

[32] Russo, I. H. and Russo, J. Pregnancy-induced changes in breast cancer risk. *J. Mammary Gland Biol. Neoplasia* 16: 221–233, 2011.

[33] Koshimizu, T. A., Fujiwara, Y., Sakai, N., Shibata, K. and Tsuchiya, H. Oxytocin stimulates expression of a noncoding RNA tumor marker in a human neuroblastoma cell line. *Life Sci.* 86: 455–460, 2010.

[34] Matthew, G. G. and Young, R. A. Repressive transcription. *Science* 329: 150–151, 2010.

[35] Barton, M. Lnc-epcam and lnc-bhlhe41 as RNA regulators of breast cancer and breast cancer prevention. Dissertation, Doctor of Philosophy, Temple University Graduate School Board, May, 2017.

[36] Wilson, B. J. and Giguere, V. Meta-analysis of human cancer microarrays reveals GATA3 is integral to the estrogen receptor alpha pathway. *Mol. Cancer* 7: 49–54, 2008.

[37] Chou, J., Provot, S. and Werb, Z. GATA3 in development and cancer differentiation: cells GATA have it! *J. Cell Physiol.* 222: 42–49, 2010.

[38] Pei, X. H., Bai, F., Smith, M. D., Usary, J., Fan, C., Pai, S. Y., Ho, I. C., Perou, C. M. and Xiong, Y. CDK inhibitor p18(INK4c) is a downstream target of GATA3 and restrains mammary luminal progenitor cell proliferation and tumorigenesis. *Cancer Cell.* 15: 389–401, 2009.

[39] Kouros-Mehr, H., Bechis, S. K., Slorach, E. M., Littlepage, L. E., Egeblad, M., Ewald, A. J., Pai, S. Y., Ho, I. C. and Werb, Z. GATA-3 links tumor differentiation and dissemination in a luminal breast cancer model. *Cancer Cell.* 13: 141–152, 2008.

[40] Fischer, J., Klein, P. J., Farrar, G. H., Hanisch, F. G. and Uhlenbruck, G. Isolation and chemical and immunochemical characterization of the peanut-lectin-binding glycoprotein from human milk-fat-globule membranes. *Biochem. J.* 224: 581–589, 1984.

[41] Chen, L., O'Bryan, J. P., Smith, H. S. and Liu, E. Overexpression of matrix Gla protein mRNA in malignant human breast cells: isolation by differential cDNA hybridization. *Oncogene.* 5: 1391–1395, 1990.

[42] Holmes, M. D., Pollak, M. N. and Hankinson, S. E. Lifestyle correlates of plasma insulin-like growth factor I and insulin-like growth factor binding

protein 3 concentrations. *Cancer Epidemiol. Biomarkers Prev.* 11: 862–867, 2002.

[43] Key, T. J., Appleby, P. N., Reeves, G. K. and Roddam, A. W. Insulin-like growth factor 1 (IGF1), IGF binding protein 3 (IGFBP3), and breast cancer risk: pooled individual data analysis of 17 prospective studies. *Lancet Oncol.* 11: 530–542, 2010.

[44] Santucci-Pereira, J., *et al.* (eds). Gene expression profile induced by pregnancy in the breast of premenopausal women. *Proc. Am. Assoc. Cancer Res.* 2294a, 2014.

[45] Russo, J., Santucci-Pereira, J. and Russo, I. H. The genomic signature of breast cancer prevention. *Genes* 5: 65–83, 2014.

[46] Csanaky, K., Doppler, W., Tamas, A., Kovacs, K., Toth, G. and Reglodi, D. Influence of terminal differentiation and PACAP on the cytokine, chemokine, and growth factor secretion of mammary epithelial cells. *J. Mol. Neurosci.* 52: 28–36, 2014.

[47] Rotunno, M., *et al.* Parity-related molecular signatures and breast cancer subtypes by estrogen receptor status. *Breast Cancer Res.* 16: R74, 2014.

[48] Callihan, E. B., *et al.* Postpartum diagnosis demonstrates a high risk for metastasis and merits an expanded definition of pregnancy-associated breast cancer. *Breast Cancer Res. Treat.* 138: 549–559, 2013.

[49] Kubicek, S., *et al.* The role of histone modifications in epigenetic transitions during normal and perturbed development. *Ernst Schering Res. Found. Workshop* 57: 1–27, 2006.

[50] Lin, W. and Dent, S. Y. Functions of histone-modifying enzymes in development. *Curr. Opin. Genet. Dev.* 16: 137–142, 2006.

[51] Zuo, T., Tycko, B., Liu, T. M., Lin, H. J. and Huang, T. H. Methods in DNA methylation profiling. *Epigenomics* 1: 331–345, 2009.

[52] Robinson, J. T., Thorvaldsdottir, H., Winckler, W., Guttman, M., Lander, E.S., Getz, G. and Mesirov, J. P. Integrative genomics viewer. *Nat. Biotechnol.* 29: 24–26, 2011.

[53] Thorvaldsdottir, H., Robinson, J. T. and Mesirov, J. P. Integrative Genomics Viewer (IGV): High-performance genomics data visualization and exploration. *Brief Bioinform.* 14: 178–192, 2013.

[54] Rakyan, V. K., *et al.* An integrated resource for genome-wide identification and analysis of human tissue-specific differentially methylated regions (tDMRs). *Genome Res.* 18: 1518–1529, 2008.

[55] Aiyar, S. E., Cho, H., Lee, J. and Li, R. Concerted transcriptional regulation by BRCA1 and COBRA1 in breast cancer cells. *Int. J. Biol. Sci.* 3: 486–492, 2007.

[56] Habas, R. and Dawid, I. B. Dishevelled and Wnt signaling: Is the nucleus the final frontier? *J. Biol.* 4: 2, 2005.

[57] Wang, X., *et al.* Association of genetic variation in genes implicated in the beta-catenin destruction complex with risk of breast cancer. *Cancer Epidemiol. Biomarkers Prev.* 17: 2101–2108, 2008.

[58] Ratcliffe, M. J., Itoh, K. and Sokol, S. Y. A positive role for the PP2A catalytic subunit in Wnt signal transduction. *J. Biol. Chem.* 275: 35680–35683, 2000.

[59] Cheyette, B. N., Waxman, J. S., Miller, J. R., Takemaru, K., Sheldahl, L. C., Khlebtsova, N., Fox, E. P., Earnest, T. and Moon, R. T. Dapper, a Dishevelled-associated antagonist of beta-catenin and JNK signaling, is required for notochord formation. *Dev. Cell* 2: 449–461, 2002.

[60] Zhao, L., *et al.* Mammary gland remodeling depends on gp130 signaling through Stat3 and MAPK. *J. Biol. Chem.* 279: 44093–44100, 2004.

[61] Chang, P. H., Hwang-Verslues, W. W., Chang, Y. C., Chen, C. C., Hsiao, M., Jeng, Y. M., Chang, K. J., Lee, E. Y., Shew, J. Y. and Lee, W. H. Activation of Robo1 signaling of breast cancer cells by Slit2 from stromal fibroblast restrains tumorigenesis via blocking PI3K/Akt/beta-catenin pathway. *Cancer Res.* 72: 4652–4661, 2012.

[62] Bertucci, M. C. and Mitchell, C. A. Phosphoinositide 3-kinase and INPP4B in human breast cancer. *Ann. NY Acad. Sci.* 1280: 1–5, 2013.

[63] Nusse, R. and Varmus, H. Three decades of Wnts: A personal perspective on how a scientific field developed. *EMBO J.* 31: 2670–2684, 2012.

[64] Turashvili, G., Bouchal, J., Burkadze, G. and Kolar, Z. Wnt signaling pathway in mammary gland development and carcinogenesis. *Pathobiology* 73: 213–223, 2006.

[65] Toniolo, P., *et al.* Human chorionic gonadotropin in pregnancy and maternal risk of breast cancer. *Cancer Res.* 70: 6779–6786, 2010.

[66] Bernstein, L., *et al.* Treatment with human chorionic gonadotropin and risk of breast cancer. *Cancer Epidemiol. Biomarkers Prev.* 4: 437–440, 1995.

[67] Tay, L. K. and Russo, J. 7, 12-Dimethylbenz (a) anthracene (DMBA) induced DNA binding and repair synthesis in susceptible and non-susceptible mammary epithelial cells in culture. *J. Natl. Cancer Inst.* 67: 155–161, 1981.

[68] Srivastava, P., Russo, J. and Russo, I. H. Chorionic gonadotropin inhibits rat mammary carcinogenesis through activation of programmed cell death. *Carcinogenesis* 18: 1799–1808, 1997.

[69] Medina, D. and Kittrell, F. S. p53 function is required for hormone-mediated protection of mouse mammary tumorigenesis. *Cancer Res.* 63: 6140–6143, 2003.

[70] Qi, J., *et al.* HDAC8 Inhibition Specifically Targets Inv (16) Acute Myeloid Leukemic Stem Cells by Restoring p53 Acetylation. *Cell Stem Cell* 17: 597–610, 2015.

[71] Qi, J., *et al.* Inhibition of HDAC8 Reactivates p53 and Abrogates Leukemia Stem Cell Activity in CBF -SMMHC Associated Acute Myeloid Leukemia. *Blood* 124: 363–363, 2014.

[72] Ryu, H. W., *et al.* HDAC6 deacetylates p53 at lysines 381/382 and differentially coordinates p53-induced apoptosis. *Cancer Lett.* 391: 162–171, 2017.

[73] Thakur, A., *et al.* Aberrant expression of X-linked genes RbAp46, Rsk4, and Cldn2 in breast cancer. *Mol. Cancer Res.* 5: 171–181, 2007.

[74] Sirchia, S. M., *et al.* Loss of the inactive X chromosome and replication of the active X in BRCA1-defective and wild-type breast cancer cells. *Cancer Res.* 65: 2139–2146, 2005.

[75] Wang, X., *et al.* HUWE1 interacts with BRCA1 and promotes its degradation in the ubiquitin-proteasome pathway. *Biochem. Biophys. Res. Commun.* 444: 290–295, 2014.

[76] Chen, G. C., *et al.* Rb-associated protein 46 (RbAp46) inhibits transcriptional transactivation mediated by BRCA1. *Biochem. Biophys. Res. Commun.* 284: 507–514, 2001.

[77] Chen, X., *et al.* BRCC36 is essential for ionizing radiation-induced BRCA1 phosphorylation and nuclear foci formation. *Cancer Res.* 66: 5039–5046, 2006.

[78] Jenuwein, T. and Allis, C. D. Translating the histone code. *Science* 293: 1074–1080, 2001.

[79] Cao, R., *et al.* Role of histone H3 lysine 27 methylation in Polycomb-group silencing. *Science* 298: 1039–1043, 2002.

[80] Holm, K., *et al.* Global H3K27 trimethylation and EZH2 abundance in breast tumor subtypes. *Mol. Oncol.* 6: 494–506, 2012.

[81] Yan, N., Xu, L., Wu, X., Zhang, L., Fei, X., Cao, Y. and Zhang, F. GSKJ4, an H3K27me3 demethylase inhibitor, effectively suppresses the breast cancer stem cells. *Exp. Cell Res.* 359: 405–414, 2017.

[82] Russo, I. H., Koszalka, M., Gimotty, P. A. and Russo, J. Protective effect of chorionic gonadotropin on DMBA-induced mammary carcinogenesis. *Br. J. Cancer* 62: 243–247, 1990.

[83] Morbeck, D. E., Roche, P. C., Keutmann, H. T. and McCormick, D. J. A receptor binding site identified in the region 81-95 of the beta-subunit of human luteinizing hormone (LH) and chorionic gonadotropin (hCG). *Mol. Cell. Endocrinol.* 97: 173–181, 1993.

[84] Noronha, S. M. R., Correa-Noronha, S. A. A., Russo, I., de Cicco, R. L., Santucci-Pereira, J. and Russo, J. Human chorionic gonadotropin and a 15 aminoacid hCG fragment of the hormone induce downregulation of the cytokine IL-8 receptor in normal breast epithelial cells. *Horm. Mol. Biol. Clin. Investig.* 6: 241–245, 2011.

[85] Waugh, D. J. and Wilson, C. The interleukin-8 pathway in cancer. *Clin. Cancer Res.* 14: 6735–6741, 2008.

[86] Ginestier, C., Liu, S., Diebel, M. E., Korkaya, H., Luo, M., Brown, M., Wicinski, J., Cabaud, O., Charafe-Jauffret, E., Birnbaum, D., Guan, J. L., Dontu, G. and Wicha, M. S. CXCR1 blockade selectively targets human breast cancer stem cells in vitro and in xenografts. *J. Clin. Invest.* 120: 485–497, 2010.

[87] Russo, J., Russo, I., Calaf, G., Zhang, P-L and Barnabas, N. Breast Susceptibility to Carcinogenesis. In: Li, J. J., Li, S., Gustafsson, J-Å., Nandi, S., Sekely, L., (eds), *Hormonal Carcinogenesis II*, Springer, New York. 1996, 120–131.

[88] Kocdor, H., *et al.* Human chorionic gonadotropin (hCG) prevents the transformed phenotypes induced by 17 β-estradiol in human breast epithelial cells. *Cell Biol. Int.* 33: 1135–1143, 2009.

[89] Russo, J., Fernandez, S. V., Russo, P. A., Fernbaugh, R., Sheriff, F. S., Lareef, H. M., Garber, J. and Russo, I. H. 17-Beta-estradiol induces transformation and tumorigenesis in human breast epithelial cells. *FASEB J.* 20:1622–1634, 2006.

[90] Russo, J., Lareef, H., Tahin, Q. and Russo, I. H. Pathways of carcinogenesis and prevention in the human breast. *Eur. J. Cancer* 38(6): S31–S32, 2002.

[91] Russo, J., Lareef, M. H., Tahin, Q., Hu, Y. F., Slater, C., Ao, X. and Russo, I. H. 17Beta-estradiol is carcinogenic in human breast epithelial cells. *J. Steroid Biochem. Mol. Biol.* 80: 149–162, 2002.

[92] Dufau, M. L., Liao, M. and Zhang, Y. Participation of signaling pathways in the derepression of luteinizing hormone receptor transcription. *Mol. Cell. Endocrinol.* 314: 221–227, 2010.

[93] Fan, Q. R. and Hendrickson, W. A. Structure of human follicle-stimulating hormone in complex with its receptor. *Nature* 433: 269–277, 2005.

[94] Canutescu, A. A., Shelenkov, A. A. and Dunbrack, R. L. Jr. A graph-theory algorithm for rapid protein side-chain prediction. *Protein Sci.* 12: 2001–2014, 2003.

[95] Wang, Q., Canutescu, A. A., Dunbrack, R. L. Jr. SCWRL and MolIDE: computer programs for side-chain conformation prediction and homology modeling. *Nat. Protoc.* 3: 1832–1847, 2008.

[96] Shapovalov, M. V., Wang, Q., Xu, Q., Andrake, M. and Dunbrack, R. L. Jr. BioAssemblyModeler (BAM): user-friendly homology modeling of protein homo- and heterooligomers. *PLoS One* 9: e98309, 2014.

[97] Leaver-Fay, A., O'Meara, M. J., Tyka, M., Jacak, R., Song, Y., Kellogg, E. H., Thompson, J., Davis, I. W., Pache, R. A., Lyskov, S., Gray, J. J., Kortemme, T., Richardson, J. S., Havranek, J. J., Snoeyink, J., Baker, D. and Kuhlman, B. Scientific benchmarks for guiding macromolecular energy function improvement. *Methods Enzymol.* 523: 109–143, 2013.

[98] Narod, S. A., Brunet, J. S., Ghadirian, P., Robson, M., Heimdal, K., Neuhausen, S. L., Stoppa-Lyonnet, D., Lerman, C., Pasini, B., de los Rios, P., Weber, B. and Lynch, H. Hereditary Breast Cancer Clinical Study G. Tamoxifen and risk of contralateral breast cancer in BRCA1 and BRCA2 mutation carriers: a case-control study. Hereditary Breast Cancer Clinical Study Group. *Lancet* 356: 1876–1881, 2000.

[99] Baum, M. and Grp, A. T. The ATAC (Arimidex, Tamoxifen, Alone or in Combination) adjuvant breast cancer trial in postmenopausal (PM) women. *Breast Cancer Res. Treat.* 69: 218, 2001.

[100] King, M. C., Wieand, S., Hale, K., Lee, M., Walsh, T., Owens, K., Tait, J., Ford, L., Dunn, B. K., Costantino, J., Wickerham, L., Wolmark, N., Fisher, B and National Surgical Adjuvant Breast and Bowel Project. Tamoxifen and breast cancer incidence among women with inherited mutations in BRCA1 and BRCA2: National Surgical Adjuvant Breast and Bowel Project (NSABP-P1) Breast Cancer Prevention Trial. *J. Am. Med. Assoc.* 286: 2251–2256, 2001.

[101] Jordan, V. C. Tamoxifen: the herald of a new era of preventive therapeutics. *J. Natl. Cancer Inst.* 89: 747–749, 1997.

[102] Gottardis, M. M. and Jordan, V. C. Antitumor actions of keoxifene and tamoxifen in the N-nitrosomethylurea-induced rat mammary carcinoma model. *Cancer Res.* 47: 4020–4024, 1987.

[103] Mouridsen, H. Superior efficacy of letrozole versus tamoxifen as first-line therapy for postmenopausal women with advanced breast cancer: Results of a phase III study of the International Letrozole Breast Cancer Group. *J. Clin. Oncol.* 19: 2596–2599, 2001.

[104] Mouridsen, H., Gershanovich, M., Sun, Y., Perez-Carrion, R., Boni, C., Monnier, A., Apffelstaedt, J., Smith, R., Sleeboom, H. P., Janicke, F., Pluzanska, A., Dank, M., Becquart, D., Bapsy, P. P., Salminen, E., Snyder, R., Lassus, M., Verbeek, J. A., Staffler, B., Chaudri-Ross, H. A. and Dugan, M. Superior efficacy of letrozole versus tamoxifen as first-line therapy for

postmenopausal women with advanced breast cancer: Results of a phase III study of the international letrozole breast cancer group. *J. Clin. Oncol.* 19: 2596–2606, 2001.

[105] Robertson, J. F., Nicholson, R. I., Bundred, N. J., Anderson, E., Rayter, Z., Dowsett, M., Fox, J. N., Gee, J. M., Webster, A., Wakeling, A. E., Morris, C. and Dixon, M. Comparison of the short-term biological effects of 7alpha-[9-(4,4,5,5,5-pentafluoropentylsulfinyl)-nonyl]estra-1,3,5, (10)-triene-3,17beta-diol (Faslodex) versus tamoxifen in postmenopausal women with primary breast cancer. *Cancer Res.* 61: 6739–6746, 2001.

[106] Soiland, H., Skaland, I., Varhaug, J. E., Korner, H., Janssen, E. A., Gudlaugsson, E., Baak, J. P. and Soreide, J. A. Co-expression of estrogen receptor alpha and Apolipoprotein D in node positive operable breast cancer—possible relevance for survival and effects of adjuvant tamoxifen in postmenopausal patients. *Acta Oncol.* 48: 514–521, 2009.

[107] Dowsett, M. Future uses for aromatase inhibitors in breast cancer. *J. Steroid Biochem. Mol. Biol.* 61: 261–266, 1997.

[108] Leunen, K., Drijkoningen, M,, Neven, P., Christiaens, M. R., Van Ongeval, C., Legius, E., Amant, F., Berteloot, P. and Vergote, I. Prophylactic mastectomy in familial breast carcinoma. What do the pathologic findings learn us? *Breast Cancer Res. Treat.* 107: 79–86, 2008.

[109] Fatouros, M., Baltoyiannis, G. and Roukos, D. H. The predominant role of surgery in the prevention and new trends in the surgical treatment of women with BRCA1/2 mutations. *Ann. Surg. Oncol.* 15: 21–33, 2008.

[110] Hoogerbrugge, N., Bult, P., de Widt-Levert, L. M., Beex, L. V., Kiemeney, L. A., Ligtenberg, M. J., Massuger, L. F., Boetes, C., Manders, P. and Brunner, H. G. High prevalence of premalignant lesions in prophylactically removed breasts from women at hereditary risk for breast cancer. *J. Clin. Oncol.* 21: 41–45, 2003.

[111] Arun, B., Vogel, K. J., Lopez, A., Hernandez, M., Atchley, D., Broglio, K. R., Amos, C. I., Meric-Bernstam, F., Kuerer, H., Hortobagyi, G. N. and Albarracin, C. T. High prevalence of preinvasive lesions adjacent to BRCA1/2-associated breast cancers. *Cancer Prev. Res. (Phila.)* 2: 122–127, 2009.

[112] Russo, I. H., Koszalka, M. and Russo, J. Human chorionic gonadotropin and rat mammary cancer prevention. *J. Natl. Cancer Inst.* 82: 1286–1289, 1990.

[113] Janssens, J. P., Russo, J., Russo, I., Michiels, L., Donders, G., Verjans, M., Riphagen, I., Van den Bossche, T., Deleu, M. and Sieprath, P. Human chorionic gonadotropin (hCG) and prevention of breast cancer. *Mol. Cell. Endocrinol.* 269: 93–98, 2007.

[114] Kliesch, S., Behre, H. M. and Nieschlag, E. High efficacy of gonadotropin or pulsatile gonadotropin-releasing hormone treatment in hypogonadotropic hypogonadal men. *Eur. J. Endocrinol.* 131: 347–354,1994.

[115] Chen, C., Jones, W. R., Fern, B. and Forde, C. Monitoring embryos after in vitro fertilization using early pregnancy factor. In: Seppala, M., Edwards, R. G., (ed), In Vitro Fertilization and Embryo Transfer. *Ann. NY Acad. Sci.* 442: 428, 1985.

[116] The European Recombinant Human Chorionic Gonadotrophin Study Group Induction of final follicular maturation and early luteinization in women undergoing ovulation induction for assisted reproduction treatment— recombinant HCG versus urinary HCG. *Hum. Reprod.* 15: 1446–1451, 2000.

[117] Chang, P., Kenley, S., Burns, T., Denton, G., Currie, K., DeVane, G. and O'Dea, L. Recombinant human chorionic gonadotropin (rhCG) in assisted reproductive technology: results of a clinical trial comparing two doses of rhCG (Ovidrel) to urinary hCG (Profasi) for induction of final follicular maturation in in vitro fertilization-embryo transfer. *Fertil. Steril.* 76: 67–74, 2001.

[118] Russo, I. H., Russo, J., DeLuca, G. and Janssens, J. hCG therapy for the treatment of breast cancer. Google Patents, 2007.

[119] Breasted, J. H., (ed). *The Edwin Smith Surgical Papyrus.* Published in facsimile and hieroglyphic transliteration with translation and commentary in two volumes, Vol. 1, University of Chicago Press, Chicago. 1991.

[120] Mustacchi, P. Ramazzini and Rigoni-Stern on parity and breast cancer. Clinical impression and statistical corroboration. *Arch. Intern. Med.* 108: 639–642, 1961.

Index